MW01615765

Springer Texts in Statistics

Series Editors

G. Allen, Department of Statistics, Rice University, Houston, USA

R. De Veaux, Department of Mathematics and Statistics, Williams College, Williamstown, USA

R. Nugent, Department of Statistics, Carnegie Mellon University, Pittsburgh, USA

Springer Texts in Statistics (STS) includes advanced textbooks from 3rd- to 4th-year undergraduate levels to 1st- to 2nd-year graduate levels. Exercise sets should be included. The series editors are currently Genevera I. Allen, Richard D. De Veaux, and Rebecca Nugent. Stephen Fienberg, George Casella, and Ingram Olkin were editors of the series for many years.

Paul R. Rosenbaum

An Introduction to the Theory of Observational Studies

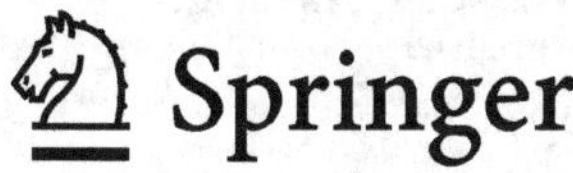

Paul R. Rosenbaum
The Wharton School
University of Pennsylvania
Philadelphia, PA, USA

ISSN 1431-875X ISSN 2197-4136 (electronic)
Springer Texts in Statistics
ISBN 978-3-031-90493-6 ISBN 978-3-031-90494-3 (eBook)
https://doi.org/10.1007/978-3-031-90494-3

Mathematics Subject Classification: 62-xx, 90-xx

© The Editor(s) (if applicable) and The Author(s), under exclusive license to Springer Nature Switzerland AG 2025

This work is subject to copyright. All rights are solely and exclusively licensed by the Publisher, whether the whole or part of the material is concerned, specifically the rights of translation, reprinting, reuse of illustrations, recitation, broadcasting, reproduction on microfilms or in any other physical way, and transmission or information storage and retrieval, electronic adaptation, computer software, or by similar or dissimilar methodology now known or hereafter developed.
The use of general descriptive names, registered names, trademarks, service marks, etc. in this publication does not imply, even in the absence of a specific statement, that such names are exempt from the relevant protective laws and regulations and therefore free for general use.
The publisher, the authors and the editors are safe to assume that the advice and information in this book are believed to be true and accurate at the date of publication. Neither the publisher nor the authors or the editors give a warranty, expressed or implied, with respect to the material contained herein or for any errors or omissions that may have been made. The publisher remains neutral with regard to jurisdictional claims in published maps and institutional affiliations.

This Springer imprint is published by the registered company Springer Nature Switzerland AG
The registered company address is: Gewerbestrasse 11, 6330 Cham, Switzerland

If disposing of this product, please recycle the paper.

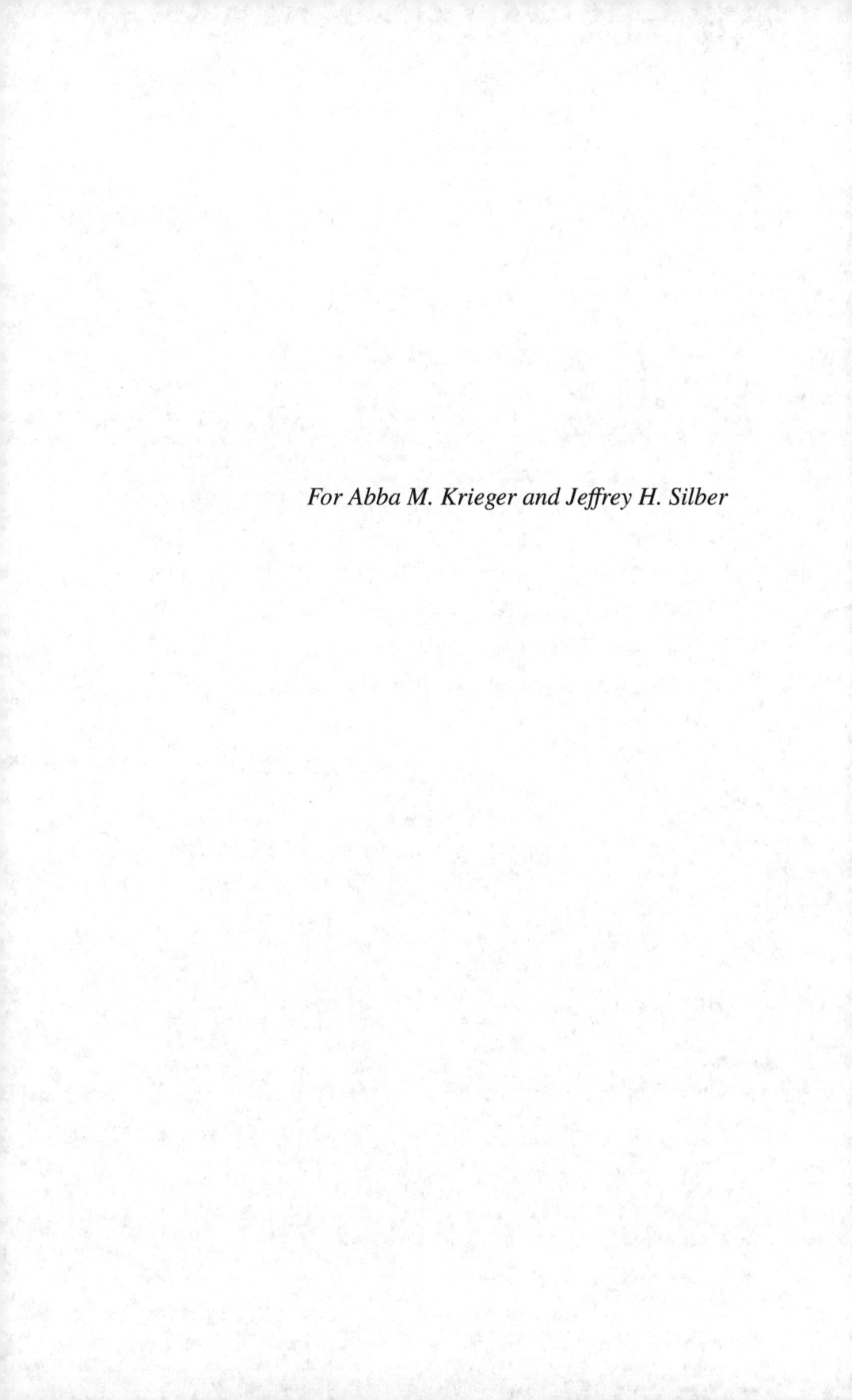

For Abba M. Krieger and Jeffrey H. Silber

The substitution of scientific for superstitious habits of inference has not been brought about by any improvement in the acuteness of the senses or in the natural workings of the function of suggestion. It is the result of regulation of the conditions under which observation and inference take place.

John Dewey
How We Think, 1910

Every time we let ourselves believe for unworthy reasons, we weaken our powers of self-control, of doubting, of judicially and fairly weighing evidence . . . The danger to society is not merely that it should believe wrong things, though that is great enough; but that it should become credulous, and lose the habit of testing things and inquiring into them.

William Kingdon Clifford
The Ethics of Belief, 1877

Preface

A Quick Jog over Hills by the Sea

This book is a quick jog along one useful and attractive path offering brief but good views of the theory of causal inference in observational studies. It is tour of an island, with an invitation to stay, but if you choose to stay, then there is more to see.

The path is attractive: I pick topics and methods that offer easy access to grand vistas. The path is useful: you could conduct excellent observational studies while staying on this path. The path quickly gets us out of base-camp into the hills; we quickly move beyond defining causal effects and making adjustments for observed covariates, to face the real challenges. That said, we will not reach all the points of interest, nor discuss all the useful methods. There are always ways to extract a bit more from data, to see a bit deeper into data, to design a better study, as well as many nearly equivalent ways to do any one thing; so, our path will not pass every site worth seeing. Chapters end with suggestions for Further Reading.

Why does our path through the southeast corner of the island go up to summit A rather than to adjacent summit B? Here are some answers, and hopefully one will satisfy. (i) If you become obsessed with such questions, you will miss some fine views. (ii) The answers to such questions are often much more difficult than the climb to summit A, and the answers are always less attractive than the view from summit A. (iii) I have taken people up summit A and summit B, and there is a short scramble over boulders on the way up to the top of B—someone always sprains their ankle on the way up to B, needs urgent care, and is carried out of the woods screaming on a stretcher. This happens all the time in statistics courses. (iv) If we go up both summit A and summit B, then our quick tour will not have time for the very different views on the north and west of the island. The southeast corner is great, but there is so much more. (v) Trust me, not forever, just until we reach the discussion of Further Reading.

The book stays focused on causal inference in observational studies, that is, on issues that arise because individuals were not assigned at random to treatment or control. In any large, complex empirical investigation, other issues will arise too, but

I leave such issues to other books that focus on topics other than causal inference in observational studies.

This book is an *introduction* to the *theory* of its subject. It is aimed at someone who wants to know how and why things are true, not someone who wants to be told what is true. As a consequence, basic knowledge of mathematical statistics, at the undergraduate level, is the prerequisite background. The proofs in the text and the problems at the end of chapters are aimed at someone who has taken an undergraduate course in mathematical statistics. In contrast, a proof in an appendix to a chapter is typically not difficult, but it may use slightly more technical tools. Appendices and sections or subsections with an asterisk may be skipped without encountering problems later in the book; however, appendices differ from sections with an asterisk. A section with an asterisk offers you more than you need to continue, something interesting but optional. By and large, an appendix demonstrates some specific technical fact needed in the text for which a reference is not available in the literature.

An `R` package `iTOS` was created as a companion to this book. It is publicly available at CRAN. The package contains the data sets and reproduces selected analyses. Some of the problems ask you to do analyses using the `iTOS` package.

What Should an Example Exemplify?

To avoid mistaking mere association for causation in an observational study, one needs to be familiar with the context, to know one's way about. One needs to have a sense of how the treatment is supposed to work, how and why some people are exposed to the treatment and others are not, what attributes of people predict their outcomes and their treatments, what various outcomes the treatment should and should not affect, what other treatments should or should not affect the outcome of interest, and on and on.

A specialist would have specialized knowledge, but this is not a book aimed at a single specialty. A health economist studying the effects of deductibles and co-payments on healthcare expenditures needs to know the strengths and limitations of medical billing and claims data, the factors that lead one person to choose an expensive, comprehensive medical plan and another person to choose inexpensive, catastrophic coverage, and so on. A psychiatrist studying the causes of ADHD in children needs to understand the social environment in which one child with symptoms receives a diagnosis and another child with similar symptoms does not. An epidemiologist asking whether coffee is a cause of pancreatic cancer needs to know to measure cigarette smoking, because smoking is a cause of pancreatic cancer, and caffeine and nicotine are both addictive stimulants. Knowledge of context is helpful, also, in designing randomized experiments for causal inference, but it is less essential—one can have a context-free statistical theory of randomized experiments, but not of observational studies.

In light of the role of context in observational studies, ask: What sort of example is helpful in an introductory book? Presumably, it is an example in which the context is at least somewhat familiar to most readers. For this reason, I focus on two simple examples involving the consumption of alcohol, one asking whether a daily glass of wine causes a desirable increase in HDL cholesterol levels (the so-called "good" cholesterol), the other asking whether five or more drinks on most days causes an undesirable increase in blood pressure. Imagine person A who drinks one glass of wine each day, and person B who consumes seven alcoholic drinks on most days. Suppose A or B has not been to a dentist in more than a year. Is it A or B? Do you have a hunch? Suppose one of these two people eats fish several days a week and the other rarely eats fish. Is it A or B who eats fish frequently? Would your guess beat a coin flip? Imagine two controls, C and D, where C is 40 years old and has consumed fewer than 10 drinks of alcohol in 40 years, while D used to drink heavily but with great effort has managed to quit. One of C and D is a smoker. Would you be willing to bet whether C or D is the smoker? If you have a hunch or are willing to guess, it is because the context is familiar: you have known people who never drink alcohol, people who drink in moderation, and people who drink to excess, and you have a sense of what else is going on in their lives. Hunches, guesses, and bets are not scientific evidence, but they can point to scientific evidence that should be examined, suggest comparisons that might enlighten, or focus attention on data that is both available and relevant.

Data from the two alcohol examples is available in the `R` package `iTOS`.

The alcohol examples discuss just a small corner of the relationship between alcohol consumption and health. In particular, there is an important concern that I do not address, namely, the abundant evidence that alcohol is a carcinogen; so, harm from its cancer-causing effects might easily outweigh any desirable increase in HDL cholesterol levels. Alcohol also causes liver diseases, accidents, and violence, and it is addictive for some people. The examples in this book are important as aids to understanding statistical concepts in a familiar context; they are not contributions to the major open questions concerning alcohol and health.

My hope is that the reader will find these commonplace examples helpful in learning general principles, and then can take the principles back to a specialized context closer to the reader's own interests or research. The examples are not intended to be an exhaustive discussion of the effects caused by alcohol, nor are they ultimately about alcohol—they are intended to exemplify the role of context in causal inference.

A Word About Notation

Notation is defined as it is introduced. There is no need to think about notation now. This paragraph is for future reference. It answers a question that you may have later on: "I forgot the meaning of a symbol—where can I find it?" In the index, a **bold** page number indicates a definition. Notation is summarized at the back of the book,

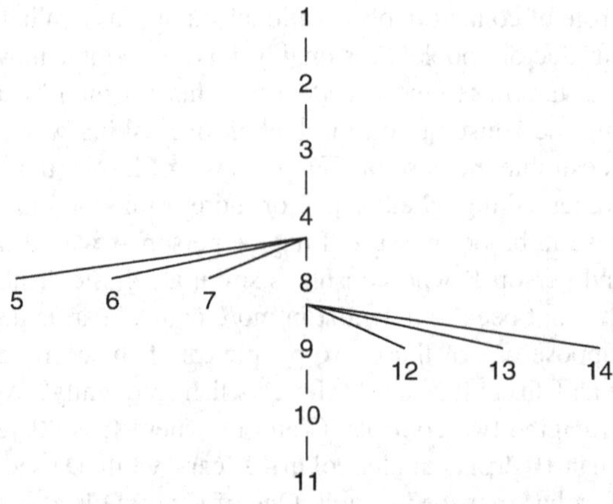

Fig. 1 Dependence among chapters

but you should turn to this section only when you are puzzled; hopefully, you will not need it.

Dependence Among Chapters

Figure 1 shows the dependence among Chaps. 1–14. Chapter 15 may be read at any time. Of course, sections or subsections of a chapter with an asterisk may be skipped.

Bits and pieces of Chaps. 12 and 13 refer to Chaps 9–11, but these bits and pieces can be skipped.

A Word About Technical Terms

As noted, the prerequisite knowledge is an undergraduate course in mathematical statistics. The Glossary at the back of the book contains reminders of some standard terminology from such a course. If you encounter an unfamiliar term while reading, look in the glossary.

Quotations

If a quotation appears inside of a chapter, its source is in the reference list for that chapter. If a quotation appears outside of a chapter, its source is in the reference list for the subsequent chapter.

A Sequence of Problems Using Binomial Distributions

Most chapters end with several problems. In particular, there is one sequence of problems involving the binomial distribution that begins in Chap. 2 and ends in Chap. 11. If you decide to do these problems, it may be best to view them as a sequence, because later problems in the sequence depend upon earlier problems.

Many technical topics in causal inference in observational studies can be illustrated with a very simple family of test statistics introduced in 1973 by Gottfried Noether. The statistics are used to test the null hypothesis of no treatment effect using I independent treated-minus-control matched-pair differences. These statistics have a binomial distribution under the null hypothesis of no treatment effect, with the consequence that a variety of technical topics may be illustrated while staying very close to the binomial distribution. Though useful, the statistics in this family are not the ultimate weapon; however, they often illustrate concepts in the simplest nontrivial case.

The simplest test statistic for I matched pairs is the sign test statistic: it counts the number of positive pair differences and compares that count to the binomial distribution with sample size I and probability of success 1/2. Unhappy with the poor efficiency of the sign test for Normally distributed matched-pair differences, Noether proposed a family of test statistics, and each member of this family has a binomial distribution under the null hypothesis of no treatment effect. Noether's statistic looks at the $I' \leq I$ pairs with the largest absolute pair differences, counting the number of positive differences among these I' pairs, and comparing that count to the binomial distribution with sample size I' and probability of success 1/2. Noether noted that taking $I' = 2I/3$ meaningfully increases the efficiency of the sign test for Normally distributed matched-pair differences; however, taking $I' = I/3$ turns out to be better in observational studies.

Problem 2.2 introduces Noether's statistic in a randomized experiment, where its randomization distribution is binomial with probability of success 1/2. Problem 8.3 shows that in a sensitivity analysis in an observational study, the sensitivity bound is again provided by a binomial distribution, but not with probability 1/2. If some people are fated to receive treatment or control—they receive treatment with probability 0 or 1—then there is a sense in which the binomial bound for Noether's statistic allows for this and is, at worst, a bit conservative; see Problem 8.4 and the caveat in Problem 8.5. Performance of test statistics in a sensitivity analysis depends upon both null and alternative hypotheses, but in simple cases involving Noether's statistic this is a comparison of two binomial distributions. It is here that Noether's family with $I' < I$ becomes interesting; see Sect. 9.2 and Problems 9.2 and 9.3, where focusing on the $I' = I/3$ largest absolute pair differences produces a statistic with good properties in a sensitivity analysis. The efficiency of certain sensitivity analyses using Noether's statistic reduces to the efficiency of certain comparisons of two binomial distributions; see Problem 11.2. Adaptive inference using two of Noether's statistics again reduces to calculations involving two independent binomial distributions; see Problem 11.4.

Pennsylvania, PA, USA
February 2025

Paul R. Rosenbaum

Acknowledgments

In writing this book, I am in debt to many colleagues or coauthors whose work is described here, including: Linda H. Aiken, Katrina Armstrong, Michael Baiocchi, Sydney Brown, Katherine Brumberg, Magdalena Cerda, Amy S. Clark, Shoshana R. Daniel, Roderic G. Eckenhoff, Darcy E. Ellis, Ashkan Ertefaie, Orit Even-Shoshan, Lee A. Fleisher, Colin B. Fogarty, Kevin R. Fox, Joseph L. Gastwirth, Bruce J. Giantonio, Robert Greevy, Xing Sam Gu, M. Elizabeth Halloran, Ben B. Hansen, Raiden Hasegawa, Sean Hashemi, Amelia Haviland, Ruth Heller, Siyu Heng, Sean Hennessy, Alex S. Hill, Paul W. Holland, Robert Hornik, Jesse Y. Hsu, Guido W. Imbens, Caleb Ing, Siddharth Jain, Marshall M. Joffe, Hyunseung Kang, Bikram Karmakar, Luke Keele, Rachel R. Kelz, Abba M. Krieger, Kwonsang Lee, Xinran Li, Yunfei Paul Li, Justin M. Ludwig, Scott Lorch, Bo Lu, Sue M. Marcus, Matt McHugh, Kewei Ming, Daniel S. Nagin, Mark D. Neuman, Bijan A. Niknam, Mark Olfson, Ricardo D. Paredes, Samuel D. Pimentel, Daniel Polsky, Kate J. Propert, Caroline E. Reinke, Joseph G. Reiter, Richard N. Ross, Donald B. Rubin, Alan J. Salzberg, Jeffrey H. Silber, Dylan S. Small, Herbert L. Smith, Sindhu Srinivas, Tom R. Ten Have, Wei Wang, David A. Wolk, Dan Yang, Ting Ye, Frank Yoon, Ruoqi Yu, Elaine Zanutto, Bo Zhang, Kai Zhang, Qingyuan Zhao, and José R. Zubizarreta. I am grateful to Judith A. McDonald and José R. Zubizarreta for many helpful suggestions.

Contents

Part I First Steps

Part III Sensitivity of Inferences to Covariates That Were Not Observed

Part IV Quasi-Experimental Devices

Acronyms

BMI	Body mass index, a measure of obesity: mass in kilograms divided by the square of height in meters
CDC	US Centers for Disease Control
CLT	Central limit theorem
NHANES	US National Health and Nutrition Examination Survey
USDA	US Department of Agriculture
WHO	World Health Organization
HDL	High-density lipoprotein cholesterol

Part I
First Steps

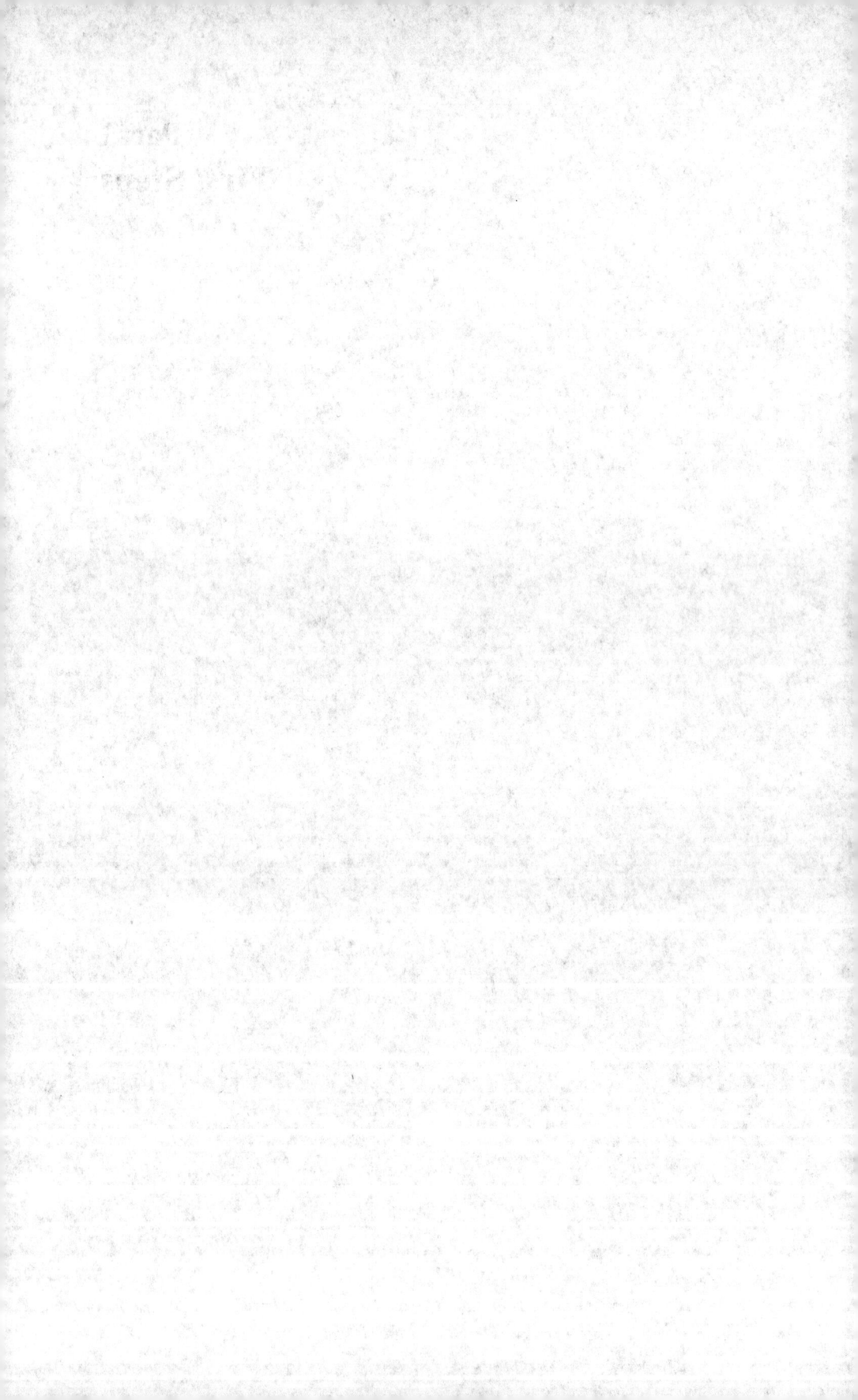

Chapter 1
Examples of Observational Studies

Abstract An observational study is an attempt to infer the effects caused by treatments when it is unethical or impractical to assign individuals to treatments at random, as would be done in a randomized experiment. Three observational studies are described. The first, from the medical literature, concerns the possible effects of general anesthesia on the risk of dementia. Of medium size, this study matched each of 54,996 treated individuals to 5 untreated controls in blocks of size six, making $329{,}976 = 6 \times 54{,}996$ individuals in total. The other two studies are of similar structure, but they are simpler and smaller, with public data that is available to the reader for reanalysis in the `R` package `iTOS`. These two smaller studies will illustrate concepts throughout the book. Both studies concern the effects of consuming alcohol. One study asks whether light daily alcohol consumption causes a desirable increase in HDL cholesterol, the so-called "good cholesterol." The second study asks whether frequent binge drinking causes an undesirable increase in blood pressure. These examples exemplify methodology, and that is their sole function. They do not address the most important effects of alcohol, such as its role in causing cancer, and its total effect on longevity, effects that are mentioned here only briefly.

1.1 Observational Studies: A Definition

William G. Cochran [9] defined an observational study as an attempt to infer the effects caused by treatments, interventions, policies or exposures, in circumstances that preclude random assignment of treatments to individuals [10, 24, 49]. So, an observational study is defined by what it lacks. It is a study with a purpose—inference about treatment effects—in which randomization is absent. The words "causal" and "observational" are common in English, with several distinct and several overlapping uses; so, one cannot be justly critical of someone who uses these words in some other way. Nonetheless, if someone speaks of "causal" without reference to the effects

© The Author(s), under exclusive license to Springer Nature Switzerland AG 2025

P. R. Rosenbaum, *An Introduction to the Theory of Observational Studies*,
Springer Texts in Statistics, https://doi.org/10.1007/978-3-031-90494-3_1

of interventions or preventable exposures, or of "observational" without reference to the absence of randomization, then she is, by definition, talking about something else.

A lack, an absence, is understood, at least initially and in part, by considering how things would be if that lack were not there. An absence is understood in comparison with a presence. Expecting to meet his friend, Pierre, at a Parisian café at 4 o'clock and finding him not there, Sartre [50, p. 42] says: "Pierre, absent, *haunts* this café;" as, indeed, the absence of randomization *haunts* an observational study. An initial and partial understanding of observational studies begins with the role of randomization in experiments, as developed in Chap. 2. With deeper understanding of the absence of randomization in observational studies comes a deeper understanding of the importance of randomization in experiments. And round and round, in widening spirals. As Michael Oakeshott [28, p. 1] expressed the thought: "... understanding is an exertion; it is the resolve to inhabit an ever more intelligible, or an ever less mysterious world. ... It is an engagement to abate mystery rather than to achieve definitive understanding."

Situations often preclude random assignment of treatments. Randomized experimentation on people cannot breach ethical norms: It cannot study the damage done by toxins and infectious agents, the psychological effects caused by trauma, or the effects of child abuse. Experimentation cannot interfere with a person's rights: In most circumstances, even beneficial treatments cannot be imposed on people who do not want them. In a democratic republic, the law cannot randomize treatments among similarly situated citizens: It cannot randomize the level of the minimum wage, the duration of compulsory schooling, or the degree of progressivity of the income tax. Much that is important in life is beyond the scope of randomized experimentation.

It is sometimes claimed that randomized experimentation is the "gold standard" for causal inference. Look for support for this claim in the major statistical journals, and you will search in vain for a "gold standard" for anything. These journals do not offer the authoritative judgments of experts but rather reasoned arguments, empirical evidence, and mathematical proof that certain research designs and analytical methods have certain desirable or undesirable properties under certain circumstances. The journals offer what Habermas[1] [17, p. 140] called "the curiously unforced force of the better argument." The journal's reader is responsible for what she makes of arguments, evidence, and proof and cannot escape responsibility by transferring it to some authority. In fields that often employ observational studies—in epidemiology and public health, in economics and public affairs, in medicine and in health outcomes research, in clinical psychology and psychiatry—the goal is to enhance human health, prosperity, and well-being without harming the people under study. Indeed, very much in this spirit, Bernanke [3] questioned whether the gold standard is the "gold standard" for currencies.

In statistics, randomized experimentation plays two roles. First, it is a highly reliable method for inference about the effects caused by those treatments that are

[1] More fully, Habermas wrote: "The proponent of a truth claim is obliged to provide justifications, while the opponent has the right to object ... It is part of the meaning of the rights and obligations within argumentation that they bring into play the curiously unforced force of the better argument."

either harmless or that offer the realistic prospect of benefit for the person treated. Randomization is important and practical in clinical medicine, and in evaluations of vaccination and screening programs in public health [31, 47]; moreover, it is sometimes practical in evaluating the effects of social programs [4, 15, 48]. Second, randomized experimentation is a leading case[2] for causal inference in general, a case in which sound methodology alone can almost mechanically ensure success in causal inference.

1.2 Does General Anesthesia Accelerate Dementia?

Laboratory work suggests that common forms of general anesthesia produce certain biological transformations at the cellular level similar to those associated with Alzheimer's disease [13, 63, 67]. Does general anesthesia materially accelerate dementia in humans? As I write in 2025, this is an open and debated question, with insufficient evidence either to demand or to alleviate concern. Even if general anesthesia affects the risk of dementia, does an hour or 2 every 10 years meaningfully increase risk? Or are ongoing risk factors, such as obesity and physical inactivity [26, 56], of much greater concern?

It is not ethical to randomly assign individuals undergoing surgery to general anesthesia or no anesthesia. Nor is it ethical to randomly assign healthy individuals not undergoing surgery to general anesthesia or no anesthesia, simply to determine whether anesthesia increases the risk of dementia. For certain types of surgery, it is ethical to randomly assign patients to either general anesthesia or regional anesthesia, and this has been done [29], but very large trials with many years of follow-up are not currently available.

An observational study of general anesthesia and dementia faces several difficulties. Anesthesia accompanies surgery, and surgery addresses some disease or injury. Certain forms of surgery—neurosurgery or coronary bypass surgery—may pose direct risks to the brain, apart from any risk that might be produced by anesthesia. Some forms of surgery may improve health or reduce suffering without curing the underlying disease; for instance, cancer surgery may be followed by chemotherapy that may affect the brain.

A natural experiment—a type of observational study—is an attempt to find a setting in which treatment assignment, though not randomized, is less affected by systematic biases in treatment assignment [1, 25, 41, 51]. Using data from the US Medicare program, Jeffrey Silber and colleagues [54] focused on appendectomy for appendicitis. They wrote:

> The present study is a natural experiment. Appendicitis occurs haphazardly in elderly individuals who are otherwise not necessarily extremely ill; moreover, with appropriate surgery, recovery is expected without continuing morbidity or treatment. In this sense, appendectomy is quite unlike surgery to remove a malignancy or surgery to transplant

[2] The *Oxford English Dictionary* says: "**leading case**: n. *Law*. a case that has settled some important point and is frequently cited as a precedent."

> a kidney. The typical case of appendicitis in Medicare resembles the typical person in Medicare but likely received about an hour of additional general anesthesia . . . Surgery for appendicitis is not elective, so there is no ambiguity from self-selection, as there would be with many forms of orthopedic surgery. Unlike most diseases that may require surgery, appendicitis does not disproportionately target people who have serious, enduring health problems, so it does not come packaged with major risk factors for ADRD [Alzheimer's disease and related disorders].

The study examined 54,996 patients aged 68 to 77 in Medicare who underwent appendectomy for appendicitis between 2002 and 2012. Medicare is a US government program that provides health care for the elderly. Each such appendicitis patient was matched to five similar controls, yielding 54,996 blocks of size six with one treated patient and five controls. Follow-up continued until 2017. Follow-up ranged from 5 to 15 years after appendectomy.

A *covariate* is a variable that describes a person prior to treatment assignment; hence, a covariate is unaffected by the treatment that the person has not yet received. In sharp contrast, an *outcome* is a variable that describes a person after treatment assignment, so it may or may not be affected by the treatment. If a patient has cognitive impairment before appendectomy, then that is a covariate, but if a patient has cognitive impairment after appendectomy, then that is an outcome, and only the latter might be affected by appendectomy. Failure to distinguish covariates and outcomes is a conceptual mistake with substantial consequences [14, 35]. When treated individuals receive treatment at different times, as in the case of appendectomy, some care is needed to compare treated individuals and controls who were similar prior to treatment.

The study used a tactic called "risk-set matching" [20, 22]. Simplifying slightly, this means that the first patient undergoing appendectomy for appendicitis in 2002 was matched to five controls who were the same age in 2002 and who looked similar to the treated patient prior to the moment that the treated patient had surgery. At a later moment in 2002, a second patient had an appendectomy and was matched to five as yet unmatched controls, again matching patients so that they are similar prior to this later moment when this second treated patient had surgery. So, matched patients were similar in terms of measured covariates prior to the moment of surgery, but the matching carefully avoided using information about the future status of patients. In particular, at the moment of surgery, all patients in a block had no prior history recording evidence of cognitive decline, neurodegeneration, or dementia. Any of the six individuals in a block might develop dementia later, but that is an outcome, not a covariate. Also, after matching, a control might later have an appendectomy for appendicitis, and this did happen for 71 of the 274,980 controls, where 71/274,980 = 0.000026. Additionally, in both treated and control groups, many patients died over the follow-up period, before or after developing dementia, but dementia and death after treatment are both outcomes.

In each block, the match used a three-year look-back from the date of surgery to characterize the health of the six patients prior to surgery, and the match tried to form blocks of people who were similar prior to the date of surgery for the patient with appendicitis. Specifics follow. All patients in the same block were the same in terms of: year of birth, race, sex, history of inflammatory bowel or diverticular disease. For many other covariates, the match defined a distance between two people reflecting how similar they were prior to the moment of appendectomy for the patient with appendicitis, and the match picked controls to make that distance small. See Chap. 5 for discussion of covariate distances and other aspects of constructing a matched observational study. Specifically, the match controlled for age as a continuous variable, for the number of surgical procedures in the previous 3 years, for the minutes of anesthesia in those previous surgeries, for the number of inpatient hospital visits in the prior 3 years, for the number of emergency department visits in the prior 3 years, for measures of poverty in a person's home neighborhood, for whether the patient was eligible for Medicaid as well as Medicare, for histories of numerous health problems including liver disorders, colon and gastrointestinal cancers and other categories of cancer, stroke and cerebrovascular diseases, specific categories of cardiac disease, lung disorders, diabetes, endocrine disorders, kidney disorders, and many other covariates. See [54, Table 1] for details, including measures of the degree of success in producing a treated and a control group comparable in terms of these covariates. Chapter 6 evaluates the degree to which a match has succeeded in producing a treated group and a control group that are similar in terms of observed covariates.

Matching for observed covariates may make the groups comparable in terms of these observed covariates, but it does little or nothing to make the groups comparable in terms of covariates that were not observed. This is a key issue in observational studies. A treated group and a control group that are visibly similar in terms of observed covarates may nonetheless differ in terms of unmeasured covariates. A difference in outcomes in treated and control groups that could plausibly be an effect caused by the treatment could instead reflect the possibility that the treated and control groups were not comparable after all. This possibility is raised in the critical discussion of most, if not all, observational studies.

The comparison of appendicitis patients and matched controls was thought to be a "natural experiment," in which the most obvious unmeasured biases were small or absent. What unmeasured biases might nonetheless be present? Here is one. The study characterized a patient's medical history using a 3-year look-back in Medicare records, but for almost everyone, entry into Medicare cannot begin before age 65. Individuals in the study were all at least 68 years old, and they all had been in Medicare for at least 3 years before they were matched. For almost everyone, Medicare provides no information about health care in youth or middle age. No doubt, some controls had their appendix removed before entering Medicare; however, aside from rare surgical errors, this could not happen in the treated group. So, there is one unmeasured difference between treated and control groups. Silber et al. [54] discuss this issue, and several unrelated but similar issues involving possible unmeasured biases, and they include sensitivity and stability analyses. Chapter 8 discusses sensitivity and stability analyses.

Most people are spared dementia by dying first. Silber et al. [54] found a similar incidence of death before dementia in treated and control groups, and actually a very slightly lower incidence of dementia before death in the treated group than in the control group. So, the study provided no sign of excess dementia in the group that had anesthesia and appendectomy when compared to untreated controls.

Does a study like this settle the matter? No. By itself, this one study is a piece of a jigsaw puzzle whose true meaning will emerge as the puzzle is assembled from additional studies with different strengths and limitations. Ultimately, causal inference from observational studies depends upon concurrence among different studies with different strengths and limitations [19, 40, 42].

A related study of children asked whether anesthesia increases the risk of subsequent neurobehavioral disorders [55]. This study also used appendectomy in a risk-set match, now with $I = 134{,}388$ exposed children, each matched to five controls in blocks of size $J = 6$, making $I \times J = 806{,}328$ children in total. Like the small example that will be discussed in Sect. 1.4, this study investigated unmeasured biases using a second control group and two unaffected outcomes.

1.3 Is Alcohol Good for You?

In 2009, the *New York Times* published an essay entitled "Alcohol's good for you? Some scientists doubt it." In it, Roni Rabin [32] wrote:

> By now, it is a familiar litany. Study after study suggests that alcohol in moderation may promote heart health and even ward off diabetes and dementia. The evidence is so plentiful that some experts consider moderate drinking—about one drink a day for women, about two for men—a central component of a healthy lifestyle.
>
> But what if it's all a big mistake? . . . It may be that moderate drinking is just something healthy people tend to do, not something that makes people healthy.

It is sometimes suggested that light alcohol consumption reduces the risk of death from cardiovascular disease, perhaps by increasing high-density lipoprotein (HDL) cholesterol, the so-called "good cholesterol" [57]; however, there is growing, perhaps justified, scepticism about a net benefit from alcohol. In a statement on behalf of the American Society of Clinical Oncology in 2018, Noelle Locante and colleagues [21, pp. 84, 88] wrote:

> The International Agency for Research on Cancer (IARC), a branch of WHO, has assessed the evidence and [. . . concluded. . .] that alcohol is a cause of cancers of the oral cavity, pharynx, larynx, esophagus, colorectum, liver (i.e., hepatocellular carcinoma), and female breast. . . . [T]he risk of cancer is increased even with low levels of alcohol consumption, so the net effect of alcohol is harmful. Thus, alcohol consumption should not be recommended to prevent cardiovascular disease or all-cause mortality.

A statement by a committee formed by the American Heart Association does not disagree [16]. It is generally recognized that heavy drinking causes many deaths from various cancers, liver diseases, accidents, and violence. Some people intend to drink lightly but end up drinking heavily. Even light alcohol consumption by pregnant women is believed to place the fetus at risk of developmental defects, the risk being present before the pregnancy is known [7].

In Sects. 1.4 and 1.5, two examples are introduced concerning the effects caused by alcohol. These examples of observational studies are simpler than the anesthesia example in Sect. 1.2, and they will serve to illustrate theoretical ideas in later chapters. The example in Sect. 1.4 concerns a possibly beneficial effect of light alcohol consumption in the form of increased HDL cholesterol levels. In contrast, the example in Sect. 1.5 concerns the possibly harmful effect of frequent binge drinking in the form of increased blood pressure. There is, in fact, fairly strong evidence in the literature for both effects [34, 57]. Neither effect speaks to the central question raised by Locante et al. [21, pp. 84, 88] concerning the net benefit or harm of alcohol on longevity [44, Ch. 9] and [46]. As noted in the Preface, the examples serve to illustrate methodology in a familiar context, not to advance the study of alcohol and its effects on health.

The data in Sect. 1.4 and Sect. 1.5 are available to the reader in the `R` package `iTOS` that is associated with this book.

1.4 Light Daily Alcohol and HDL Cholesterol

Does light daily alcohol consumption cause a desirable increase in high-density lipoprotein (HDL) cholesterol? We will look at a comparison in $I = 406$ blocks, $i = 1, \ldots, I$, where each block i contains $J = 4$ individuals, $j = 1, \ldots, J$, one of whom currently drinks a moderate amount of alcohol on most days, while the other three currently drink infrequently or not at all. The data are from the US National Health and Nutrition Examination Surveys (NHANES) for 2013-2014 and 2015-2016.[3]

Each block i contains one treated individual or "daily drinker" (D) who drank a moderate amount of alcohol on most days. Specifically, individual D drank alcohol on at least $260 = 5 \times 52$ days, typically consuming between one and three drinks on drinking days. This individual has $Z_{ij} = 1$ signifying a "treated individual" and belongs to group $G_{ij} = \text{D}$, signifying "daily drinking." The other three individuals are controls, with $Z_{ij} = 0$; so, $1 = \sum_{j=1}^{4} Z_{ij}$ for each block i. The three controls are different. The groups are defined using several variables in NHANES. To force consistency on the responses of a couple of people who responded inconsistently, the definitions that follow sound a bit redundant. One control is a "never drinker," signified by $G_{ij} = \text{N}$. This never-drinking control had fewer than 12 drinks in their life, fewer than 12 drinks in the past year, and no period in their life when they engaged in binge drinking on most days. A second control was a "rare drinker," signified by $G_{ij} = \text{R}$. The rare drinker had 12 or more drinks in their life, but fewer than 12 in the past year, with no period in their life of binge drinking on most days. The third control was a "past binge drinker," signified by $G_{ij} = \text{B}$. A past binge drinker did have a history of binge drinking, that is, a past period of drinking at least

[3] The data are in the `aHDL` data frame in the `iTOS` package in `R`.

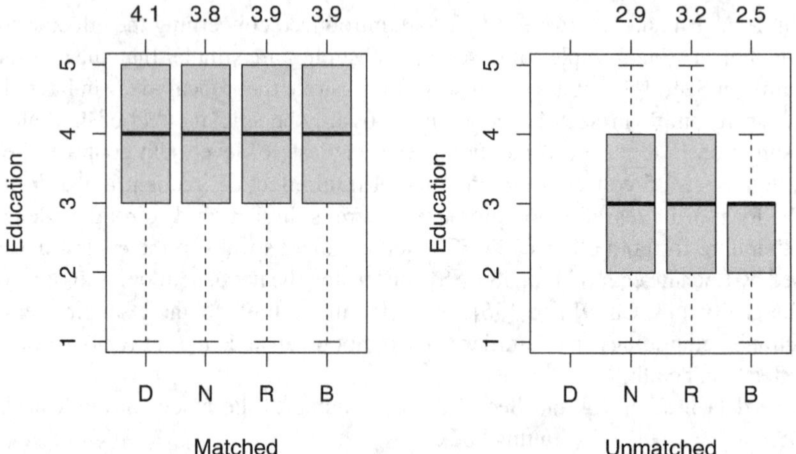

Fig. 1.1 Balance of the covariate "education" for matched and unmatched individuals, in the study of HDL cholesterol and light daily alcohol consumption. The mean education appears above each boxplot. D = daily drinking, N = never drinking, R = rare drinking, B = past binge drinking. 1 = less than 9th grade, 3 = high school, 5 = BA degree

four or five drinks per day on most days, but currently drinks at most once a week, that is, on at most 52 days in the past year.

The blocks were matched for age, sex, and education. Education is recorded in five categories, 1 for less than 9th grade, 2 for 9th to 11th grade without a high school degree, 3 for a high school or equivalent degree, 4 for some college such as a 2-year associates degree, and 5 for at least a 4-year BA college degree. For instance, block $i = 1$ contained four men with BA degrees aged between 40 and 43. This is a simple type of matching that attempts to form blocks that are quite homogeneous in terms of a few observed covariates. Matching methods are described in Chap. 5. Write $\mathbf{x}_{ij}$ for the observed covariates—here, age, sex, and education—for the jth individual in block i.

Table 1.1 describes age, sex, and education, before and after matching, and Fig. 1.1 depicts education for matched and unmatched individuals. In the conventional way, the boxes in the boxplots in Fig. 1.1 have horizontal lines at the median and quartiles, where extreme individuals, if any, are plotted as individual points [60]. All $I = 406$ treated individuals—that is, all daily light drinkers D—were matched, each to one control of each type, N = never drinkers, R = rare drinkers and B = past binge drinkers. In terms of the three observed covariates, the four groups are quite different before matching, quite similar after matching. It is (i) important that the groups were similar in terms of observed covariates after matching; (ii) important, also, that the groups were dissimilar before matching; and (iii) important, finally that, before matching, the three control groups differed in different ways from the treated group.

Table 1.1 Sample sizes and covariate means or percents Before and After matching in the study of light alcohol and HDL cholesterol. The unmatched individuals (Not) combine with the matched individuals After matching to form the group Before matching. All 406 treated individuals in group D were matched, so none were unmatched. D=daily, N=never, R=rarely, B=past binger

	Sample Size			Female %			Age			Education		
	Before	After	Not	Before	After	Not	Before	After	Not	Before	After	Not
D	406	406	0	34	34		57	57		4.1	4.1	
N	1536	406	1130	71	34	84	51	57	50	3.2	3.8	2.9
R	1237	406	831	72	34	90	53	56	51	3.4	3.9	3.2
B	914	406	508	29	34	25	54	56	53	3.1	3.9	2.5

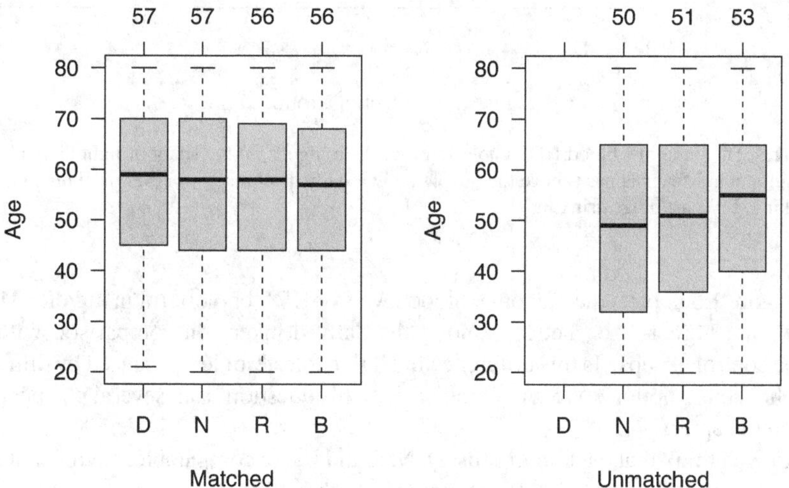

Fig. 1.2 Balance of the covariate "age" for matched and unmatched individuals, in the study of HDL cholesterol and light daily alcohol consumption. The mean age appears above each boxplot. D = daily drinking, N = never drinking, R = rare drinking, B = past binge drinking

Before matching, most daily drinkers were men, as were most past binge drinkers, whereas most never drinkers or rare drinkers were women. Daily drinkers were older than controls and had more education. See also Figs. 1.1 and 1.2. Problems 1.1–1.3 consider the sample sizes in Table 1.1.

Multiplying "drinking days per year" by "drinks on drinking days" to obtain a crude approximation to "drinks in the past year," the medians in the matched groups are 520 drinks in group D, 0 in group N, 0 in group R, and 4 in group B. The upper quartiles or 75th percentiles are 728 drinks in group D, 0 in group N, 3 in group R, and 36 in group B. The 90th percentiles are 1008 drinks in group D, 0 in group N, 6 in group R and 104 in group B. Despite drinking lightly, group D consumed much more alcohol than the other groups.

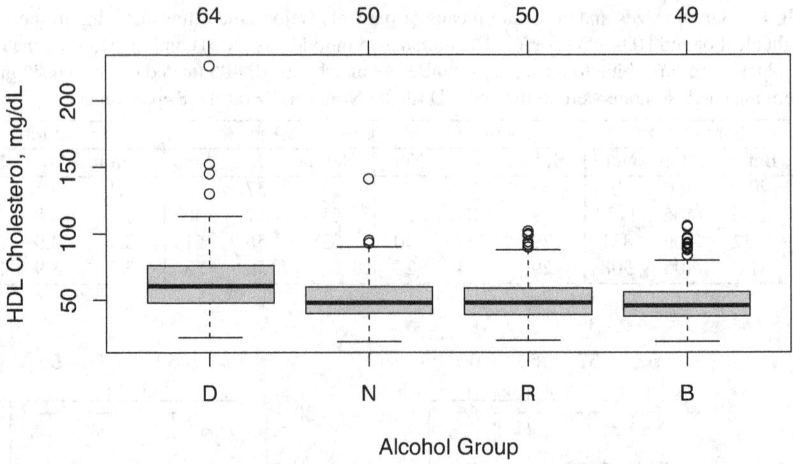

Fig. 1.3 The outcome, blood HDL cholesterol levels in mg/dL, in the study of light daily alcohol consumption. Means appear above the boxplots. D = daily drinking, N = never drinking, R = rare drinking, B = past binge drinking

Figure 1.3 depicts the outcome, blood levels of HDL cholesterol in mg/dL. These levels are higher—i.e., better—among the daily drinkers, in comparison with all three control groups. Is this difference in HDL cholesterol levels caused by differing alcohol consumption? We will come back to this question from several perspectives in later chapters.

Do you think that the four groups, D, N, R and B, are comparable, having matched for age, sex, and education? If not, how might they differ?

Participants in NHANES between ages 18 and 59 were asked: "Have you ever, even once, used marijuana or hashish?" The 404 blocks were matched fairly closely for age. Recall that the data used here required an age of at least 20 but included people aged 60 or more; so, in the matched analysis, only 860 people between 20 and 59 were asked this question, while the remaining $4 \times 404 - 860 = 1624 - 860 = 764$ were not asked, because they were at least 60 years old. Of the 860 people who were asked, 24 declined to respond, so there were 836 responses. Do you think that groups D, N, R, and B gave similar or dissimilar responses? If dissimilar, what pattern do you expect? Please think for a moment before continuing.

Among responders in the matched groups, the percentages who had tried marijuana or hashish were 73% in group D, 9% in group N, 25% in group R, and 75% in group B. In this respect, the groups are very different, despite matching for three measured covariates. In terms of having tried marijuana or hashish, former bingers B are more similar to daily drinkers D than groups N and R, but there is nothing to ensure this is true of other covariates. By itself, having tried marijuana or hashish once probably means little for health; however, this pattern of responses suggests, as perhaps you already guessed, that the four groups have led different lives, quite apart from age, sex, and education. We will see more evidence of their different lifestyles in later chapters. This is one reason why it is interesting to have three control groups, with different histories, rather than one [2, 6, 25, 37, 38, 45]; see Chap. 13.

We often look for problems in an observational study by examining outcomes that the treatment is expected to not affect [5, 23, 33, 36, 39, 53, 58]. If, after matching for observed covariates, a treatment is associated with outcomes that it should not affect, then this is often taken as indicating that treatment groups differ in terms of some unmeasured covariate.

Methylmercury is a neurotoxin. Pedersen et al. [30] looked for methylmercury in alcoholic beverages but did not find detectable levels; see also [12]. The World Health Organization [64] says that "People are mainly exposed to methylmercury, an organic compound, when they eat fish and shellfish that contain the compound;" see also [61]. Shark, swordfish, and tuna contain relatively high levels of methylmercury. So, it seems unlikely that alcohol causes a meaningful increase in methylmercury levels in the blood, and more likely that a difference in methylmercury levels indicates different dietary preferences.

For a subsample, NHANES obtained blood methylmercury levels. The 406 blocks in Table 1.1 were formed to contain either four individuals from the sample with methylmercury levels or four individuals without methylmercury levels. The 406 blocks are composed of 200 blocks with methylmercury levels and 206 blocks without methylmercury levels.

Figure 1.4 depicts the level of methylmercury in blood for the $800 = 4 \times 200$ individuals in the 200 blocks for which methylmercury was measured. To make the central portion of the boxplot visible, the right panel of Fig. 1.4 uses a square root scale, meaning that the vertical axis is labeled with methylmercury levels, but the plotting positions of points are determined by their square roots.

Compare Fig. 1.4 for methylmercury to Fig. 1.3 for HDL cholesterol. Parallel boxplots appear in Fig. 1.5. What should we make of Figs. 1.3, 1.4 and 1.5? We have reason to doubt that Fig. 1.4 depicts an effect on methymercury caused by consuming alcohol. Should the pattern in Fig. 1.4 make us doubt that Fig. 1.3 depicts an effect on HDL cholesterol caused by consuming alcohol? We will return to this question in Chap. 12.

1.5 Binge Drinking and Blood Pressure

Does frequent binge drinking cause an undesirable increase in blood pressure?

The data are from NHANES 2017-2020 (which was interrupted by COVID-19 and so is not a survey). In NHANES, binge drinking is defined as four or more drinks per day for a woman or five or more drinks per day for a man. The study compares people at least 20 years old, forming a treated group and two control groups based on responses to questions about alcohol consumption. The three groups are named:

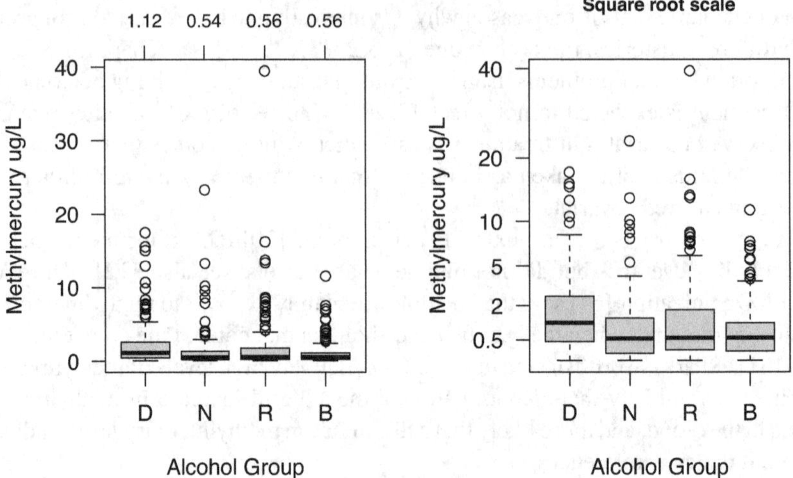

Fig. 1.4 An outcome, methylmercury, for which no effect was expected. Medians appear above the boxplots on the left plot. The plot on the right uses a square root scale, so that the central portion of the boxplot is visible. D = daily drinking, N = never drinking, R = rare drinking, B = past binge drinking

group B for "binge," group N for "never," and group P for "past." On at least 3 days each week in the past year, group B engaged in binge drinking. Group N did not binge at all in the past year, drank alcohol on at most 1 day a week in the last year, and there was no time in their lives when they binged almost every day. Group P used to engage in binge drinking but quit. Specifically, people in group P did have a period in their lives when they engaged in binge drinking almost every day, but they did not engage in binge drinking at any time in the past year and drank alcohol on at most 1 day a week during the past year. Pause for a moment to imagine one person in each group. In an observational study, your imagination is a poor guide to what is true, but it might help you decide how and where to look in the data.

The outcomes are measures of diastolic and systolic blood pressure, plus a combination of the two. The values for diastolic and systolic blood pressure are each the average of between one and three blood pressure readings for a person; so, they are somewhat more stable than individual readings. The combined measure, `bpCombined`, adds together robustly standardized versions of diastolic and systolic blood pressure; so, `bpcombined` is especially elevated when both diastolic and systolic blood pressure are elevated.[4]

[4] This is discussed in detail in the documentation for the `R` package `iTOS` that is associated with this book. Specifically, as discussed in the documentation for `binge` in the `R` package `iTOS`: "bpCombined is the sum of two standardized measures, one for systolic blood pressure and one for diastolic blood pressure. We often standardize a quantity by subtracting its mean and dividing

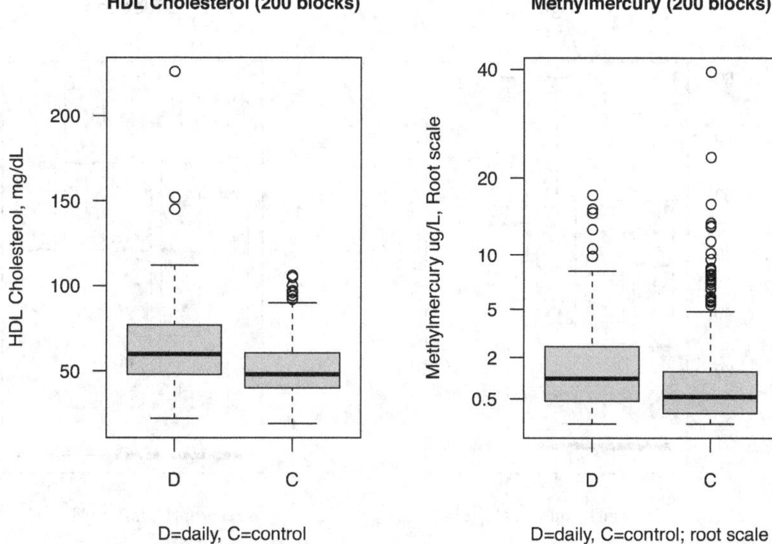

Fig. 1.5 Parallel boxplots for HDL cholesterol and methylmercury, for the same 200 blocks. The three control groups, N, R, and B, are merged into one group C. The plot on the right uses a square root scale. Should we believe the left plot for HDL cholesterol is an effect caused by alcohol if we do not believe the plot on the right for methylmercury is an effect caused by alcohol?

The groups are matched for nine covariates: age, sex, education, body-mass-index (BMI), waist-to-hip ratio, engagement in vigorous activity in recreation or at work, current smoking, having quit smoking (for current nonsmokers), and currently taking medication for blood pressure (bpRX). Body-mass-index and waist-to-hip ratio are two indices of obesity. Before matching, ask: What do you expect to see? Are most binge drinkers in their 20's? Are binge drinkers fat or skinny? Do they abstain from vigorous activity? Do binge drinkers also smoke? Are past bingers similar to current bingers or to never bingers?

In Sect. 1.4 for HDL cholesterol, an attempt was made to match closely for three covariates, age, sex, and education, but the current match for high blood pressure has nine covariates. This is largely for expository purposes: matching for nine covariates

---

the result by its standard deviation. The mean and standard deviation are distorted by outliers; so, the standardization will replace the mean by the median, and the standard deviation by the "mad" (=median absolute deviation from the median). In the larger NHANES data set of individuals at least 20 years of age who are not pregnant, the median and the mad were determined separately for systolic and diastolic blood pressure, producing a standardized systolic blood pressure and a standardized diastolic blood pressure. The variable `bpCombined` is the sum of these two standardized measures. The calculation used the median and mad functions in the `stats` package, so the mad was by default scaled to resemble the standard deviation for a Normal distribution.

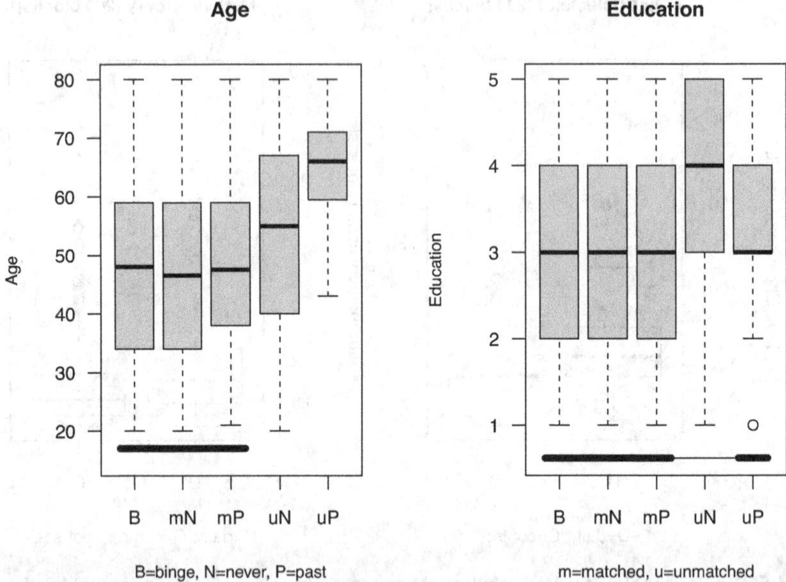

Fig. 1.6 Covariates age and education in the study of binge drinking and blood pressure. The five groups do not overlap, as "u" signifies the unmatched individuals excluded from the matched comparison

requires slightly different concepts and tools, as will be examined in detail in Chaps. 5 and 6. Typical examples have many more covariates, as in Sect. 1.2.

As was discussed in Sect. 1.2, if you match or adjust for an outcome because you are under the mistaken impression that it is a covariate—if you adjust for a variable that may have been affected by the treatment—then you may distort or bias estimates of the effect of the treatment on the outcome that interests you [35]. Issues of this kind can be quite subtle: a variable that bears the name of a covariate may in fact be an outcome, because the manner in which the variable is measured is affected by the treatment [27]. Are measures of obesity—BMI and waist/hip ratio—actually covariates? On the one hand, alcohol is a source of calories, so binge drinking could conceivably cause obesity; however, the situation is complex, and the evidence is mixed [59, 62]. If binge drinking causes an increase in blood pressure, might it consequentially cause someone to take blood pressure medication? We will reconsider this issue and the list of covariates in Chap. 7 and Sect. 14.2.

Table 1.2 shows covariate means or percents, before and after matching, for groups B, N, and P. Education is as in Sect. 1.4, with 1 for less than ninth grade, 3 for high school degree or equivalent, and 5 for at least a BA degree. The groups look similar after matching. Before matching, never bingers were mostly female, while current and past bingers were mostly male. Before matching, past bingers were older

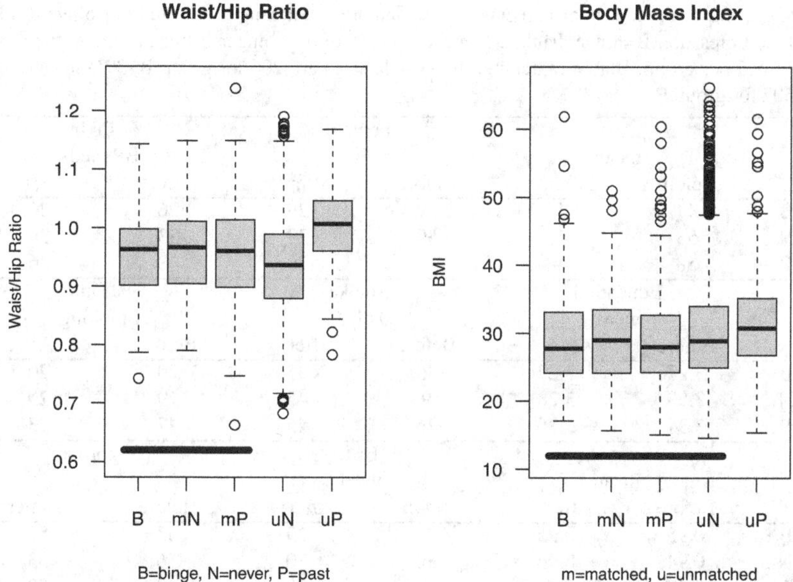

Fig. 1.7 Covariates waist/hip ratio and body mass index (BMI) in the study of binge drinking and blood pressure. The five groups do not overlap, as "u" signifies the unmatched individuals excluded from the matched comparison

and more likely to be taking medication for high blood pressure (bpRX). Before matching, current bingers were more likely to be daily smokers, while past bingers were more likely to have quit smoking as well as binge drinking. Before matching, vigorous activity was more common among current bingers.

Figures 1.6 and 1.7 depict four covariates in matched (m) and unmatched (u) groups. Unlike Table 1.2, the unmatched groups (u) in Figs. 1.6 and 1.7 show who was *excluded* from the match. For example, a person appears in one and only one boxplot for age in Fig. 1.6. Notably, the excluded past bingers were much older than the matched groups, and the excluded never bingers had more education than the matched groups. The measures of obesity in Fig. 1.7 were not very dissimilar before matching; nonetheless, the excluded never bingers had lower waist-to-hip ratios than the matched groups, while the excluded past bingers had higher waist-to-hip ratios. The BMI was slightly higher among excluded past bingers.

People are good at finding patterns, even patterns that are not there. Which wiggles in boxplots might deserve attention, and which wiggles look like sampling noise? One way to think about this is discussed in Chap. 6. Here, let's take a quick but informal look. For age in Fig. 1.6, the lower quartile for matched past binge drinkers (denoted mP in Fig. 1.6) is higher than in matched groups B and mN. Is that difference about as big as expected by chance? What about the two boxplots of

Table 1.2 Covariate means or percents, before and after matching in the study of binge drinking and blood pressure. B=binge drinker, N=never binger, P=past binger. After matching, the sample size is 206 per group. Before matching, the sample sizes are 206 for group B, 3919 for group N, and 502 for group P

	Age mean		Female %		% Taking BP meds	
	Before	After	Before	After	Before	After
B	47	47	29	29	26	26
N	53	47	59	29	33	26
P	58	48	24	29	43	26
	Education mean		Smoke Daily %		% Quit Smoking	
	Before	After	Before	After	Before	After
B	3.27	3.27	45	45	20	20
N	3.59	3.28	9	45	19	20
P	3.24	3.26	26	45	47	23
	Waist/Hip mean		BMI mean		Vigorous %	
	Before	After	Before	After	Before	After
B	0.95	0.95	29	29	53	53
N	0.94	0.96	30	30	36	53
P	0.98	0.96	31	30	40	50

age for the individuals who were not matched, uN and uP? If the five groups had been formed by randomly assigning individuals to groups, what sort of difference among the boxplots would be expected to result from random assignment and what sort of difference is too large to be produced in that way? The five boxplots of age were compared pairwise, in all $(5\times 4)/(2\times 1) = 10$ possible ways, using Wilcoxon's rank sum test, and the ten P-values were adjusted for multiple testing using Holm's procedure [18, 65]; so, the chance is at most 0.05 that random assignment to the five groups would misleadingly produce an adjusted P-value ≤ 0.05.[5] In Figs. 1.6 and 1.7, boxplots underlined by a thick horizontal line have adjusted P-values above 0.05 compared to other boxplots with a thick horizontal line—i.e., they form a group of boxplots that do not differ significantly—whereas a thin line or the absence of a line indicates an isolated boxplot that differs significantly from *every* other boxplot. The adjusted P-values that are ≤ 0.05 are all quite small, the largest being 0.0074. The adjusted P-values that are > 0.05 are all quite large, the smallest being 0.36. Some of the unmatched groups are clearly different from the rest, unlike the matched groups. Particularly in Fig. 1.7, the P-values make distinctions that are not obvious to the eye. Again, a better way of assessing covariate balance is discussed in Chap. 6.

[5] Of course, we know that treatments were not randomly assigned; so, we are not actually testing whether treatments were randomly assigned. We are using the test informally to ask: Would the imbalance in a covariate seen in boxplots seem out of place if it were observed in a randomized experiment? If you are interested, Holm's procedure and adjusted P-values are described in the Glossary at the back of the book. General graphical displays of multiple comparisons are discussed by Xi and Bretz [66].

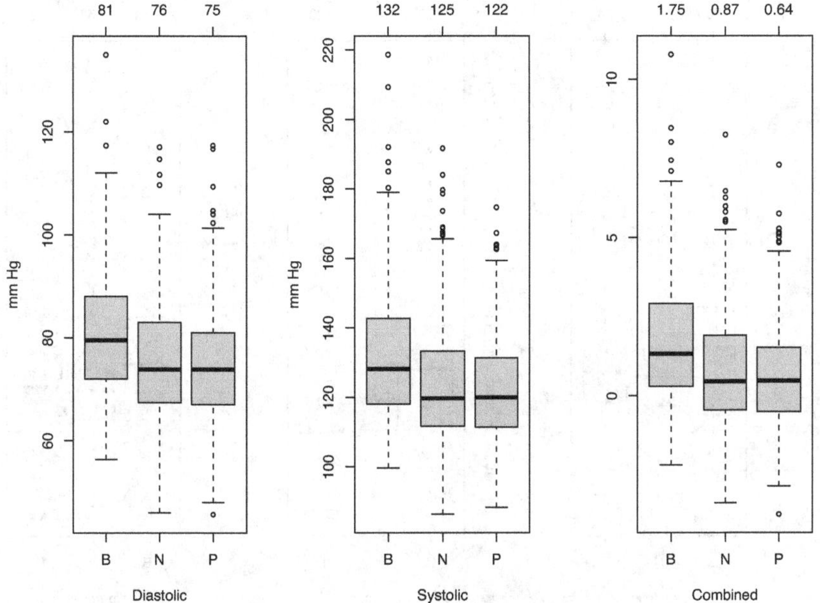

Fig. 1.8 Matched blood pressure outcomes in the study of binge drinking. Group means appear above the boxplots

Figure 1.8 depicts the three blood pressure outcomes, diastolic, systolic, and their standardized combination for matched individuals. The group of current bingers, group B, has somewhat higher blood pressure than groups N or P.

In 54 of the 206 blocks of 3 individuals, all 3 individuals said they were currently taking medication to control high blood pressure. Figure 1.9 depicts the remaining 152 blocks, in which no one said they were currently taking blood pressure medication. Figures 1.8 and 1.9 look fairly similar. Is the pattern in Figs. 1.8 and 1.9 an effect caused by binge drinking? We will return to this question in later chapters.

Problems

1.1 Standard Errors in Unbalanced and Balanced Designs
(a) Suppose that $Y_{ij} = \mu_j + \epsilon_{ij}$, for $i = 1, \ldots, n_i$ and $j = 1, \ldots, J$, where the ϵ_{ij}'s are independent random variables with the same distribution, with expectation 0 and variance σ^2. Give a formula for the least squares unbiased estimate of the contrast $\mu_1 - (\mu_2 + \cdots + \mu_J)/(J-1)$, and give a formula for the variance of this estimate.

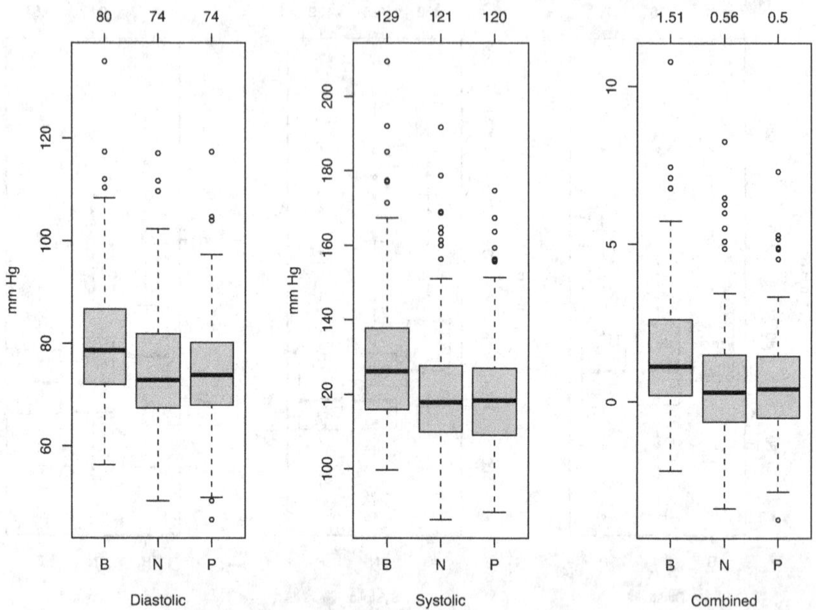

Fig. 1.9 Matched blood pressure outcomes in the study of binge drinking, excluding the 54 blocks in which individuals were currently taking medication to control blood pressure. Group means appear above the boxplots

(b) What is the variance of the estimate in (a) if $J = 4$ and $n_1 = n_2 = n_3 = n_4 = 406$, in parallel with Table 1.1? (The answer will involve the unknown parameter σ^2.)
(c) What is the variance of the estimate in (a) if $J = 4$ and $n_1 = 406$, $n_2 = 1536$, $n_3 = 1237$, $n_4 = 914$, in parallel with Table 1.1?
(d) The standard error of an estimate is its standard deviation or equivalently the square root of its variance. Determine the ratio formed as the standard error in part (b) divided by the standard error in part (c). (The answer will not involve σ^2; it will be a number.) Remark: Under simple Gaussian (i.e., Normal) models, when the sample sizes are large, this ratio will approximate the ratio of the lengths of the confidence intervals for the contrast.
(e) What is the ratio of the total sample size, $n_1 + n_2 + n_3 + n_4$, in part (b) divided by the total sample size in part (c)?
(f) Comment about the disparity in the sizes of the two ratios you computed in parts (d) and (e). Why is the sample size much larger in (c) than in (b), but the standard error is only modestly smaller in (c) than in (b)?
(g) Redo part (d) with $n_2 = 812$ and $n_1 = n_3 = n_4 = 406$. (This would happen if two N's were matched to each D.)

1.2 Suppose the model in Problem 1.1 were $Y_{ij} = \beta_i + \mu_j + \epsilon_{ij}$, so that the model includes I block terms, β_i, with $I = n_1 = \cdots = n_J$. If the β_i were independent random variables, independent of the ϵ_{ij}, with variance $\sigma_\beta^2 > 0$, then the variance of

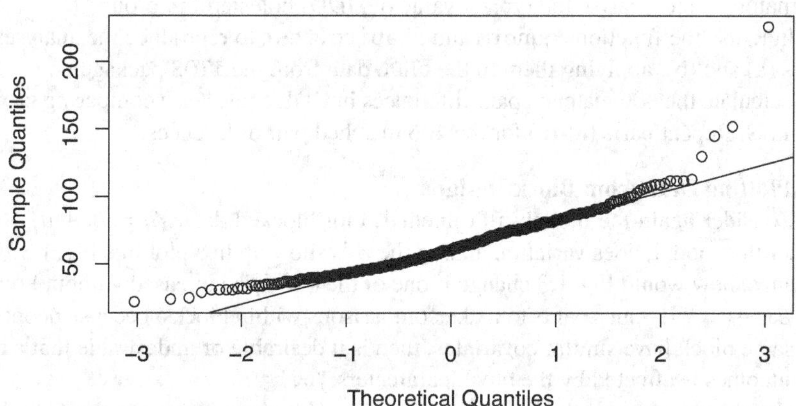

Fig. 1.10 A Normal quantile-quantile plot of HDL cholesterol levels in group D

Y_{ij} is $\sigma^2 + \sigma_\beta^2 > \sigma^2$. Is the contrast estimator you proposed in Problem 1.1(a) still an unbiased estimate? How does σ_β^2 affect its variance?

1.3 Infinite Sample Sizes in Unbalanced Designs
(a) In part (c) of Problem 1.1, the sample size was $n_2 = 1536$. What is the answer to part (c) of Problem 1.1 in the limit as $n_2 \to \infty$ with the other n_j's fixed? (That is, $n_1 = 406$, $n_3 = 1237$, $n_4 = 914$, but $n_2 \to \infty$.)
(b) Answer parts (d) through (f) of Problem 1.1 in the limit as $n_2 \to \infty$ with the other n_j's fixed.
(c) Consider two designs, one with $n_1 = n'$, $n_2 = 1536$, $n_3 = 1237$, $n_4 = 914$, the other with $n_1 = 406$, $n_2 = \infty$, $n_3 = 1237$, $n_4 = 914$. How large would n' have to be for the first design to have a smaller standard error than the second design?

1.4 Is It Wise to Use the Mean?
(a) Figure 1.3 reported a mean HDL cholesterol level of 64 for the daily drinkers or group D. Figure 1.10 is a Normal quantile-quantile plot of the $n = 406$ HDL cholesterol levels in group D. That is, the 406 HDL cholesterol levels are sorted into increasing order and are plotted as "y" against quantiles of the Normal distribution as "x," with the ith largest cholesterol level plotted against $\Phi^{-1}\{(i-0.5)/n\}$, where $\Phi(\cdot)$ is the standard Normal cumulative distribution. In a large sample from the Normal distribution, we expect to see a fairly straight line in a Normal quantile plot. Do the HDL cholesterol levels in group D look like a sample from a Normal distribution? If not, how does the sample seem to differ from a Normal distribution?
(b) The Shapiro-Wilk [52] test has as its null hypothesis that the data are a sample from the Normal distribution, and in essence, it asks whether a Normal quantile plot looks "straight enough." The P-value from the Shapiro-Wilk test is 1.265×10^{-14}. How does this affect your conclusion in part (a)?

(c) In light of parts (a) and (b), discuss the relative merits of using the mean or other estimators to summarize the typical value of HDL cholesterol in group D.
(d) In R, use the functions `qqnorm` and `shapiro.test` to reproduce the analyses in parts (a) and (b), applying them to the `aHDL` data from the `iTOS` package.
(e) Calculate the 406 matched pair differences in HDL cholesterol comparing groups D and N. Repeat parts (a)-(d) for the 406 matched pair differences.

1.5 Plotting Data from Block Designs
(a) Consider again the model in Problem 1.3 for blocked data, $Y_{ij} = \beta_i + \mu_j + \epsilon_{ij}$. Under this model, does variation among the β_i's show up in a plot like Fig. 1.3? For instance, how would Fig. 1.3 change if one of the 406 β_i's increased without bound, say $\beta_{97} \rightarrow \infty$? If your goal is to make comparisons within blocks, because people in the same block have similar covariates, then is it desirable or undesirable that a plot of outcomes is affected by the block parameters, β_i?
(b) How could you plot the four groups in Fig. 1.3 while eliminating the β_i? (Hint: The simplest way uses six boxplots for four groups [43, Figure 2]. There are also subtler ways to plot blocked data eliminating block effects: One compares treated-control differences in one boxplot to symmetrized $\pm$ control-control differences in a second boxplot [68, Figure 1]; another symmetrically transforms both tails to reduce the visual impact of outliers [43, Figures 3 & 5].)
(c) Suppose the ϵ_{ij}'s were independent observations from the same Normal distribution, but the β_i's were independent observations from a long-tailed distribution. How would that affect your interpretation of the analysis in Problem 1.4? Could $Y_{i1} - Y_{i2}$, comparing groups D and N, be Normally distributed when neither Y_{i1} nor Y_{i2} is Normally distributed? Given the appearance of Fig. 1.3, do you expect that $Y_{i1} - Y_{i2}$ will be approximately Normal in the actual data from the HDL cholesterol data?
(d) In the HDL cholesterol data in `aHDL` in the `iTOS` package in R, plot $Y_{i1} - Y_{i2}$ for groups D=1 and N=2. Do a boxplot, a Normal quantile plot and the Shapiro-Wilk test. Do block terms, β_i, explain the deviations from a Normal distribution that you observed in Problem 1.4?

1.6 Reading Exercise: The Weight of Evidence
Read either Locante et al. [21] or Goldberg et al. [16] to see how evidence from many observational studies is integrated into an argument for a particular policy or conclusion.

References

1. Angrist, J.D., Krueger, A.B.: Empirical strategies in labor economics. In: Ashenfelter, O., Card, D. (eds.) Handbook of Labor Economics, vol. 3, pp. 1277–1366. Elsevier, New York (1999)
2. Battistin, E., Rettore, E.: Ineligibles and eligible non-participants as a double comparison group in regression-discontinuity designs. J. Econ. **142**(2), 715–730 (2008)

3. Bernanke, B.S.: The macroeconomics of the Great Depression: a comparative approach. In: Essays on the Great Depression, pp. 5–37. Princeton University Press, Princeton, NJ (2009). Reprinted from the Journal of Money, Credit and Banking (1995)
4. Boruch, R.F.: Randomized Experiments for Planning and Evaluation: A Practical Guide, vol. 44. Sage, New York (1997)
5. Brumberg, K., Ellis, D.E., Small, D.S., Hennessy, S., Rosenbaum, P.R.: Using natural strata when examining unmeasured biases in an observational study of neurological side effects of antibiotics. J. R. Stat. Soc. C (Appl. Stat.) **72**(2), 314–329 (2023)
6. Campbell, D.T.: Prospective: Artifact and control. In: Rosenthal, R., Rosnow, R. (eds.) Artifacts in Behavioral Research. Academic Press, New York (1969). Reprinted in Campbell 1988, pp. 167–190
7. CDC: Alcohol Use in Pregnancy. US Centers for Disease Control, www.cdc.gov/ncbddd/fasd/alcohol-use.html (2021)
8. Clifford, W.K.: The Ethics of Belief and Other Essays. Prometheus Books, Amherst, NY (1999). The quote is from page 76. The essay was first published in the Contemporary Review in 1877
9. Cochran, W.G.: The planning of observational studies of human populations (with Discussion). J. R. Stat. Soc. A **128**(2), 234–266 (1965)
10. Dempster, A.P.: Reflections on W. G. Cochran, 1909–1980. Int. Stat. Rev. **51**, 321–322 (1983)
11. Dewey, J.: How We Think. D. C. Heath and Co, Boston (1910)
12. Dressler, V.L., Santos, C.M.M., Antes, F.G., Bentlin, F.R.S., Pozebon, D., Flores, E.M.M.: Total mercury, inorganic mercury and methyl mercury determination in red wine. Food Anal. Methods **5**, 505–511 (2012)
13. Eckenhoff, R.G., Johansson, J.S., Wei, H., Carnini, A., Kang, B., Wei, W., Pidikiti, R., Keller, J.M., Eckenhoff, M.F.: Inhaled anesthetic enhancement of amyloid-β oligomerization and cytotoxicity. Anesthesiology **101**(3), 703–709 (2004)
14. Gail, M.H.: Does cardiac transplantation prolong life? A reassessment. Ann. Intern. Med. **76**(5), 815–817 (1972)
15. Gerber, A.S., Green, D.P.: Field Experiments: Design, Analysis, and Interpretation. W. W. Norton & Company, New York (2012)
16. Goldberg, I.J., Mosca, L., Piano, M.R., Fisher, E.A.: Wine and your heart: a science advisory for healthcare professionals from the Nutrition Committee, Council on Epidemiology and Prevention, and Council on Cardiovascular Nursing of the American Heart Association. Circulation **103**(3), 472–475 (2001)
17. Habermas, J.: Truth and Justification. MIT Press, Cambridge, MA (2003)
18. Holm, S.: A simple sequentially rejective multiple test procedure. Scand. J. Stat. **6**, 65–70 (1979)
19. Lawlor, D.A., Tilling, K., Davey Smith, G.: Triangulation in aetiological epidemiology. Int. J. Epidemiol. **45**(6), 1866–1886 (2016)
20. Li, Y.P., Propert, K.J., Rosenbaum, P.R.: Balanced risk set matching. J. Am. Stat. Assoc. **96**(455), 870–882 (2001)
21. LoConte, N.K., Brewster, A.M., Kaur, J.S., Merrill, J.K., Alberg, A.J.: Alcohol and cancer: a statement of the American Society of Clinical Oncology. J. Clin. Oncol. **36**(1), 83–93 (2018)
22. Lu, B., Greevy, R.A.: Risk set matching. In: Zubizarreta, J.R., Stuart, E.A., Small, D.S., Rosenbaum, P.R. (eds.) Handbook of Matching and Weighting Adjustments for Causal Inference, pp. 169–184. Chapman and Hall/CRC, Boca Raton, FL (2023)
23. McKillip, J.: Research without control groups: a control construct design. In: Methodological Issues in Applied Social Psychology, pp. 159–175. Springer, Berlin (1992)
24. Meier, P.: William G. Cochran and public health. In: Rao, P.S.R.S., Sedransk, J. (eds.) W. G. Cochran's Impact on Statistics, pp. 73–81. Wiley, New York (1984)
25. Meyer, B.D.: Natural and quasi-experiments in economics. J. Bus. Econ. Stat. **13**(2), 151–161 (1995)
26. Nianogo, R.A., Rosenwohl-Mack, A., Yaffe, K., Carrasco, A., Hoffmann, C.M., Barnes, D.E.: Risk factors associated with Alzheimer disease and related dementias by sex and race and ethnicity in the US. JAMA Neurol. **79**(6), 584–591 (2022)

27. Niknam, B.A., Arriaga, A.F., Rosenbaum, P.R., Hill, A.S., Ross, R.N., Even-Shoshan, O., Romano, P.S., Silber, J.H.: Adjustment for atherosclerosis diagnosis distorts the effects of percutaneous coronary intervention and the ranking of hospital performance. J. Am. Heart Assoc. **7**(11), e008366 (2018)
28. Oakeshott, M.: On Human Conduct. Oxford University Press, Oxford (1975)
29. O'Brien, K., Feng, R., Sieber, F., Marcantonio, E.R., Tierney, A., Magaziner, J., Carson, J.L., Dillane, D., Sessler, D.I., Menio, D., Stone, T., Papp, S., Schwenk, E.S., Marshall, M., Jaffe, J.D., Luke, C., Sharma, B., Azim, S., Hymes, R., Chin, K., Sheppard, R., Perlman, B., Sappenfield, J., Hauck, E., Hoeft, M.A., Karlawish, J., Mehta, S., Donegan, D.J., Horan, A., Ellenberg, S.S., Neuman, M.D.: Outcomes with spinal versus general anesthesia for patients with and without preoperative cognitive impairment: secondary analysis of a randomized clinical trial. Alzheimer's & Dementia **19**(9), 4008–4019 (2023). https://doi.org/10.1002/alz.13132
30. Pedersen, G.A., Mortensen, G.K., Larsen, E.H.: Beverages as a source of toxic trace element intake. Food Addit. Contam. **11**(3), 351–363 (1994)
31. Piantadosi, S.: Clinical Trials: A Methodologic Perspective. Wiley, New York (2017)
32. Rabin, R.C.: Alcohol's good for you? Some scientists doubt it. The New York Times **158**(54708), D1–L (2009)
33. Reynolds, K.D., West, S.G.: A multiplist strategy for strengthening nonequivalent control group designs. Eval. Rev. **11**(6), 691–714 (1987)
34. Roerecke, M., Kaczorowski, J., Tobe, S.W., Gmel, G., Hasan, O.S., Rehm, J.: The effect of a reduction in alcohol consumption on blood pressure: a systematic review and meta-analysis. Lancet Public Health **2**(2), e108–e120 (2017)
35. Rosenbaum, P.R.: The consequences of adjustment for a concomitant variable that has been affected by the treatment. J. R. Stat. Soc. A **147**(5), 656–666 (1984)
36. Rosenbaum, P.R.: From association to causation in observational studies: the role of tests of strongly ignorable treatment assignment. J. Am. Stat. Assoc. **79**(385), 41–48 (1984)
37. Rosenbaum, P.R.: The role of a second control group in an observational study. Stat. Sci. **2**(3), 292–306 (1987)
38. Rosenbaum, P.R.: On permutation tests for hidden biases in observational studies. Ann. Stat. **17**(2), 643–653 (1989)
39. Rosenbaum, P.R.: The role of known effects in observational studies. Biometrics **45**, 557–569 (1989)
40. Rosenbaum, P.R.: Replicating effects and biases. Am. Stat. **55**(3), 223–227 (2001)
41. Rosenbaum, P.R.: Observation and Experiment: An Introduction to Causal Inference. Harvard University Press, Cambridge, MA (2017)
42. Rosenbaum, P.R.: Replication and Evidence Factors in Observational Studies. Chapman and Hall/CRC, New York (2021)
43. Rosenbaum, P.R.: A new transformation of treated-control matched-pair differences for graphical display. Am. Stat. **76**(4), 346–352 (2022)
44. Rosenbaum, P.R.: Causal Inference. MIT Press, New York (2023)
45. Rosenbaum, P.R.: A second evidence factor for a second control group. Biometrics **79**, 3968–3980 (2023)
46. Rosenbaum, P.R.: Does a daily glass of wine prolong life? Insight from a second control group. Chance **38**(1), 25–30 (2025)
47. Rosenberger, W.F., Lachin, J.M.: Randomization in Clinical Trials: Theory and Practice. Wiley, New York (2015)
48. Rossi, P.H., Lipsey, M.W., Henry, G.T.: Evaluation: A Systematic Approach. Sage Publications, New York (2018)
49. Rubin, D.: William G. Cochran's contributions to the design, analysis and interpretation of observational studies. In: Rao, P.S.R.S., Sedransk, J. (eds.) W. G. Cochran's Impact on Statistics, pp. 37–69. Wiley, New York (1984)
50. Sartre, J.P.: Being and Nothingness. Washington Square Press, New York (2022)
51. Sekhon, J.S., Titiunik, R.: When natural experiments are neither natural nor experiments. Am. Polit. Sci. Rev. **106**(1), 35–57 (2012)

52. Shapiro, S.S., Wilk, M.B.: An analysis of variance test for normality. Biometrika **52**(3/4), 591–611 (1965)
53. Shi, X., Miao, W., Tchetgen Tchetgen, E.: A selective review of negative control methods in epidemiology. Curr. Epidemiol. Rep. **7**, 190–202 (2020)
54. Silber, J.H., Rosenbaum, P.R., Reiter, J.G., Hill, A.S., Jain, S., Wolk, D.A., Small, D., Hashemi, S., Niknam, B.A., Neuman, M.D., Fleisher, L.A., Eckenhoff, R.: Alzheimer's dementia after exposure to anesthesia and surgery in the elderly: a matched natural experiment using appendicitis. Ann. Surg. **276**(5), e377–e385 (2022)
55. Silber, J.H., Rosenbaum, P.R., Reiter, J.G., Jain, S., Hill, A.S., Hashemi, S., Brown, S., Olfson, M., Ing, C.: Exposure to operative anesthesia in childhood and subsequent neurobehavioral diagnoses: A natural experiment using appendectomy. Anesthesiology **141**(3), 489–499 (2024)
56. Slomski, A.: Obesity is now the top modifiable dementia risk factor in the US. J. Am. Med. Assoc. **328**(1), 10–10 (2022)
57. Suh, I., Shaten, B.J., Cutler, J.A., Kuller, L.H.: Alcohol use and mortality from coronary heart disease: the role of high-density lipoprotein cholesterol. Ann. Intern. Med. **116**(11), 881–887 (1992)
58. Tchetgen Tchetgen, E.: The control outcome calibration approach for causal inference with unobserved confounding. Am. J. Epidemiol. **179**(5), 633–640 (2014)
59. Traversy, G., Chaput, J.P.: Alcohol consumption and obesity: an update. Curr. Obes. Rep. **4**, 122–130 (2015)
60. Tukey, J.W.: Exploratory Data Analysis. Addison-Wesley, Boston (1977)
61. US Centers for Disease Control: Mercury (2009). https://www.cdc.gov/biomonitoring/pdf/Mercury-FactSheet.pdf (Accessed 3 July 2023)
62. Wang, L., Lee, I.M., Manson, J.E., Buring, J.E., Sesso, H.D.: Alcohol consumption, weight gain, and risk of becoming overweight in middle-aged and older women. Arch. Intern. Med. **170**(5), 453–461 (2010)
63. Whittington, R.A., Virág, L., Marcouiller, F., Papon, M.A., Khoury, N.B.E., Julien, C., Morin, F., Emala, C.W., Planel, E.: Propofol directly increases tau phosphorylation. PloS One **6**(1), e16648 (2011)
64. World Health Organization: Mercury and Health (2017). https://www.who.int/news-room/fact-sheets/detail/mercury-and-health (Accessed 3 July 2023)
65. Wright, S.P.: Adjusted p-values for simultaneous inference. Biometrics **48**, 1005–1013 (1992)
66. Xi, D., Bretz, F.: Graphical approaches for multiple comparison procedures. In: Handbook of Multiple Comparisons, pp. 91–119. Chapman and Hall/CRC, Boca Raton, FL (2021)
67. Xie, Z., Dong, Y., Maeda, U., Alfille, P., Culley, D.J., Crosby, G., Tanzi, R.E.: The common inhalation anesthetic isoflurane induces apoptosis and increases amyloid β protein levels. Anesthesiology **104**(5), 988–994 (2006)
68. Ye, T., Small, D.S., Rosenbaum, P.R.: Dimensions, power and factors in an observational study of behavioral problems after physical abuse of children. Ann. Appl. Stat. **16**(4), 2732–2754 (2022)

Chapter 2
Causal Inference in Randomized Experiments

Abstract Causal inference in randomized experiments is introduced as one leading case for causal inference in observational studies. The goal is to understand precisely what is missing in an observational study and to put in place certain structures that will prove useful in later chapters. Fisher argued that randomization forms "the reasoned basis" for causal inference in randomized experiments, and a goal of the chapter is to develop a clear view of what that means. This leading case sets a precedent: Causal inference in randomized experiments does not require assumptions; rather, it depends upon the fact that the experimenter randomly assigned individuals to treatment or control. The causal effect on a single person cannot be estimated even in a randomized trial—it is not identified by the data from such a trial—and yet causal inference for the finite population of people in a randomized trial is possible, almost routine. So, even in a randomized trial, we are drawing inferences about causal effects that are only partially identified, and this lack of complete identification becomes more complex and challenging as we move from experiments to observational studies.

2.1 The Simplest Randomized Block Design

Blocks and Covariates

There are I blocks, $i = 1, \ldots, I$, and J people in each block, $j = 1, \ldots, J$; so, ij refers to a specific person. Person j in block i has a vector $\mathbf{x}_{ij}$ of observed covariates. Typically, the blocks were formed with the hope and intention that two people, j and j', in the same block i have similar values of the observed covariates, so that $\mathbf{x}_{ij}$ and $\mathbf{x}_{ij'}$ are close. In practice, these hopes and intentions are imperfectly realized. In Sect. 1.4, $\mathbf{x}_{ij}$ consisted of the age, sex, and education of person j in block i, and block $i = 1$ contained four men with BA degrees aged between 40 and 43. In brief

© The Author(s), under exclusive license to Springer Nature Switzerland AG 2025
P. R. Rosenbaum, *An Introduction to the Theory of Observational Studies*,
Springer Texts in Statistics, https://doi.org/10.1007/978-3-031-90494-3_2

moments, to crisply make a theoretical point, it may be assumed that our hopes and intentions were perfectly realized, that $\mathbf{x}_{ij} = \mathbf{x}_{ij'}$ for every i, j, and j'; however, outside such brief moments of theoretical euphoria, we need to be realistic about our inability to match exactly for a large number of observed covariates. This inability is not a disability: Causal inference does not require the comparison of individuals who are the same on many observed covariates. At present, and unless explicitly stated otherwise, it is *not* assumed that $\mathbf{x}_{ij} = \mathbf{x}_{ij'}$ for every i, j, and j'.

In observational studies, we always end up discussing some covariate or covariates that were not observed, and it helps to make a place in the notation for such a covariate. Participation in the discussion of unmeasured covariates is not voluntary: The possibility of bias from failure to control for an unobserved covariate is raised by referees and critics of most, if not all, observational studies [6]. Let u_{ij} denote a covariate, or perhaps a vector of covariates, that were not observed. In Sect. 1.4, the difference in methylmercury levels for daily light drinkers and controls led us to suspect that daily drinkers ate more fish than controls, so u_{ij} might describe, among other things, the consumption of fish. Because u_{ij} is not observed, there is no reason to expect that people in the same block are the same or similar with respect to u_{ij}. At various points later on, we will have occasion to ponder whether, of necessity, u_{ij} represents many covariates that could most appropriately be written as a vector, or whether, of necessity, u_{ij} is a single covariate that could most appropriately be written as a scalar; see, in particular, Sect. 4.5.

Treatment Assignments

Write $Z_{ij} = 1$ if the treated person in block i is person j, and write $Z_{ij} = 0$ otherwise, for $i = 1, \ldots, I$ and $j = 1, \ldots, J$. In this chapter, one person in each block is treated, so that $1 = \sum_{j=1}^{J} Z_{ij}$ for $i = 1, \ldots, I$. Write $\mathbf{Z}$ for the $I \times J$ array containing the Z_{ij}.

In how many ways can treatments be assigned? There are J possible treatment assignments for the first block, $i = 1$, and J possible treatment assignments for the second block, $i = 2$, and any assignment in the first block could occur together with any assignment in the second block; so there are $J \times J = J^2$ possible assignments for the first two blocks taken together. For $I = 2$ blocks of size $J = 3$, there are $J^I = 3^2 = 9$ possible treatment assignments, as listed in the nine arrays in (2.1). In the same way, there are J possible assignments for each of I blocks, and each assignment in any one block is compatible with any assignment in the other blocks, so there are J^I possible treatment assignments in total. A treatment assignment $\mathbf{z}$ is a possible value of $\mathbf{Z}$, and each of these J^I possible $\mathbf{z}$'s is an $I \times J$ array with a single one and $J - 1$ zeros in each of its I rows. Collect the J^I possible $I \times J$ arrays $\mathbf{z}$ in a set $\mathcal{Z}$; so each $\mathbf{z}$ is an element of $\mathcal{Z}$. If $\mathcal{S}$ is a finite set, write $|\mathcal{S}|$ for the number of elements in $\mathcal{S}$, that is, for the cardinality of the set. Then $|\mathcal{Z}| = J^I$ because the set $\mathcal{Z}$ contains J^I different arrays $\mathbf{z}$. For example, with $I = 2$ blocks of size $J = 3$, there are $J^I = 3^2 = 9 = |\mathcal{Z}|$ elements $\mathbf{z} \in \mathcal{Z}$, namely:

$$\mathcal{Z} = \left\{ \begin{array}{ccc} \begin{bmatrix} 1\,0\,0 \\ 1\,0\,0 \end{bmatrix}, & \begin{bmatrix} 1\,0\,0 \\ 0\,1\,0 \end{bmatrix}, & \begin{bmatrix} 1\,0\,0 \\ 0\,0\,1 \end{bmatrix}, \\ \\ \begin{bmatrix} 0\,1\,0 \\ 1\,0\,0 \end{bmatrix}, & \begin{bmatrix} 0\,1\,0 \\ 0\,1\,0 \end{bmatrix}, & \begin{bmatrix} 0\,1\,0 \\ 0\,0\,1 \end{bmatrix}, \\ \\ \begin{bmatrix} 0\,0\,1 \\ 1\,0\,0 \end{bmatrix}, & \begin{bmatrix} 0\,0\,1 \\ 0\,1\,0 \end{bmatrix}, & \begin{bmatrix} 0\,0\,1 \\ 0\,0\,1 \end{bmatrix} \end{array} \right\}. \tag{2.1}$$

A first thought is that random assignment of treatments means picking the actual treatment assignment $\mathbf{Z}$ as one $\mathbf{z}$ in $\mathcal{Z}$ with equal probabilities attached to every $\mathbf{z}$ in $\mathcal{Z}$, that is, with $\Pr(\mathbf{Z} = \mathbf{z}) = J^{-I}$ for each $\mathbf{z} \in \mathcal{Z}$. For instance, in (2.1), this entails picking as the treatment assignment $\mathbf{Z}$ one of the nine possibilities $\mathbf{z}$ in $\mathcal{Z}$, each with probability $J^{-I} = 3^{-2} = 1/9$. Can you see what is wrong with this first thought?

The correct definition of random assignment looks superficially similar but is actually a much stronger condition. This mistaken first thought restricts the marginal distribution of the treatment assignment, $\Pr(\mathbf{Z} = \mathbf{z})$, but the work is done by restricting a certain conditional distribution, not the marginal distribution. In a sense, that is obvious. If randomization is going to do work for us, it is going to have to connect treatment assignment $\mathbf{Z}$ to the other things we care about, and the marginal distribution of $\mathbf{Z}$ just doesn't do that. A fair coin flip doesn't just come up heads half the time; it comes up heads half the time for everyone, rich or poor, male or female, fated to develop dementia or to die without dementia. No matter what genes you inherited, no matter what preferences you may have, no matter which of your cells have been damaged by toxins, no matter what you secretly desire or fear, no matter how your neurons are connected, no matter what your parents said to you as a child, no matter what your future holds in store under treatment, no matter what your future holds in store under control, no matter what—a fair coin comes up heads for you half the time. A fair coin flip achieves a peculiar perfection: It predicts nothing we care about, by virtue of predicting nothing at all. A fair coin flip can predict the future only if it is endowed with the power to alter the future. In causal inference, a fair coin flip can do some amazing things. But to make this clear, we need a bit more notation.

2.2 The Effects Caused by a Treatment

A Causal Effect Compares Two Potential Outcomes of the Same Person

The jth person in block i has two potential responses, r_{Tij} if assigned to treatment with $Z_{ij} = 1$, or r_{Cij} if assigned to the control with $Z_{ij} = 0$. In Sect. 1.4, r_{Tij} was the HDL cholesterol level for the jth person in block i if this person—for brevity, person ij–drank small amounts of alcohol daily, and r_{Cij} was the HDL cholesterol level if this same person, ij, currently refrained from drinking alcohol.

The effect on person ij caused by the treatment is a comparison of r_{Tij} and r_{Cij}, commonly $r_{Tij} - r_{Cij}$. Write $\delta_{ij} = r_{Tij} - r_{Cij}$ for the causal effect on person ij. To say that daily drinking caused person ij to have a higher HDL cholesterol level is to say $r_{Tij} - r_{Cij} > 0$ or $\delta_{ij} > 0$, and to say daily drinking had no effect on person ij is to say $r_{Tij} - r_{Cij} = 0$ or $r_{Tij} = r_{Cij}$ or $\delta_{ij} = 0$. To say that daily drinking increases HDL cholesterol level for some people but does nothing for other people is to say $\delta_{ij} > 0$ for some people ij but $\delta_{i'j'} = 0$ for other people $i'j'$. The average treatment effect—also called the average causal effect—is $\overline{\delta} = (IJ)^{-1} \sum_{i=1}^{I} \sum_{j=1}^{J} \delta_{ij}$. This notation expresses causal effects as comparisons of the potential outcomes of individuals under alternative treatments, and it is due to Jerzy Neyman [50] and Donald Rubin [81, 82]; see also [13, 26, 37, 87, 103, 105]. Neyman introduced the notation for use in randomized experiments, and Rubin developed its important uses in observational studies; so, it is reasonable to refer to it as the Neyman-Rubin notation for causal effects.

Write R_{ij} for the response we actually observe from person ij. If person ij is picked for treatment with $Z_{ij} = 1$, then we observe $R_{ij} = r_{Tij}$, but if ij is picked for control with $Z_{ij} = 0$, then we observe $R_{ij} = r_{Cij}$. Saying this with symbols rather than words,

$$R_{ij} = Z_{ij}\, r_{Tij} + \left(1 - Z_{ij}\right) r_{Cij} = r_{Cij} + \delta_{ij}\, Z_{ij}. \tag{2.2}$$

The central problem in causal inference is that we observe r_{Tij} if $Z_{ij} = 1$ or r_{Cij} if $Z_{ij} = 0$—that is, we observe $\left(R_{ij}, Z_{ij}\right)$—but we do not observe $\left(r_{Tij}, r_{Cij}\right)$ jointly; so, we never observe a causal effect $\delta_{ij} = r_{Tij} - r_{Cij}$. Causal inference is inference about something we cannot observe. This central problem is a manageable problem, perhaps even a small problem, when treatments are randomly assigned, but it is a substantial problem in observational studies.

Write $\mathcal{F}$ for the potential outcomes, $\left(r_{Tij}, r_{Cij}\right)$, observed and unobserved covariates, $\left(\mathbf{x}_{ij}, u_{ij}\right)$, for the IJ people under study, or

$$\mathcal{F} = \left\{\left(r_{Tij}, r_{Cij}, \mathbf{x}_{ij}, u_{ij}\right),\ i = 1, \ldots, I,\ j = 1, \ldots, J\right\}. \tag{2.3}$$

Notably, much of $\mathcal{F}$ is not observed. Were $\mathcal{F}$ observed, causal inference would reduce to arithmetic: From $\mathcal{F}$, were $\mathcal{F}$ observed, we could calculate the causal effects, δ_{ij}, describe the patterns in their behavior, and we could calculate the average treatment effect, $\overline{\delta}$. In a sense, $\mathcal{F}$ contains everything we care about in a causal inference, everything people talk about, including the potential outcomes, the causal effects, and the unobserved covariates that are the source of most of the debate in a causal inference. The calligraphic F symbol, $\mathcal{F}$, is used, because these are quantities *f*ixed by conditioning in *F*isher's [21] theory of randomization inference.

Interference Between Units

Is it simply true that person ij has two responses, r_{Tij} if assigned to treatment with $Z_{ij} = 1$ or r_{Cij} if assigned to control with $Z_{ij} = 0$? It does seem that one response will be seen if ij is assigned to treatment and another if ij is assigned to control, so it seems, at first, that there are just two responses for ij. How could that be false?

Implicit in this notation is the idea that my response is affected by the treatment I receive, and your response is affected by the treatment you receive. That is why I have two potential responses, and so do you. In certain contexts, however, it can happen that I am affected not only by the treatment I receive but also by the treatment you receive.

The traditional example is vaccination, say vaccination for flu or placebo. If I am assigned to placebo (i.e., my Z is 0), whether or not I catch flu may depend upon whether I catch it from you, and whether I catch it from you may depend upon whether you are assigned to vaccine or placebo—that is, my outcome may depend upon both my Z and on your Z. Contagion does not seem unlikely, given that you and I play poker every Thursday. So, that makes $2 \times 2 = 4$ responses for me, based your treatment assignment and on mine. And of course you too have four responses, depending upon my Z and your Z.

Actually, it is much worse than this. It is not just you and me at the poker game. There are three other people every Thursday at the poker game, and whether I catch flu may depend upon whether each of the five of us is vaccinated, and there are $2^5 = 32$ ways that the five of us may be vaccinated or not; so, I have 32 possible responses, and so do you, and so do the other poker players.

Actually, it is much worse than this. Each of the poker players has a family, so the outcome of every poker player may be affected by the vaccination or placebo assignment Z for every member of the five families. And on and on.

David Cox [14, §2.4] says there is "no interference between units" if the response of one unit is "unaffected by the particular assignment of treatments to the other units." Over several pages, he discusses a variety of examples in which interference is either likely or unlikely. If there is no interference between units, then each unit has two potential responses depending upon the treatment given to that unit. Rubin [84] speaks of this as the "stable unit-treatment-value assumption" or SUTVA. In principle, if there is interference between units, then each individual ij has a different potential outcome for each $\mathbf{z} \in \mathcal{Z}$ rather than two potential outcomes [64, §2.5.2]. With $I = 2$ blocks of $J = 3$ people in a randomized block design in (2.1), each of the $IJ = 6$ individuals has $J^I = 3^2 = 9$ potential outcomes that correspond with the $J^I = 3^2 = 9$ treatment assignments $\mathbf{z}$ that have positive probability in this experiment.

Causal inference is possible in randomized experiments with interference between units [2, 34, 57, 68, 93, 98]. Many of the issues that arise when interference is present are the same or similar to issues that arise when there is no interference, but the notation for interference is more elaborate, and the conclusions are a bit less satisfying; so, these methods are not discussed in this book.

In the simplest possible type of interference, there are I matched pairs of $J = 2$ individuals, one of whom is treated, $1 = Z_{i1} + Z_{i2}$, and interference may occur within a pair but not across different pairs; that is, the two individuals, $i1$ and $i2$, in each pair i have four potential outcomes depending upon both treatment assignments in that pair, (Z_{i1}, Z_{i2}), but not depending upon treatment assignments in other pairs, $Z_{\ell j}$, $\ell \neq i$. For instance, imagine vaccinating one randomly chosen spouse in each of I married couples who live in different cities; then, interference is likely within a couple but not across different couples. Because the randomization enforces $1 = Z_{i1} + Z_{i2}$, this randomized experiment can exhibit only two of the four possible outcomes for each individual. If attention shifts from the effect on individuals to the effect on couples of vaccinating one spouse and not the other, then certain conventional analyses of matched pair differences are correct but acquire a new and different interpretation [65, §6]. Taking a step beyond this case, the simplest case considered by Hudges and Halloran [34] also has interference within but not across pairs but randomly assigns four treatment patterns to the pairs, namely, $(Z_{i1}, Z_{i2}) = (1, 1), (1, 0), (0, 1), (0, 0)$; so, one can then estimate, for instance, the effect of being unvaccinated with a vaccinated spouse versus unvaccinated with an unvaccinated spouse. These simplest situations are helpful stepping stones en route to general situations that permit any individual in the experiment to interfere with any other individual [34, 68].

2.3 What Is Randomized Treatment Assignment?

Recall from Sect. 2.1 that $\mathcal{Z}$ is the set containing the $|\mathcal{Z}| = J^I$ possible values $\mathbf{z}$ of the treatment assignment $\mathbf{Z}$, where each $\mathbf{z} \in \mathcal{Z}$ is an $I \times J$ array with a single one and $J - 1$ zeros in each of its I rows. By definition, the randomized block design in Sect. 2.1 always has $\mathbf{Z} \in \mathcal{Z}$. To distinguish this situation from certain other situations that will be discussed later, when speaking of a block design, a probability that $\mathbf{Z}$ does this or that will always condition upon the event $\mathbf{Z} \in \mathcal{Z}$, and for brevity this will be denoted as conditioning upon $\mathcal{Z}$ rather than conditioning upon $\mathbf{Z} \in \mathcal{Z}$. In particular, we are about to discuss $\Pr(\mathbf{Z} = \mathbf{z} \mid \mathcal{F}, \mathcal{Z})$, which is read as the conditional probability that the treatment assignment $\mathbf{Z}$ takes a particular value $\mathbf{z}$ given the values of the quantities in $\mathcal{F}$ and the fact that $\mathbf{Z} \in \mathcal{Z}$. Admittedly, conditioning upon $\mathcal{Z}$ rather $\mathbf{Z} \in \mathcal{Z}$ is a slight abuse of notation, but it will simplify the appearance of notation that appears frequently.

So, the expression $\Pr(\mathbf{Z} = \mathbf{z} \mid \mathcal{F}, \mathcal{Z})$ has two aspects, a boring aspect and a startling aspect. The boring aspect says $\mathbf{Z}$ is compatible with the block design, that is, $\mathbf{Z} \in \mathcal{Z}$. The startling aspect is that $\Pr(\mathbf{Z} = \mathbf{z} \mid \mathcal{F}, \mathcal{Z})$ conditions upon everything we care about in causal inference, namely, $\mathcal{F}$, and most of what we care about in $\mathcal{F}$ is not observed. Usually, when we employ a conditional probability, say $\Pr(A \mid B)$, to do something, we have the quantities that are conditioned upon, here B, and we use what we have to predict a quantity we do not have, here A. For instance, a poker player might ask: What is the conditional probability of drawing an ace when drawing two cards (event A) given that she has an ace in her hand and can see another ace face-up on the table (event B)? The probability $\Pr(\mathbf{Z} = \mathbf{z} \mid \mathcal{F}, \mathcal{Z})$ is unusual and startling, because it conditions on something we do not have and can never have, namely, $\mathcal{F}$. Of what possible use is such an unusual conditional probability?

Randomization in an experiment is not about a probability that we found in the world. Randomization is about a probability that we create, that we bring into the world, as we are designing the experiment. If we are going to create a probability, we might as well create a good one, or even better, a startlingly good one. So, in Sect. 2.1, we randomize treatment assignment by setting

$$\Pr(\mathbf{Z} = \mathbf{z} \mid \mathcal{F}, \mathcal{Z}) = \frac{1}{J^I} = \frac{1}{|\mathcal{Z}|} \text{ for each } \mathbf{z} \in \mathcal{Z}. \tag{2.4}$$

Expression (2.4) says: If someone gave you the key elements in causal inference, namely, $\mathcal{F}$, they would be of no help in predicting the treatment assignment, $\mathbf{Z}$.

How does one create the probability (2.4)? It is easy. Obtain a fair, J-sided die, and role it independently I times to assign treatments in the I blocks. In practice, this J-sided die would exist only in some computer's imagination.[1]

How is $\Pr(\mathbf{Z} = \mathbf{z} \mid \mathcal{F}, \mathcal{Z}) = J^{-I}$ in (2.4) different from the mistaken notion, $\Pr(\mathbf{Z} = \mathbf{z}) = J^{-I}$, in Sect. 2.1? The following example shows that $\Pr(\mathbf{Z} = \mathbf{z}) = J^{-I}$ is compatible with extremely biased treatment assignment. Suppose that (i) the IJ unobserved covariate values u_{ij} were independently sampled from a continuous distribution, such as the Normal, (ii) the J people in each block i were sorted into a random order, independently for $i = 1, \ldots, I$, (iii) we set $Z_{ij} = 1$ for the person in block i with the largest value of u_{ij}. In this case, $\Pr(\mathbf{Z} = \mathbf{z}) = J^{-I}$ is true, but $\Pr(\mathbf{Z} = \mathbf{z} \mid \mathcal{F}, \mathcal{Z}) = J^{-I}$ is as false as it can be. That is, every position ij has probability $1/J$ of being the treated position in block i, but we can use $\mathcal{F}$, which contains the u_{ij}, to perfectly predict the identity of the treated person in every block. Indeed, $\Pr(\mathbf{Z} = \mathbf{z} \mid \mathcal{F}, \mathcal{Z}) = 1$ for one $\mathbf{z} \in \mathcal{Z}$ determined by the u_{ij}, and $\Pr(\mathbf{Z} = \mathbf{z} \mid \mathcal{F}, \mathcal{Z}) = 0$ for all other $\mathbf{z} \in \mathcal{Z}$.

Lemma 2.1 is often useful. Its proof makes use of the notation and requires counting the number of ways various events may occur, but the proof is little more than the definition of conditional probability for discrete random variables. Denote the J-dimensional vector of treatment assignments in block i by $\mathbf{Z}_i = (Z_{i1}, Z_{i2}, \ldots, Z_{iJ})$.

Lemma 2.1 *Under randomized treatment assignment (2.4), the I vectors $\mathbf{Z}_i$ are conditionally independent of each other given $\mathcal{F}$, $\mathcal{Z}$, with* $\Pr\left(Z_{ij} = 1 \,\middle|\, \mathcal{F}, \mathcal{Z}\right) = 1/J$ *for* $i = 1, \ldots, I$, $j = 1, \ldots, J$.

---

[1] In R, for $I = 30$ blocks of size $J = 3$, pick the treated individual in block i as follows:

```
I<-30
J<-3
treated<-rep(NA,I)
for (i in 1:I) treated[i]<-sample(1:J,1)
treated
2 3 1 3 3 1 1 1 2 3
3 3 3 2 2 3 1 2 1 3
1 2 3 2 1 2 2 3 1 2 .
```

Proof Let $\mathbf{Z}_{-i}$ be the $(I-1) \times J$ matrix formed from $\mathbf{Z}$ by excluding its ith row, $\mathbf{Z}_i = (Z_{i1}, Z_{i2}, \ldots, Z_{iJ})$, and let $\mathbf{z}_{-i}$ be any one of the J^{I-1} possible values of $\mathbf{Z}_{-i}$. Let $\mathbf{a}_j$ be the J-tuple with a one in coordinate j and zeros in the remaining $J-1$ coordinates; so $\mathbf{a}_j$ is one of the J possible values of $\mathbf{Z}_i$. The problem is to show $\Pr\left(\mathbf{Z}_i = \mathbf{a}_j \,\middle|\, \mathcal{F}, \mathcal{Z}\right) = \Pr\left(\mathbf{Z}_i = \mathbf{a}_j \,\middle|\, \mathbf{Z}_{-i} = \mathbf{z}_{-i}, \mathcal{F}, \mathcal{Z}\right) = 1/J$. If we insert $\mathbf{a}_j$ into $\mathbf{z}_{-i}$ after row $i-1$, we make a complete treatment assignment $\mathbf{z} \in \mathcal{Z}$ with probability J^{-I} by (2.4). Fixing $\mathbf{a}_j$ and summing over the J^{I-1} completions $\mathbf{z}$ with $\mathbf{a}_j$ as row i gives a total probability $\Pr\left(\mathbf{Z}_i = \mathbf{a}_j \,\middle|\, \mathcal{F}, \mathcal{Z}\right) = J^{-I} + \cdots + J^{-I} = J^{I-1} \times J^{-I} = 1/J$. Fixing $\mathbf{z}_{-i}$ and summing over the J completions $\mathbf{z}$ having $\mathbf{a}_1, \ldots, \mathbf{a}_J$ as row i gives a total probability $\Pr\left(\mathbf{Z}_{-i} = \mathbf{z}_{-i} \mid \mathcal{F}, \mathcal{Z}\right) = J^{-I} + \cdots + J^{-I} = J \times J^{-I} = J^{-(I-1)}$. Then, from the definition of conditional probability,

$$\begin{aligned}\Pr\left(\mathbf{Z}_i = \mathbf{a}_j \,\middle|\, \mathbf{Z}_{-i} = \mathbf{z}_{-i}, \mathcal{F}, \mathcal{Z}\right) &= \frac{\Pr\left(\mathbf{Z}_i = \mathbf{a}_j \text{ and } \mathbf{Z}_{-i} = \mathbf{z}_{-i} \,\middle|\, \mathcal{F}, \mathcal{Z}\right)}{\Pr\left(\mathbf{Z}_{-i} = \mathbf{z}_{-i} \mid \mathcal{F}, \mathcal{Z}\right)} \\ &= \frac{J^{-I}}{J^{-(I-1)}} = \frac{1}{J},\end{aligned}$$

as required. □

2.4 Unbiased Estimation of the Average Treatment Effect

The General Result

There is one treated person in block i, identified by $Z_{ij} = 1$, and the observed response of this one treated person is $\sum_{j=1}^{J} Z_{ij} R_{ij}$, which equals $\sum_{j=1}^{J} Z_{ij} r_{Tij}$ because $R_{ij} = r_{Tij}$ if $Z_{ij} = 1$. So, the mean response of the I individuals who are actually treated is

$$\overline{R}_t = \frac{1}{I} \sum_{i=1}^{I} \sum_{j=1}^{J} Z_{ij} R_{ij}. \tag{2.5}$$

In parallel, the mean observed response of the $I(J-1)$ controls is

$$\overline{R}_c = \frac{1}{I(J-1)} \sum_{i=1}^{I} \sum_{j=1}^{J} \left(1 - Z_{ij}\right) R_{ij}. \tag{2.6}$$

Both $\overline{R}_t$ and $\overline{R}_c$ are quantities that we can calculate from the observed values of R_{ij} and Z_{ij}.

Recall from Sect. 2.2 that the central problem in causal inference is that we never see any causal effects δ_{ij}, yet we want to draw inferences about them, for instance, by estimating the average $\overline{\delta}$ of the IJ causal effects. How can we estimate the average of IJ quantities that we can never see? In a randomized experiment, there is a simple solution.

Proposition 2.1 *In a randomized experiment defined by (2.4), the difference in sample means, $\overline{R}_t - \overline{R}_c$, is an unbiased estimate of the average treatment effect, $\overline{\delta}$; that is,*

$$\mathrm{E}\left(\overline{R}_t - \overline{R}_c \,\middle|\, \mathcal{F}, \mathcal{Z}\right) = \overline{\delta};$$

moreover,

$$\mathrm{E}\left(\overline{R}_t \,\middle|\, \mathcal{F}, \mathcal{Z}\right) = \frac{1}{IJ}\sum_{i=1}^{I}\sum_{j=1}^{J} r_{Tij} \text{ and } \mathrm{E}\left(\overline{R}_c \,\middle|\, \mathcal{F}, \mathcal{Z}\right) = \frac{1}{IJ}\sum_{i=1}^{I}\sum_{j=1}^{J} r_{Cij}. \tag{2.7}$$

Proof Using the fact that $R_{ij} = r_{Tij}$ if $Z_{ij} = 1$ and $R_{ij} = r_{Cij}$ if $Z_{ij} = 0$, we have from (2.5) and (2.6)

$$\overline{R}_t - \overline{R}_c = \frac{1}{I}\sum_{i=1}^{I}\sum_{j=1}^{J} Z_{ij}\, r_{Tij} - \frac{1}{I(J-1)}\sum_{i=1}^{I}\sum_{j=1}^{J}\left(1 - Z_{ij}\right) r_{Cij}.$$

Now, r_{Tij} and r_{Cij} are part of $\mathcal{F}$, and they are fixed by conditioning of $\mathcal{F}$; so, conditionally given $\mathcal{F}$, $\mathcal{Z}$, only the Z_{ij} are random variables in $\overline{R}_t - \overline{R}_c$, and their distribution is given by (2.4). By Lemma 2.1, $\mathrm{E}\left(Z_{ij} \,\middle|\, \mathcal{F}, \mathcal{Z}\right) = \Pr\left(Z_{ij} = 1 \,\middle|\, \mathcal{F}, \mathcal{Z}\right) = 1/J$, and $\mathrm{E}\left(1 - Z_{ij} \,\middle|\, \mathcal{F}, \mathcal{Z}\right) = (J-1)/J$. Then,

$$\begin{aligned}\mathrm{E}\left(\overline{R}_t - \overline{R}_c \,\middle|\, \mathcal{F}, \mathcal{Z}\right) &= \frac{1}{I}\sum_{i=1}^{I}\sum_{j=1}^{J}\frac{1}{J} r_{Tij} - \frac{1}{I(J-1)}\sum_{i=1}^{I}\sum_{j=1}^{J}\frac{J-1}{J} r_{Cij} \\ &= \frac{1}{IJ}\sum_{i=1}^{I}\sum_{j=1}^{J}\left(r_{Tij} - r_{Cij}\right) = \frac{1}{IJ}\sum_{i=1}^{I}\sum_{j=1}^{J}\delta_{ij} = \overline{\delta}.\end{aligned}$$

The proof of (2.7) is the same, except that it considers $\overline{R}_t$ and $\overline{R}_c$ separately. □

*Application to Cumulative Distribution Functions

There is a sense in which a cumulative distribution function is a collection of expectations, and an empirical distribution function is a collection of sample means. Can we apply Proposition 2.1 to distribution functions? In one sense, yes; in another sense, no.

Define $w_{Tijv} = 1$ if $r_{Tij} \le v$ and $w_{Tijv} = 0$ otherwise. Also, define $w_{Cijv} = 1$ if $r_{Cij} \le v$ and $w_{Cijv} = 0$ otherwise. We may write $F_T(v)$ for $(IJ)^{-1}\sum_{i=1}^{I}\sum_{j=1}^{J} w_{Tijv}$, so $F_T(v)$ is the proportion of the IJ values r_{Tij} that are no larger than v. The function $F_T(\cdot)$ is the cumulative distribution of the r_{Tij} in the finite population of IJ individuals. In parallel, $F_C(v) = (IJ)^{-1} \sum_{i=1}^{I} \sum_{j=1}^{J} w_{Cijv}$ is the cumulative distribution r_{Cij} in the finite population of IJ individuals. In words, $F_T(\cdot)$ is the distribution of responses r_{Tij} if all IJ individuals received treatment, and $F_C(\cdot)$ is the distribution of responses r_{Cij} if all IJ individuals received control.

Applying Proposition 2.1 to (w_{Tij}, w_{Cij}) rather than (r_{Tij}, r_{Cij}) says that a randomized block experiment yields unbiased estimates of $F_T(v)$, $F_C(v)$ and $F_T(v) - F_C(v)$ for every v. From estimates of $F_T(v)$, we may estimate properties of $F_T(\cdot)$, such as its median, quartiles or standard deviation, and the same goes for $F_C(\cdot)$.

It is easy to see that the median of $F_T(\cdot)$ minus the median of $F_C(\cdot)$ is not generally the median of the IJ causal effects δ_{ij}. More generally, write $F_\delta(v)$ for the proportion of the IJ causal effects δ_{ij} that are $\leq v$. In general, the functions $F_T(\cdot)$ and $F_C(\cdot)$ do not determine $F_\delta(\cdot)$. Proposition 2.1 provides estimates of $F_T(\cdot)$ and $F_C(\cdot)$, but not of $F_\delta(\cdot)$. It is possible to estimate the causal effect, δ_{ij}, at the median response to control, r_{Cij}, but only by adding assumptions [61] connecting r_{Tij} and r_{Cij} that are not needed in Proposition 2.1.

Internal and External Validity

It is important that Proposition 2.1 is true without sampling assumptions. If we randomly assigned treatments, then (2.4) is a fact, not an assumption. Proposition 2.1 says nothing about situations in which we did not randomly assign treatments, and nothing about situations in which individuals lack potential outcomes, (r_{Tij}, r_{Cij}), under competing treatments. Several aspects of Proposition 2.1 merit elaboration.

- Proposition 2.1 describes an inference from the observed responses and treatment assignments, (R_{ij}, Z_{ij}), to an aspect, $\overline{\delta}$, of the causal effects, δ_{ij}, none of which were observed. Proposition 2.1 describes a statistical inference, arguably one of the most important statistical inferences.
- The average treatment effect, $\overline{\delta}$, in Proposition 2.1 refers to IJ specific people, the participants in the randomized experiment. This is neither a problem that needs to be fixed, nor a notational convention that needs to be assumed away; it is, instead, a reality that needs to be acknowledged.[2] If we wanted to say something about people who were not in the experiment, then we would need more than (2.4). Perhaps the imagined ideal is a randomized experiment performed on a random sample from a population, but in any society that respects the rights of the individual, that doubtful ideal remains idle: Participation in a randomized

[2] About several specific issues, I will make this distinction between a problem that should be solved and a reality that should be acknowledged. I am keen to resist the temptation to address a challenging or insoluble problem by assuming the problem is not there. I am also keen to persuade the reader to resist this same temptation and to notice when someone else has fallen victim to it. I owe this distinction to Richard Foley [22, p. 19] who wrote: "Our lack of … guarantees of our reliability is not a failing that needs to be corrected. It is a reality that needs to be acknowledged."

experiment requires informed consent; so, experiments rely on convenient volunteers, not random samples. Pretending that IJ convenient volunteers constitute a random sample from a population is pretending. Donald Campbell [7] expressed this by saying that a randomized trial has internal validity—that is, it can estimate $\overline{\delta}$ for the IJ people in the experiment—but a randomized trial might or might not have external validity, that is, $\overline{\delta}$ might not be relevant to some other group of people. Campbell is recognizing an important problem that randomized treatment assignment solves, and acknowledging another important problem that it does not address. Campbell argued that internal validity had priority: If you cannot estimate the effect of the treatment on the IJ people in the experiment, then good luck using those IJ people to estimate the effect on other people. Once internal validity is secured, ideas for also securing a degree of external validity are discussed by Shadish, Cook and Campbell [91], Stuart et al. [95] and Dahabreh et al. [16].

- Statistical calculations often use asymptotic approximations. For instance, we may be unable to compute the exact distribution of a statistic when I is large, but we may have an excellent large sample approximation to that distribution, perhaps one that uses some form of central limit theorem. The most common large sample approximations imagine an ever larger sample, $I \to \infty$, from a population that neither changes as I increases nor becomes depleted or completely sampled as I increases. These genuinely useful and often necessary approximations occur so often in statistical theory that they sometimes appear to be reasonable descriptions of some actual situation in the real world. There is a disconnect between a reasonable concern about external validity in the previous bullet point and a reasonable concern about practical approximations to the distributions of certain statistics. Again, this disconnect is not a problem that needs to be fixed but a reality that needs to be acknowledged. If we study IJ people and IJ is not small, then a central limit theorem may provide a useful and accurate approximation at this large IJ to an exact distribution we are unable to compute. So far, so good; we have what we need at that point. At the same time, there may be no intelligible reality that corresponds to letting $I \to \infty$, and abstract talk of letting $I \to \infty$ may snuff out a needed discussion of ways the treatment may have a different effect on the people in the experiment and other very different people who were not in the experiment.

2.5 Seeing Evidence Against a Hypothesis About Causal Effects

The Distinction Between δ_{ij} and δ

The effect $\delta_{ij} = r_{Tij} - r_{Cij}$ of a treatment on person ij will never be known, because person ij either received treatment with $Z_{ij} = 1$, so that $R_{ij} = r_{Tij}$ is observed, or person ij received control with $Z_{ij} = 0$, so that $R_{ij} = r_{Cij}$ is observed, but in either case, we cannot calculate $\delta_{ij} = r_{Tij} - r_{Cij}$. Given this, it might seem at first that we can never learn about the $I \times J$ matrix $\boldsymbol{\delta}$ containing δ_{ij} in row i and column j, which is, after all, just a collection of quantities δ_{ij} that we can never see. In this section, a few boxplots will show that certain particular $\boldsymbol{\delta}$'s would be implausible in light of data from a randomized experiment, while other $\boldsymbol{\delta}$'s are not rendered implausible by the data. We can say this despite our inability to say much at all about any single δ_{ij}. We can say this based on randomized treatment assignment, with no additional assumptions. Much of the rest of this chapter will develop statistical tests and confidence intervals that expand on this simple theme, but the tests and confidence intervals repeat with greater precision what you have already seen in the boxplots.

Expressed differently, the parameter $\boldsymbol{\delta}$ is not identified in a randomized block experiment—there is no consistent estimate of $\boldsymbol{\delta}$ as $I \to \infty$—and yet for moderately large I, it is often possible to recognize that a candidate $\boldsymbol{\delta}$ is not actually compatible with the observed data.

Simple Hypotheses About Causal Effects

A simple null hypothesis H_0 about treatment effects specifies a value δ_{0ij} for each treatment effect δ_{ij}, and this is written as $H_0 : \delta_{ij} = \delta_{0ij}$, $i = 1, \ldots, I$, $j = 1, \ldots, J$, or more concisely as $H_0 : \boldsymbol{\delta} = \boldsymbol{\delta}_0$ where $\boldsymbol{\delta}$ and $\boldsymbol{\delta}_0$ are the $I \times J$ matrices of δ_{ij} and δ_{0ij}, respectively.[3] Do the data from a randomized block experiment provide evidence against $H_0 : \boldsymbol{\delta} = \boldsymbol{\delta}_0$?

Fisher's "hypothesis of no effect" is the special case $H_0 : \boldsymbol{\delta} = \mathbf{0}$, where $\boldsymbol{\delta}_0 = \mathbf{0}$ is the $I \times J$ matrix of zeros. In his 1935 book, *Design of Experiments*, Fisher [21, pp. 12–21] developed his claim that randomized experimentation provides the "reasoned basis" for inference about causal effects, and "the physical basis of the validity of the test." He discussed this with specific reference to the experiment of the "lady tasting tea," in which the lady had claimed that she could tell, from taste alone, whether tea or milk had been added first to the cup. Fisher [21, p. 19] wrote:

> The element in the experimental procedure which contains the essential safeguard is that the two modifications of the test beverage are to be prepared in "random order." In fact, this is the only point in the experimental procedure in which the laws of chance, which are to be in exclusive control of our frequency distribution, have been explicitly introduced . . . by which the validity of the test of significance may be guaranteed against corruption by the causes of disturbance which have not been eliminated.

[3] The distinction between a simple and a composite null hypothesis is discussed in the Glossary. Section 2.8 will test simple null hypotheses; then Sect. 2.9 will test composite null hypotheses. Stated informally, a simple null hypothesis asserts something very specific, and a composite null hypothesis asserts something less specific, namely, that the truth is some one simple hypothesis in a possibly infinite set of simple hypotheses.

Of the null hypothesis of no treatment effect, Fisher [21, p. 16] wrote:

> In relation to any experiment, we may speak of this hypothesis as the "null hypothesis," and it should be noted that the null hypothesis is never proved or established but is possibly disproved, in the course of experimentation.

He claimed that no assumptions of any kind are needed to test $H_0 : \boldsymbol{\delta} = \mathbf{0}$ in a randomized experiment. As will be seen in Sect. 2.8, Fisher's logic applies unchanged to testing any simple hypothesis $H_0 : \boldsymbol{\delta} = \boldsymbol{\delta}_0$ about causal effects; it need not assert $H_0 : \boldsymbol{\delta} = \mathbf{0}$.[4]

At about the time that Fisher [21] published the *Design of Experiments*, Karl Popper published in Vienna in 1934 his *Logik der Forschung*, translated in 1959 as *The Logic of Scientific Discovery* [56]. Popper also claimed that scientific theories are not proved or established but rather tested. He said a theory that had survived many severe tests was "corroborated"–a technical term—immediately mentioning that the next severe test might overturn the theory. He wrote [56, p. 50]:

> If you insist on strict proof or strict disproof in the empirical sciences, then you will never benefit from experience and never learn from it how wrong you are.

Almost a century later, statistical hypothesis tests and Popper's philosophical ideas remain influential, perhaps dominant, yet controversial for a variety of reasons. It is difficult today to draw a bright red line that would separate hypothesis tests and Popper's ideas, although they meet only in a narrow region. For us in this book, it is important that there may be (i) strong evidence against one hypothesis $H_0 : \boldsymbol{\delta} = \boldsymbol{\delta}_0$ about causal effects; (ii) no evidence against two other hypotheses, $H_0 : \boldsymbol{\delta} = \boldsymbol{\delta}_0^{'}$ and $H_0 : \boldsymbol{\delta} = \boldsymbol{\delta}_0^{''}$, where $\boldsymbol{\delta}_0^{'} \neq \boldsymbol{\delta}_0^{''}$; and (iii) no prospect that this situation would change if the sample size, I, increased without bound, $I \longrightarrow \infty$. In technical language, there can be compelling and useful evidence in a sampling situation that is not identified.

Before thinking about formal hypothesis tests, let us think about how causal effects show up when we plot data from a randomized experiment.

[4] What is the relationship between "interference between units" in Sect. 2.2 and Fisher's claim that $H_0 : \boldsymbol{\delta} = \mathbf{0}$ can be tested without assumptions? It might seem that talk of $\delta_{ij} = 0$ assumes the existence of $\delta_{ij} = r_{Tij} - r_{Cij}$, and it therefore assumes "no interference between units"; however, that is not correct. Hypotheses are not assumptions: We do not assume them to be true, we are in the midst of investigating whether they are false, and we are often content to find strong evidence that they are false. The hypothesis $H_0 : \boldsymbol{\delta} = \mathbf{0}$ implies no interference between units, so if there is interference, then the null hypothesis $H_0 : \boldsymbol{\delta} = \mathbf{0}$ is simply false. The hypothesis $H_0 : \boldsymbol{\delta} = \mathbf{0}$ says that **R** does not change if **Z** changes, and that implies both no treatment effect and no interference between units in the magnitude of the treatment effect. In parallel, the hypothesis $H_0 : \boldsymbol{\delta} = \boldsymbol{\delta}_0$ says that **R** changes in a specific way as **Z** changes, and this hypothesis implies no interference between units, so if there is interference then $H_0 : \boldsymbol{\delta} = \boldsymbol{\delta}_0$ is simply false. If H_0 is false, then of course we are happy to reject it. Nonetheless, the test statistic that we would use to detect that $H_0 : \boldsymbol{\delta} = \mathbf{0}$ is false would depend upon what we thought might be true instead; so, we would use a different test statistic to discover interference than to discover that $\delta_{ij} > 0$ for many ij.

What Can We See About Causal Effects by Plotting the Data?

While thinking about whether $H_0 : \boldsymbol{\delta} = \boldsymbol{\delta}_0$ is true, we have certain things and don't have others: We have the hypothesized values, δ_{0ij}, and the observed data, R_{ij} and Z_{ij}, but we don't have the actual causal effects, δ_{ij}. If we adjust the observed response, R_{ij}, for the hypothesized effect, δ_{0ij}, by calculating $R_{ij} - Z_{ij}\,\delta_{0ij}$, then using (2.2), we would obtain $r_{Cij} = R_{ij} - Z_{ij}\,\delta_{ij}$ if $\delta_{0ij} = \delta_{ij}$; moreover, we would obtain something else—not r_{Cij}—if $\delta_{0ij} \neq \delta_{ij}$ and $Z_{ij} = 1$. Randomization means that treatment assignment Z_{ij} is unrelated to r_{Cij}, because r_{Cij} is part of $\mathcal{F}$, and (2.4) says that Z_{ij} given $\mathcal{F}$, $\mathcal{Z}$ is simply random. So, if the hypothesis $H_0 : \boldsymbol{\delta} = \boldsymbol{\delta}_0$ were true, we expect no relationship between treatment assignment Z_{ij} and something we can calculate, namely, $R_{ij} - Z_{ij}\,\delta_{0ij}$. Can we use that to judge that $H_0 : \boldsymbol{\delta} = \boldsymbol{\delta}_0$ is untrue? Does it look like there is no relationship between Z_{ij} and $R_{ij} - Z_{ij}\,\delta_{0ij}$?

Write $\mathbf{R}$ for the $I \times J$ matrix containing the observed responses, R_{ij}, and write $\mathbf{r}_C$ for the $I \times J$ matrix containing the potential responses under control, r_{Cij}. Also, write $\mathbf{R}^{\boldsymbol{\delta}_0}$ for the $I \times J$ matrix containing the values $R_{ij}^{\delta_0} = R_{ij} - Z_{ij}\,\delta_{0ij}$.[5] From the definitions of R_{ij} and δ_{ij} in (2.2), we have the elementary but important fact:

$$\mathbf{R}^{\boldsymbol{\delta}_0} = \mathbf{r}_C \text{ if } H_0 : \boldsymbol{\delta} = \boldsymbol{\delta}_0 \text{ is true; that is, } \mathbf{R}^{\boldsymbol{\delta}} = \mathbf{r}_C. \tag{2.8}$$

Though elementary, the equality $\mathbf{R}^{\boldsymbol{\delta}} = \mathbf{r}_C$ in (2.8) is remarkable and useful. As you can see from (2.2), R_{ij} generally depends upon Z_{ij}, and consequently $\mathbf{R}$ generally depends upon $\mathbf{Z}$; that is, whenever the treatment has an effect, those effects may show up in some of the observed responses, $\mathbf{R}$. Intuitively, if there is a nonzero treatment effect, then you expect $\mathbf{R}$ to track $\mathbf{Z}$, in some sense that still needs to be made clear. Is this useful?

Of course, we do not know or see $\delta_{ij} = r_{Tij} - r_{Cij}$—that is the central problem in causal inference in Sect. 2.2. Can we see evidence against the hypothesis $H_0 : \boldsymbol{\delta} = \boldsymbol{\delta}_0$? We can certainly calculate $\mathbf{R}^{\boldsymbol{\delta}_0}$; that calculation is just arithmetic using the data we have and our hypothesis, $H_0 : \boldsymbol{\delta} = \boldsymbol{\delta}_0$. If the hypothesis were true, then (2.8) says $\mathbf{R}^{\boldsymbol{\delta}_0} = \mathbf{r}_C$, where $\mathbf{r}_C$ is in $\mathcal{F}$ and hence is fixed in (2.4) by conditioning on $\mathcal{F}$, $\mathcal{Z}$. In other words, we expect the random variable $\mathbf{R}$ to track the random variable $\mathbf{Z}$ when there is a nonzero treatment effect, but if $H_0 : \boldsymbol{\delta} = \boldsymbol{\delta}_0$ is true, the adjusted response $\mathbf{R}^{\boldsymbol{\delta}_0} = \mathbf{r}_C$ is a constant that does not track the treatment assignment $\mathbf{Z}$; rather, $\mathbf{r}_C$ just sits there as $\mathbf{Z}$ moves about. In a randomized experiment, the problem of reaching a judgment about the hypothesis $H_0 : \boldsymbol{\delta} = \boldsymbol{\delta}_0$ has become the problem of reaching a judgment about whether $\mathbf{R}^{\boldsymbol{\delta}_0}$ tracks $\mathbf{Z}$, and that is a problem about two quantities we do observe.

---

[5] If you prefer, you may write this calculation in terms of matrices. Given any two $I \times J$ matrices, $\mathbf{a}$ and $\mathbf{b}$, with entries a_{ij} and b_{ij}, their Hadamard product, $\mathbf{a} \odot \mathbf{b}$, is the $I \times J$ matrix with entries $a_{ij}\,b_{ij}$. In matrix notation, by definition, $\mathbf{R}^{\boldsymbol{\delta}_0} = \mathbf{R} - \mathbf{Z} \odot \boldsymbol{\delta}_0$. By (2.2), if $H_0 : \boldsymbol{\delta} = \boldsymbol{\delta}_0$ is true, then $\mathbf{R}^{\boldsymbol{\delta}_0} = \mathbf{R}^{\boldsymbol{\delta}} = \mathbf{R} - \mathbf{Z} \odot \boldsymbol{\delta} = \mathbf{r}_C$. Whether or not $H_0 : \boldsymbol{\delta} = \boldsymbol{\delta}_0$ is true, it is always true that $\mathbf{R}^{\boldsymbol{\delta}_0} = \mathbf{R} - \mathbf{Z} \odot \boldsymbol{\delta}_0 = \mathbf{r}_C + \mathbf{Z} \odot (\boldsymbol{\delta} - \boldsymbol{\delta}_0)$.

Better still, even if $H_0 : \boldsymbol{\delta} = \boldsymbol{\delta}_0$ is false—that is, whether or not $\delta_{0ij} \neq \delta_{ij}$ for some ij—we find, using (2.2), that

$$R_{ij} - Z_{ij}\,\delta_{0ij} = r_{Cij} + Z_{ij}\left(\delta_{ij} - \delta_{0ij}\right). \tag{2.9}$$

In words, (2.9) gives one sense in which the observed outcome adjusted for the hypothesized treatment effect, $R_{ij} - Z_{ij}\,\delta_{0ij}$, tracks the assigned treatment, Z_{ij}, when $\delta_{0ij} \neq \delta_{ij}$ because $H_0 : \boldsymbol{\delta} = \boldsymbol{\delta}_0$ is false. So, we ask of the data: Does $R_{ij} - Z_{ij}\,\delta_{0ij}$ track Z_{ij}?

Let us consider some cases. If the hypothesized δ_{0ij}'s are too small—if $\delta_{ij} > \delta_{0ij}$ for all ij—then all individuals ij will have a larger value of $R_{ij} - Z_{ij}\,\delta_{0ij}$ under treatment, with $Z_{ij} = 1$, than under control, with $Z_{ij} = 0$, and perhaps we could see that in a pair of boxplots of $R_{ij} - Z_{ij}\,\delta_{0ij}$ for $Z_{ij} = 1$ and $Z_{ij} = 0$; that is, for treated individuals and randomized controls, the treated boxplot is expected to be higher than the control boxplot. For instance, had the two HDL cholesterol boxplots on the left in Fig. 1.5 been from a blocked randomized experiment, then this pair of boxplots would look incompatible with Fisher's hypothesis $H_0 : \boldsymbol{\delta} = \mathbf{0}$, because $\delta_{0ij} = 0$ looks too small to be the true value of all the δ_{ij}'s. If almost but not all of δ_{0ij}'s are too small—if $\delta_{ij} > \delta_{0ij}$ for almost all ij—then that too might be visible in the same pair of boxplots of $R_{ij} - Z_{ij}\,\delta_{0ij}$. Perhaps nothing we could see in the data from a randomized experiment will distinguish "*all* $\delta_{ij} > \delta_{0ij}$" from "*almost all* $\delta_{ij} > \delta_{0ij}$," but perhaps that subtle distinction might be less important than the things we can see, such as "mostly, $\delta_{ij} > \delta_{0ij}$." Similarly, if the δ_{0ij}'s are too small for men and too large for women, then we should see that in four parallel boxplots, for treated and control men, and for treated and control women.

Consider another case. Suppose the δ_{ij}'s and δ_{0ij}'s are both centered at the same positive number, so the δ_{0ij} are neither always too high nor always too low, but the δ_{ij}'s are more dispersed than the δ_{0ij}'s, in the sense that $\delta_{ij} - \delta_{0ij}$ tends to be positive when δ_{0ij} is positive, and $\delta_{ij} - \delta_{0ij}$ tends to be negative when δ_{0ij} is negative. In this situation, the treated or $Z_{ij} = 1$ boxplot of $R_{ij} - Z_{ij}\,\delta_{0ij} = r_{Cij} + Z_{ij}\left(\delta_{ij} - \delta_{0ij}\right)$ should be more dispersed than the corresponding control or $Z_{ij} = 0$ boxplot.

Admittedly, $H_0 : \boldsymbol{\delta} = \boldsymbol{\delta}_0$ might be false in some subtle way, and we might miss this subtlety through inattention, through lack of skill in graphing data, or even because the subtle failure of $H_0 : \boldsymbol{\delta} = \boldsymbol{\delta}_0$ is not a discernible failure. Indeed, as is evident from simple theoretical examples, in any randomized experiment, many false hypotheses $H_0 : \boldsymbol{\delta} = \boldsymbol{\delta}_0$ about treatment effects $\boldsymbol{\delta}$ are not discernibly different from true hypotheses about treatment effects; see Problem 2.9 and Sect. 3.2. Still, in a randomized block experiment, a specific hypothesis, $H_0 : \boldsymbol{\delta} = \boldsymbol{\delta}_0$, is often plainly contradicted by visible patterns in data. Recall Fisher's remark Sect. 2.5 about the possibility of strong evidence against a null hypothesis about treatment effects, $H_0 : \boldsymbol{\delta} = \boldsymbol{\delta}_0$, even if there is no way to determine, even approximately, the true value of the IJ-dimensional effect $\boldsymbol{\delta}$, even in the limit as the size of the experiment increases without bound, $I \to \infty$. Because we never see r_{Tij} and r_{Cij} for the same person ij, and because $\delta_{ij} = r_{Tij} - r_{Cij}$, there are definite limits to what we can know about an individual δ_{ij}; nonetheless, an experiment can provide strong evidence against many hypotheses, $H_0 : \boldsymbol{\delta} = \boldsymbol{\delta}_0$, that specify IJ causal effects.

Plots of Systolic Blood Pressure for a Few Hypotheses

To illustrate, return to the example of binge drinking and blood pressure in Sect. 1.5, briefly (and no doubt unwisely) neglecting the absence of randomization to treatment or control. Figure 2.1 depicts adjusted systolic blood pressure, $R_{ij} - Z_{ij}\,\delta_{0ij}$, for three hypotheses, $H_0 : \boldsymbol{\delta} = \boldsymbol{\delta}_0$, comparing frequent binge drinkers (B) to matched controls who never engaged in frequent binge drinking and rarely drink now (N). Panel (i) of Fig. 2.1 refers to Fisher's hypothesis of no effect, $H_0 : \boldsymbol{\delta} = \mathbf{0}$ or $\delta_{0ij} = 0$ for all i and j. Had we seen Panel (i) of Fig. 2.1 in a randomized block experiment, we would regard $H_0 : \boldsymbol{\delta} = \mathbf{0}$ as implausible, because group B has higher systolic blood pressure than group N. Panel (ii) of Fig. 2.1 plots $R_{ij} - Z_{ij}\,\delta_{0ij}$ with $\delta_{0ij} = 8.17$ for all i and j or equivalently $\boldsymbol{\delta}_0 = 8.17 \times \mathbf{1}$ where $\mathbf{1}$ is an $I \times J$ matrix of ones. Where did the value 8.17 come from? It is, in fact, an estimate of the type proposed by Hodges and Lehmann [29], in which a test of no effect is inverted to obtain an estimate; however, we will come to all that in Sect. 2.10. For now, the hypothesis in Panel (ii) is just one of infinitely many hypotheses about the $2 \times 206 = 412$-dimensional vector $\boldsymbol{\delta}$ of causal effects. Unlike Panel (i), the B and N boxplots look similar in Panel (ii), suggesting that we have little evidence against this null hypothesis. Panel (iii) refers to a multiplicative effect, $\delta_{0ij} = 0.0676 \times r_{Cij}$ or $r_{Tij} = 1.0676 \times r_{Cij}$, where again the value 1.0676 is a Hodges-Lehmann estimate. As in Panel (ii), the B and N boxplots look similar in Panel (iii), so there appears to be little evidence against either of two hypotheses that are mathematically different, namely, $\delta_{0ij} = 8.17$ in Panel (ii) or $\delta_{0ij} = 0.0676 \times r_{Cij}$ in Panel (iii). It cannot be true that $\delta_{0ij} = 8.17$ for all i and j and $\delta_{0ij} = 0.0676 \times r_{Cij}$ for all i and j; yet, Panels (ii) and (iii) provide little reason to prefer one hypothesis over the other. No doubt, there are many hypotheses, $H_0 : \boldsymbol{\delta} = \boldsymbol{\delta}_0$, that would seem to remove the ostensible treatment effect, in the sense that $R_{ij} - Z_{ij}\,\delta_{0ij}$ does not track Z_{ij}, and no doubt some of these hypotheses are very different from the hypotheses in Panels (ii) and (iii) of Fig. 2.1. This is, yet again, Fisher's comment in Sect. 2.5 that experiments provide evidence against certain hypotheses, not evidence in support of hypotheses.

Figure 2.2 examines the same two hypotheses, $\delta_{0ij} = 8.17$ or $\delta_{0ij} = 0.0676 \times r_{Cij}$, separately for women and men. The $I = 206$ pairs consist of 60 pairs of 2 women and 146 pairs of 2 men. The boxplots in Fig. 2.2 wiggle a bit more than the boxplots in Fig. 2.1, perhaps because each boxplot represents fewer people. The Bf and Nf boxplots look similar to each other, and the Bm and Nm boxplots look similar to each other, suggesting again that there is little evidence against these hypotheses.

How can this line of reasoning be developed to provide a formal test of the hypothesis $H_0 : \boldsymbol{\delta} = \boldsymbol{\delta}_0$? For that, we will need a test statistic in Sect. 2.6, and the distribution of that test statistic when $H_0 : \boldsymbol{\delta} = \boldsymbol{\delta}_0$ is true in Sect. 2.8.

2.6 A Few Test Statistics

A test statistic T is a function of observed quantities, such as R_{ij}, Z_{ij}, $\mathbf{x}_{ij}$, and quantities specified in the null hypothesis, such as δ_{0ij}; so, T is a quantity we can compute. In the current section, $T = t(\cdot, \cdot)$ is a function of two $I \times J$ arrays, but in Chap. 7, the statistic T is also a function of observed covariates, $\mathbf{x}_{ij}$. Also, in the current section, the statistic is written as a function, $T = t(\mathbf{Z}, \mathbf{R})$, of the treatment assignments $\mathbf{Z}$ and the observed responses $\mathbf{R}$, as would be appropriate for testing the hypothesis of no effect, $H_0 : \boldsymbol{\delta} = \mathbf{0}$, but in Sect. 2.8, this becomes $T = t\left(\mathbf{Z}, \mathbf{R}^{\delta_0}\right)$ when testing any simple hypothesis, $H_0 : \boldsymbol{\delta} = \boldsymbol{\delta}_0$.

What are some possible test statistics? One thought is suggested by Proposition 2.1, namely, the difference $\overline{R}_t - \overline{R}_c$ between the mean response $\overline{R}_t$ observed among treated individuals and the mean response $\overline{R}_c$ observed among controls, and using their definitions, (2.5) and (2.6), it is clear that $\overline{R}_t - \overline{R}_c$ can be calculated from $\mathbf{R}$ and $\mathbf{Z}$, so it can be written as a function $\overline{R}_t - \overline{R}_c = T = t(\mathbf{Z}, \mathbf{R})$.

A sturdy old statistic for randomized block designs is essentially due to Wilcoxon [104], and its use in block designs is discussed by Lehmann [40, §3.3] and Noether [51]. The blocked Wilcoxon rank sum statistic ranks the R_{ij} in each block i from

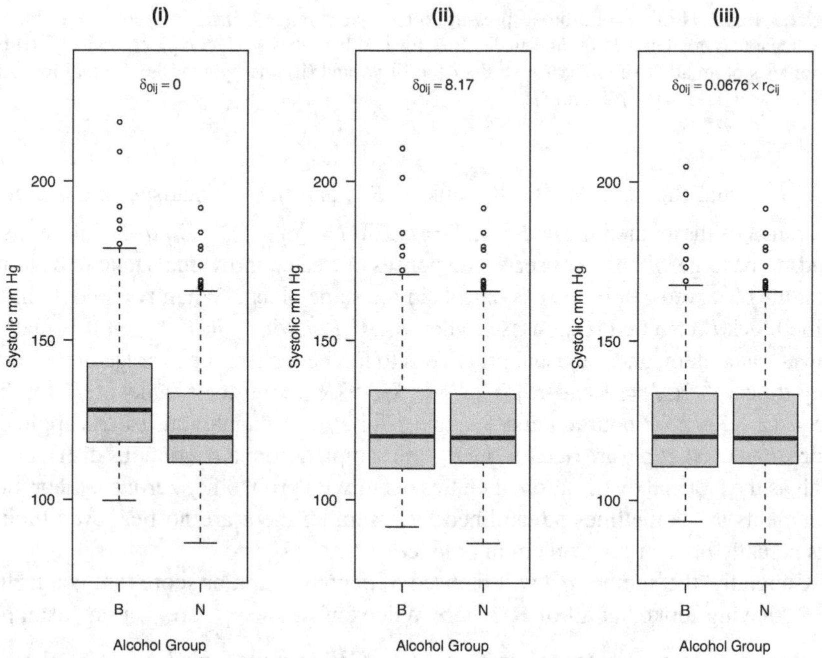

Fig. 2.1 Boxplots of systolic blood pressure for frequent binge drinkers (B) and never bingers (N), for three hypotheses $H_0 : \boldsymbol{\delta} = \boldsymbol{\delta}_0$ about causal effects δ_{ij}, namely: (i) the hypothesis of no effect, $\delta_{ij} = 0$ for all ij, (ii) one hypothesis of an additive effect, $\delta_{ij} = 8.17$ for all ij, and (iii) one hypothesis of a multiplicative effect, $\delta_{ij} = 0.0676\, r_{Cij}$, for all ij.

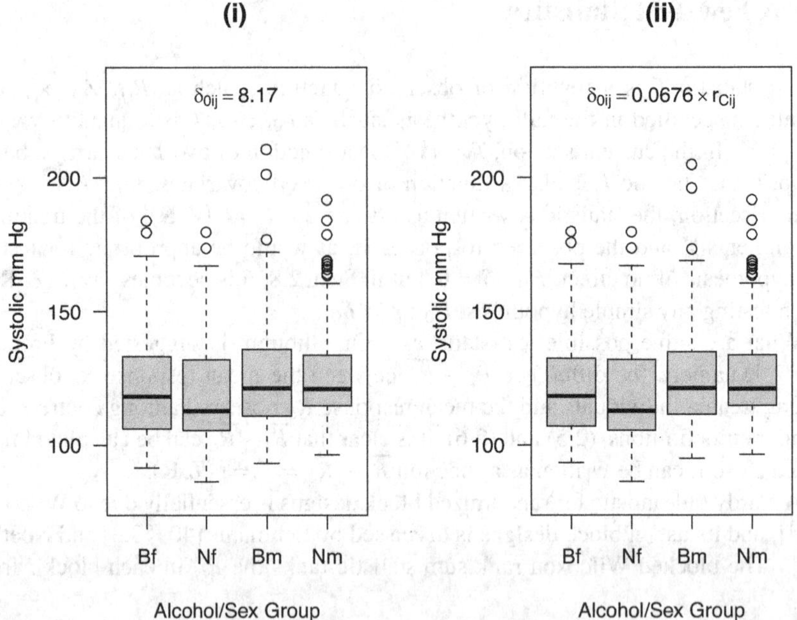

Fig. 2.2 Boxplots of systolic blood pressure for frequent binge drinkers (B) and never bingers (N), separately for females (f) and males (m), for two hypotheses $H_0 : \boldsymbol{\delta} = \boldsymbol{\delta}_0$, namely: (i) one hypothesis of an additive effect, $\delta_{ij} = 8.17$ for all ij, and (ii) one hypothesis of a multiplicative effect, $\delta_{ij} = 0.0676\, r_{Cij}$, for all ij.

1 to J, giving the name q^*_{ij} to the rank of R_{ij}, and the test statistic is the sum of the ranks of the treated individuals, $T = t(\mathbf{Z}, \mathbf{R}) = \sum_{i=1}^{I} \sum_{j=1}^{J} Z_{ij}\, q^*_{ij}$. This statistic tends to be large when the observed responses of treated individuals tend to be larger than the observed responses of controls in the same block. When two people in the same block i have tied responses—when $R_{ij} = R_{ij'}$ with $j \neq j'$—then it is unclear how to rank them, and the usual practice is to let them share the average of the ranks they deserve. If $J = 4$ and $R_{i1} > R_{i2} = R_{i3} > R_{i4}$, then their ranks are 4 for R_{i1}, $2.5 = (2 + 3)/2$ for both R_{i2} and R_{i3}, and 1 for R_{i4}. An analogous rule is applied if more than two people are tied. If the R_{ij} are sampled from a continuous distribution, such as the Normal distribution, then ties occur with probability zero; so, theoretical arguments are sometimes streamlined by assuming there are no ties, even though ties actually present no problem in practice.

Generally, the symbol q_{ij} will be used to denote a rank or score that is attached to R_{ij} having looked at all of $\mathbf{R}$, where Wilcoxon's ranks q^*_{ij} are just one example. Another rank is simply some function $\phi(\cdot)$ of Wilcoxon's ranks, $q_{ij} = \phi\left(q^*_{ij}\right)$; see

Lehmann [40, §3.5D] or Puri [58]. Instead, if you take

$$q_{ij} = \frac{1}{I}\left(R_{ij} - \frac{1}{J-1}\sum_{\ell \neq j} R_{i\ell}\right), \tag{2.10}$$

then $T = t(\mathbf{Z}, \mathbf{R}) = \sum_{i=1}^{I} \sum_{j=1}^{J} Z_{ij}\, q_{ij}$ equals the difference in means $\overline{R}_t - \overline{R}_c$ in Proposition 2.1.

Quade [59] and Tardif [97] improved the performance of the blocked Wilcoxon rank sum statistic when used in randomized block experiments with a small block size J, say $2 \leq J \leq 6$. For each block i, they calculated a within-block range,

$$w_i = \max_{1 \leq j \leq J} R_{ij} - \min_{1 \leq j \leq J} R_{ij}, \tag{2.11}$$

and ranked these from 1 to I, again using average ranks for ties. The idea here is that a block in which w_i is small cannot exhibit strong evidence of a treatment effect and should therefore be given less weight. The test statistic is again $T = t(\mathbf{Z}, \mathbf{R}) = \sum_{i=1}^{I} \sum_{j=1}^{J} Z_{ij}\, q_{ij}$, except q_{ij} is now the product of Wilcoxon's within-block rank q_{ij}^{*} and the rank, say b_i, of the ranges in (2.11), so $q_{ij} = q_{ij}^{*}\, b_i$.[6] For matched treated-control pairs—equivalently for a block size of $J = 2$—Quade's statistic $\sum_{i=1}^{I} \sum_{j=1}^{J} Z_{ij}\, q_{ij}$ is essentially the same as Wilcoxon's [104] second statistic, his signed rank statistic, in the sense that the two statistics differ by an additive constant and give the same P-values, confidence intervals and point estimates; see Problems 2.6–2.7. Tardif [97] generalizes Quade's statistic in several ways: for instance, the range in (2.11) might be replaced by some other measure of dispersion.

In general, a weighted rank statistic [79] is defined to be any statistic of the form $T = t(\mathbf{Z}, \mathbf{R}) = \sum_{i=1}^{I} \sum_{j=1}^{J} Z_{ij}\, q_{ij}$ with $q_{ij} = \phi\left(q_{ij}^{*}\right) \varphi\{b_i/(I+1)\}$, where $\phi(\cdot)$ and $\varphi(\cdot)$ are two nonnegative, monotone increasing functions, and b_i is a rank of some within-block dispersion measure such as the range w_i in (2.11). Quade's statistic is essentially the same as taking $\phi(q) = q$ for all q and $\varphi(a) = a$ for all a; again, see Problem 2.7 for more about test statistics that are "essentially the same." The blocked Wilcoxon rank sum statistic is the trivial case of a weighted rank sum statistic in which $\phi(q) = q$ for all q and $\varphi(a) = 1$ for all a, whereas Puri's [58] statistic is the case in which $\varphi(a) = 1$ for all a.[7]

---

[6] The motivation for these statistics comes, in part, from the heavily studied case of randomized matched pairs, $J = 2$, where w_i in (2.11) simplifies to $|R_{i1} - R_{i2}|$. For $J = 2$, the blocked Wilcoxon statistic becomes the sign test, and Quade's [59] statistic becomes Wilcoxon's other statistic, his signed rank statistic for matched pairs. For matched pairs from a Normal distribution, the signed rank statistic is almost as efficient as the t-test and is much more efficient than the sign test, though both tests are much more efficient than the t-test for long-tailed distributions. This is nicely discussed by Lehmann [40, §4.3]. As we will see in Chap. 9, other considerations govern the relative performance of test statistics when used in observational studies—their relative performance in randomized experiments is a poor guide.

[7] Sometimes, with long-tailed distributions, it is useful to permit $\phi(\cdot)$ or $\varphi(\cdot)$ to rise and then descend [71, 74], but score functions that rise and descend are not discussed in this book.

2.7 *Many More Test Statistics

There are many other statistics in use in randomized block experiments, but they are not discussed in this book. As will be seen in Sect. 2.8, randomization inference works in a similar way with any test statistic; so, a development in terms of other statistics would parallel and mostly repeat what is said about the rank statistics in Sect. 2.6. Indeed, the same is true throughout this book: Rank statistics can be replaced by other types of statistics [64, 73, 76]. This brief section, which may be skipped, mentions some other test statistics and then explains the small advantages of the rank statistics in Sect. 2.6 for an introductory text.

A large, robust, attractive, and flexible class of statistics is comprised of Huber's [32, 33] M-statistics, which are a generalization of maximum likelihood statistics, of efficient score test statistics, and of least squares statistics. With a slight adjustment due to Maritz [46], M-statistics can be used in exact randomization inferences in matched pairs, and this adjustment also works in blocks larger than $J = 2$, including blocks of unequal sizes [69] or weighted blocks [73]. These M-statistics still have the form $\sum_{i=1}^{I} \sum_{j=1}^{J} Z_{ij}\, q_{ij}$, but with a different definition of the score q_{ij}; see [77, §2.8] for an elementary example. The method is implemented in several R packages, including `sensitivitymult` and `sensitivityfull`; see [75]. Rank statistics and M-statistics can accomplish the same things: In a certain sense, for any statistic in one class, there is a statistic in the other class that is asymptotically equivalent [36, Ch. 7].

Although the examples in this book have continuous outcomes, randomization inference for binary outcomes is entirely standard. For blocked binary outcomes, $\left(r_{Tij}, r_{Cij}\right)$ and R_{ij}, the familiar Mantel-Haenszel test is the large sample approximation to a randomization test [3] of $H_0 : \boldsymbol{\delta} = \mathbf{0}$ based on $\sum_{i=1}^{I} \sum_{j=1}^{J} Z_{ij}\, R_{ij}$; moreover, it can also test $H_0 : \boldsymbol{\delta} = \boldsymbol{\delta}_0$ and be inverted for confidence intervals [63].

Randomization inference can instead be developed in terms of quantiles or order statistics [60, 61, 96]. Many if not most tests for censored survival times are randomization or permutation tests; so, with a few caveats, they can be developed in parallel [45, 53]. This is true also for tests about multivariate outcomes [27, 89, 108]. A parallel development of a variety of tests and contexts is available in my *Observational Studies* monograph [64, Ch. 2–Ch 5].

To keep things simple in this introductory book, I will restrict attention to means and a few rank statistics. This focus reflects ease of exposition, nothing more. In the first place, it is simpler to discuss one class of statistics rather than to discuss many classes in parallel. The Wilcoxon statistics and Hodges-Lehmann estimates may be familiar from introductory courses, particularly courses that use the basic `stats` package in R, and Quade's [59] statistic is simply the generalization of the signed-rank statistic from pairs, $J = 2$, to small blocks, $J \geq 2$. The rank statistics have exact randomization distributions, and this simplification appears in some of the problems at the end of chapters. More importantly, the rank statistics have an exact moment generating function in sensitivity analyses, and this simplifies the efficiency calculations in Chap. 11. Certain evidence factors in Chap. 13 are exactly independent for rank statistics, and only approximately so for other statistics [72, 78].

2.8 Testing a Simple Hypothesis About Causal Effects

The General Method

Consider testing the simple null hypothesis $H_0 : \boldsymbol{\delta} = \boldsymbol{\delta}_0$ using a test statistic $t(\cdot, \cdot)$. Section 2.5 considered ways to plot the data to see whether the treatment assignment, $\mathbf{Z}$, tracked the response after removing the hypothesized effect, $\mathbf{R}^{\boldsymbol{\delta}_0}$. Now, we let $t(\cdot, \cdot)$ ask the same question.

Specifically, we calculate $T^{\boldsymbol{\delta}_0} = t\left(\mathbf{Z}, \mathbf{R}^{\boldsymbol{\delta}_0}\right)$ and ask whether $T^{\boldsymbol{\delta}_0}$ would seem surprisingly large were $H_0 : \boldsymbol{\delta} = \boldsymbol{\delta}_0$ true. To answer that question, we need the null distribution of $T^{\boldsymbol{\delta}_0}$, that is, the distribution of $T^{\boldsymbol{\delta}_0}$ when $H_0 : \boldsymbol{\delta} = \boldsymbol{\delta}_0$ is true. For any constant a, we want the probability that $T^{\boldsymbol{\delta}_0} \geq a$ when $H_0 : \boldsymbol{\delta} = \boldsymbol{\delta}_0$ is true, and happily Proposition 2.2 says the null distribution has an extremely simple form for every test statistic, $t(\cdot, \cdot)$. The simple form calculates $\mathbf{r}_C = \mathbf{R}^{\boldsymbol{\delta}_0}$ under the presumption that $H_0 : \boldsymbol{\delta} = \boldsymbol{\delta}_0$ is true and then holds this $\mathbf{r}_C$ fixed while calculating $t(\mathbf{z}, \mathbf{r}_C)$ for every treatment assignment $\mathbf{z} \in \mathcal{Z}$; finally, the probability we want is simply the proportion treatment assignments $\mathbf{z} \in \mathcal{Z}$ such that $t(\mathbf{z}, \mathbf{r}_C) \geq a$. The probability is just a proportion, because every $\mathbf{z} \in \mathcal{Z}$ has the same probability in a randomized block experiment.

It is important that Proposition 2.2 is true without assumptions. In a randomized block experiment, (2.3) is true, because the investigator assigned treatments using random numbers; so (2.3) is simply true not an assumption. A null hypothesis, $H_0 : \boldsymbol{\delta} = \boldsymbol{\delta}_0$, is not an assumption, not least because we are content to reject it. Recall from Sect. 2.1 that, if $\mathcal{S}$ is a finite set, then the number of elements in $\mathcal{S}$ is denoted $|\mathcal{S}|$.

Proposition 2.2 *If $H_0 : \boldsymbol{\delta} = \boldsymbol{\delta}_0$ is true in a randomized block experiment (2.3), then (i) $\mathbf{r}_C = \mathbf{R}^{\boldsymbol{\delta}_0}$, and (ii) given $\mathcal{F}$, $\mathcal{Z}$, the distribution of $T^{\boldsymbol{\delta}_0} = t\left(\mathbf{Z}, \mathbf{R}^{\boldsymbol{\delta}_0}\right)$ is:*

$$\Pr\{t(\mathbf{Z}, \mathbf{r}_C) \geq a \mid \mathcal{F}, \mathcal{Z}\} = \frac{|\{\mathbf{z} \in \mathcal{Z} : t(\mathbf{z}, \mathbf{r}_C) \geq a\}|}{|\mathcal{Z}|}. \tag{2.12}$$

Proof We did all the hard work in Sect. 2.5, showing that $\mathbf{r}_C = \mathbf{R}^{\boldsymbol{\delta}_0}$ if $H_0 : \boldsymbol{\delta} = \boldsymbol{\delta}_0$ is true, and in this case $\mathbf{r}_C$ is known and is fixed by conditioning on $\mathcal{F}$. So, $t(\mathbf{Z}, \mathbf{r}_C)$ is a random variable given $\mathcal{F}$, $\mathcal{Z}$ only because $\mathbf{Z}$ is a random variable, and $\Pr(\mathbf{Z} = \mathbf{z} \mid \mathcal{F}, \mathcal{Z}) = 1/|\mathcal{Z}|$ by (2.3). □

In summary, to test $H_0 : \boldsymbol{\delta} = \boldsymbol{\delta}_0$ at level α using statistic $t(\cdot, \cdot)$ in a randomized block design, do the following.[8] Use the null hypothesis $H_0 : \boldsymbol{\delta} = \boldsymbol{\delta}_0$ and the observed responses R_{ij} to calculate the adjusted responses, $R_{ij}^{\boldsymbol{\delta}_0} = R_{ij} - Z_{ij}\,\delta_{0ij}$ and the corresponding array $\mathbf{R}^{\boldsymbol{\delta}_0}$, which is $\mathbf{R}^{\boldsymbol{\delta}_0} = \mathbf{r}_C$ when $H_0 : \boldsymbol{\delta} = \boldsymbol{\delta}_0$ is true. Assuming H_0 is true for the purpose of testing it, obtain (2.12) by evaluating $t(\mathbf{z}, \mathbf{r}_C)$ for all J^I elements $\mathbf{z} \in \mathcal{Z}$. Find the smallest a such that $\Pr\{t(\mathbf{Z}, \mathbf{r}_C) \geq a \mid \mathcal{F}, \mathcal{Z}\} \leq \alpha$.

[8] If the "level of a test" is unfamiliar, see the entry in the Glossary. Conventionally, $\alpha = 0.05$, but that is just a convention.

Reject $H_0 : \delta = \delta_0$ at level α if $t\left(\mathbf{Z}, \mathbf{R}^{\delta_0}\right) \geq a$. This test has level α, meaning that the chance is at most α that it rejects $H_0 : \delta = \delta_0$ when H_0 is true.

Testing Terminology: Size of a Test; *P*-Value

Closely related to the level α of the test is the size of the test. The distribution (2.12) is discrete: Its probability mass function $\Pr\{t(\mathbf{Z}, \mathbf{r}_C) = a \mid \mathcal{F}, \mathcal{Z}\}$ deposits all of its probability on a finite set of numbers a. Consequently, for fixed α, it is possible that $\Pr\{t(\mathbf{Z}, \mathbf{r}_C) \geq a \mid \mathcal{F}, \mathcal{Z}\} \neq \alpha$ for every a. The size of a level α test that rejects when $T^{\delta_0} \geq a$ is $\Pr\{t(\mathbf{Z}, \mathbf{r}_C) \geq a \mid \mathcal{F}, \mathcal{Z}\}$, and it may be strictly less than α. If the size of a level α test is strictly less than α, then the test is often said to be conservative.[9]

The P-value is a random variable that is a function of the random variable T^{δ_0}: It is the smallest α such that T^{δ_0} leads to rejection of H_0. First, we find the null distribution (2.12) at every a that can occur with positive probability as a possible value of T^{δ_0}; that is, we make a table whose first row is a and whose second row is the probability in (2.12). For the a's in this table, size and level are equal, because every a in this table occurs as a possible value of T^{δ_0} with positive probability. The second row is the level α of a test that rejects when $T^{\delta_0} \geq a$. The probabilities, α, in the second row decline as a increases, that is, as we move to the right in the table. The smallest α that leads us to reject H_0 on the basis of the observed values of T^{δ_0} is the α in the column of the table with $a = T^{\delta}$, because a larger a would not lead us to reject H_0 and a smaller a would have a larger α than we need to reject H_0. In brief, the P-value looks up α in our table of the null distribution (2.12) at the random location $a = T^{\delta}$.

Discreteness of a probability distribution can lead a test with level $\alpha = 0.05$ to be conservative with size strictly (but typically only very slightly) smaller than $\alpha = 0.05$. This does not affect P-values; discreteness does not make them conservative. If a level $\alpha = 0.05$ test is conservative due to discreteness, then you will never see a P-value of 0.05; however, the P-values you do see will not be conservative.

Exact Calculation of the Null Distribution

The set $\mathcal{Z}$ contains J^I treatment assignments, $\mathbf{z}$, so Proposition 2.2 is proposing quite a bit of computation to test one hypothesis, $H_0 : \delta = \delta_0$, and in practice we must test many hypotheses to form a confidence interval. Even the small example of binge drinking in Sect. 1.5 has $I = 206$ and $J = 3$, so $|\mathcal{Z}| = J^I = 3^{206} = 1.94 \times 10^{98}$. Is exact computation feasible? Is exact computation needed? The answers are

[9] This terminology of level and size is from Lehmann and Romano [41, p. 57]. Fraser [23, pp. 71–72] speaks instead of exact size and size. The terminology is adjusted slightly for tests of composite null hypotheses in Sect. 2.9.

"sometimes" and "no". "Sometimes" is interesting and is discussed here, but "no" is more useful and is discussed in the next subsection.

The blocked Wilcoxon rank sum statistic in Sect. 2.6 ranks the responses in each block from 1 to J and sums the ranks for the I treated individuals. In the absence of ties, the statistic takes integer values and could be as small as I if treated individuals always had rank one, or as large as IJ if treated individuals always had rank J. Consequently, the statistic takes values I, $I+1, \ldots, IJ$, so it takes $IJ - I + 1$ possible values. Computing the exact null distribution entails computing $IJ - I + 1$ probabilities, or $206 \times 3 - 206 + 1 = 413$ probabilities in the case of binge drinking in Sect. 1.5. Can we compute 413 probabilities without computing $t(\mathbf{z}, \mathbf{r}_C)$ for 1.94×10^{98} values of $\mathbf{z}$?

Lemma 2.1 is helpful: It says the I blocks are independent. If we knew the distribution of T^{δ_0} for I blocks, then we would obtain the distribution of T^{δ_0} for $I+1$ blocks by convolving the distribution of T^{δ_0} for I blocks with the distribution of a random variable that take values $1, 2, \ldots, J$ with probabilities $1/J$. This is illustrated in Problem 2.4. Perhaps better, we could convolve the distribution of T^{δ_0} for I blocks with itself to obtain the distribution for $2I$ blocks. Pagano and Tritchler [54] obtain very quickly some null distributions of the kind in Proposition 2.2 using the fast Fourier transform to convolve integer-valued discrete distributions. This is easy to do in R; see Problem 2.4.

Obtaining the exact distribution of Quade's statistic in Sect. 2.6 is only slightly harder. The block whose range has rank 1 contributes $1, 2, \ldots, J$, each with probability $1/J$. The block whose range has rank 2 contributes $2 \times 1, 2 \times 2, \ldots, 2 \times J$, each with probability $1/J$. The block whose range has rank i contributes $i \times 1, i \times 2, \ldots, i \times J$, each with probability $1/J$. So, again the problem is to convolve I integer-valued random variables.

None of this is of any help for a test statistic $t(\mathbf{z}, \mathbf{r}_C)$ that takes on $|\mathcal{Z}| = J^I$ distinct values as $\mathbf{z}$ varies over $\mathcal{Z}$. For instance, the difference in means, $\overline{R}_t - \overline{R}_c$, can take on J^I values for $\mathbf{z} \in \mathcal{Z}$. Fortunately, it is easy to use Lemma 2.1 in a different way to approximate the null distribution of $t(\mathbf{Z}, \mathbf{r}_C)$.

Approximating the Null Distribution

Consider testing $H_0 : \delta = \delta_0$ using a statistic $T^{\delta_0} = t\left(\mathbf{Z}, \mathbf{R}^{\delta_0}\right) = \sum_{i=1}^{I} \sum_{j=1}^{J} Z_{ij}\, q_{ij}$ where q_{ij} is a function of $\mathbf{R}^{\delta_0}$. For instance, all of the statistics in Sect. 2.6 had this form. Because q_{ij} is a function of $\mathbf{R}^{\delta_0}$, we should write $q_{ij}^{\delta_0}$ rather than q_{ij} to indicate the dependence of q_{ij} on the hypothesis, $H_0 : \delta = \delta_0$; however, to avoid cumbersome notation, this dependence is left implicit, with reminders now and then, as needed.

Importantly, if $H_0 : \delta = \delta_0$ is true, then $q_{ij}^{\delta_0} = q_{ij}$ is a function of $\mathbf{R}^{\delta_0} = \mathbf{r}_C$, which is part of $\mathcal{F}$. So, if $H_0 : \delta = \delta_0$ is true, then q_{ij} is fixed by conditioning on $\mathcal{F}, \mathcal{Z}$ in Proposition 2.2.

Proposition 2.3 *If $H_0 : \delta = \delta_0$ is true in a randomized block experiment (2.4), then conditionally given $\mathcal{F}$, $\mathcal{Z}$: (i) the statistic $T^{\delta_0} = \sum_{i=1}^{I} \sum_{j=1}^{J} Z_{ij}\, q_{ij}$ is the sum of I independent random variables, (ii) the ith of these I independent random variables, $\sum_{j=1}^{J} Z_{ij}\, q_{ij}$, is one of the J fixed scores, $q_{i1}, \ldots, q_{iJ}$, picked at random with probability $1/J$, (iii) the expectation and variance of $T^{\delta_0} = \sum_{i=1}^{I} \sum_{j=1}^{J} Z_{ij}\, q_{ij}$ are:*

$$\mathrm{E}\left(T^{\delta_0} \mid \mathcal{F}, \mathcal{Z}\right) = \sum_{i=1}^{I} \mu_i, \text{ where } \mu_i = \frac{1}{J} \sum_{j=1}^{J} q_{ij}, \tag{2.13}$$

and

$$\operatorname{var}\left(T^{\delta_0} \mid \mathcal{F}, \mathcal{Z}\right) = \frac{1}{J} \sum_{i=1}^{I} \sum_{j=1}^{J} \left(q_{ij} - \mu_i\right)^2. \tag{2.14}$$

Proof As just noted, q_{ij} is fixed when $H_0 : \delta = \delta_0$ is true, so Lemma 2.1 implies the I random variables $\sum_{j=1}^{J} Z_{ij}\, q_{ij}$, $i = 1, \ldots, I$, are conditionally independent given $\mathcal{F}$, $\mathcal{Z}$, proving (i) and (ii). Then (2.13) is $\mathrm{E}\left(\sum_{i=1}^{I} \sum_{j=1}^{J} Z_{ij}\, q_{ij} \,\middle|\, \mathcal{F}, \mathcal{Z}\right) = \sum_{i=1}^{I} \sum_{j=1}^{J} q_{ij}\, \mathrm{E}\left(Z_{ij} \mid \mathcal{F}, \mathcal{Z}\right)$, where $\mathrm{E}\left(Z_{ij} \mid \mathcal{F}, \mathcal{Z}\right) = 1/J$ from Lemma 2.1, proving (2.13). The variance of the sum of independent random variables is the sum of their variances, so $\operatorname{var}\left(T^{\delta_0} \mid \mathcal{F}, \mathcal{Z}\right) = \sum_{i=1}^{I} \operatorname{var}\left(\sum_{j=1}^{J} Z_{ij}\, q_{ij} \,\middle|\, \mathcal{F}, \mathcal{Z}\right)$. Also, the equality, $\operatorname{var}\left(\sum_{j=1}^{J} Z_{ij}\, q_{ij} \,\middle|\, \mathcal{F}, \mathcal{Z}\right) = \frac{1}{J} \sum_{j=1}^{J} \left(q_{ij} - \mu_i\right)^2$, is simply the definition of the variance of the random variable $\sum_{j=1}^{J} Z_{ij}\, q_{ij}$, proving (2.14). □

Write $\Phi(\cdot)$ for the standard Normal cumulative distribution function, so that the chance that a standard Normal random variable is less than or equal to d is $\Phi(d)$. It is natural to hope that a central limit theorem of some sort applies to $T^{\delta_0} = \sum_{i=1}^{I} \sum_{j=1}^{J} Z_{ij}\, q_{ij}$, in the sense that for each d,

$$\Pr\left\{ \frac{T^{\delta_0} - \mathrm{E}\left(T^{\delta_0} \mid \mathcal{F}, \mathcal{Z}\right)}{\sqrt{\operatorname{var}\left(T^{\delta_0} \mid \mathcal{F}, \mathcal{Z}\right)}} \geq d \right\} \rightarrow 1 - \Phi(d) \text{ as } I \rightarrow \infty, \tag{2.15}$$

$$\text{under } H_0 : \delta = \delta_0 \text{ and (2.3).}$$

When is (2.15) true?

The simple case is the blocked Wilcoxon rank sum statistic. In this case, the q_{ij} are $1, \ldots, J$ for every i, so the I random variables $\sum_{j=1}^{J} Z_{ij}\, q_{ij}^{*}$ are not only independent under $H_0 : \delta = \delta_0$ and (2.3) but also identically distributed with finite variance. In this case, (2.15) follows from the most familiar central limit theorem, the one for independent and identically distributed random variables. All this is true also if q_{ij}^{*} is replaced by a function $\phi(\cdot)$ of Wilcoxon's ranks, $q_{ij} = \phi\left(q_{ij}^{*}\right)$, as in Puri [58].

Quade's [59] statistic in Sect. 2.6 has the form $q_{ij} = q^*_{ij}\, b_i$ where b_i is the rank of the within-block range w_i in (2.11). In this case, Proposition 2.3 says the I random variables $\sum_{j=1}^{J} Z_{ij}\, q_{ij}$ are independent; however, they are not identically distributed. Somewhat more generally, consider a statistic with $q_{ij} = \phi\left(q^*_{ij}\right) a_i$ for some function $\phi(\cdot)$ and some block scores a_i that are functions of $R^{\delta_0}_{ij}$, so that Quade's statistic is a special case. A "special" central limit theorem due to Hajek, Sidak and Sen [25, §6.1.2] says that (2.15) is true provided

$$\frac{\sum_{i=1}^{I} a_i^2}{\max_{1\le i\le I} a_i^2} \rightarrow \infty \text{ as } I \rightarrow \infty. \tag{2.16}$$

Stated informally, condition (2.16) says that, as the number of blocks increases, $I \rightarrow \infty$, no one block a_i dominates the statistic; i.e., $\sum_{i=1}^{I} a_i^2$ is large compared with $\max_{1\le i\le I} a_i^2$. In particular, (2.16) holds for Quade's statistic with $a_i = b_i$. This "special" central limit theorem is proved [25, §6.1.2] by verifying the Lindeberg condition of the Lindeberg-Feller central limit theorem [10, §9.1].

Is (2.15) true in general? No, for two reasons. First, it is not true in particular cases, so it is not true in general, and second it is too vague to be true in general. Let us consider these two reasons in turn.

For the first reason, as a particular case, suppose the r_{Cij} are independently sampled from a Cauchy distribution.[10] This is a sampling model that might have produced a part of $\mathcal{F}$. A single Cauchy random variable and the average of I independent Cauchy random variables have the same distribution, so neither the law of large numbers nor the central limit theorem apply to the mean of independent Cauchy random variables [90, Example 11.16]. In this case, the central limit theorem (2.15) does not apply when testing $H_0 : \boldsymbol{\delta} = \mathbf{0}$ using the difference in means, $T^{\mathbf{0}} = \overline{R}_t - \overline{R}_c$, which has the form $T^{\mathbf{0}} = \sum_{i=1}^{I}\sum_{j=1}^{J} Z_{ij}\, q_{ij}$ with q_{ij} given by (2.10). So, (2.15) is not true in general, because it is not true in a particular case. In contrast, this Cauchy model presents no problems for testing $H_0 : \boldsymbol{\delta} = \mathbf{0}$ using the blocked Wilcoxon rank sum statistic.

The particular case that we just considered lent expression (2.15) more coherence than it has. The quantity $\mathcal{F}$ changes as $I \rightarrow \infty$, with more and more $\left(r_{Tij}, r_{Cij}\right)$ and $\delta_{ij} = r_{Tij} - r_{Cij}$ as $I \rightarrow \infty$. Whether or not (2.15) is true depends upon how these new fixed quantities behave as I increases. The Cauchy case in the previous paragraph took the r_{Cij} to be independent observations from the same distribution before conditioning upon them. It is reasonable to add assumptions to obtain a

---

[10] If that seems like the wrong model for a block design, then you obtain the same result from a conventional additive linear model for a block design, $R_{ij} = \beta_i + Z_{ij}\tau + \varepsilon_{ij}$ where the ε_{ij} are IJ independent Cauchy distributed random variables and $\delta_{ij} = r_{Tij} - r_{Cij} = \tau$ for all ij. If $\delta_{ij} = \tau$ seems too restrictive, then you obtain the same result from an unconventional linear model for a block design with $R_{ij} = \beta_i + Z_{ij}\delta_{ij} + \varepsilon_{ij}$ where the ε_{ij} are IJ independent Cauchy distributed random variables. The key but familiar point is that a mean of Cauchy random variables does not converge in probability to a constant with increasing sample size, so $\overline{R}_t - \overline{R}_c$ does not converge in probability to a limit as $I \rightarrow \infty$. Proposition 2.1 says $\overline{R}_t - \overline{R}_c$ is an unbiased estimate for each I, but this property does not guarantee acceptable performance for long-tailed ε_{ij}.

counterexample but, as stated, expression (2.15) is simply too vague to be true in general.

What are the options? What are the options for obtaining or approximating the distribution (2.12)? There are several. One good option is to use statistics such that (2.15) is simply true, such as the blocked Wilcoxon statistic, Quade's statistic, a wide variety of weighted rank statistics, and some other rank statistics [40, Ch. 3]. A second good option is to use robust statistics, such as robust Huber-Maritz M-statistics [46, 69], so that (2.15) is simply true except in the most bizarre circumstances. Robust statistics, including certain rank and quantile statistics, limit the influence of individual blocks i regardless of the behavior of the (r_{Tij}, r_{Cij}), thereby permitting the use of the Lindeberg-Feller central limit theorem [10, §9.1] for I independent but not identically distributed random variables $\sum_{j=1}^{J} Z_{ij}\, q_{ij}$, $i = 1, \ldots, I$. Statistics that are robust are also attractive simply because they are robust, quite apart from the applicability of the central limit theorem. A third option does not require the statistic to be robust but rather makes assumptions about the behavior of (r_{Tij}, r_{Cij}) as $I \to \infty$ [43]. A fourth option, sometimes possible, is to obtain the exact null distribution, as discussed in the previous subsection. Before randomization, a fourth option is to reduce the size of the set $\mathcal{Z}$ of possible treatment assignments from J^I to, say, 10,000, and then to implement Proposition 2.2 by direct calculation [99].

Tukey's Advice About Assumptions

John Tukey [100, p. 72] offered the following advice about assumptions:

> Reduce dependence on assumptions, in particular by (1) using assumptions as leading cases, not truths ... (2) being explicit about using alternative assumptions (robustness; Chamberlain's definition, "Science is the holding of multiple working hypotheses"); and (3) when possible, using randomization to ensure validity—leaving to assumptions the task of helping with stringency.

Commenting about a specific method of adjusting for selection bias in either nonresponse or causal inference, Tukey [101, p. 108] wrote:

> Some of my deepest discomfort stems from the feeling that the authors equate 'assumption' to 'truth.' If we assume it, it is so—if we don't, it isn't!

In a similar context, Roderick Little [44] describes a similar discomfort.

To follow Tukey's suggestion, to "use assumptions as leading cases, not truths," and to "work with multiple alternative assumptions" is to hold each assumption at arm's length and without conviction, to understand its role in an inference by varying it, relaxing it, omitting it, and attempting to corroborate it. If this is to work—if it is going to be possible to subject important assumptions to close scrutiny—then the inference cannot depend on many assumptions.

Commonly, validity refers to the level of a hypothesis test or the coverage rate of a confidence interval. A valid 0.05-level test of hypothesis H_0 rejects H_0 with probability at most 5% when H_0 is true. A valid 95% confidence interval for a scalar parameter τ is a random interval $[A, B]$ that will cover the fixed number τ with probability at least 0.95. The test or confidence interval is valid if it has its defining property. To use "randomization to ensure validity" means that treatments were randomly assigned and a theorem like Proposition 2.2 ensures the level of the test or the coverage rate of the confidence interval. We can only use "randomization to ensure validity" in randomized experiments. In an observational study, we titrate the addition of assumptions that affect validity, so these few assumptions may be varied, relaxed (in sensitivity analyses in Chap. 8), omitted (in evidence factors in Chap. 13), corroborated or corrected (with known effects in Chap. 12 or multiple control groups in Chap. 13), and constrained by observed data in Sect. 12.3.

Validity is not enough. We want hypothesis tests to be valid, but also powerful. We want confidence intervals to be valid, but also short. We want powerful tests and short confidence intervals over a variety of sampling situations, not in just one sampling situation, such as the Normal distribution. This is what Tukey means by his informal use of the word stringency.[11] He advocates "leaving to assumptions the task of helping with stringency," after randomization has ensured validity. This entails evaluating the performance of competing valid tests or confidence intervals under several assumed sampling models, preferring tests with high power across models, and confidence intervals that are short across models. These sampling models are not used for inference but rather as a basis for recommending one broadly valid test instead of another, because the first test exhibits better performance across several sampling models. For instance, in Chapter 3 of his book *Nonparametrics*, Lehmann [40] discusses several tests that are broadly valid in randomized block designs, and then in his Chapter 4, he compares the performance of these broadly valid tests under several simple and specific sampling models, such as a linear model for a block design with Normal errors or Cauchy errors. Assumptions are titrated when evaluating validity, but not when evaluating stringency. We want methods that are broadly valid and that exhibit good performance in several sampling models.

Tukey mentions "multiple working hypotheses," with reference to an article by Thomas C. Chamberlain [8] published in *Science* in 1890. Chamberlain's ideas are discussed by John Platt [55] in connection with what he calls "strong inference."

This book follows Tukey's advice, titrating the addition of assumptions that affect validity,[12] but freely using various fully specified models either to generate needed counterexamples or to compare the relative performance of statistical procedures in several settings. Assumptions about violations of random assignment (2.4) are titrated, but the relative performance of two test statistics in Sect. 2.6 may be evaluated using, for example, a linear model with various error distributions. For instance, eventually we will decide against using the blocked Wilcoxon rank sum statistic, because it performs poorly in a variety of models, but those models will not be used to draw inferences about treatment effects.

---

[11] There are related formal concepts: a "most stringent test," as discussed by Lehmann and Romano [41, §8.6], and a "maximin robust test or estimate," as discussed by Gastwirth [24].

[12] Oxford English Dictionary: **Titrate**: To regulate ... by means of incremental changes in dose ... Also in extended use and figurative: to adjust or control (something) carefully.

2.9 Testing a Composite Hypothesis About Causal Effects

The General Method

As discussed in Sect. 2.8, a simple null hypothesis about causal effects has the form $H_0 : \boldsymbol{\delta} = \boldsymbol{\delta}_0$ for an $I \times J$ array $\boldsymbol{\delta}_0$, and Proposition 2.2 gives the unique null distribution of any statistic $t\left(\mathbf{Z}, \mathbf{R}^{\boldsymbol{\delta}_0}\right)$ when this hypothesis is true. To test $H_0 : \boldsymbol{\delta} = \boldsymbol{\delta}_0$ at level α, we determine the smallest a such that $\Pr\{t(\mathbf{Z}, \mathbf{r}_C) \geq a \mid \mathcal{F}, \mathcal{Z}\} \leq \alpha$ in (2.12) and reject $H_0 : \boldsymbol{\delta} = \boldsymbol{\delta}_0$ if $t\left(\mathbf{Z}, \mathbf{R}^{\boldsymbol{\delta}_0}\right) \geq a$.

A composite null hypothesis considers not one $\boldsymbol{\delta}_0$ but rather a set Δ_0 containing two or more $\boldsymbol{\delta}_0$'s. Often, Δ_0 contains infinitely many $\boldsymbol{\delta}_0$'s. Each $\boldsymbol{\delta}_0$ in Δ_0 is one component of the composite hypothesis. A composite null hypothesis, $H_0 : \boldsymbol{\delta} \in \Delta_0$, is true if the true $\boldsymbol{\delta}$ is in Δ_0; otherwise, the composite null hypothesis $H_0 : \boldsymbol{\delta} \in \Delta_0$ is false.

One procedure for testing $H_0 : \boldsymbol{\delta} \in \Delta_0$ at level α is conceptually simple in a randomized block experiment (2.4). Test each simple component $\boldsymbol{\delta}_0$ in Δ_0, one at a time, using the method in Proposition 2.2 for testing a simple null hypothesis at level α. If every $\boldsymbol{\delta}_0$ in Δ_0 is rejected at level α, then reject at level α the composite hypothesis, $H_0 : \boldsymbol{\delta} \in \Delta_0$; otherwise, do not reject the composite hypothesis.

It is easy to see that this simple procedure rejects a true composite null hypothesis $H_0 : \boldsymbol{\delta} \in \Delta_0$ with probability at most α. If $H_0 : \boldsymbol{\delta} \in \Delta_0$ is true, then the true value of $\boldsymbol{\delta}$, say $\boldsymbol{\delta}^*$, is in Δ_0. The simple procedure tests every $\boldsymbol{\delta} \in \Delta_0$; so, in particular, it tests the true simple hypothesis, $H_0 : \boldsymbol{\delta} = \boldsymbol{\delta}^*$, and when it does that, it falsely rejects with probability at most α. So, rejecting the composite hypothesis $H_0 : \boldsymbol{\delta} \in \Delta_0$ when it is true entails rejecting the simple hypothesis $H_0 : \boldsymbol{\delta} = \boldsymbol{\delta}^*$, and the latter event happens with probability at most α.

Examples of Composite Hypotheses About Causal Effects

What are some examples of composite null hypotheses? Here are a few. To be definite, a positive causal effect $\delta_{ij} = r_{Tij} - r_{Cij} > 0$ is understood to be a benefit for person ij.

(i) No benefit from treatment: Let Δ_0 consist of all $I \times J$ arrays $\boldsymbol{\delta}_0$ with IJ nonpositive coordinates, $\delta_{0ij} \leq 0$ for all ij. The composite null hypothesis $H_0 : \boldsymbol{\delta} \in \Delta_0$ says that no individual would benefit from treatment, though some individuals may be harmed. Here, Δ_0 is a quadrant in an IJ-dimensional space, and Fisher's hypothesis of no effect, $H_0 : \boldsymbol{\delta} = \mathbf{0}$, is the boundary corner point of this quadrant.

(ii) At most, small benefits from treatment: Let $\kappa \geq 0$ be a specified magnitude of benefit judged too small to justify the expense, and perhaps the risks, of treatment. Let Δ_0 consist of all $I \times J$ arrays $\boldsymbol{\delta}_0$ with IJ coordinates $\delta_{0ij} \leq \kappa$. The composite null hypothesis $H_0 : \boldsymbol{\delta} \in \Delta_0$ says that no individual would experience benefits large enough to justify use of the treatment. Under this composite null hypothesis, some people might experience small benefits, while others might experience substantial harms. If $\kappa > 0$, then this composite null hypothesis includes Fisher's hypothesis of no effect, $H_0 : \boldsymbol{\delta} = \mathbf{0}$, as an interior point.

(iii) Effects are all close to zero: Let $\kappa > 0$ be an absolute magnitude of effect thought to be too small in magnitude to matter, and let Δ_0 consist of all $I \times J$ arrays $\boldsymbol{\delta}_0$ with IJ coordinates $-\kappa \leq \delta_{0ij} \leq \kappa$ for all ij. The composite null hypothesis $H_0 : \boldsymbol{\delta} \in \Delta_0$ says that some or all individuals may experience small effects, but none of these is large enough to matter. Stated informally, it says that Fisher's simple hypothesis of no effect, $H_0 : \boldsymbol{\delta} = \mathbf{0}$, may be false, but it is nearly true. In this composite null hypothesis, the set Δ_0 is an IJ-dimensional cube, $\Delta_0 = [-\kappa, \kappa] \times \cdots \times [-\kappa, \kappa]$, centered at Fisher's hypothesis of no effect, $H_0 : \boldsymbol{\delta} = \mathbf{0}$.

*Testing a Composite Hypothesis Using the Wilcoxon Statistic

Fix a real number κ, and consider the composite null hypothesis that $\delta_{ij} \leq \kappa$ for all ij, so Δ_0 consists of all $I \times J$ arrays $\boldsymbol{\delta}_0$ with IJ coordinates $\delta_{0ij} \leq \kappa$. Consider testing $H_0 : \boldsymbol{\delta} \in \Delta_0$ using the blocked Wilcoxon rank sum statistic.

Hypothesis $H_0 : \boldsymbol{\delta} \in \Delta_0$ allows an individual coordinate δ_{0ij} to take any value in the half line $(-\infty, \kappa]$. For a control with $Z_{ij} = 0$, changing δ_{0ij} does not change the adjusted response, $R_{ij} - Z_{ij}\,\delta_{0ij}$; rather, $R_{ij} - Z_{ij}\,\delta_{0ij} = R_{ij}$ because $Z_{ij} = 0$. In contrast, for the one treated individual in block i with $Z_{ij} = 1$, the adjusted response $R_{ij} - Z_{ij}\,\delta_{0ij} = R_{ij} - \delta_{0ij}$ decreases as δ_{0ij} increases to κ.

As a consequence, the within-block rank q^*_{ij} computed from $R_{ij} - Z_{ij}\,\delta_{0ij}$ for the treated individual in block i is smallest when it is computed with $\delta_{0ij} = \kappa$; that is, q^*_{ij} is smallest at $\boldsymbol{\delta}_0 = \kappa\mathbf{1} \in \Delta_0$, where $\mathbf{1}$ is an $I \times J$ array of ones. This is true for every block i, and the ranks in one block do not affect the ranks in another block. So, for $\boldsymbol{\delta}_0 \in \Delta_0$, Wilcoxon's statistic, $T^{\boldsymbol{\delta}_0} = t\left(\mathbf{Z}, \mathbf{R}^{\boldsymbol{\delta}_0}\right) = \sum_{i=1}^{I} \sum_{j=1}^{J} Z_{ij}\, q^*_{ij}$ is smallest when computed from $\boldsymbol{\delta}_0 = \kappa\mathbf{1} \in \Delta_0$; that is,

$$T^{\kappa\mathbf{1}} \leq T^{\boldsymbol{\delta}_0} \text{ for all } \boldsymbol{\delta}_0 \in \Delta_0. \tag{2.17}$$

We want to say something like: $t\left(\mathbf{Z}, \mathbf{R}^{\boldsymbol{\delta}_0}\right)$ is as small as it can be when computed from $\boldsymbol{\delta}_0 = \kappa\mathbf{1} \in \Delta_0$, and if that smallest value is still too large, then we can reject not only the simple hypothesis $H_0 : \boldsymbol{\delta} = \kappa\mathbf{1}$ but also the entire composite hypothesis $H_0 : \boldsymbol{\delta} \in \Delta_0$ of which this is merely one component. Can we say this? We are tantalizingly close to being able to say this, and we will ultimately say this, but unfortunately there is still some work to do.

In what sense are we tantalizingly close to a solution? If $\mathbf{R}^{\boldsymbol{\delta}_0}$ had no ties in any of the I blocks, then the distribution in (2.12) of $t\left(\mathbf{Z}, \mathbf{R}^{\boldsymbol{\delta}_0}\right)$ under the simple null hypothesis $H_0 : \boldsymbol{\delta} = \boldsymbol{\delta}_0$ would always be the same: It would be the distribution of the sum of I independent random variables, where the ith random variable is one of the numbers, $1, 2, \ldots, J$ picked with equal probabilities $1/J$. Because the null distribution of $t\left(\mathbf{Z}, \mathbf{R}^{\delta_0}\right)$ is always the same if there are no ties, rejection of $H_0 : \boldsymbol{\delta} = \boldsymbol{\delta}_0$, $\boldsymbol{\delta}_0 \in \Delta_0$, depends only on the test statistic, $t\left(\mathbf{Z}, \mathbf{R}^{\delta_0}\right)$, and this is minimized at $H_0 : \boldsymbol{\delta} = \kappa\mathbf{1}$. This means that we can reject every component $H_0 : \boldsymbol{\delta} = \boldsymbol{\delta}_0$ that does not induce ties in $\mathbf{R}^{\delta_0}$ provided we can reject $H_0 : \boldsymbol{\delta} = \kappa\mathbf{1}$ and provided $\mathbf{R}^{\kappa\mathbf{1}}$ does not have ties. Indeed, Δ_0 is composed of infinitely many $\boldsymbol{\delta}_0$, and only finitely many $\boldsymbol{\delta}_0$ induce ties. Alas, none of this helps, because Wilcoxon's statistic $t\left(\mathbf{Z}, \mathbf{R}^{\delta_0}\right)$ is not continuous as a function of $\boldsymbol{\delta}_0$, and ties make it jump. So we need to take a different approach.

The computational procedure is very simple, but it takes a moment to understand why it works. We compute the blocked Wilcoxon statistic $T^{\delta_0} = t\left(\mathbf{Z}, \mathbf{R}^{\delta_0}\right)$ in the usual way using average ranks for ties, and we use the central limit theorem (2.15) to obtain an approximate P-value for each simple hypothesis, $H_0 : \boldsymbol{\delta} = \boldsymbol{\delta}_0$, but in Proposition 2.3, we always use the expectation and variance for untied q_{ij}^*, even when there are ties in $\mathbf{R}^{\delta_0}$; i.e., we use the "wrong" variance when there are ties. In the untied situation, the q_{ij}^* are a permutation of $1, 2, \ldots, J$ for each block i, and some algebra [40, Appendix §1] yields in Proposition 2.3 the simplified untied formulas:

$$\mathrm{E}\left(T^{\delta_0} \,\middle|\, \mathcal{F}, \mathcal{Z}\right) = I \times \frac{J+1}{2}, \tag{2.18}$$

and

$$\mathrm{var}\left(T^{\delta_0} \,\middle|\, \mathcal{F}, \mathcal{Z}\right) = I \times \frac{(J-1)(J+1)}{12}. \tag{2.19}$$

Define the deviate, D^{δ_0}, by

$$D^{\delta_0} = \frac{T^{\delta_0} - \frac{I(J+1)}{2}}{\sqrt{I(J-1)(J+1)/12}}. \tag{2.20}$$

The simple procedure is: Reject at level α the composite hypothesis, $H_0 : \boldsymbol{\delta} \in \Delta_0$, if $D^{\kappa\mathbf{1}} \geq \Phi^{-1}(1-\alpha)$. In other words, we compute just one deviate, namely, $D^{\kappa\mathbf{1}}$, and it decides the fate of all components $\boldsymbol{\delta}_0 \in \Delta_0$ of the composite hypothesis. Conventionally, $\alpha = 0.05$ and $\Phi^{-1}(1-\alpha) = 1.645$, but the procedure can be used with any $\alpha < \frac{1}{2}$. Why does this work?

In this chapter's Appendix Sect. 2.12, it is shown that the expectation is unaffected by ties and the variance is reduced by ties; so, for each $\boldsymbol{\delta}_0$, if $H_0 : \boldsymbol{\delta} = \boldsymbol{\delta}_0$ is true in a randomized block experiment (2.4) then:

$$\mathrm{E}\left(T^{\delta_0} \,\middle|\, \mathcal{F}, \mathcal{Z}\right) = I \times \frac{J+1}{2}, \tag{2.21}$$

$$\mathrm{var}\left(T^{\delta_0} \,\middle|\, \mathcal{F}, \mathcal{Z}\right) \leq I \times \frac{(J-1)(J+1)}{12}, \tag{2.22}$$

so that

$$\left|D^{\delta_0}\right| = \frac{\left|T^{\delta_0} - \frac{I(J+1)}{2}\right|}{\sqrt{I\,(J-1)\,(J+1)\,/12}} \leq \frac{\left|T^{\delta_0} - \mathrm{E}\left(T^{\delta_0} \mid \mathcal{F}, \mathcal{Z}\right)\right|}{\sqrt{\mathrm{var}\left(T^{\delta_0} \mid \mathcal{F}, \mathcal{Z}\right)}}. \tag{2.23}$$

Using (2.17) and (2.23), if $D^{\kappa\mathbf{1}} \geq \Phi^{-1}(1-\alpha)$ then $D^{\delta_0} \geq \Phi^{-1}(1-\alpha)$ for all $\delta_0 \in \Delta_0$. This is what we wanted all along: Rejecting the one hypothesis $H_0 : \boldsymbol{\delta} = \kappa\mathbf{1}$ by this computationally simple procedure entails rejecting every component hypothesis $H_0 : \boldsymbol{\delta} = \boldsymbol{\delta}_0$, $\boldsymbol{\delta}_0 \in \Delta_0$, and consequently it entails rejecting the composite hypothesis $H_0 : \boldsymbol{\delta} \in \Delta_0$.[13]

The argument here works for Wilcoxon's within-block ranks, q_{ij}^*, but it also works for the statistic of Puri [58] in which q_{ij}^* is replaced by $\phi\left(q_{ij}^*\right)$ for some function $\phi(\cdot)$. The formulas for the untied expectation and variance in (2.18) would change, but that is the only change. For $\phi\left(q_{ij}^*\right)$, the untied expectation and variance formulas are given by Proposition 2.3 with scores q_{ij} given by a permutation of $\phi(1)$, $\phi(2)$, $\ldots$, $\phi(J)$. Despite using the untied variance, the statistic T^{δ_0} itself is computed using average ranks for ties, meaning $\phi(j)$'s are averaged for tied $R_{ij} - \kappa Z_{ij}$.

*Example: Binge Drinking and Blood Pressure

Consider again the example of binge drinking and blood pressure in Sect. 1.5, again unwisely neglecting the absence of randomization to treatment or control. Consider the composite null hypothesis that asserts that for every individual ij, frequent binge drinking did not increase systolic blood pressure by more than 5 mmHg; i.e., the hypothesis that asserts $\delta_{ij} \leq 5$ for $i = 1, \ldots, I = 206$, $j = 1, \ldots, J = 3$. This is the composite hypothesis $H_0 : \boldsymbol{\delta} \in \Delta_0$ where Δ_0 contains all $I \times J$ matrices $\boldsymbol{\delta}_0$ with IJ coordinates $\delta_{0ij} \leq 5$.

We test the composite hypothesis by testing just one of its components, namely, the extreme hypothesis $H_0 : \boldsymbol{\delta} = 5\times\mathbf{1}$, where $\mathbf{1}$ is an $I \times J$ matrix of ones. If we reject

[13] In typical applications, the set Δ_0 contains infinitely many δ_0's, and only a finite number of δ_0's induce ties in $\mathbf{R}^{\delta_0}$; so, (2.23) is an equality except for a finite number of $\boldsymbol{\delta}_0 \in \Delta_0$. The stated procedure for testing $H_0 : \boldsymbol{\delta} \in \Delta_0$ may be slightly conservative, but only at the finitely many $\boldsymbol{\delta}_0 \in \Delta_0$ such that (2.23) is a strict inequality. If we were particularly interested in one or a few $\boldsymbol{\delta}_0 \in \Delta_0$ that do induce ties in $\mathbf{R}^{\delta_0}$, then we could switch from (2.23) to (2.14) when testing these few $\boldsymbol{\delta}_0$. For example, when testing $H_0 : \delta_{ij} \leq 0$ for all ij, one could very easily test Fisher's hypothesis, $H_0 : \delta_{ij} = 0$, using (2.14) and all other $\boldsymbol{\delta}_0 \in \Delta_0$ using (2.23). Also, when testing $H_0 : \delta_{ij} \leq \kappa$ for all ij, one could very easily test $H_0 : \delta_{ij} = \kappa$ for all ij using (2.14) and all other $\boldsymbol{\delta}_0 \in \Delta_0$ using (2.23). Issues of this sort are of little importance when testing a composite hypothesis, $H_0 : \boldsymbol{\delta} \in \Delta_0$, in isolation. In principle, however, if (2.14) is used to determine a confidence interval, and (2.23) is used to test $H_0 : \boldsymbol{\delta} \in \Delta_0$, then different judgments might be reached about the hypothesis $H_0 : \boldsymbol{\delta} = \kappa\mathbf{1}$ that determines whether the confidence interval is open or closed. As was just indicated, compatible inferences are easily available by testing the endpoint, $H_0 : \delta_{ij} = \kappa$ for all ij, using (2.14) in both cases.

the hypothesis that the treatment effect is always 5 in favor of larger effects, then we can reject the hypothesis that the effect is never greater than 5; that is, if we can reject $\delta_{ij} = 5$ for $i = 1, \ldots, I = 206$, $j = 1, \ldots, J = 3$, then we can reject $\delta_{ij} \leq 5$ for $i = 1, \ldots, I = 206$, $j = 1, \ldots, J = 3$. The one detail is that in performing this test, we need to test using the untied variance formula (2.21), because some $\boldsymbol{\delta}_0 \in \Delta_0$ create ties and others don't, and we want to reject every $\boldsymbol{\delta}_0 \in \Delta_0$.

First, we calculate the adjusted responses, $R_{ij} - 5Z_{ij}$ or $\mathbf{R}^{\boldsymbol{\delta}_0^*} = \mathbf{R} - 5\mathbf{Z}$, where $\boldsymbol{\delta}_0^* = 5 \times \mathbf{1}$. As it turns out, in five of the $I = 206$ blocks, two individuals have the same $R_{ij} - 5Z_{ij}$; that is, they are tied. We compute the blocked Wilcoxon rank sum statistic using average ranks for ties, and its value is $T^{\boldsymbol{\delta}_0^*} = t\left(\mathbf{Z}, \mathbf{R}^{\boldsymbol{\delta}_0^*}\right) = 441$. In an $I \times J = 206 \times 3$ randomized block design (2.4) in which the true $\boldsymbol{\delta}$ actually is $\boldsymbol{\delta}_0^*$, the value of Wilcoxon's statistic, $T^{\boldsymbol{\delta}_0^*} = 441$, is somewhat high; the expected rank of the treated individual in each block is $(J + 1)/2 = (3 + 1)/2 = 2$, so the null expectation is $206 \times 2 = 412$, whether or not there are ties. If we were solely testing the simple hypothesis $H_0 : \boldsymbol{\delta} = \boldsymbol{\delta}_0^*$, then we would allow for ties in computing the variance (2.14) of the Wilcoxon statistic, obtaining a variance of 136.5. However, we want to test the composite null hypothesis $H_0 : \boldsymbol{\delta} \in \Delta_0$, and for most $\boldsymbol{\delta}_0 \in \Delta_0$, there are no ties among the $\mathbf{R}^{\boldsymbol{\delta}_0}$, and then the null variance of Wilcoxon's statistic is larger than 136.5, making it harder to reject such a $\boldsymbol{\delta}_0$. We use (2.18) to compute the variance of the Wilcoxon statistic in the absence of ties as $I(J - 1)(J + 1)/12 = 206 \times 2 \times 4/12 = 137.3333 > 136.5$. Using the untied variance, the deviate is $D^{\boldsymbol{\delta}_0^*} = (441 - 412)/\sqrt{137.3333} = 2.47$ with approximate P-value of 0.00676 from (2.15), whereas using the variance formula (2.14) that allows for ties yields a deviate of $(441 - 412)/\sqrt{136.5} = 2.48$ with a smaller approximate P-value of 0.00657. Evidently, had the data in Sect. 1.5 been from a randomized experiment, it would be quite implausible that binge drinking never caused an increase in systolic blood pressure of more than 5 mmHg.

We have been fussing about two issues that trade-off against one another, and we have been seeing that one of the issues is often trivial, while the other is of value, so the trade-off is very clear. The difference between P-values of 0.00657 and 0.00676 is not worth serious attention. On the other hand, it is attractive to be able to interpret rejection of $H_0 : \delta_{ij} = 5$ for all ij as rejection of $H_0 : \delta_{ij} \leq 5$ for all ij.

*Testing a Composite Hypothesis Using a Weighted Rank Statistic

As noted in Sect. 2.6, for randomized experiments with small block sizes, say $J \leq 5$, Quade [59] and Tardif [97] improved the performance of the blocked Wilcoxon rank sum statistic by replacing Wilcoxon's within-block ranks, q_{ij}^*, by $q_{ij} = q_{ij}^*\, b_i$ where b_i is the rank of the within-block range,

$$w_i^{\delta_0} = \max_{1 \leq j \leq J} R_{ij}^{\delta_0} - \min_{1 \leq j \leq J} R_{ij}^{\delta_0}. \tag{2.24}$$

These and closely related statistics may also be used to test composite hypotheses. As with Wilcoxon's statistic, one uses the untied variance, because different but nearly identical components, $\boldsymbol{\delta}_0 \in \Delta_0$, of the composite hypothesis, $\Delta_0 = \left\{\boldsymbol{\delta}_0 : \delta_{0ij} \leq \kappa,\ i = 1, \ldots, I,\ j = 1, \ldots, J\right\}$, will have different patterns of ties. The appendix to this chapter, Sect. 2.12, shows that the untied variance is never smaller than the tied variance, so a calculation parallel to (2.23) is, again, slightly conservative for just a few $\boldsymbol{\delta}_0 \in \Delta_0$. The null expectation and variance of the weighted rank statistic will have a different simple form (2.34) than in (2.23), but a single null expectation and variance are used to test every $\boldsymbol{\delta}_0 \in \Delta_0$.

One issue remains, however. It was important that Wilcoxon's blocked rank sum statistic $T^{\boldsymbol{\delta}_0} = t\left(\mathbf{Z}, \mathbf{R}^{\boldsymbol{\delta}_0}\right)$ never increases as the IJ coordinates δ_{0ij} increase in the half line $(-\infty, \kappa]$ that defines Δ_0. That fact allowed us to reject all $\boldsymbol{\delta}_0 \in \Delta_0$ when we rejected as too small a single $\boldsymbol{\delta}_0$, namely, $\boldsymbol{\delta}_0 = \kappa \times \mathbf{1}$, where $\mathbf{1}$ is an $I \times J$ matrix of ones. As in the case of Wilcoxon's statistic, for a control with $Z_{ij} = 0$, the adjusted response, $R_{ij} - Z_{ij}\,\delta_{0ij}$ does not change as δ_{0ij} increases, but for a treated individual with $Z_{ij} = 1$, the adjusted response $R_{ij} - Z_{ij}\,\delta_{0ij}$ decreases as δ_{0ij} increases. This implies that the rank of the treated response, $\sum_{j=1}^{J} Z_{ij}\, q_{ij}^*$, in block i declines or stays the same as the δ_{0ij} increase in $(-\infty, \kappa]$. So far, so good, but what about b_i?

The new issue is that an increase in δ_{0ij} may change the range $w_i^{\boldsymbol{\delta}_0}$ in (2.24) and its rank b_i. With ranks, a decline in one b_i means an increase in $b_{i'}$ for some $i' \neq i$. It takes a moment to realize that this is not a problem, as seen in Proposition 2.4. The proofs of Proposition 2.4 and Corollary 2.1 are in Appendix Sect. 2.13.

Proposition 2.4 *Let $q_{ij\boldsymbol{\delta}_0}^*$ and $b_{i\boldsymbol{\delta}_0}$ be the values of the within-block rank q_{ij}^* and the rank of the block range b_i when computed from $\mathbf{R}^{\boldsymbol{\delta}_0}$. Viewed as a function of $\boldsymbol{\delta}_0$ for fixed $\mathbf{Z}$, the weighted rank statistic $T^{\boldsymbol{\delta}_0} = t\left(\mathbf{Z}, \mathbf{R}^{\boldsymbol{\delta}_0}\right) = \sum_{i=1}^{I} \sum_{j=1}^{J} Z_{ij}\, q_{ij\boldsymbol{\delta}_0}^*\, b_{i\boldsymbol{\delta}_0}$ achieves its minimum value over $\Delta_0 = \left\{\boldsymbol{\delta}_0 : \delta_{0ij} \leq \kappa,\ i = 1, \ldots, I,\ j = 1, \ldots, J\right\}$ at $\boldsymbol{\delta}_0 = \kappa \times \mathbf{1}$.*

Corollary 2.1 *Proposition 2.4 remains true if $b_{i\boldsymbol{\delta}_0}$ is replaced by $\varphi\{b_{i\boldsymbol{\delta}_0}/(I+1)\}$ for a monotone increasing function $\varphi(\cdot)$.*

2.10 Confidence Sets and Point Estimates for Causal Effects

The General Method

Instead of testing one simple null hypothesis about causal effects, suppose that we test at level α every simple hypothesis, $H_0 : \boldsymbol{\delta} = \boldsymbol{\delta}_0$, using Proposition 2.2, for every $I \times J$ matrix $\boldsymbol{\delta}_0$, collecting those $\boldsymbol{\delta}_0$ that are not rejected into a set $\mathcal{D}$.

Proposition 2.5 *The random set $\mathcal{D}$ will contain the fixed parameter $\boldsymbol{\delta}$ with probability at least $1-\alpha$; that is, $\mathcal{D}$ is a $1-\alpha$ confidence set for the unknown parameter $\boldsymbol{\delta}$.*

Proof The elementary proof is from first principles [41, §3.5], that is, from the definition of the set $\mathcal{D}$. Let $\boldsymbol{\delta}^*$ be the unknown but true value of $\boldsymbol{\delta}$. The procedure for constructing $\mathcal{D}$ tests every hypothesis $H_0 : \boldsymbol{\delta} = \boldsymbol{\delta}_0$, so eventually, unbeknownst to the procedure, it happens to test the one true hypothesis, namely, $H_0 : \boldsymbol{\delta} = \boldsymbol{\delta}^*$. By Proposition 2.2, the test of this true hypothesis $H_0 : \boldsymbol{\delta} = \boldsymbol{\delta}^*$ falsely rejects $\boldsymbol{\delta}^*$ with probability at most α. So, with probability at least $1 - \alpha$, the random set $\mathcal{D}$ will contain $\boldsymbol{\delta}^*$. □

For example, in Fig. 2.1, the $\boldsymbol{\delta}_0 = \mathbf{0}$ that produces panel (i) is rejected at the two-sided 0.05-level by Wilcoxon's blocked rank sum test; so, $\mathbf{0} \notin \mathcal{D}$. In contrast, $\delta_{0ij} = 8.17$ for all ij in panel (ii) and $\delta_{0ij} = 0.0676 \times r_{Cij}$ in panel (iii) are not rejected, so $\boldsymbol{\delta}_0 \in \mathcal{D}$ for these two $\boldsymbol{\delta}_0$'s.

In the binge drinking example in Sect. 2.9, we tested the composite hypothesis, $H_0 : \boldsymbol{\delta} \in \Delta_0$, for the set Δ_0 of all $I \times J$ matrices $\boldsymbol{\delta}_0$ such that $\delta_{0ij} \leq 5$ for all ij, and it rejected $H_0 : \boldsymbol{\delta} \in \Delta_0$ at level $\alpha = 0.00676$. Consequently, the 95% confidence set $\mathcal{D}$ (and indeed even the larger $1 - \alpha = 1 - 0.00676 = 0.99324$ confidence set) contains no $\boldsymbol{\delta}$ with $\delta_{0ij} \leq 5$ for all ij, that is, $\emptyset = \mathcal{D} \cap \Delta_0$. Moreover, this $\mathcal{D}$ does not contain the one $\boldsymbol{\delta}$ with $\delta_{0ij} = 5$ for all ij; so, it seems that many δ_{ij} are larger than five.

This confidence set $\mathcal{D}$ is not consistent: as the number of blocks increases, $I \to \infty$, the set $\mathcal{D}$ does not collapse toward a single matrix $\boldsymbol{\delta}$. Indeed: (i) as $I \to \infty$, the dimension of $\boldsymbol{\delta}$ and $\mathcal{D}$ increases, and as always (ii) there is no consistent confidence set for the causal effect δ_{ij} for any single individual ij.

Although $\mathcal{D}$ is not consistent, it is informative and useful. This is, again, Fisher's comment as quoted in Sect. 2.5. The set $\mathcal{D}$ excludes many $\boldsymbol{\delta}_0$ that have been rejected at level α, and so it is informative about $\boldsymbol{\delta}$.

The $1 - \alpha$ confidence set $\mathcal{D}$ for $\boldsymbol{\delta}$ is a set of infinitely many $I \times J$ matrices $\boldsymbol{\delta}_0$. The main problem with $\mathcal{D}$ is not a technical problem with $\mathcal{D}$ itself but rather a problem with our own cognitive limitations: We have a limited ability to conceive of a set $\mathcal{D}$ of infinitely many $I \times J$ matrices $\boldsymbol{\delta}_0$. How can we make sense of such a set? If we could digest and interpret $\mathcal{D}$, then we would know what the data from a randomized block experiment tell us about the IJ causal effects, $\boldsymbol{\delta}$. As we just saw, a test of a composite hypothesis, $H_0 : \boldsymbol{\delta} \in \Delta_0$, is the same as asking whether $\mathcal{D} \cap \Delta_0$ is empty; so, findings of that sort are easy to understand, despite the dimensionality of $\mathcal{D}$.

*Parametric Models as Devices for Exploring a Nonparametric Confidence Set $\mathcal{D}$

The next subsection discusses the most common approach to understanding $\mathcal{D}$, namely, limiting attention to one or several parametric models in which $\boldsymbol{\delta}$ is a function $\boldsymbol{\delta}(\eta)$ of a scalar parameter, say η, so this function maps $\Re \to \Re^{IJ}$, returning an $I \times J$ matrix $\boldsymbol{\delta}$ in exchange for a scalar η. Parametric models are, of course, widely used throughout statistics; however, they can seem out of place in randomization inference, because they introduce assumptions that are otherwise not needed. How should we think about confidence intervals for scalar parameters when the parameter of interest, $\boldsymbol{\delta}$, is an $I \times J$ array?

We can think of a parametric model as merely a way of becoming acquainted with the nonparametric confidence set $\mathcal{D}$. By Proposition 2.5, the confidence set $\mathcal{D}$ is valid without resort to parametric models. We ask: What part of the curve $\boldsymbol{\delta}(\eta)$ lies in $\mathcal{D}$, what set of values of $\eta \in \Re$ give rise to $\boldsymbol{\delta}(\eta)$'s in $\mathcal{D}$, and what is the shortest interval in $\Re$ that contains all the η's that give rise to $\boldsymbol{\delta}(\eta)$'s in $\mathcal{D}$? Those $\boldsymbol{\delta}(\eta)$'s that are *not* in $\mathcal{D}$ have been rejected by a level-α test; so, those $\boldsymbol{\delta}(\eta)$'s, together with their η's, are not especially plausible, and that is news and insight into the structure of $\mathcal{D}$. Of course, $\mathcal{D}$ typically contains many $\boldsymbol{\delta}$'s that are not on the parameterized curve that do not equal $\boldsymbol{\delta}(\eta)$ for any η; so, $\mathcal{D}$ does not endorse the parameterized model or the values of $\boldsymbol{\delta}(\eta)$ that have not been rejected. However, that is always true of hypothesis tests and consequently of confidence sets: They tell us what isn't plausible, not what is. This is again Fisher's comment quoted in Sect. 2.5: "the null hypothesis is never proved or established, but is possibly disproved, in the course of experimentation."

When testing values $\boldsymbol{\delta}(\eta)$ for $\eta \in \Re$, it is impossible to falsely reject the true $\boldsymbol{\delta}$ if the true $\boldsymbol{\delta}$ does not equal $\boldsymbol{\delta}(\eta)$ for any η. To falsely reject a true null hypothesis, you must test a true null hypothesis. Depending upon the nature of the parametric model, $\boldsymbol{\delta}(\eta)$, and the test statistic, $T^{\boldsymbol{\delta}_0}$, the nonparametric confidence set $\mathcal{D}$ could reject the entire parametric model; that is, it could reject $H_0 : \boldsymbol{\delta} = \boldsymbol{\delta}(\eta_0)$ for every $\eta_0 \in \Re$.

Having traced the portion of one parameterized curve, $\boldsymbol{\delta}(\eta)$, that lies in $\mathcal{D}$, we can set that curve aside and look at another. Indeed, we began to do this in Fig. 2.1, where panel (ii) looked at one additive effect, $\delta_{ij} = \tau$ with $\tau = 8.17$, and panel (iii) looked at one multiplicative effect $\delta_{ij} = \eta \times r_{Cij}$ with $\eta = 0.0676$. There is no multiple testing problem when exploring several or many parametric models, providing that we always test $H_0 : \boldsymbol{\delta} = \boldsymbol{\delta}_0$ using the same test statistic, $T^{\boldsymbol{\delta}_0}$, perhaps the blocked Wilcoxon statistic. This is evident from the proof of Proposition 2.5. The nonparametric confidence set $\mathcal{D}$ has coverage at least $1 - \alpha$, because the true $\boldsymbol{\delta}$ is rejected with probability at most α. The true $\boldsymbol{\delta}$ may be in several parametric models and hence may be tested several times, but the decision about it is always the same.

Parametric models are not the only way to produce a one-dimensional confidence interval that summarizes the IJ-dimensional confidence set $\mathcal{D}$. It is often possible to characterize $\mathcal{D}$ in terms of a one-dimensional quantity, called an "attributable effect," such that a one-dimensional interval for the attributable effect completely determines which $\boldsymbol{\delta}_0$ are in $\mathcal{D}$ and which are not [62,63,66]; see Sect. 2.11.

Inference About Scalar Parameters

The treatment has an additive constant effect if there is some number τ such that $\delta_{ij} = \tau$ for all ij, or equivalently if $\boldsymbol{\delta} \in \{\tau \times \mathbf{1} : \tau \in \Re\}$, where $\mathbf{1}$ is an $I \times J$ array of 1's and $\Re$ is the real line.

Proposition 2.6 *If $\mathcal{D}$ is a $1-\alpha$ confidence set for $\boldsymbol{\delta}$ and the treatment has an additive effect τ, then $C = \{\tau : \tau \times \mathbf{1} \in \mathcal{D}\}$ is a $1-\alpha$ confidence set for τ.*

Proof Let $\boldsymbol{\delta}^*$ be the true value of $\boldsymbol{\delta}$. By assumption, $\boldsymbol{\delta}^* \in \{\tau \times \mathbf{1} : \tau \in \Re\}$. By Proposition 2.5, $\mathcal{D}$ will contain $\boldsymbol{\delta}^*$ with probability at least $1-\alpha$. So $\mathcal{D} \cap \{\tau \times \mathbf{1} : \tau \in \Re\}$ will contain $\boldsymbol{\delta}^*$ with probability at least $1-\alpha$. □

Of confidence intervals derived from randomization tests, by far the most widely used are confidence intervals for an additive or shift effect found by inverting either the Wilcoxon signed rank test or the Wilcoxon rank sum test [27, 30, 38, 40], as implemented in R in the `wilcox.test` function in the `stats` package. That confidence interval is the same as the interval in Proposition 2.6, as discussed in Lehmann and Romano [41, §5.12]; however, it may also be derived from a population sampling model [40], as discussed later in Sect. 3.2. Proposition 2.6 also provides confidence intervals by inverting tests based on other test statistics, for instance, tests based on (i) the blocked Wilcoxon rank sum test, (ii) weighted rank statistics like Quade's [59, 97] statistic, and (iii) M-statistics [46, 69, 73].

In a randomized block experiment (2.4), the confidence interval is found using Proposition 2.2 by testing $H_0 : \boldsymbol{\delta} = \tau_0 \times \mathbf{1}$ for $\tau_0 \in \Re$ and retaining for C the values of τ_0 that are not rejected at level α. For a scalar parameter like τ, a $1-\alpha$ confidence set C is associated with a $1-\alpha$ confidence interval: The $1-\alpha$ confidence interval is, by definition, the shortest interval that contains C. Because the interval contains C, and C will contain τ with probability at least $1-\alpha$, the interval also contains τ with probability at least $1-\alpha$. For some test statistics, the set C and its associated confidence interval always coincide, so finding C reduces to a binary search for the endpoints of the confidence interval.

As $\alpha \to 1$, the confidence interval becomes shorter, typically collapsing to a point or short interval, which is the Hodges-Lehmann [29] point estimate $\widehat{\tau}$ of τ. Taking $\boldsymbol{\delta}_0 = \tau_0 \times \mathbf{1}$, the Hodges-Lehmann point estimate $\widehat{\tau}$ of τ is the solution, τ_0, to the equation $T^{\tau_0 \times \mathbf{1}} = \mathrm{E}\left(T^{\tau_0 \times \mathbf{1}} \mid \mathcal{F}, \mathcal{Z}\right)$, where $\mathrm{E}\left(T^{\boldsymbol{\delta}_0} \mid \mathcal{F}, \mathcal{Z}\right)$ is given in Proposition 2.3. Sometimes this equation has a short interval of values, τ_0, that solve the equation, in which case the estimate $\widehat{\tau}$ is any point in this short interval, conventionally its midpoint. Sometimes, $T^{\tau_0 \times \mathbf{1}}$ is strictly above the expectation, but the smallest increase, from τ_0 to $\tau_0 + \epsilon$ with $\epsilon > 0$, makes $T^{(\tau_0+\epsilon)\times \mathbf{1}}$ strictly below the expectation; then, the point estimate $\widehat{\tau}$ is defined to be this value τ_0 where $T^{\tau_0 \times \mathbf{1}}$ passes $\mathrm{E}\left(T^{\tau_0 \times \mathbf{1}} \mid \mathcal{F}, \mathcal{Z}\right)$.

For matched pairs, $J = 2$, the median of the I treated-minus-control pair differences is one very simple Hodges-Lehmann estimate. Specifically, for matched pairs, $J = 2$, the median matched pair difference is the Hodges-Lehmann estimate associated with the blocked Wilcoxon rank sum test, which sums I independent scores, 1 or 2, where a 2 score indicates that the treated individual in block or pair i had a higher response than the control, and a 1 score indicates that the control had the higher response.[14] If $H_0 : \boldsymbol{\delta} = \tau_0 \times \mathbf{1}$ is true in the absence of tied responses,

[14] For $J = 2$, the blocked Wilcoxon rank sum statistic is equivalent to the sign test, which uses scores 0 or 1 rather than 1 or 2; see Problem 2.7. The median pair difference is also one of Huber's M-statistics, with influence function equal to the sign, -1, 0, or 1, of the pair difference.

then $\mathrm{E}\left(T^{\tau_0 \times \mathbf{1}} \mid \mathcal{F}, \mathcal{Z}\right) = I(1+2)/2$, and the Hodges-Lehmann estimated $\widehat{\tau}$ "solves" the equation $T^{\tau_0 \times \mathbf{1}} = I(1+2)/2$. If I is even, then $\widehat{\tau}$ is any value between the two middle order statistics. If I is odd, then the equation has no solution, but we pass from $T^{\tau_0 \times \mathbf{1}} > I(1+2)/2$ to $T^{\tau_0 \times \mathbf{1}} < I(1+2)/2$ at the middle order statistic.

For matched pairs, $J = 2$, the Hodges-Lehmann estimate $\widehat{\tau}$ associated with Wilcoxon's signed rank statistic [40, §4.40] is the median of the $I(I+1)/2$ averages of two matched-pair differences from two blocks, $i \leq i'$. For pair differences that are independent observations from the same Normal distribution, $\widehat{\tau}$ is almost as efficient as the mean pair difference, and $\widehat{\tau}$ is much more efficient than the mean for pair differences from longer-tailed symmetric unimodal distributions. This Hodges-Lehmann estimate performed well in the Princeton Robustness Study [1]. Quade's statistic for small $J \geq 2$ in Sect. 2.6 becomes Wilcoxon's signed rank statistic when $J = 2$, and consequently their Hodges-Lehmann estimates are the same for $J = 2$.

Point estimates are difficult to interpret unless we have some sense of their stability. Often, an estimator is reported with a standard error. If an estimator is approximately Normally distributed about the true value of the parameter, then an estimate plus or minus its standard error is approximately a 2/3 confidence interval; i.e., an interval that is twice as likely to cover its parameter as to miss it. Michael Stoto [94] suggested reversing these concepts: view the 2/3 confidence interval as an aid to interpreting a point estimate, and view an estimate plus or minus its standard error as an approximation to the 2/3 confidence interval. This is attractive when we have a confidence interval that is derived from an exact test, as the 2/3 coverage property is exact; moreover, it is essential when the estimator is not approximately Normal in its distribution but instead is markedly skewed. Viewed in this way, Proposition 2.6 yields a point estimate, a 95% confidence interval, and the information we commonly associate with a standard error.

Return to the example of binge drinking in Sect. 2.5. Panel (i) of Fig. 2.1 compared the systolic blood pressure of frequent binge drinkers (B) and never bingers who rarely drink now (N). In a randomized experiment comparing systolic blood pressure in $I = 206$ B-N pairs or blocks of size $J = 2$, we might use Wilcoxon's signed rank test in the `stats` package in R (which is Quade's test for $J = 2$). Briefly ignoring the important fact that Fig. 2.1 is not from a randomized experiment, the randomization inference would yield a two-sided P-value of 0.0000029 testing $H_0 : \tau = 0$, a Hodges-Lehmann point estimate of $\widehat{\tau} = 8.17$, a 95% two-sided confidence interval of [5.00, 11.17], and a 2/3-confidence interval of [6.67, 9.67]. Panel (ii) of Fig. 2.1 subtracted $\widehat{\tau} = 8.17$ from the responses of treated individuals (B), whereupon the boxplots of systolic blood pressure for groups B and N look fairly similar.

Interpreting Inferences Expressed in Terms of a Scalar Effect Parameter

Of course, it is entirely possible that the effect of the treatment is not an additive constant τ, so that $\boldsymbol{\delta} \notin \{\tau \times \mathbf{1} : \tau \in \mathfrak{R}\}$. In a randomized block experiment (2.4), this is possible in two very different ways. It is possible that the data can tell us that the treatment effect is not constant, $\boldsymbol{\delta} \notin \{\tau \times \mathbf{1} : \tau \in \Re\}$, and it is possible that the data are silent about whether $\boldsymbol{\delta} \notin \{\tau \times \mathbf{1} : \tau \in \Re\}$. Saying the same thing in other words, whether $\boldsymbol{\delta} \in \{\tau \times \mathbf{1} : \tau \in \Re\}$ or $\boldsymbol{\delta} \notin \{\tau \times \mathbf{1} : \tau \in \Re\}$ may or may not be identified. For example, in a randomized block experiment with a large number I of blocks, it may be evident in boxplots that R_{ij} is both higher and more dispersed for treated individuals with $Z_{ij} = 1$ than controls with $Z_{ij} = 0$, thereby showing that $\boldsymbol{\delta} \notin \{\tau \times \mathbf{1} : \tau \in \Re\}$. As another example, it may be evident that the distribution of R_{ij} has a different shape for $Z_{ij} = 1$ and $Z_{ij} = 0$, perhaps because only some treated individuals respond to treatment, and this too may be examined [12,67]. As yet another example of an identified failure of the model $\boldsymbol{\delta} \in \{\tau \times \mathbf{1} : \tau \in \Re\}$, there may be effect modification in the sense that the magnitude of the effect, δ_{ij}, may vary systematically with the observed covariates, $\mathbf{x}_{ij}$, and of course this too may be examined [15,31,39,107], as was done in Fig. 2.2.

If the observable data provide evidence that $\boldsymbol{\delta} \notin \{\tau \times \mathbf{1} : \tau \in \Re\}$, then we would abandon the additive model and consider other models. Panel (iii) of Fig. 2.1 considered one alternative model involving a scalar parameter, namely, the multiplicative model, $r_{Tij} = \omega\, r_{Cij}$ or $\delta_{ij} = (\omega - 1)\, r_{Cij}$. Under this model, $\log\left(r_{Tij}\right) = \log\left(r_{Cij}\right) + \log(\omega)$, so the same methods as above applied to $\log\left(R_{ij}\right)$ yield a confidence interval and point estimate for $\log(\omega)$, and hence also for ω. Panel (iii) of Fig. 2.1 removed this estimated multiplicative effect, plotting $R_{ij}/\widehat{\omega}^{Z_{ij}}$ against Z_{ij} for $\widehat{\omega} = 1.0676$. Notably, there is little reason in Fig. 2.1 for preferring either the additive model or the multiplicative model.

In contrast, it is also possible that $\boldsymbol{\delta} \notin \{\tau \times \mathbf{1} : \tau \in \Re\}$, but the observable quantities, $\left(R_{ij}, Z_{ij}, \mathbf{x}_{ij}\right)$, can provide no information that can reveal this. That is, even as the number of blocks increases, $I \longrightarrow \infty$, the data from a randomized block experiment (2.4) may offer no visible evidence in $\left(R_{ij}, Z_{ij}, \mathbf{x}_{ij}\right)$ that $\boldsymbol{\delta} \notin \{\tau \times \mathbf{1} : \tau \in \Re\}$. Problem 2.9 asks you to consider such a situation. In Problem 2.9, there is a conventional randomized block model with block parameters β_i, a shift of τ in the distribution of responses to treatment, and independent bivariate Normal errors with expectation zero, variances 1 and correlation ρ,

$$\begin{aligned} r_{Tij} &= \beta_i + \tau + \epsilon_{Tij}, \\ r_{Cij} &= \beta_i + \epsilon_{Cij}, \\ \begin{pmatrix} \epsilon_{Tij} \\ \epsilon_{Cij} \end{pmatrix} &\sim N\left\{\begin{pmatrix} 0 \\ 0 \end{pmatrix}, \begin{bmatrix} 1 & \rho \\ \rho & 1 \end{bmatrix}\right\}, \end{aligned} \tag{2.25}$$

so that in a randomized block experiment,

$$\begin{aligned} R_{ij} &= Z_{ij}\, r_{Tij} + \left(1 - Z_{ij}\right) r_{Cij} \\ &= \beta_i + Z_{ij}\, \tau + \varepsilon_{ij}, \\ \varepsilon_{ij} &= Z_{ij}\, \epsilon_{Tij} + \left(1 - Z_{ij}\right) \epsilon_{Cij} \sim N(0, 1), \end{aligned} \tag{2.26}$$

where (2.4) ensures that Z_{ij} is independent of $\left(\epsilon_{Tij}, \epsilon_{Cij}\right)$, with the consequence that the ε_{ij} are independent observations from the Normal distribution with expectation zero and variance one, $N(0, 1)$. In this model, $\mathrm{E}\left(r_{Tij} - r_{Cij} \,\middle|\, \mathcal{F}, \mathcal{Z}\right) = r_{Tij} - r_{Cij} = \delta_{ij} = \tau + \epsilon_{Tij} - \epsilon_{Cij}$, which equals τ only if $\rho = 1$, but $\mathrm{E}\left\{\mathrm{E}\left(r_{Tij} - r_{Cij} \,\middle|\, \mathcal{F}, \mathcal{Z}\right) \,\middle|\, \mathcal{Z}\right\} = \tau$ is an expected treatment effect and a shift in the distribution from r_{Cij} to the distribution of r_{Tij}. In this case, the Hodges-Lehmann point estimate $\widehat{\tau}$ is a consistent estimate of the shift τ and the randomization-based $1 - \alpha$ confidence interval will cover τ with probability $1 - \alpha$; yet, the effect $r_{Tij} - r_{Cij} = \delta_{ij} = \tau + \epsilon_{Tij} - \epsilon_{Cij}$ is not constant; see also Problem 2.9 and Sect. 3.2. The distinction is not trivial: if $r_{Tij} - r_{Cij} = \tau$ for all ij, then a physician could tell every patient ij that he will benefit by τ, but if $r_{Tij} - r_{Cij} = \tau + \epsilon_{Tij} - \epsilon_{Cij}$ then the physician can only say that patients typically benefit by τ, although some patients may be harmed by treatment.

In the situation defined by (2.25), distinguishing $\delta_{ij} = \tau + \epsilon_{Tij} - \epsilon_{Cij}$ from $\delta_{ij} = \tau$ is not possible using the observable quantities $\left(R_{ij}, Z_{ij}, \mathbf{x}_{ij}\right)$. This is not a surprise: A single δ_{ij} is not identified by the observable data $\left(R_{ij}, Z_{ij}, \mathbf{x}_{ij}\right)$—that is the central problem in causal inference, and nothing is going to make that problem go away. Nonetheless, as seen in Sect. 3.2, randomization tests and confidence intervals are valid inferences about τ in (2.25), despite ambiguity about the relationship between τ and the effect of the treatment, δ_{ij}, on a specific individual ij.

In brief, randomization tests and confidence intervals for τ have at least three valid but logically distinct interpretations. (i) The tests are valid tests, and the confidence intervals concisely summarize many valid tests, about hypotheses that assert the effect is constant, $H_0 : \delta_{ij} = \tau_0$ for $i = 1, \ldots, I$, $j = 1, \ldots, J$. (ii) With a little attention to some minor technical matters, they are valid inferences about certain composite hypotheses, such as $H_0 : \delta_{ij} \leq \tau_0$ for $i = 1, \ldots, I$, $j = 1, \ldots, J$, as in Sect. 2.9. In particular, a two-sided confidence interval $\left[\tau_{\mathrm{low}}, \tau_{\mathrm{high}}\right]$ for a constant effect τ is correctly interpreted as rejecting two composite hypotheses, namely, $H_0 : \delta_{ij} < \tau_{\mathrm{low}}$ for $i = 1, \ldots, I$, $j = 1, \ldots, J$ and $H_0 : \delta_{ij} > \tau_{\mathrm{high}}$ for $i = 1, \ldots, I$, $j = 1, \ldots, J$. (iii) Finally, they are valid inferences about a shift τ in a population distribution (2.25) with no reference to causal effects on individuals, δ_{ij}. Philip Dawid [17] has pointed to (iii) as a reason for avoiding talk about causal effects at the individual level, $\delta_{ij} = r_{Tij} - r_{Cij}$. I agree with Dawid that interpretation (iii) is available, is important, and should not be neglected; however, the availability of (iii) does not strike me as a reason for ignoring the several valid interpretations of inferences about scalar or low-dimensional parameters like τ, or the often important gaps between these interpretations. To talk about these gaps, we need a language that includes $\delta_{ij} = r_{Tij} - r_{Cij}$, even though δ_{ij} is not identified for any individual ij.

2.11 *Further Reading

Confidence intervals without parametric models: In a randomized experiment, a randomization test of Fisher's hypothesis of no effect, $H_0 : \delta_{ij} = 0$ for $i = 1, \ldots, I$,

$j = 1, \ldots, J$, requires no assumptions. If treatments are assigned at random, then (2.4) is a fact not an assumption. The null hypothesis, $H_0 : \delta_{ij} = 0$ for $i = 1, \ldots, I$, $j = 1, \ldots, J$, is not an assumption—it may be true or false, and if false we are happy to reject it—but either way it is not an assumption. There is no presumption that H_0 is true. Is there a confidence interval for the magnitude of causal effects that also requires no assumptions? In a sense, $\mathcal{D}$ in Sect. 2.10 requires only the assumption that (r_{Tij}, r_{Cij}) exist and are well defined—essentially the assumption of no interference between units; however, $\mathcal{D}$ is a subset of IJ-dimensional space and is often hard to examine in detail. It is possible to produce a one-dimensional confidence for an "attributable effect" that completely characterizes the division of IJ-dimensional space into $\mathcal{D}$ and its complement [62, 63]. Stated informally: For Wilcoxon's rank sum test, the attributable effect is the number or proportion of times that a treated individual has a higher response than a control because of effects caused by the treatment. Under Fisher's hypothesis of no effect, the attributable effect is zero. There are also attributable effects for binary outcomes and for quantile displacements [64, §5.5-§5.6]. Attributable effects are also applicable in the presence of interference between units [68], or when only some treated individuals are affected by the treatment [67].

Confidence intervals with infinite-dimensional models for causal effect: Doksum [19] considered essentially the model $r_{Tij} = r_{Cij} + \Psi(r_{Cij})$ where $\Psi(\cdot)$ is an unknown, monotone increasing function; see also [20,61]. If $\Psi(\cdot)$ is constant, then Doksum's model becomes the model of a constant effect. Stated as $r_{Tij} = r_{Cij} + \Psi(r_{Cij})$, the model entails that a larger r_{Cij} means a larger effect, $\delta_{ij} = r_{Tij} - r_{Cij}$; however, as with a shift τ in distributions, $\Psi(\cdot)$ can be understood to refer to distributions in infinite populations of r_{Tij} and r_{Cij}, without constraining or referring to their joint distribution, as in Sect. 3.2.

Bayesian Methods for Causal Inference: In 1978, Donald Rubin [83] gave a Bayesian justification for randomized treatment assignment. Stated informally: Viewing the observed treatment assignment $\mathbf{Z}$ as fixed is the same as conditioning upon the observed treatment assignment if treatments were assigned by randomization; otherwise, the Bayesian who views $\mathbf{Z}$ as fixed has ignored a factor in the likelihood that cannot correctly be ignored, i.e., a needed factor is not "ignorable." As in Fisher's frequentist argument, in Rubin's Bayesian argument for randomized treatment assignment, randomization plays a critical role in the mathematics; so, the distinction between experiments and observational studies is clear with clear consequences. Fan Li, Peng Ding and Fabrizia Mealli [42] provide an extensive review of recent work on Bayesian causal inference.

Multiple Randomizations: In this chapter, treatments were randomly assigned within blocks. Many experiments involve several randomizations [5]. For instance, one set of treatments might be randomized within blocks, while another set of treatments are randomized among whole blocks, a design known as a split-plot design. Multiple randomizations are connected with evidence factors [70, 78] in Chap. 13.

Randomized Experiments and Analysis of Variance: A large literature discusses the approximation of the randomization distributions of quantities arising in the analysis of variance, such as $\overline{R}_t - \overline{R}_c$, with no sampling assumptions [13, 43, 103, 105].

Developments in Experimental Design: This chapter has viewed randomized experiments as a leading case—a precedent setting case—for causal inference in observational studies. Of course, there is much interesting work being done in experimental design unrelated to observational studies. In recent decades, important work in experimental design has considered new methods of randomization [80] or rerandomization [48], the possiblity of redesigning or terminating early an on-going clinical trial [102], deeper understandings of fractional factorial designs [4, 9, 18, 49], and computer experiments [85, 86, 106].

2.12 *Appendix: Effect of Ties on the Variance

When ranks are used in a test of $H_0 : \boldsymbol{\delta} = \boldsymbol{\delta}_0$, tied quantities derived from the $R_{ij}^{\delta_0}$ are often assigned the average of the ranks that they would have received had they differed by an infinitesimal amount; see Sect. 2.6. Propositions 2.2 and 2.3 are correct as they stand when average ranks are used for ties. When testing a simple hypothesis, $H_0 : \boldsymbol{\delta} = \boldsymbol{\delta}_0$, no special issues arise on account of ties.

When testing a composite hypothesis about causal effects $\boldsymbol{\delta}$, or when determining a confidence set for $\boldsymbol{\delta}$, by testing infinitely many simple hypotheses, $H_0 : \boldsymbol{\delta} = \boldsymbol{\delta}_0$, different $\boldsymbol{\delta}_0$'s will introduce sporadic ties of different types in different places. Conceptually, one could apply Propositions 2.2 and 2.3 to each of infinitely many $\boldsymbol{\delta}_0$'s allowing for whatever ties occur. As a practical matter, we often wish to speed up these infinitely many tests, saying, for example, that if $\mathbf{0}$ is judged too small when testing $H_0 : \boldsymbol{\delta} = \mathbf{0}$, then we can also reject infinitely many hypotheses $H_0 : \boldsymbol{\delta} = \boldsymbol{\delta}_0$ with $\delta_{0ij} \leq 0$ for all ij. In doing this, we often want to say "yes, yes, ties will appear sporadically for some of the infinitely many $\boldsymbol{\delta}_0$'s, but they are not a real problem, and in some sense we can ignore them." The current, somewhat fussy, appendix is concerned to say that, in a certain sense, ties reduce the null variance of certain test statistics, but not all test statistics.

It is easy to see that averaging two or more of the q_{ij} does not change the expectation (2.13) of $T^{\delta_0} = \sum_{i=1}^{I} \sum_{j=1}^{J} Z_{ij}\, q_{ij}$ in a randomized block design (2.4), but it often does alter its variance (2.14). If it were always true that use of average ranks for ties reduced the variance compared to the untied situation, and if we used the untied variance in (2.15), then the deviate that we look up in the Normal distribution would be tilted slightly toward zero, and the resulting approximate P-value would be slightly conservative. This was discussed in a particular case in Sect. 2.9. In other words, we could reject an infinite set of simple hypotheses $H_0 : \delta = \delta_0$ without worrying that some hypotheses removed a few sporadic ties and should not be rejected. For some statistics, ties always reduce the variance of T^{δ_0} in (2.14), but that is not true for all statistics. When we want to test an infinite set of simple hypotheses, it is conceptually tidy to use a statistic whose variance is always reduced by ties.

For some test statistics, ties can sometimes increase the variance of the statistic. To see this, consider a small example. Conover and Iman [11] assign ranks 1 to IJ to the $R_{ij}^{\delta_0}$, so that, with $I = 2$ blocks of size $J = 3$, a tie between the two smallest $R_{ij}^{\delta_0}$ might convert the $I \times J = 2 \times 3$ ranks

$$\begin{bmatrix} 1 & 3 & 4 \\ 2 & 5 & 6 \end{bmatrix} \text{ into } \begin{bmatrix} 1.5 & 3 & 4 \\ 1.5 & 5 & 6 \end{bmatrix}, \tag{2.27}$$

so that the variance (2.14) *increases* from 4.44 for the untied left array to 4.77 for the tied right array in (2.27). The pattern in (2.27) can also occur with the aligned ranks of Hodges and Lehmann [28]. The methods of Conover and Iman [11] and Hodges and Lehmann [28] have many attractive properties, but they do not have the property that average ranks always reduce the null variance of the test statistic.

Recall from Sect. 2.6 that Quade's statistic generalizes Wilcoxon's signed rank statistic from matched pairs, $J = 2$, to small blocks $J \geq 2$; see also Problem 2.7. In Quade's statistic, the untied ranks are $i \times 1, i \times 2, \ldots, i \times J$ in the block with the ith largest range ω_i in (2.11). These untied ranks can become tied in either of two ways, either a tie of adjusted responses, $R_{ij}^{\delta_0} = R_{ij'}^{\delta_0}$, inside block i, or a tie between the ranges, $\omega_i = \omega_{i'}$, in (2.11) for blocks i and i'. Consider $I = 2$ blocks of size $J = 3$, where block $i = 2$ has the larger range, $\omega_1 < \omega_2$, and hence ranks of ranges $b_1 = 1$ and $b_2 = 2$, so Quade's ranks $q_{ij} = q_{ij}^* \times b_i$ are:

$$\begin{bmatrix} 1 & 2 & 3 \\ 2 & 4 & 6 \end{bmatrix}. \tag{2.28}$$

A tie of the form $R_{21}^{\delta_0} = R_{22}^{\delta_0}$ would replace the 2 and 4 in block $i = 2$ by their average, 3 and 3:

$$\begin{bmatrix} 1 & 2 & 3 \\ 3 & 3 & 6 \end{bmatrix}. \tag{2.29}$$

In contrast, if the ranges in blocks $i = 1$ and $i = 2$ were tied, then the ranks of these ranges, namely, $b_1 = 1$ and $b_2 = 2$, would be replaced by their average, $b_1 = b_2 = 1.5$, which yields ranks $q_{ij} = q_{ij}^* \times b_i$:

$$\begin{bmatrix} 1.5 & 3 & 4.5 \\ 1.5 & 3 & 4.5 \end{bmatrix}. \tag{2.30}$$

In the untied array (2.28), the variance (2.14) is 3.333, but the variance is 2.667 for (2.29) and is 3 for (2.30). So, in the simple example in (2.28)–(2.30), the untied variance is larger than the two tied cases. Is this true in general? Is it always true for Quade's statistic? Is it always true for a larger class of statistics containing Quade's statistic?

More generally, consider a weighted rank statistic in Sect. 2.6, such as Quade's statistic. When testing $H_0 : \delta = \delta_0$, the weighted rank statistic is computed from the $R_{ij}^{\delta_0}$ and has the form $T^{\delta_0} = \sum_{i=1}^{I} \sum_{j=1}^{J} Z_{ij}\, \varphi_i\, \phi_{ij}$. In the absence of ties, ϕ_{ij} is $\phi\left(q_{ij}^*\right)$ for some function $\phi(\cdot)$, where q_{ij}^* is Wilcoxon's within-block rank, and φ_i is $\varphi\{b_i/(I+1)\}$ where b_i is the rank of the within-block dispersion measure, perhaps the range in (2.11). A tie within block i means that the corresponding ϕ_{ij} are averaged, and a tie between blocks means the corresponding φ_i are averaged. Note that it is ϕ_{ij} and φ_i that are averaged, not q_{ij}^* and b_i; these are different when $\phi(\cdot)$ or $\varphi(\cdot)$ is nonlinear. Proposition 2.7 says that the statistic $T^{\delta_0} = \sum_{i=1}^{I} \sum_{j=1}^{J} Z_{ij}\, \phi_{ij}\, \varphi_i$ that uses average ranks for ties has variance (2.14) that is at most equal to the variance of this statistic in the absence of ties; i.e., ties never increase the variance of T^{δ_0}.

Proposition 2.7 *If $H_0 : \delta = \delta_0$ is true in a randomized block experiment (2.4), then the variance (2.14) of the weighted rank statistic $T^{\delta_0} = \sum_{i=1}^{I} \sum_{j=1}^{J} Z_{ij}\, \phi_{ij}\, \varphi_i$ is at most equal to the variance of $T^* = \sum_{i=1}^{I} \sum_{j=1}^{J} Z_{ij}\, \phi(j)\, \varphi\{i/(I+1)\}$.*

Proof The proof makes use of elementary results from the theory of majorization as discussed by Marshall and Olkin [47]. To simplify notation, write $c_i = \varphi\{i/(I+1)\}$ and $d_j = \phi(j)$, so that $T^* = \sum_{i=1}^{I} \sum_{j=1}^{J} Z_{ij}\, c_i\, d_j$. Let $\mathbf{c}$ be the vector of dimension I containing the c_i in nondecreasing order, and let $\mathbf{d}$ be the vector of dimension J containing the d_j in nondecreasing order. Let $\boldsymbol{\varphi}$ be the vector of dimension I containing the φ_i, in nondecreasing order. So, $\boldsymbol{\varphi}$ was obtained from $\mathbf{c}$ by averaging adjacent coordinates of $\mathbf{c}$; e.g., if $I = 5$, with the first three and last two coordinates of $\boldsymbol{\varphi}$ tied, then

$$\boldsymbol{\varphi} = \begin{bmatrix} \frac{1}{3} & \frac{1}{3} & \frac{1}{3} & 0 & 0 \\ \frac{1}{3} & \frac{1}{3} & \frac{1}{3} & 0 & 0 \\ \frac{1}{3} & \frac{1}{3} & \frac{1}{3} & 0 & 0 \\ 0 & 0 & 0 & \frac{1}{2} & \frac{1}{2} \\ 0 & 0 & 0 & \frac{1}{2} & \frac{1}{2} \end{bmatrix} \mathbf{c}, \tag{2.31}$$

and generally $\boldsymbol{\varphi} = \mathbf{P}\mathbf{c}$ for some $I \times I$ doubly stochastic matrix like the one in (2.31); so, $\boldsymbol{\varphi}$ is majorized by $\mathbf{c}$ (Marshall and Olkin [47, Theorem 2.A.4]). The mean of the $\boldsymbol{\varphi}$ equals the mean of the $\mathbf{c}$, because $\mathbf{P}$ is doubly stochastic: If $\mathbf{1}$ is an I-dimensional vector of 1's, then from (2.31), $\mathbf{1}^T\boldsymbol{\varphi}/I = \mathbf{1}^T\mathbf{P}\mathbf{c}/I = \mathbf{1}^T\mathbf{c}/I$. In the same way, for each block i, the J-dimensional vector $\boldsymbol{\phi}_i$ of sorted ϕ_{ij} are majorized by $\mathbf{d}$, and the mean of each $\boldsymbol{\phi}_i$ equals the mean of $\mathbf{d}$. Because (i) $\mathbf{c}$ majorizes $\boldsymbol{\varphi}$ and $\mathbf{d}$ majorizes $\boldsymbol{\phi}_i$ for every i, and (ii) a sum of squares is Schur convex, we have

$$\sum_{i=1}^{I} c_i^2 \geq \sum_{i=1}^{I} \varphi_i^2 \text{ and } \sum_{j=1}^{J} d_j^2 \geq \sum_{j=1}^{J} \phi_{ij}^2, \; i = 1, \ldots, I, \tag{2.32}$$

and also

$$\overline{d} = \overline{\phi}_i, \text{ for } i = 1, \ldots, I, \text{ where } \overline{d} = \frac{1}{J}\sum_{j=1}^{J} d_j \text{ and } \overline{\phi}_i = \frac{1}{J}\sum_{j=1}^{J} \phi_{ij}. \tag{2.33}$$

Using (2.14),

$$\begin{aligned}
\operatorname{var}(T^* \mid \mathcal{F}, \mathcal{Z}) &= \frac{1}{J}\sum_{i=1}^{I}\sum_{j=1}^{J}\left(c_i\, d_j - \mu_i^*\right)^2 \text{ where } \mu_i^* = \frac{1}{J}\sum_{j=1}^{J} c_i\, d_j \qquad (2.34)\\
&= \left(\sum_{i=1}^{I} c_i^2\right)\left\{\frac{1}{J}\sum_{j=1}^{J}\left(d_j - \overline{d}\right)^2\right\}\\
&= \left(\sum_{i=1}^{I} c_i^2\right)\left\{\left(\frac{1}{J}\sum_{j=1}^{J} d_j^2\right) - \overline{d}^2\right\}
\end{aligned}$$

In parallel, using (2.14) and (2.33),

$$\begin{aligned}
\operatorname{var}\left(T^{\delta_0} \mid \mathcal{F}, \mathcal{Z}\right) &= \sum_{i=1}^{I} \varphi_i^2 \left\{\left(\frac{1}{J}\sum_{j=1}^{J} \phi_{ij}^2\right) - \overline{d}^2\right\}\\
&\leq \sum_{i=1}^{I} \varphi_i^2 \left\{\left(\frac{1}{J}\sum_{j=1}^{J} d_j^2\right) - \overline{d}^2\right\} \text{ by (2.32)}\\
&\leq \left(\sum_{i=1}^{I} c_i^2\right)\left\{\left(\frac{1}{J}\sum_{j=1}^{J} d_j^2\right) - \overline{d}^2\right\} \text{ by (2.32)}\\
&= \operatorname{var}(T^* \mid \mathcal{F}, \mathcal{Z}).
\end{aligned}$$

2.13 *Appendix: Proof of Proposition 2.4

This appendix contains a proof of Proposition 2.4 and Corollary 2.1 in Sect. 2.9.

Proof Consider moving from $\boldsymbol{\delta}_0 \in \Delta_0$ to $\kappa \times \mathbf{1}$ in a series of IJ steps, where each step increases just one δ_{0ij} to κ. Clearly, if $T^{\delta_0} = \sum_{i=1}^{I} b_{i\delta_0} \sum_{j=1}^{J} Z_{ij}\, q_{ij\delta_0}^*$ never increases in any of these steps, then T^{δ_0} achieves at $\boldsymbol{\delta}_0 = \kappa \times \mathbf{1}$ its minimum value over $\boldsymbol{\delta}_0 \in \Delta_0$. So, consider what happens as one δ_{0ij} increases. As noted in Sect. 2.9, T^{δ_0} changes with δ_{0ij} only for treated individuals, so focus on a treated individual ij with $Z_{ij} = 1$. As noted in Sect. 2.9, as δ_{0ij} increases, $\sum_{j=1}^{J} Z_{ij}\, q^*_{ij\delta_0}$ decreases or remains the same; so, we are concerned with the contributions of $b_{i\delta_0}$ and $b_{i'\delta_0}$ for $i' \neq i$. Write $A_{i\delta_0} = b_{i\delta_0} \sum_{j=1}^{J} Z_{ij}\, q^*_{ij\delta_0}$ for the contribution to T^{δ_0} from block i. As δ_{0ij} increases for the treated individual in block i, the range $w_i^{\delta_0}$ in (2.24) and its rank $b_{i\delta_0}$ change as follows. So long as the treated individual has the largest $R_{ij} - Z_{ij}\,\delta_{0ij}$ in block i—that is, while $J = \sum_{j=1}^{J} Z_{ij}\, q^*_{ij\delta_0}$—the range $w_i^{\delta_0}$ declines linearly as δ_{0ij} increases; so, $b_{i\delta_0}$ is unchanged or decreasing; moreover, $A_{i\delta_0} = J b_{i\delta_0}$ decreases when the rank $b_{i\delta_0}$ decreases. While the treated individual's $R_{ij} - Z_{ij}\,\delta_{0ij}$ has a middle rank in block i with $J > \sum_{j=1}^{J} Z_{ij}\, q^*_{ij\delta_0} > 1$, the range w_i does not change as δ_{0ij} increases; so, $b_{i\delta_0}$ is unchanging, but $A_{i\delta_0} = b_{i\delta_0} \sum_{j=1}^{J} Z_{ij}\, q^*_{ij\delta_0}$ decreases when $\sum_{j=1}^{J} Z_{ij}\, q^*_{ij\delta_0}$ decreases. While the treated individual's $R_{ij} - Z_{ij}\,\delta_{0ij}$ has the lowest rank in block i with $1 = \sum_{j=1}^{J} Z_{ij}\, q^*_{ij\delta_0}$, the range w_i increases as δ_{0ij} increases; so $A_{i\delta_0} = b_{i\delta_0} \times 1$ increases when the rank $b_{i\delta_0}$ increases. Because $b_{i\delta_0}$ is a rank, when $b_{i\delta_0}$ decreases by grabbing a lower rank, some other block $i' \neq i$ must contribute that lower rank and receive from block i its former higher rank. As just noted, $b_{i\delta_0}$ decreases only when $J = \sum_{j=1}^{J} Z_{ij}\, q^*_{ij\delta_0}$, but we always have $\sum_{j=1}^{J} Z_{i'j}\, q^*_{i'j\delta_0} \leq J$, so this swapping of ranks $b_{i\delta_0}$ and $b_{i'\delta_0}$ cannot increase $T^{\delta_0} = \sum_{i=1}^{I} b_{i\delta_0} \sum_{j=1}^{J} Z_{ij}\, q^*_{ij\delta_0}$. Conversely, when $b_{i\delta_0}$ increases by grabbing a higher rank, some other block $i' \neq i$ must contribute that higher rank and receive from block i its former lower rank. As just noted, $b_{i\delta_0}$ increases only when $1 = \sum_{j=1}^{J} Z_{ij}\, q^*_{ij\delta_0}$, but we always have $\sum_{j=1}^{J} Z_{i'j}\, q^*_{i'j\delta_0} \geq 1$, so this swapping of ranks $b_{i\delta_0}$ and $b_{i'\delta_0}$ cannot increase $T^{\delta_0} = \sum_{i=1}^{I} b_{i\delta_0} \sum_{j=1}^{J} Z_{ij}\, q^*_{ij\delta_0}$. There is one more case to consider. Just for a brief moment as $\delta_{0ij} \to \kappa$, at the δ_{0ij} that causes $b_{i\delta_0}$ to swap with $b_{i'\delta_0}$, the two between-block ranks, $b_{i\delta_0}$ and $b_{i'\delta_0}$, are tied and share their average rank; however, the same argument shows that $T^{\delta_0} = \sum_{i=1}^{I} b_{i\delta_0} \sum_{j=1}^{J} Z_{ij}\, q^*_{ij\delta_0}$ can remain the same or decrease at that brief moment. □

The proof of Corollary 2.1 consists of going back over the above proof, noting that the proof never depends upon the numerical value of $b_{i'\delta_0}$, but only on which of two $b_{i'\delta_0}$'s is larger.

Problems

2.1 Symmetry of Matched-Pair Differences

In the case of matched pairs—i.e., blocks of size $J = 2$—consider the hypothesis of a constant treatment effect, $H_\tau : r_{Tij} = r_{Cij} + \tau$, for $i = 1, \ldots, I$, $j = 1, 2$. Define Y_i

to be the treated-minus-control matched pair difference in pair i; so,

$$Y_i = (R_{i1} - R_{i2})(Z_{i1} - Z_{i2}).$$

(i) Show that if H_τ is true, then

$$Y_i = \tau + (r_{Ci1} - r_{Ci2})(Z_{i1} - Z_{i2}).$$

(ii) Write $\varepsilon_i = (r_{Ci1} - r_{Ci2})(Z_{i1} - Z_{i2})$, so that from part (i), $Y_i = \tau + \varepsilon_i$. Write $a_i = |\varepsilon_i|$. Show that a_i is fixed by conditioning upon $(\mathcal{F}, \mathcal{Z})$ but that ε_i is not generally fixed by conditioning on $(\mathcal{F}, \mathcal{Z})$. Show that ε_i is symmetrically distributed about zero, in the sense that

$$Pr(\varepsilon_i = a_i \mid \mathcal{F}, \mathcal{Z}) = Pr(\varepsilon_i = -a_i \mid \mathcal{F}, \mathcal{Z}) = \frac{1}{2} \quad \text{if} \quad a_i \neq 0,$$

and

$$Pr(\varepsilon_i = 0 \mid \mathcal{F}, \mathcal{Z}) = 1 \quad \text{if} \quad a_i = 0.$$

(iii) Show that if H_τ is true in a randomized block experiment with $J = 2$, then Y_i is symmetrically distributed about τ, in the sense that

$$Pr(Y_i - \tau = a_i \mid \mathcal{F}, \mathcal{Z}) = Pr(Y_i - \tau = -a_i \mid \mathcal{F}, \mathcal{Z}) = 1/2.$$

(iv) Use Lemma 2.1 to show that in a randomized block experiment with $J = 2$, the Y_i are conditionally independent given $(\mathcal{F}, \mathcal{Z})$.

2.2 Noether's Statistic for Matched Pairs
(This problem uses the notation and results of Problem 2.1.) In the case of matched pairs, $J = 2$, Noether [52] proposed an interesting test statistic for the hypothesis $H_\tau : r_{Tij} = r_{Cij} + \tau$, for $i = 1, \ldots, I$, $j = 1, 2$. Let $0 \leq f < 1$. Noether [52] favored $f = 1/3$, but $f = 2/3$ has some interesting properties in observational studies that will be considered in Chap. 9. Rank the $|Y_i - \tau|$ from 1 to I with average ranks for ties, and define $\mathcal{N} \subseteq \{1, 2, \ldots, I\}$ as the set of pair indices i such that (1) the rank of $|Y_i - \tau|$ is greater than or equal to fI, and (2) $|Y_i - \tau| \neq 0$. (Typically, f is large enough that (2) happens automatically as a consequence of (1); however, explicitly requiring both (1) and (2) means that the test statistic is well defined in all cases.) Denote the number of elements of $\mathcal{N}$ by $|\mathcal{N}|$.
(i) Assuming H_τ is true for the purpose of testing it, show that the set $\mathcal{N}$ is fixed by conditioning upon $(\mathcal{F}, \mathcal{Z})$.
(ii) Define Noether's test statistic T to be the number of positive $Y_i - \tau$ among the $|\mathcal{N}|$ pairs $i \in \mathcal{N}$. Show that under H_τ in a randomized block experiment with $J = 2$, the statistic T has a binomial distribution with probability of success 1/2 and sample size $|\mathcal{N}|$.
(iii) If $f = 0$, then Noether's statistic is the number of positive Y_i among the nonzero Y_i; so, it is the sign test procedure. Noether proposed his statistic as an improvement upon the sign test. Your task is to use simulation to compare the performance of the

sign test, $f = 0$, and Noether's test with his suggested $f = 1/3$. In R, simulate 1000 samples of size 50 from a Normal distribution with expectation 1/2 and variance 1. In your 1000 samples, compare the test statistics with $f = 0$ and $f = 1/3$ when used in a two-sided 0.05-level test of the null hypothesis that the Y_i are symmetric about zero. In how many of the 1000 samples is the null hypothesis rejected by each of the two tests? What are the medians of the 1000 P-values from the two tests? In how many of the 1000 samples is the P-value from Noether's test with $f = 1/3$ smaller than the P-value from the sign test?
(iv) From first principles, you can build a confidence interval for τ by testing every H_τ, retaining the values that are not rejected. Noether [52] gives an explicit form for this confidence interval. If interested, try to produce Noether's explicit form.
(v) Your simulation in part (iii) should conclude that Noether's test with $f = 1/3$ has greater power to reject $\tau = 0$ than does the sign test in the situation that you simulated. If Noether's test is more likely to reject $\tau = 0$ than the sign test, then ask: Which test is more likely to produce a confidence interval that excludes $\tau = 0$?

2.3 Unbiased Estimation of the Average Treatment Effect
Return to Proposition 2.1, and consider the performance of $\overline{R}_t - \overline{R}_c$ as an estimate of $\overline{\delta}$. Suppose that $\delta_{ij} = \tau$ for $i = 1, \ldots, I$, $j = 1, \ldots, J$, but the IJ responses to control, r_{Cij}, are independently sampled from a Cauchy distribution. Let the number of blocks increase, $I \to \infty$. Is $\overline{R}_t - \overline{R}_c$ a consistent estimate of $\overline{\delta} = \tau$? In other words, does $\overline{R}_t - \overline{R}_c$ converge in probability to τ? How can Proposition 2.1 be true if r_{Cij} could be a sample of size IJ from a Cauchy distribution?

2.4 Exact Randomization Distribution of the Blocked Wilcoxon Rank Sum Statistic
(i) For $I = 2$ and $J = 3$, use (2.1) and Proposition 2.2 to determine the exact randomization distribution of the blocked Wilcoxon rank sum statistic under Fisher's hypothesis of no treatment effect. (Assume there are no ties, so tied ranks do not occur.)
(ii) Repeat part (i), but use the gconv function in the iTOS package in R.
(iii) Repeat part (ii), but with $I = 4$ and $J = 3$.

2.5 Exact Randomization Distribution of Quade's statistic
Repeat (i)-(iii) for Problem 2.4 but with Quade's statistic from Sect. 2.6 as the test statistic in place of Wilcoxon's statistic. The documentation for gconv includes examples for ($I = 2$, $J = 3$) and ($I = 3$, $J = 3$).

2.6 Wilcoxon's signed rank statistic
In the article in which he introduced the rank sum statistic, Wilcoxon [104] also introduced another statistic, his signed rank statistic for matched pairs, or equivalently for blocks of size $J = 2$. In this statistic, Wilcoxon ranked the I absolute pair differences, $|R_{i1} - R_{i2}|$, from 1 to I, and the signed rank statistic is the sum of the ranks of the pairs in which the treated individual had the larger response. Assume there are no ties of any kind. For matched pairs, $J = 2$, show that Wilcoxon's signed rank statistic and Quade's [59]'s statistic $\sum_{i=1}^{I} \sum_{j=1}^{J} Z_{ij}\, q_{ij}$ in Sect. 2.6 differ by an additive constant involving I.

2.7 Test Statistics That Are Essentially the Same

(i) Reexamine Proposition 2.2. In a randomized block experiment, consider testing the simple null hypothesis $H_0 : \delta = \delta_0$ using a test statistic $T = t\left(\mathbf{Z}, \mathbf{R}^{\delta_0}\right)$. Let $a > 0$ and b be two constants. Suppose that you tested the same null hypothesis with the test statistic $a\,T + b$ in place of T. Suppose that you reject H_0 for large values of the test statistic. How would the P-values using T or $aT + b$ in place of T differ?
(ii) Suppose that $a > 0$ and b were not constant but were functions of $\mathcal{F}$, $\mathcal{Z}$ and of I and J. How would that change your answer to part (i)?
(iii) Reexamine Problem 2.6. In a randomized block design with $J = 2$, how do the P-values from Wilcoxon's signed rank statistic and from Quade's statistic compare?

2.8 Alternatives to the Range in Quade's Statistic

(i) When testing Fisher's null hypothesis of no effect, Quade's statistic in Sect. 2.6 ranked the I within-block ranges in (2.11) from 1 to I. Suppose that you substituted a different measure of dispersion within blocks, such as the sample standard deviation of the J responses $R_{i1}, \ldots, R_{iJ}$ in block i, ranking the standard deviations from 1 to I. Assume ties never occur, so average ranks are never needed. How would that change in the measure of dispersion alter the exact distribution of Quade's statistic in Proposition 2.2 under Fisher's null hypothesis of no effect?
(ii) Are the two versions of Quade's statistic in part (i) equivalent statistics in the sense of Problem 2.7? Would you obtain the same P-values from these two versions of Quade's statistic?

2.9 Distinct Hypotheses That Are Not Discernibly Different

Consider throughout this problem the following very simple situation: randomized treatment assignment (2.4), $r_{Tij} = \beta_i + \tau + \epsilon_{Tij}$ and $r_{Cij} = \beta_i + \epsilon_{Cij}$, for $i = 1, \ldots, I$, $j = 1, \ldots, J$, where the IJ bivariate vectors $(\epsilon_{Tij}, \epsilon_{Cij})$ are independent with the same bivariate Normal distribution with expectation, variance, and correlation given by: $0 = \mathrm{E}(\epsilon_{Tij}) = \mathrm{E}(\epsilon_{Cij})$; $1 = \mathrm{var}(\epsilon_{Tij}) = \mathrm{var}(\epsilon_{Cij})$; $\rho = \mathrm{cor}\left(\epsilon_{Tij}, \epsilon_{Cij}\right)$. Here, τ, ρ, and the β_i's are unknown fixed parameters. Once we condition upon $\mathcal{F}$, the origin of r_{Tij}, and r_{Cij} in this linear model is no longer relevant, so that δ and $\overline{\delta}$ are fixed. Before we condition upon $\mathcal{F}$ in this model, δ is an IJ-dimensional random vector and $\overline{\delta}$ is a random variable, with distributions determined by their origin in a particular Gaussian linear model. This problem asks you to consider the situation *before* we condition on $\mathcal{F}$; that is, it asks you to consider what happens if you run a randomized experiment on data having its origin in a Gaussian linear model and if you analyze the data under the assumptions of a Gaussian linear model. A particular case with added assumptions allows you to say more, but it should not sharply contradict what you are entitled to say in general without the added assumptions of the particular case. Adding assumptions—here, the Gaussian linear model—will allow you to say more, for instance, to obtain a t-test of the hypothesis that τ equals zero, but additional assumptions should not undermine what you were already entitled to say without those assumptions. For example, if $\overline{R}_t - \overline{R}_c$ is unbiased without additional assumptions, it should not become biased with additional assumptions. Also, if a parameter is not identified with additional assumptions, it should not become identified without those additional assumptions.

(i) Show that $\tau = \mathrm{E}(\overline{\delta})$.

(ii) If $\rho = 1$, what is the probability that $\tau = \overline{\delta}$?

(iii) If $\rho < 1$, what is the probability that $\tau = \overline{\delta}$?

(iv) Is there anything you can see in the observable data—i.e., in (R_{ij}, Z_{ij})—that can distinguish $\rho = 1$ from $\rho < 1$?

(v) Does $\overline{\delta}$ converge in probability to τ as the number of blocks increases, $I \to \infty$?

(vi) What is the distribution of the difference in sample means, $\overline{R}_t - \overline{R}_c$? What is its expectation? What is its variance? Does the distribution of $\overline{R}_t - \overline{R}_c$ depend upon ρ? (As throughout this problem, all of these questions refer to the linear model, before you make that model irrelevant by conditioning on $\mathcal{F}$.)

(vii) Proposition 2.1 says $\overline{R}_t - \overline{R}_c$ is unbiased for $\overline{\delta}$ given $\mathcal{F}$, and in part (vi) you found that $\overline{R}_t - \overline{R}_c$ is unconditionally unbiased for τ. Also, part (i) showed that $\tau = \mathrm{E}(\overline{\delta})$. How can all of this be true at the same time?

(viii) Which is larger, $\mathrm{var}(\overline{R}_t - \overline{R}_c \mid \mathcal{Z})$ or $\mathrm{E}\{\mathrm{var}(\overline{R}_t - \overline{R}_c \mid \mathcal{F}, \mathcal{Z}) \mid \mathcal{Z}\}$? Is there a value of ρ such that $\mathrm{var}(\overline{R}_t - \overline{R}_c \mid \mathcal{Z}) = \mathrm{E}\{\mathrm{var}(\overline{R}_t - \overline{R}_c \mid \mathcal{F}, \mathcal{Z}) \mid \mathcal{Z}\}$? If you used the bootstrap to estimate the variance of $\overline{R}_t - \overline{R}_c$ by repeated with-replacement sampling of I of the I blocks, then would you be estimating $\mathrm{var}(\overline{R}_t - \overline{R}_c \mid \mathcal{Z})$ or $\mathrm{E}\{\mathrm{var}(\overline{R}_t - \overline{R}_c \mid \mathcal{F}, \mathcal{Z}) \mid \mathcal{Z}\}$?

(ix) Give the linear model t-statistic testing the linear model hypothesis, $H_0 : \tau = 0$. Is $H_0 : \overline{\delta} = 0$ a hypothesis about parameters of the linear model?

(x) Consider, first, the blocked Wilcoxon rank sum statistic as a test of $H_0 : \tau = \tau_0$ in the Gaussian linear model. Obviously, you do not *need* Normally distributed errors to apply Wilcoxon's statistic, but you can apply that statistic to data with Normal errors. Consider, second, the blocked Wilcoxon rank sum randomization statistic as a test given $\mathcal{F}$, $\mathcal{Z}$ of the hypothesis $H_0 : \boldsymbol{\delta} = \tau_0 \mathbf{1}$, where $\mathbf{1}$ is an $I \times J$ matrix of 1's, as in Sect. 2.8. Is the numerical value of the test statistic the same in both cases? Is its null distribution the same in both cases? Will the same data sets lead to acceptance or rejection of both hypotheses? If you inverted both tests to obtain confidence intervals, would the confidence intervals for these different parameters be the same?

(xi) Suppose that there are $I + M$ blocks with $M \geq 1$ and the linear model holds for all $I + M$ blocks. You pick I of the $I + M$ blocks at random, run the randomized experiment on those I blocks, and use the experimental results to advise the MJ people in the remaining M blocks about the best treatment for them. As always, the average treatment effect $\overline{\delta}$ is the average of δ_{ij} for the IJ people in the experiment;

however, you have avoided the problem of external validity by sampling I of $I + M$ blocks for the experiment. Compare the linear model hypothesis $H_0 : \tau = 0$ and the hypothesis $H_0 : \overline{\delta} = 0$. In light of part (iii), which of these two hypotheses is more relevant to advising the MJ people in the remaining M blocks about the best treatment for them? Consider also part (v) and part (viii). Compare with part (x).

(xii) As $I \to \infty$ in the Gaussian linear model with $|\rho| < 1$, is there a consistent estimate of δ_{11}? Is there a consistent estimate of the vector $\boldsymbol{\delta}$? Is there a consistent test of $H_0 : \delta_{11} = 0$? How does this relate to the quote from Fisher in Sect. 2.5?

(xiii) In a randomized block experiment (2.4), consider a different linear model, namely $R_{ij} = \beta_i + Z_{ij}\,\tau + \varepsilon_{ij}$ where ε_{ij} are independently sampled from a Normal distribution with expectation zero and variance one. Would the observable data—(R_{ij}, Z_{ij})—from this linear model (with no counterfactual interpretation) be discernibly different from the observable data from the linear model with bivariate Normal errors (for which there is an explicit counterfactual interpretation)?

(xiv) Read Donald B. Rubin's [83] "Bayesian inference for causal effects: The role of randomization," and A. Philip Dawid's [17] article, "Causal inference without counterfactuals." Reconsider your work on this problem in light of their views. In Rubin's Bayesian formulation, a causal inference depends explicitly on the joint distribution of (r_{Tij}, r_{Cij}), even though (R_{ij}, Z_{ij}) provides no information about what is joint in that joint distribution, namely, the copula [35, 88, 92]. Dawid expresses skepticism about statistical methods that depend upon the copula when there is no information about the copula. What do you think?

References

1. Andrews, D.F., Hampel, F.R., Bickel, P.J., Huber, P.J., Rogers, W.H., Tukey, J.W.: Robust Estimates of Location: Survey and Advances. Princeton University Press, Princeton, NJ (1972)
2. Basse, G.W., Feller, A., Toulis, P.: Randomization tests of causal effects under interference. Biometrika **106**(2), 487–494 (2019)
3. Birch, M.W.: The detection of partial association, I: the 2×2 case. J. R. Stat. Soc. B **26**(2), 313–324 (1964)
4. Box, G., Tyssedal, J.: Projective properties of certain orthogonal arrays. Biometrika **83**(4), 950–955 (1996)
5. Brien, C.J., Bailey, R.A.: Multiple randomizations. J. R. Stat. Soc. Ser. B **68**(4), 571–609 (2006)
6. Bross, I.D.J.: Statistical criticism. Cancer **13**(2), 394–400 (1960). Reprinted in *Observational Studies*, vol. 4(2), 2018, with Discussion by William B. Fairley, William A. Huber, Joseph L. Gastwirth, Andrew Gelman, Jennifer Hill, Katherine J. Hoggatt, Daniel E. Ho, Charles S. Reichardt, David Rindskopf, Paul R. Rosenbaum and Dylan S. Small
7. Campbell, D.T.: Relabeling internal and external validity for applied social scientists. New Directions for Program Evaluation **1986**(31), 67–77 (1986)

8. Chamberlain, T.C.: The method of multiple working hypotheses. Science **15**(366), 92–96 (1890). Reprinted in Science **148**, 754–759 (1965)
9. Cheng, C.S.: Theory of Factorial Design. Chapman & Hall/CRC Press, Boca Raton, FL (2013)
10. Chow, Y.S., Teicher, H.: Probability Theory: Independence, Interchangeability, Martingales, 2nd edn. Springer Science & Business Media, New York (1988)
11. Conover, W.J., Iman, R.L.: Rank transformations as a bridge between parametric and nonparametric statistics. Am. Stat. **35**(3), 124–129 (1981)
12. Conover, W.J., Salsburg, D.S.: Locally most powerful tests for detecting treatment effects when only a subset of patients can be expected to "respond" to treatment. Biometrics **44**, 189–196 (1988)
13. Cox, D.R.: The interpretation of the effects of non-additivity in the latin square. Biometrika **45**(1/2), 69–73 (1958)
14. Cox, D.R.: Planning of Experiments. Wiley, New York (1958)
15. Crump, R.K., Hotz, V.J., Imbens, G.W., Mitnik, O.A.: Nonparametric tests for treatment effect heterogeneity. Rev. Econ. Stat. **90**(3), 389–405 (2008)
16. Dahabreh, I.J., Robertson, S.E., Tchetgen, E.J., Stuart, E.A., Hernán, M.A.: Generalizing causal inferences from individuals in randomized trials to all trial-eligible individuals. Biometrics **75**(2), 685–694 (2019)
17. Dawid, A.P.: Causal inference without counterfactuals. J. Am. Stat. Assoc. **95**(450), 407–424 (2000)
18. Deng, L.Y., Tang, B.: Generalized resolution and minimum aberration criteria for Plackett-Burman and other nonregular factorial designs. Statistica Sinica **9**, 1071–1082 (1999)
19. Doksum, K.A.: Empirical probability plots and statistical inference for nonlinear models in the two-sample case. Ann. Stat. **2**, 267–277 (1974)
20. Doksum, K.A., Sievers, G.L.: Plotting with confidence: Graphical comparisons of two populations. Biometrika **63**(3), 421–434 (1976)
21. Fisher, R.A.: Design of Experiments. In: Oliver and Boyd, Edinburgh (1935). (Quotations are from the 6th, the 1951, edition)
22. Foley, R.: Intellectual Trust in Oneself and Others. Cambridge University Press, Cambridge (2001)
23. Fraser, D.A.S.: Nonparametric Methods in Statistics. Wiley, New York (1957)
24. Gastwirth, J.L.: On robust procedures. J. Am. Stat. Assoc. **61**(316), 929–948 (1966)
25. Hajek, J., Sidak, Z., Sen, P.K.: Theory of Rank Tests. Academic Press, New York (1999)
26. Hamilton, M.A.: Choosing the parameter for a 2× 2 table or a 2 × 2 × 2 table analysis. Am. J. Epidemiol. **109**(3), 362–375 (1979)
27. Hettmansperger, T.P., McKean, J.W.: Robust Nonparametric Statistical Methods. Chapman & Hall/CRC Press, Boca Raton, FL (2010)
28. Hodges, J., Lehmann, E.: Rank methods for combination of independent experiments in analysis of variance. Ann. Math. Stat. **33**(2), 482–497 (1962)
29. Hodges, J., Lehmann, E.: Estimates of location based on rank tests. Ann. Math. Stat. **34**(2), 598–611 (1963)
30. Hollander, M., Wolfe, D.A., Chicken, E.: Nonparametric Statistical Methods, 3rd edn. Wiley, New York (2013)
31. Hsu, J., Zubizarreta, J.R., Small, D., Rosenbaum, P.R.: Strong control of the familywise error rate in observational studies that discover effect modification by exploratory methods. Biometrika **102**(4), 767–782 (2015)
32. Huber, P.J.: Robust estimation of a location parameter. Ann. Math. Stat. **35**(1), 73–101 (1964)
33. Huber, P.J.: Robust regression: Asymptotics, conjectures and Monte Carlo. Ann. Stat. **1**(5), 799–821 (1973)
34. Hudgens, M.G., Halloran, M.E.: Toward causal inference with interference. J. Am. Stat. Assoc. **103**(482), 832–842 (2008)
35. Joe, H.: Dependence Modeling with Copulas. Chapman & Hall/CRC, Boca Raton, FL (2014)
36. Jurečková, J., Sen, P.K., Picek, J.: Methodology in Robust and Nonparametric Statistics. Chapman and Hall/CRC, Boca Raton, FL (2012)

37. Kempthorne, O.: The Design and Analysis of Experiments. Wiley, New York (1952)
38. Kloke, J., McKean, J.W.: Nonparametric Statistical Methods Using R. CRC Press, Boca Raton, FL (2014)
39. Lee, K., Small, D.S., Rosenbaum, P.R.: A powerful approach to the study of moderate effect modification in observational studies. Biometrics **74**(4), 1161–1170 (2018)
40. Lehmann, E.L.: Nonparametrics. Holden-Day, San Francisco (1975)
41. Lehmann, E.L., Romano, J.P.: Testing Statistical Hypotheses, 3rd edn. Springer, New York (2005)
42. Li, F., Ding, P., Mealli, F.: Bayesian causal inference: a critical review. Phil. Trans. R. Soc. A **381**(2247), 1–23 (2023). https://doi.org/10.1098/rsta.2022.0153
43. Li, X., Ding, P.: General forms of finite population central limit theorems with applications to causal inference. J. Am. Stat. Assoc. **112**(520), 1759–1769 (2017)
44. Little, R.J.A.: A note about models for selectivity bias. Econometrica **53**, 1469–1474 (1985)
45. Mantel, N.: Ranking procedures for arbitrarily restricted observation. Biometrics **23**, 65–78 (1967)
46. Maritz, J.S.: A note on exact robust confidence intervals for location. Biometrika **66**(1), 163–170 (1979)
47. Marshall, A.W., Olkin, I.: Inequalities: Theory of Majorization and Its Applications. Academic Press, New York (1979)
48. Morgan, K.L., Rubin, D.B.: Rerandomization to improve covariate balance in experiments. Ann. Stat. **40**(2), 1263–1282 (2012)
49. Mukerjee, R., Wu, C.F.J.: A Modern Theory of Factorial Design. Springer, Berlin (2006)
50. Neyman, J.: On the application of probability theory to agricultural experiments. Stat. Sci. **5**, 465–472 (1923). Republication in English in 1990 of a paper published in Polish in 1923.
51. Noether, G.E.: Efficiency of the Wilcoxon two-sample statistic for randomized blocks. J. Am. Stat. Assoc. **58**(304), 894–898 (1963)
52. Noether, G.E.: Some simple distribution-free confidence intervals for the center of a symmetric distribution. J. Am. Stat. Assoc. **68**(343), 716–719 (1973)
53. O'Brien, P.C., Fleming, T.R.: A paired Prentice-Wilcoxon test for censored paired data. Biometrics **43**, 169–180 (1987)
54. Pagano, M., Tritchler, D.: On obtaining permutation distributions in polynomial time. J. Am. Stat. Assoc. **78**(382), 435–440 (1983)
55. Platt, J.R.: Strong inference. Science **146**(3642), 347–353 (1964)
56. Popper, K.R.: The Logic of Scientific Discovery. Basic Books, New York (1959)
57. Puelz, D., Basse, G., Feller, A., Toulis, P.: A graph-theoretic approach to randomization tests of causal effects under general interference. J. R. Stat. Soc. Ser. B **84**(1), 174–204 (2022)
58. Puri, M.L.: On the combination of independent two sample tests of a general class. Revue de l'Institut International de Statistique **33**, 229–241 (1965)
59. Quade, D.: Using weighted rankings in the analysis of complete blocks with additive block effects. J. Am. Stat. Assoc. **74**(367), 680–683 (1979)
60. Rosenbaum, P.R.: Quantiles in nonrandom samples and observational studies. J. Am. Stat. Assoc. **90**(432), 1424–1431 (1995)
61. Rosenbaum, P.R.: Reduced sensitivity to hidden bias at upper quantiles in observational studies with dilated treatment effects. Biometrics **55**(2), 560–564 (1999)
62. Rosenbaum, P.R.: Effects attributable to treatment: inference in experiments and observational studies with a discrete pivot. Biometrika **88**(1), 219–231 (2001)
63. Rosenbaum, P.R.: Attributing effects to treatment in matched observational studies. J. Am. Stat. Assoc. **97**(457), 183–192 (2002)
64. Rosenbaum, P.R.: Observational Studies, 2nd edn. Springer, New York (2002)
65. Rosenbaum, P.R.: Exact confidence intervals for nonconstant effects by inverting the signed rank test. Am. Stat. **57**(2), 132–138 (2003)
66. Rosenbaum, P.R.: Attributable effects in case^2 studies. Biometrics **61**(1), 246–253 (2005)
67. Rosenbaum, P.R.: Confidence intervals for uncommon but dramatic responses to treatment. Biometrics **63**(4), 1164–1171 (2007)

68. Rosenbaum, P.R.: Interference between units in randomized experiments. J. Am. Stat. Assoc. **102**(477), 191–200 (2007)
69. Rosenbaum, P.R.: Sensitivity analysis for M-estimates, tests, and confidence intervals in matched observational studies. Biometrics **63**(2), 456–464 (2007)
70. Rosenbaum, P.R.: Evidence factors in observational studies. Biometrika **97**(2), 333–345 (2010)
71. Rosenbaum, P.R.: A new U-statistic with superior design sensitivity in matched observational studies. Biometrics **67**(3), 1017–1027 (2011)
72. Rosenbaum, P.R.: Some approximate evidence factors in observational studies. J. Am. Stat. Assoc. **106**(493), 285–295 (2011)
73. Rosenbaum, P.R.: Weighted M-statistics with superior design sensitivity in matched observational studies with multiple controls. J. Am. Stat. Assoc. **109**(507), 1145–1158 (2014)
74. Rosenbaum, P.R.: Bahadur efficiency of sensitivity analyses in observational studies. J. Am. Stat. Assoc. **110**(509), 205–217 (2015)
75. Rosenbaum, P.R.: Two R packages for sensitivity analysis in observational studies. Observational Studies **1**(2), 1–17 (2015)
76. Rosenbaum, P.R.: Sensitivity analysis for stratified comparisons in an observational study of the effect of smoking on homocysteine levels. Ann. Appl. Stat. **12**(4), 2312–2334 (2018)
77. Rosenbaum, P.R.: Design of Observational Studies, 2nd edn. Springer, New York (2020)
78. Rosenbaum, P.R.: Replication and Evidence Factors in Observational Studies. Chapman and Hall/CRC, New York (2021)
79. Rosenbaum, P.R.: Bahadur efficiency of observational block designs. J. Am. Stat. Assoc. **119**(547), 1871–1881 (2024)
80. Rosenberger, W.F., Lachin, J.M.: Randomization in Clinical Trials: Theory and Practice. Wiley, New York (2015)
81. Rubin, D.B.: Estimating causal effects of treatments in randomized and nonrandomized studies. J. Educ. Psychol. **66**(5), 688 (1974)
82. Rubin, D.B.: Assignment to treatment group on the basis of a covariate. J. Educ. Stat. **2**(1), 1–26 (1977)
83. Rubin, D.B.: Bayesian inference for causal effects: the role of randomization. Ann. Stat. **6**, 34–58 (1978)
84. Rubin, D.B.: Comment: Which ifs have causal answers? J. Am. Stat. Assoc. **81**(396), 961–962 (1986)
85. Sacks, J., Schiller, S.B., Welch, W.J.: Designs for computer experiments. Technometrics **31**(1), 41–47 (1989)
86. Santner, T.J., Williams, B.J., Notz, W.I.: The Design and Analysis of Computer Experiments, vol. 1. Springer, New York (2003)
87. Scheffe, H.: The Analysis of Variance. Wiley, New York (1959)
88. Schweizer, B., Wolff, E.F.: On nonparametric measures of dependence for random variables. Ann. Stat. **9**(4), 879–885 (1981)
89. Sen, P.K., Puri, M.L.: Nonparametric Methods in Multivariate Analysis. Wiley, New York (1971)
90. Severini, T.A.: Elements of Distribution Theory. Cambridge University Press, New York (2005)
91. Shadish, W., Cook, T.D., Campbell, D.T.: Experimental and Quasi-experimental Designs for Generalized Causal Inference. Houghton Mifflin Boston, MA (2002)
92. Sklar, A.: Random variables, joint distribution functions, and copulas. Kybernetika **9**(6), 449–460 (1973)
93. Sobel, M.E.: What do randomized studies of housing mobility demonstrate? Causal inference in the face of interference. J. Am. Stat. Assoc. **101**(476), 1398–1407 (2006)
94. Stoto, M.A.: The accuracy of population projections. J. Am. Stat. Assoc. **78**(381), 13–20 (1983)
95. Stuart, E.A., Cole, S.R., Bradshaw, C.P., Leaf, P.J.: The use of propensity scores to assess the generalizability of results from randomized trials. J. R. Stat. Soc. Ser. A: Stat. Soc. **174**(2), 369–386 (2011)

96. Su, Y., Li, X.: Treatment effect quantiles in stratified randomized experiments and matched observational studies. Biometrika **111**(1), 235–254 (2024)
97. Tardif, S.: Efficiency and optimality results for tests based on weighted rankings. J. Am. Stat. Assoc. **82**(398), 637–644 (1987)
98. Tchetgen-Tchetgen, E.J., VanderWeele, T.J.: On causal inference in the presence of interference. Stat. Methods Med. Res. **21**(1), 55–75 (2012)
99. Tukey, J.W.: Improving crucial randomized experiments—especially in weather modification—by double randomization and rank combination. In: Proceedings of the Berkeley Conference in Honor of Jerzy Neyman and Jack Kiefer, pp. 79–108. Wadsworth Belmont (1985)
100. Tukey, J.W.: Sunset salvo. Am. Stat. **40**(1), 72–76 (1986)
101. Tukey, J.W.: Comments. In: Wainer, H. (ed.) Drawing Inferences from Self-Selected Samples, pp. 108–110. Routledge, New York (2013). Reprint of a book first published by Lawrence Erlbaum Associates in 1986.
102. Wassmer, G., Brannath, W.: Group Sequential and Confirmatory Adaptive Designs in Clinical Trials. Springer, New York (2016)
103. Welch, B.L.: On the z-test in randomized blocks and Latin squares. Biometrika **29**(1/2), 21–52 (1937)
104. Wilcoxon, F.: Individual comparisons by ranking methods. Biometrics **1**(6), 80–83 (1945)
105. Wilk, M.B.: The randomization analysis of a generalized randomized block design. Biometrika **42**(1/2), 70–79 (1955)
106. Wu, C.F.J., Hamada, M.S.: Experiments: Planning, Analysis, and Optimization. Wiley, New York (2021)
107. Xu, Y., Ignatiadis, N., Sverdrup, E., Fleming, S., Wager, S., Shah, N.: Treatment heterogeneity with survival outcomes. In: Zubizarreta, J.R., Stuart, E.A., Small, D.S., Rosenbaum, P.R. (eds.) Handbook of Matching and Weighting Adjustments for Causal Inference, pp. 445–482. Chapman and Hall/CRC, Boca Raton, FL (2023)
108. Ye, T., Small, D.S., Rosenbaum, P.R.: Dimensions, power and factors in an observational study of behavioral problems after physical abuse of children. Ann. Appl. Stat. **16**(4), 2732–2754 (2022)

Chapter 3
Some Background Topics in Statistics

Abstract This chapter reviews two topics from mathematical statistics, where the second topic is slightly technical and may be skipped. In Sect. 3.1, A. P. Dawid's notation for conditional independence is reviewed. This material is used in later chapters, is brief, and is not difficult. The notation is introduced in the context of two toy models, one for randomized experiments and the other for observational studies. In contrast, Sect. 3.2 connects randomization inference in experiments and permutation inference in population models. Under many conditions, randomization inferences based on randomized treatment assignment in Chap. 2 are identical to permutation tests in population models, and seeing this connection is helpful in understanding both perspectives. That said, the material in Sect. 3.2 is mentioned only briefly in later parts of the book; so, it is not essential reading.

3.1 Conditional Independence and Dawid's Notation

A Toy Model for a Randomized Experiment

Imagine a random sample from an infinite population of people, one quarter young men, denoted $\mathbf{X} = (0, 0)$, one quarter young women, denoted $\mathbf{X} = (0, 1)$, one quarter old men, denoted $\mathbf{X} = (1, 0)$, and one quarter old women, denoted $\mathbf{X} = (1, 1)$. Treatment ($Z = 1$) or control ($Z = 0$) is assigned to people by independent flips of a fair coin.[1] In this case, the probability of treatment is $\Pr(Z = 1) = \frac{1}{2}$ for everyone, and the probability that a randomly selected person is female is $\Pr\{\mathbf{X} = (0, 1) \text{ or } \mathbf{X} = (1, 1)\} = \frac{1}{2}$. Moreover, the conditional probability of treatment given age and sex, $\Pr(Z = z \mid \mathbf{X} = \mathbf{x})$, is $\Pr(Z = z \mid \mathbf{X} = \mathbf{x}) = \frac{1}{2}$ for $z = 0$ and

[1] As discussed in Sect. 2.4 in connection with the topics of internal and external validity, this is a toy model for a randomized experiment, because it is nearly impossible, if not impossible, to conduct a randomized experiment on a random sample of people.

© The Author(s), under exclusive license to Springer Nature Switzerland AG 2025
P. R. Rosenbaum, *An Introduction to the Theory of Observational Studies*,
Springer Texts in Statistics, https://doi.org/10.1007/978-3-031-90494-3_3

$z = 1$, and for $\mathbf{x} = (0, 0),\ (0, 1),\ (1, 0)$, and $(1, 1)$. Philip Dawid [2] writes

$$Z \perp\!\!\!\perp \mathbf{X} \text{ if } \Pr(Z = z \mid \mathbf{X} = \mathbf{x}) = \Pr(Z = z \mid \mathbf{X} = \mathbf{x}') \text{ for all } z, \mathbf{x}, \mathbf{x}'; \tag{3.1}$$

so, as it stands, (3.1) says that the chance of being assigned to treatment is the same for young men, young women, old men, and old women, a property that we can ensure for each person by using a fair coin to assign treatments.[2] That is, as it stands, (3.1) says that $\Pr(Z = z \mid \mathbf{X} = \mathbf{x})$ is the same for all $\mathbf{x}$, but whether $\mathbf{X}$ is a random variable or a fixed quantity, perhaps a fixed parameter, is left slightly ambiguous. If we go beyond what (3.1) says and interpret $\mathbf{X}$ as the age and sex of a randomly selected person, then a straightforward application of Bayes theorem demonstrates

$$Z \perp\!\!\!\perp \mathbf{X} \implies \mathbf{X} \perp\!\!\!\perp Z, \tag{3.2}$$

which Dawid [2, Theorem 2.1] states as a theorem. To say that $\mathbf{X} \perp\!\!\!\perp Z$ is to say $\Pr(\mathbf{X} = \mathbf{x} \mid Z = 1) = \Pr(\mathbf{X} = \mathbf{x} \mid Z = 0)$ for each $\mathbf{x}$, so that, for instance, old females occur with the same probability, namely, $\frac{1}{4}$, in the treated and control groups. Expressing the same thought in different words, if $\mathbf{X} \perp\!\!\!\perp Z$ then the probability distribution of $\mathbf{X}$ is the same in treated and control groups, or the distribution of $\mathbf{X}$ is balanced across treated and control groups. In this toy situation, (3.2) says that random assignment results in covariate balance. This toy description of an experiment does not distinguish properties of probability distributions and properties of the observed data; rather, it is all about probability distributions. That is one of several senses in which this description is just a toy.

A Toy Model for an Observational Study

Continuing the toy example, define an event D by (i) $D = 1$ if $\mathbf{X} = (0, 1)$ or $\mathbf{X} = (1, 0)$ and (ii) $D = 0$ if $\mathbf{X} = (1, 1)$ or $\mathbf{X} = (0, 0)$. So, $D = 1$ for young women and old men, and $D = 0$ for old women and young men. If $D = 0$, we assign treatments by the flip of a fair coin, so $\Pr(Z = 1 \mid \mathbf{X} = \mathbf{x}) = \frac{1}{2}$ if $\mathbf{X} = (1, 1)$ or $\mathbf{X} = (0, 0)$, or equivalently

$$\Pr(Z = 1 \mid \mathbf{X} = \mathbf{x}) = \Pr(Z = 1 \mid D = 0, \mathbf{X} = \mathbf{x}) = \Pr(Z = 1 \mid D = 0) = \frac{1}{2}$$
$$\text{if } \mathbf{X} = (1, 1) \text{ or } \mathbf{X} = (0, 0)\,.$$

[2] In a measure-theoretic development of probability, $\Pr(Z = z \mid X = x)$ is defined not for all x but for almost all x. If you would like to see Dawid's notation introduced in this way, see his paper Dawid [3].

Table 3.1 Covariate imbalance in a toy observational study formed by rolling a die for some covariate values and flipping a coin for others. The covariate distributions are imbalanced—i.e., not the same—for treated and control groups

$\mathbf{x}$	D	$\Pr(\mathbf{X}=\mathbf{x})$	$\Pr(Z=1 \mid \mathbf{X}=\mathbf{x})$	$\Pr(\mathbf{X}=\mathbf{x} \mid Z=1)$	$\Pr(\mathbf{X}=\mathbf{x} \mid Z=0)$
01	1	0.25	1/6	0.1250	0.3125
10	1	0.25	1/6	0.1250	0.3125
11	0	0.25	1/2	0.3750	0.1875
00	0	0.25	1/2	0.3750	0.1875
Total				1.0000	1.0000

Table 3.2 Covariate balance in a toy observational study having stratified on D. These are conditional probabilities of $\mathbf{X} = \mathbf{x}$ given Z and D derived from Table 3.1. The treated and control distributions of $\mathbf{X}$ are the same within strata or blocks defined by D

$\mathbf{x}$	D	Stratum $D = 1$		Stratum $D = 0$	
		$\Pr(\mathbf{X} \mid Z=1, D=1)$	$\Pr(\mathbf{X} \mid Z=0, D=1)$	$\Pr(\mathbf{X} \mid Z=1, D=0)$	$\Pr(\mathbf{X} \mid Z=0, D=0)$
01	1	0.5	0.5	0.0	0.0
10	1	0.5	0.5	0.0	0.0
11	0	0.0	0.0	0.5	0.5
00	0	0.0	0.0	0.5	0.5

If $D = 1$, then we roll a fair die and assign an individual to treatment if the die turns up 1; otherwise, the individual is assigned to control.[3] Then

$$\Pr(Z = 1 \mid \mathbf{X} = \mathbf{x}) = \Pr(Z = 1 \mid D = 1, \mathbf{X} = \mathbf{x}) = \Pr(Z = 1 \mid D = 1) = \frac{1}{6}$$
$$\text{if } \mathbf{X} = (0, 1) \text{ or } \mathbf{X} = (1, 0).$$

In this small departure from a completely randomized experiment, (3.1) is no longer true, so covariate balance in (3.2) cannot be deduced from (3.1). In particular, old women and young men, $\mathbf{X} = (1, 1)$ or $\mathbf{X} = (0, 0)$, are overrepresented in the treated group, while young women and old men, $\mathbf{X} = (0, 1)$ or $\mathbf{X} = (1, 0)$, are overrepresented in the control group. Covariate imbalance is shown in Table 3.1. Notably, the distribution of $\mathbf{X}$ in Table 3.1 is not the same in treated, $Z = 1$, and control, $Z = 0$, groups.

In group $D = 0$, there is a completely randomized experiment, so if we confined attention to group $D = 0$, then there would be covariate balance. Similarly, in group $D = 1$, there is a completely randomized experiment, albeit one with 5/6 of the population assigned to control, and again there would be covariate balance if we confined attention to group $D = 1$; see Table 3.2. The problem in Table 3.1 is produced by combining groups $D = 1$ and $D = 0$ where $\Pr(Z = 1 \mid D = 1) = \frac{1}{6} \neq \frac{1}{2} = \Pr(Z = 1 \mid D = 0)$.

If A is conditionally independent of B given C, then Dawid [2] writes

$$A \perp\!\!\!\perp B \mid C \text{ if } \Pr(A = a \mid B = b, C = c) = \Pr(A = a \mid C = c) \text{ for all } a, b, c. \quad (3.3)$$

[3] This toy example is used in [16, Ch. 4] to introduce propensity scores with minimal notation.

It is often convenient to write (3.3) concisely as $\Pr(A \mid B, C) = \Pr(A \mid C)$. As with independence in (3.2), if B is a random variable, then

$$A \perp\!\!\!\perp B \mid C \implies B \perp\!\!\!\perp A \mid C, \tag{3.4}$$

which Dawid [2, Theorem 3.1] states as a theorem. In particular, in the toy observational study,

$$Z \perp\!\!\!\perp \mathbf{X} \mid D$$

because

$$\Pr(Z = 1 \mid D = 1, \mathbf{X} = \mathbf{x}) = \Pr(Z = 1 \mid D = 1) = \frac{1}{6},$$

$$\Pr(Z = 1 \mid D = 0, \mathbf{X} = \mathbf{x}) = \Pr(Z = 1 \mid D = 0) = \frac{1}{2}.$$

Using (3.4), $Z \perp\!\!\!\perp \mathbf{X} \mid D$ implies covariate balance within groups $D = 1$ and $D = 0$ separately, namely, $\mathbf{X} \perp\!\!\!\perp Z \mid D$.

If this toy model of an observational study were true, and if we picked a treated individual and $J - 1$ controls with the same value of $\mathbf{X}$, then we would have picked J individuals for a block with the same chance of treatment, so that, conditioning on the known fact that one of them received treatment, the conditional probability that each of them received treatment would be $1/J$, as in Chap. 2. Even simpler, this would all be true if we picked a treated individual and $J - 1$ controls with the same value of D, even if these individuals had different values of $\mathbf{X}$. So, life would be extremely simple if this toy model of an observational study were true. Of course, it is not true. It is a toy model that provides a little motivating insight, but life is not so simple. In particular, observational studies are not built by flipping a coin and rolling a die, so the treatment assignment probabilities are not known and may also depend upon covariates that were not measured. All of this will be discussed in later chapters.

Dawid's Calculus

Dawid's [2] paper about conditional independence offers a conceptual argument and a calculus. The conceptual argument claims that theories or hypotheses framed in terms of conditional independence are more likely to approximate scientific hypotheses than theories that append assumptions of convenience, such as Gaussian distributions or errors with constant variance or similar structures. The conceptual argument encourages thinking in terms of conditional independence, and other general structures like stochastic order, rather than in terms of highly specific models like the Gaussian linear model. One might reasonably compare this conceptual argument with Tukey's conceptual argument about assumptions, as quoted in Sect. 2.8. As you recall, Tukey argued that extensive assumptions were useful only when evaluating the relative performance of statistical procedures in terms of "stringency." Dawid's conceptual argument is closely related to Little's [12] claim that assumptions of convenience cannot safely be used as a substitute for randomized treatment assignment or random sampling.

Dawid [2, Lemma 4] then offers a simple lemma in three parts that serves as a calculus for arguments involving conditional independence. His claim is that long arguments involving conditional independence can often be shorter and clearer with reference to the lemma. Here, the lemma is stated in terms of general symbols A, B, C, D, and E that have not been reserved for specific uses in this book.

Lemma 3.1 (Dawid's Lemma 4.1) $A \perp\!\!\!\perp B \mid C$ *if and only if* $(A, C) \perp\!\!\!\perp (B, C) \mid C$.

Lemma 3.2 (Dawid's Lemma 4.2) *If* $A \perp\!\!\!\perp B \mid C$ *and* D *is a function of* A, *then (i)* $D \perp\!\!\!\perp B \mid C$ *and (ii)* $A \perp\!\!\!\perp B \mid (C, D)$.

Lemma 3.3 (Dawid's Lemma 4.3) *If* $A \perp\!\!\!\perp B \mid C$ *and* $A \perp\!\!\!\perp E \mid (B, C)$, *then*

$$A \perp\!\!\!\perp (B, E) \mid C.$$

The proofs of these lemmas are almost immediate, and their value lies in their compression. For example, for Lemma 3.3: if $\Pr(A \mid B, C) = \Pr(A \mid C)$ and $\Pr(A \mid E, B, C) = \Pr(A \mid B, C)$, then combining these gives $\Pr(A \mid E, B, C) = \Pr(A \mid C)$.

3.2 *Permutation Tests and Distributional Symmetry

Two Questions About the Assumptions Underlying a Statistical Method

When trying to understand the assumptions that underlie a statistical method, M, we may ask two questions: (i) Under assumption A, is method M valid? (ii) Under what assumptions is method M valid? Knowing the answer to (i) but not (ii) leaves you in doubt about the importance of assumption A to the validity of method M. Perhaps assumption A is very important, and dropping it invalidates method M. Or perhaps A is not particularly important, and dropping A merely requires small adjustments to the interpretation of conclusions from method M. Question (ii) is the deeper question and the one that is more relevant to statistical practice. If you only understand method M under only one set of assumptions, then you don't understand much about method M.

Take the simplest example, from a freshman course in statistics. Wilcoxon's two sample rank sum statistic is commonly presented in elementary textbooks with assumptions that one continuous distribution has been shifted by a constant τ to produce a second continuous distribution. Are these assumptions important? The assumption that the distributions are continuous is entirely unimportant: It precludes ties when ranking the outcomes, so formulas look pretty in a textbook, but the method is valid without continuous distributions, and the `wilcox.test` function in the basic `stats` package in R correctly handles ties with no effort on the part of the analyst. Who would worry whether the computer uses a pretty or a less pretty formula?

The model of a control distribution shifted by τ to produce a treated distribution plays a slightly larger role in Wilcoxon's statistic: It permits the test to be inverted to yield a compatible confidence interval for τ and a Hodges-Lehmann [6, 8] point estimate of τ. The `wilcox.test` function also calculates the estimate and confidence interval. It is easy to check a pair of boxplots to see if the treated and control distributions of outcomes look shifted, that is, to check whether the distributions have similar dispersion and similar shape. If the boxplots look compatible with a shift, then it may be convenient to compare the distributions in terms of a shift. If not, the Wilcoxon test remains valid as a test of the equality of two distributions against the alternative that one distribution is stochastically larger than the other. Moreover, abandoning the shift model, the test can be understood to refer to a nonparametric parameter, the probability that a treated response exceeds a control response, and this nonparametric parameter can replace τ in estimates and confidence intervals [7, §4.2.18]. With small adjustments, this nonparametric parameter can be understood in terms of potential outcomes [14, §4]. So far as the validity of the Wilcoxon test is concerned, the shift is not so important either; moreover, a discovery that the distributions under treatment and control do not look shifted may be of scientific importance, for it may suggest that only some people respond to the treatment [1, 15].

Goal of This Section

The current section revisits the methods in Chap. 2 under different assumptions.

In Chap. 2, randomization tests were derived from the random assignment of treatments (2.4). These tests are often identical to permutation tests derived from null hypotheses that assert that the observed responses R_{ij} have distributions with certain symmetries. It is helpful to be familiar with both views of these tests and to view one test from two perspectives.

This section contains a selective, brief, and informal summary of important but standard material from Fraser [4, 5], Lehmann and Romano [10, Ch. 5] and Lehmann and Stein [11]. The section ends with an elementary exposition of a celebrated theorem [10, Theorem 5.8.1] that uses the complete sufficiency of the order statistics to show that the *only* valid nonparametric tests of no effect are permutation tests, essentially the randomization tests of Chap. 2; *every* other test requires distributional assumptions—e.g., Normal errors or whatever—to be valid.

The Hypothesis of Symmetry Within Blocks

Associated with the block design in Chap. 2 is the following hypothesis of symmetry.

Definition 3.1 (Hypothesis of Symmetry, $H_0^\dagger$) For $i = 1, \ldots, I$, the observations $R_{i1}, R_{i2}, \ldots, R_{iJ}$ in block i are independently sampled from the same continuous distribution $F_i(\cdot)$ with density, $f_i(\cdot)$. Distinct blocks are independent.

Notably in Definition 3.1, the I blocks may be very different in the sense that $f_i(\cdot)$ and $F_i(\cdot)$ may vary with i. In experiments and observational studies, individuals in the same block are typically similar in terms of some measured covariates, and they are different from people in some other blocks in terms of these measured covariates. To the extent that the blocking was worthwhile—to the extent that the measured covariate matters—it is plausible, indeed likely, that the $F_i(\cdot)$'s will vary from block to block.

The hypothesis of symmetry $H_0^\dagger$ is a different way of expressing the thought that the treatment has no effect. Under the hypothesis of symmetry, if we pick one person at random in each block for treatment with $Z_{ij} = 1$, assigning the rest to control with $Z_{ij} = 0$, then the response of the treated person in block i, namely, $\sum_{j=1}^{J} Z_{ij} R_{ij}$, has the same distribution as the responses of the $J - 1$ controls in block i.

Fisher's hypothesis of no effect, $H_0 : \boldsymbol{\delta} = \mathbf{0}$, and the hypothesis of symmetry, $H_0^\dagger$, are quite different, but each has its advantages. Fisher's hypothesis speaks about the effects of treatments on particular people, ij, and that hypothesis is a constant reminder of the limits to what randomized experiments can say about the causal effects on individuals. In contrast, the hypothesis of symmetry, $H_0^\dagger$, concerns probability distributions, not individual people. Perhaps more can be said about $H_0^\dagger$ than about $H_0 : \boldsymbol{\delta} = \mathbf{0}$, and perhaps that fact can be put to constructive use. As seen in (2.25) and Problem 2.9, there are models for (r_{Tij}, r_{Cij}) such that the hypothesis of symmetry $H_0^\dagger$ is true, but Fisher's hypothesis $H_0 : \boldsymbol{\delta} = \mathbf{0}$ is false: A treatment may harm your spouse and benefit your child, but there may be no way to see this in the data $(R_{ij}, Z_{ij}, \mathbf{x}_{ij})$ that is provided by a randomized block experiment. A few people who write about causal inference believe that spouses and children are not real, that only probability distributions are real, but happily due to progress in psychopharmacology, with proper daily medication, it is often possible for such people to lead relatively normal lives. It is important to understand both $H_0^\dagger$ and $H_0 : \boldsymbol{\delta} = \mathbf{0}$: how they are similar, how they are different, and how to put each to its appropriate use.

A Sufficient Statistic Under the Hypothesis of Symmetry

The hypothesis of symmetry $H_0^\dagger$ does not specify the I continuous distributions $F_i(\cdot)$, $i = 1, \ldots, I$. The hypothesis $H_0^\dagger$ has an unknown parameter, $\mathbb{F} = \{F_1(\cdot), \ldots, F_I(\cdot)\}$, where $\mathbb{F}$ is comprised of I unknown continuous cumulative distribution functions.

The practical question is: How do we test $H_0^\dagger$ given that we do not know the $F_i(\cdot)$? At first, the problem appears daunting, because we have IJ observations where J may be 2 or 3 or 4, yet we have I completely unspecified distributions $F_i(\cdot)$, and as the sample size increases, as $I \to \infty$, the unknown $\mathbb{F}$ expands to include more and more unknown distributions $F_i(\cdot)$.

What is a sufficient statistic? A statistic $\mathbf{S}$ is a function of the data $\mathbf{R}$. By definition [10, §1.9], a statistic $\mathbf{S}$ is sufficient for the unknown parameter, $\mathbb{F}$, of the distribution of $\mathbf{R}$ if the conditional distribution of $\mathbf{R}$ given $\mathbf{S}$ does not depend upon $\mathbb{F}$. With some license, we might express this in symbols as $\Pr(\mathbf{R} \mid \mathbb{F}, \mathbf{S}) = \Pr(\mathbf{R} \mid \mathbf{S})$ or $\mathbf{R} \perp\!\!\!\perp \mathbb{F} \mid \mathbf{S}$. When $H_0^\dagger$ is true, is there a sufficient statistic for the unknown parameter $\mathbb{F}$?

Sort the J responses in each block i into nondecreasing order to obtain the within-block order statistics, $R_{i(1)} \leq R_{i(2)} \leq \cdots \leq R_{i(J)}$, and let $\overrightarrow{\mathbf{R}}$ be the $I \times J$ matrix whose ith row is $\left\{R_{i(1)}, \ldots, R_{i(J)}\right\}$. Because $F_i(\cdot)$ is continuous when $H_0^\dagger$ is true, ties occur with probability zero, so we may presume that $R_{i(1)} < R_{i(2)} < \cdots < R_{i(J)}$ for each i. What is the distribution of $\overrightarrow{\mathbf{R}}$ under the hypothesis of symmetry, $H_0^\dagger$? Is $\overrightarrow{\mathbf{R}}$ a sufficient statistic for $\mathbb{F}$? Proposition 3.1 is well known [10, §5.8].

Proposition 3.1 *When the hypothesis of symmetry $H_0^\dagger$ is true:*

(i) the probability density of $\left\{R_{i(1)}, \ldots, R_{i(J)}\right\}$ at $r_{i(1)} < \ldots < r_{i(J)}$ is $J!\prod_{j=1}^{J} f_i\left\{r_{i(j)}\right\}$,
(ii) if $\mathbf{r}$ is an $I \times J$ matrix whose ith row is $r_{i(1)} < \ldots < r_{i(J)}$, then the probability density of $\overrightarrow{\mathbf{R}}$ at $\mathbf{r}$ is $(J!)^I \prod_{i=1}^{I}\prod_{j=1}^{J} f_i\left\{r_{i(j)}\right\}$, so that, in particular, the I rows $\left\{R_{i(1)}, \ldots, R_{i(J)}\right\}$ of $\overrightarrow{\mathbf{R}}$ are independent of each other, and
(iii) the conditional density of $\mathbf{R}$ given $\overrightarrow{\mathbf{R}} = \mathbf{r}$ does not depend upon

$$\mathbb{F} = \{F_1(\cdot), \ldots, F_I(\cdot)\}$$

and attaches equal probability $1/(J!)^I$ to each of the $(J!)^I$ ways of permuting the $r_{i(1)} < \ldots < r_{i(J)}$ in the I rows of $\mathbf{r}$, so that, in particular, $\overrightarrow{\mathbf{R}}$ is a sufficient statistic for $\mathbb{F}$.

Proof Assume $H_0^\dagger$ is true. Consider, first, the distribution of $\left\{R_{i(1)}, \ldots, R_{i(J)}\right\}$. For each possible value $r_{i(1)} < \ldots < r_{i(J)}$ of $\left\{R_{i(1)}, \ldots, R_{i(J)}\right\}$, there are $J!$ distinct points in $\mathfrak{R}^J$ that produce this same value of the order statistic, and these points are formed by permuting $\left\{r_{i(1)}, \ldots, r_{i(J)}\right\}$ in all $J!$ ways. Because the R_{ij} are independent with the same density $f_i(\cdot)$, each of these $J!$ points has the same density $\prod_{j=1}^{J} f_i\left\{r_{i(j)}\right\}$, so that adding these $J!$ terms gives the density of $\left\{R_{i(1)}, \ldots, R_{i(J)}\right\}$ at $\left\{r_{i(1)}, \ldots, r_{i(J)}\right\}$ as $J!\prod_{j=1}^{J} f_i\left\{r_{i(j)}\right\}$, proving (i). Under $H_0^\dagger$, the $(R_{i1}, \ldots, R_{iJ})$ for distinct blocks are independent, and $\left\{R_{i(1)}, \ldots, R_{i(J)}\right\}$ is a function of $(R_{i1}, \ldots, R_{iJ})$; so, distinct rows $\left\{R_{i(1)}, \ldots, R_{i(J)}\right\}$ of $\overrightarrow{\mathbf{R}}$ are independent, and using (i) their joint density is $\prod_{i=1}^{I}\left[J!\prod_{j=1}^{J} f_i\left\{r_{i(j)}\right\}\right] =$

$(J!)^I \prod_{i=1}^{I} \prod_{j=1}^{J} f_i \left\{r_{i(j)}\right\}$, proving (ii). There are $(J!)^I$ matrices $\mathbf{r}^*$ that can be formed by permuting the $r_{i(j)}$ within each of the I rows of $\mathbf{r}$, and each of these has the same density $\prod_{i=1}^{I} \prod_{j=1}^{J} f_i \left\{r_{i(j)}\right\}$, so

$$\Pr\left(\mathbf{R} = \mathbf{r}^* \mid \overrightarrow{\mathbf{R}} = \mathbf{r}\right) = \frac{\prod_{i=1}^{I} \prod_{j=1}^{J} f_i \left\{r_{i(j)}\right\}}{(J!)^I \prod_{i=1}^{I} \prod_{j=1}^{J} f_i \left\{r_{i(j)}\right\}} = \frac{1}{(J!)^I}, \tag{3.5}$$

proving (iii). □

Testing the Hypothesis of Symmetry in a Randomized Experiment

The test statistics $t(\mathbf{Z}, \mathbf{R})$ in Sect. 2.6 are indifferent to the numbering j of individuals in the same block i. That is, if we interchanged individuals ij and ij' in block i, so $\left(Z_{ij}, R_{ij}\right)$ was renumbered to swap it with $\left(Z_{ij'}, R_{ij'}\right)$, then the value of $t(\mathbf{Z}, \mathbf{R})$ is unchanged. In saying this, it is important that Z_{ij} and R_{ij} are both assigned the same new index j'. Throughout Sect. 3.2, it is *assumed without further mention* that the test statistic $t(\mathbf{Z}, \mathbf{R})$ has this property of being invariant to renumbering individuals j inside the same block i.

Suppose that the hypothesis of symmetry, $H_0^{\dagger}$, is true, and suppose that a randomized block experiment was defined not by (2.4) but instead by

$$\Pr\left(\mathbf{Z} = \mathbf{z} \mid \overrightarrow{\mathbf{R}}, \mathcal{Z}\right) = \frac{1}{J^I} = \frac{1}{|\mathcal{Z}|} \text{ for each } \mathbf{z} \in \mathcal{Z}. \tag{3.6}$$

Here, (3.6) says that the treatment assignments $\mathbf{Z}$ are independent of the order statistics, $\overrightarrow{\mathbf{R}}$. As in Chap. 2, randomization (3.6) precludes biased assignment of treatments $\mathbf{Z}$ within each block i. As honest investigators, we could easily make both (2.4) and (3.6) true: Roll a fair J-sided die independently I times to pick the one treated person in each block i. One could imagine a deceitful investigator who knows the treatment is worthless, who knows that $H_0^{\dagger}$ is true, but who can partly predict $\mathbf{R}$ from a patient's pallor, and who assigns to control anyone who looks especially sickly, thereby making both (2.4) and (3.6) untrue.

If $H_0^{\dagger}$ and (3.6) were both true, then

$$\Pr\left\{t(\mathbf{Z}, \mathbf{R}) \geq a \mid \overrightarrow{\mathbf{R}}, \mathcal{Z}\right\} = \Pr\left\{t\left(\mathbf{Z}, \overrightarrow{\mathbf{R}}\right) \geq a \,\middle|\, \overrightarrow{\mathbf{R}}, \mathcal{Z}\right\} \tag{3.7}$$

$$= \frac{\left|\left\{\mathbf{z} \in \mathcal{Z} : t\left(\mathbf{z}, \overrightarrow{\mathbf{R}}\right) \geq a\right\}\right|}{|\mathcal{Z}|}, \tag{3.8}$$

where the first equality in (3.7) follows from two facts: (i) $t(\mathbf{Z}, \mathbf{R})$ is invariant to renumbering individuals within block i; (ii) using (3.6), renumbering individuals does not change the conditional distribution of $\mathbf{Z}$ given $\overrightarrow{\mathbf{R}}$.

The null distribution for testing $H_0^{\dagger}$ in (3.8) is exactly the same as the null distribution for testing Fisher's null hypothesis of no effect $H_0 : \boldsymbol{\delta} = \mathbf{0}$ in (2.12), so these two null distributions report the same P-value for every $(\mathbf{Z}, \mathbf{R})$. This is slightly surprising, because both the null hypothesis and the definition of randomization have changed. The distribution in (3.8) refers to the hypothesis of symmetry of an unknown probability distribution involving the unknown $f_i(\cdot)$ and makes no reference to potential outcomes, (r_{Tij}, r_{Cij}). The hypothesis $H_0 : \boldsymbol{\delta} = \mathbf{0}$ refers to the causal effect $\boldsymbol{\delta}$ of the treatment on IJ specific people and makes no reference to a stochastic model that might produce $\mathcal{F}$. The definition of randomization in (2.4) makes explicit reference to potential outcomes, (r_{Tij}, r_{Cij}), as they are part of $\mathcal{F}$, but there are no potential outcomes in (3.6), just observable order statistics, $\overrightarrow{\mathbf{R}}$. The definition (3.6) presumes $H_0^{\dagger}$ is true, but the definition of randomization (2.4) in Chap. 2 does not presume the truth of Fisher's hypothesis of no effect, $H_0 : \boldsymbol{\delta} = \mathbf{0}$.

In brief, whether you insist on expressing treatment effects in terms of potential outcomes, (r_{Tij}, r_{Cij}), or refuse to do so; whether you find the hypothesis $H_0 : \boldsymbol{\delta} = \mathbf{0}$ too specific or the hypothesis $H_0^{\dagger}$ too vague and removed from human concerns with particular people; whether you define randomization by (2.4) or (3.6); whatever your view of these issues, you still have to admit that the absence of a treatment effect is implausible if $t(\mathbf{Z}, \mathbf{R}) \geq a$ for an a such that (2.12) and (3.8) give this event a very small probability. Moreover, (2.12) and (3.8) always attached exactly the same probability to the event $t(\mathbf{Z}, \mathbf{R}) \geq a$.[4]

Inference About a Shift in Distribution

Suppose that $H_0^{\dagger}$ may be false in the following way. The responses R_{ij} of controls, $Z_{ij} = 0$, in block i are independently sampled from $F_i(r) = \Pr(R_{ij} \leq r)$, but the response R_{ij} of the treated person, $Z_{ij} = 1$, in block i is sampled from $G_i(r) = F_i(r - \tau)$. In this case, all of the distributions $G_i(r)$ of treated responses are shifted up by τ compared to the distributions $F_i(r)$ of control responses in the same block i, although the $F_i(r)$ may be entirely different in different blocks. Define the hypothesis $H_{\tau_0}^{\dagger} : \tau = \tau_0$ to combine the stated structure, $G_i(r) = F_i(r - \tau)$, with a specified value, τ_0, for τ.

The hypothesis $H_{\tau_0}^{\dagger} : \tau = \tau_0$ is reminiscent of the hypothesis $H_0 : \boldsymbol{\delta} = \tau_0 \times \mathbf{1}$ from Sect. 2.10, where $\mathbf{1}$ is an $I \times J$ matrix of ones. These hypotheses differ in much the

[4] In several ways in several places, Erich Lehmann [8–10] views one mathematical structure from two complementary perspectives. In his nonparametric textbook, adjacent parallel chapters [8, Ch. 1–4] contrast randomization-based nonparametrics with population-based nonparametrics. Elsewhere, he and Joseph Romano [10, §5.8–§5.12] develop the close connection between inference based on randomized treatment assignment and permutation inference based on hypotheses of distributional symmetry. Elsewhere, Lehmann [8] reconciles the sometimes diverging views of Fisher and Neyman about hypothesis testing. In general, my sense is that viewing one mathematical structure from two or more complementary perspectives is not a process of noting minor inconsistencies among perspectives but rather a process of deepening an understanding of a single structure.

same way that $H_0^\dagger$ and $H_0 : \boldsymbol{\delta} = \mathbf{0}$ differ; one hypothesis avoids potential outcomes, $\delta_{ij} = r_{Tij} - r_{Cij}$, while the other is stated in terms of them. As seen in Problem 2.9, there are models for $\left(r_{Tij}, r_{Cij}\right)$ such that $H_{\tau_0}^\dagger : \tau = \tau_0$ is true but $H_0 : \boldsymbol{\delta} = \tau \times \mathbf{1}$ is false. Is there a relationship between the tests of $H_{\tau_0}^\dagger : \tau = \tau_0$ and $H_0 : \boldsymbol{\delta} = \tau_0 \times \mathbf{1}$?

Define $R_{ij}^{\tau_0} = R_{ij} - \tau_0 Z_{ij}$. Let $\mathbf{R}^{\tau_0}$ be the corresponding $I \times J$ matrix of $R_{ij}^{\tau_0}$, and let $\overrightarrow{\mathbf{R}}^{\tau_0}$ be the matrix of the order statistics $R_{i(j)}^{\tau_0}$ of the $R_{ij}^{\tau_0}$, that is, with $R_{i(1)}^{\tau_0} < R_{i(2)}^{\tau_0} < \cdots < R_{i(J)}^{\tau_0}$ for each i. Define R_{ij}^{τ}, $\mathbf{R}^{\tau}$, and $\overrightarrow{\mathbf{R}}^{\tau}$ similarly, so that $\overrightarrow{\mathbf{R}}^{\tau} = \overrightarrow{\mathbf{R}}^{\tau_0}$ if $H_{\tau_0}^\dagger : \tau = \tau_0$ is true. Redefine randomization, replacing (3.6) by

$$\Pr\left(\mathbf{Z} = \mathbf{z} \mid \overrightarrow{\mathbf{R}}^{\tau}, \mathcal{Z}\right) = \frac{1}{J^I} = \frac{1}{|\mathcal{Z}|} \text{ for each } \mathbf{z} \in \mathcal{Z}. \tag{3.9}$$

Of course, if $H_{\tau_0}^\dagger : \tau = \tau_0$ were true, we could again ensure that (3.9) is also true by letting Z_{ij} be determined by I independent rolls of a fair J-sided die. If $H_{\tau_0}^\dagger : \tau = \tau_0$ and (3.9) were both true, then in parallel with (3.7)–(3.8), because $\overrightarrow{\mathbf{R}}^{\tau_0} = \overrightarrow{\mathbf{R}}^{\tau}$,

$$\begin{aligned} \Pr\left\{t\left(\mathbf{Z}, \mathbf{R}^{\tau_0}\right) \geq a \mid \overrightarrow{\mathbf{R}}^{\tau_0}, \mathcal{Z}\right\} &= \Pr\left\{t\left(\mathbf{Z}, \overrightarrow{\mathbf{R}}^{\tau}\right) \geq a \,\middle|\, \overrightarrow{\mathbf{R}}^{\tau}, \mathcal{Z}\right\} \\ &= \frac{\left|\left\{\mathbf{z} \in \mathcal{Z} : t\left(\mathbf{z}, \overrightarrow{\mathbf{R}}^{\tau}\right) \geq a\right\}\right|}{|\mathcal{Z}|}. \end{aligned} \tag{3.10}$$

As in (3.7)–(3.8), the parallel form (3.10) is true, because renumbering individuals j in block i changes neither $t\left(\mathbf{Z}, \mathbf{R}^{\tau_0}\right)$ nor the distribution of $\mathbf{Z}$ in (3.9), and because $H_{\tau_0}^\dagger$ and (3.10) imply that the hypothesis of symmetry is true of the $R_{ij}^{\tau_0} = R_{ij} - \tau_0 Z_{ij}$.

The important point is that the tests of $H_{\tau_0}^\dagger : \tau = \tau_0$ and $H_0 : \boldsymbol{\delta} = \tau_0 \times \mathbf{1}$ are exactly the same, even though the hypotheses are different. More precisely, a permutation test of $H_{\tau_0}^\dagger : \tau = \tau_0$ with randomization defined by (3.9) rejects $H_{\tau_0}^\dagger$ at level α for precisely the same data $(\mathbf{Z}, \mathbf{R})$ that the randomization test from Sect. 2.10 using (2.12) rejects $H_0 : \boldsymbol{\delta} = \tau_0 \times \mathbf{1}$, where randomization was defined by (2.4). Because this is true for each τ_0, the $1 - \alpha$ confidence sets built by inverting the two tests are also the same, as are the Hodges-Lehmann point estimates [6, 13].

Although the tests of $H_{\tau_0}^\dagger : \tau = \tau_0$ and $H_0 : \boldsymbol{\delta} = \tau_0 \times \mathbf{1}$ are exactly the same, always rejecting their null hypotheses for the same data sets, the interpretations of the tests are different. In both cases, we calculate $R_{ij}^{\tau_0} = R_{ij} - \tau_0 Z_{ij}$ and test for no effect in what remains. In testing $H_{\tau_0}^\dagger : \tau = \tau_0$, the transformation $R_{ij}^{\tau_0} = R_{ij} - \tau_0 Z_{ij}$ has shifted a probability distribution by τ_0, thereby restoring the hypothesis of symmetry $H_0^\dagger$ for $R_{ij}^{\tau_0}$ when $H_{\tau_0}^\dagger : \tau = \tau_0$ is true; however, there is no thought that $R_{ij}^{\tau_0}$ says something about what would have happened to person ij had this person been assigned to control. In contrast, $R_{ij} - \tau_0 Z_{ij} = r_{Cij}$ when $H_0 : \boldsymbol{\delta} = \tau_0 \times \mathbf{1}$ is true.

Completeness of the Order Statistics

Write $\mathbf{Y}$ for the $I \times J$ matrix of R_{ij} placing the one treated response in the first column, $Y_{i1} = \sum_{j=1}^{J} Z_{ij} R_{ij}$, and the $J-1$ control responses in the subsequent columns, 2, 3, ..., J. Of course, the within-block order statistics $\overrightarrow{\mathbf{Y}}$ of $\mathbf{Y}$ equal the within-block order statistics $\overrightarrow{\mathbf{R}}$ of $\mathbf{R}$—that is, $\overrightarrow{\mathbf{Y}} = \overrightarrow{\mathbf{R}}$–because $\mathbf{Y}$ is simply a rearrangement of $\mathbf{R}$. In a randomized block experiment (2.4) under hypothesis $H_0^{\dagger}$, the symmetry of both $H_0^{\dagger}$ and randomization entail that $\mathbf{R}$ and $\mathbf{Y}$ have the same distribution; however, we do not have to look at $\mathbf{Z}$ to identify treated individuals in $\mathbf{Y}$. This shift in notation is adequate in randomized experiments but creates complexities in observational studies, because it buries treatment assignment Z_{ij} in the j subscript, making it awkward to discuss biased treatment assignment. Nonetheless, this shift in notation is needed briefly here. In a randomized block experiment, the within-block order statistic $\overrightarrow{\mathbf{Y}}$ is sufficient for the unknown parameter $\{F_1(\cdot), \ldots, F_I(\cdot)\}$ when $H_0^{\dagger}$ is true by Proposition 3.1. More than this, $\overrightarrow{\mathbf{Y}}$ is a complete sufficient statistic,[5] meaning that, for any function $h(\cdot)$,

$$\text{if E}\left\{h\left(\overrightarrow{\mathbf{Y}}\right)\right\} = 0 \text{ for all } \{F_1(\cdot), \ldots, F_I(\cdot)\}, \text{ then } h(\mathbf{r}) = 0 \text{ for all } \mathbf{r}. \tag{3.11}$$

For a proof of the completeness of the order statistics, see Fraser [5, §1.7] or Lehmann and Romano [10, Example 4.3.4]. Is completeness useful?

Size and Level of Permutation Tests

The next subsection discusses a celebrated result [10, Theorem 5.8.1] that completely characterizes all tests of the hypothesis of symmetry $H_0^{\dagger}$ that falsely reject $H_0^{\dagger}$ with probability α. Before that, we need to pause briefly to convince ourselves that a certain extremely minor issue is, indeed, extremely minor. The distributions (2.12) and (3.8) are discrete: They deposit dollops of probability at a finite number of

---

[5] Slightly more precisely, in terms of probability measures: If $h(\cdot)$ is any measurable function, if $\text{E}\left\{h\left(\overrightarrow{\mathbf{Y}}\right)\right\} = 0$ for all absolutely continuous distributions $\{F_1(\cdot), \ldots, F_I(\cdot)\}$, then $h(\mathbf{y}) = 0$ except perhaps on a set $\mathcal{S}$ of values of $\mathbf{y}$ that has probability zero for all $\{F_1(\cdot), \ldots, F_I(\cdot)\}$; see Lehmann and Romano [10, §4.3]. For example, let $\mathcal{S}$ be the set of $I \times J$ matrices that have at least one within-block tie. Then $\mathcal{S}$ has probability zero for all absolutely continuous $\{F_1(\cdot), \ldots, F_I(\cdot)\}$. Let $h(\mathbf{y})$ be the number of within-block ties in $\mathbf{y}$. Then $\text{E}\left\{h\left(\overrightarrow{\mathbf{Y}}\right)\right\} = 0$ for all absolutely continuous distributions $\{F_1(\cdot), \ldots, F_I(\cdot)\}$, and $h(\mathbf{y}) = 0$ except on the set $\mathcal{S}$ which has probability zero for all $\{F_1(\cdot), \ldots, F_I(\cdot)\}$, but $h(\mathbf{y})$ is not zero for $\mathbf{y} \in \mathcal{S}$.

possible values for $t\left(\mathbf{Z}, \overrightarrow{\mathbf{R}}\right)$. Each dollop is an integer multiple of $1/J^I$, so it is quite small.[6]

In the binge drinking example in Sect. 1.5, $I = 206$ and $J = 3$, so each dollop is an integer multiple of $1/3^{206} = 1.936\times 10^{-98}$. Suppose that we want to falsely reject $H_0^\dagger$ with probability exactly $\alpha = 0.05$ when $I = 206$ and $J = 3$. That is, suppose that we want a test of size exactly $\alpha = 0.05$. Is that possible? Clearly, if we can take steps of size 1.94×10^{-98}, then we can get very close to $\alpha = 0.05$ but can we get $\alpha = 0.05$ exactly? If $\alpha = 0.05 = 1/(4\times 5) = k/3^{206}$ then $k = 3^{206}/(4\times 5)$ is not an integer because no power of 3 is exactly divisible by 4 or 5. So, exact size $\alpha = 0.05$ is not quite possible, even though we can get extremely close. Write $\lfloor k \rfloor$ for the greatest integer less than or equal to k and $\lceil k \rceil$ for the least integer greater than or equal to k. If we set $k^* = \lfloor 3^{206}/(4\times 5)\rfloor$, then we can test with exact size $\alpha = k^*/3^{206} \leq 0.05$; moreover, this number is so close to 0.05 that the computer cannot distinguish them. If we test with exact size $\alpha = k^*/3^{206}$, then the test falsely rejects $H_0^\dagger$ with probability $k^*/3^{206} < 0.05$, so the advertised level is 0.05, even though the exact size is ever so slightly below 0.05.

Let us say that α is a possible size for a randomization test if $\alpha = k/J^I$ for some integer $k = 1, 2, \ldots, J^I - 1$. The theorem in the next section will then apply to all of these possible sizes. To repeat, in this section I have been trying to convince you that restricting attention to possible sizes, k/J^I, is an extremely minor issue, not something to worry about.[7]

Only Permutation Tests Have Size α When Testing $H_0^\dagger$

Let α be a possible size for a randomization test, as defined in the previous section. For any test of $H_0^\dagger$, there is a function $\varpi(\cdot)$ of $\mathbf{Y}$ that indicates whether $H_0^\dagger$ is rejected, with $\varpi(\mathbf{Y}) = 1$ for rejection of $H_0^\dagger$, and $\varpi(\mathbf{Y}) = 0$ otherwise. To say that this test

---

[6] Some test statistics $t\left(\mathbf{Z}, \overrightarrow{\mathbf{R}}\right)$ take J^I distinct values, while others take fewer than J^I distinct values. With probability 1 under $H_0^\dagger$, the treated-minus-control difference in mean responses takes J^I distinct values. The blocked Wilcoxon statistic takes fewer than J^I distinct values. If $t\left(\mathbf{Z}, \overrightarrow{\mathbf{R}}\right)$ takes J^I distinct values, then each dollop of probability is exactly $1/J^I$. So, there are test statistics such that the null distributions (2.12) and (3.8) can have exact size α for any $\alpha = k/J^I$ for $k = 1, \ldots, J^I - 1$.

[7] Most authors (e.g., [10, §3.1]) handle this tiny issue in a different way. We cannot have $\alpha = 0.05$ with $I = 206$ and $J = 3$ because $\lfloor 3^{206}/(4\times 5)\rfloor/3^{206} < 0.05 < \lceil 3^{206}/(4\times 5)\rceil/3^{206}$. Most authors use an irrelevant uniform random number to close the gap to 0.05, rejecting in some but not all cases in which the exact P-value from (2.12) or (3.8) is barely above 0.05. In theoretical textbooks, this problem comes up repeatedly and using an irrelevant uniform random number is a tidy way to make the problem go away once and for all; however, one would never do this in practice. In the current book, this problem comes up in the next subsection and nowhere else, so I simply restrict the possible sizes α in the next subsection.

has size α is to say that,

$$\mathrm{E}\left\{\varpi\left(\mathbf{Y}\right)\right\} = \alpha \text{ for all } \left\{F_1\left(\cdot\right), \ldots, F_I\left(\cdot\right)\right\} \text{ under } H_0^\dagger. \tag{3.12}$$

Because in general $\mathrm{E}\left(A\right) = \mathrm{E}\left\{\mathrm{E}\left(A \mid B\right)\right\}$, we have from (3.12) that a test of size α has

$$0 = \mathrm{E}\left\{\varpi\left(\mathbf{Y}\right)\right\} - \alpha = \mathrm{E}\left[\mathrm{E}\left\{\varpi\left(\mathbf{Y}\right) - \alpha \,\middle|\, \overrightarrow{\mathbf{Y}}\right\}\right] \tag{3.13}$$

$$\text{for all } \left\{F_1\left(\cdot\right), \ldots, F_I\left(\cdot\right)\right\} \text{ under } H_0^\dagger.$$

Of course, $\mathrm{E}\left\{\varpi\left(\mathbf{Y}\right) - \alpha \mid \overrightarrow{\mathbf{Y}}\right\}$ is a function of $\overrightarrow{\mathbf{Y}}$, which we may write as $h\left(\overrightarrow{\mathbf{Y}}\right) = \mathrm{E}\left\{\varpi\left(\mathbf{Y}\right) - \alpha \mid \overrightarrow{\mathbf{Y}}\right\}$. Moreover, $\overrightarrow{\mathbf{Y}}$ is a complete sufficient statistic under $H_0^\dagger$, so that using (3.11), condition (3.13) implies

$$\mathrm{E}\left\{\varpi\left(\mathbf{Y}\right) \mid \overrightarrow{\mathbf{Y}}\right\} = \alpha \text{ for all } \overrightarrow{\mathbf{Y}} \text{ and } \left\{F_1\left(\cdot\right), \ldots, F_I\left(\cdot\right)\right\} \text{ under } H_0^\dagger. \tag{3.14}$$

It takes a moment to digest (3.14), but that moment is well-spent, because (3.14) says something quite remarkable. Given the order statistic, $\overrightarrow{\mathbf{Y}}$, the only thing that is random about $\mathbf{Y}$ is the ordering of the J responses in each of the I rows; that is, $\mathbf{Y}$ must take on one of the $(J!)^I$ possible within-block permutations of $\overrightarrow{\mathbf{Y}}$. So, (3.14) says that if $\varpi\left(\mathbf{Y}\right)$ is to have level α in the sense that (3.12) holds, then $\varpi\left(\mathbf{Y}\right)$ must reject $H_0^\dagger$ for $\alpha\left(J!\right)^I$ within-block permutations of $\overrightarrow{\mathbf{Y}}$ and must fail to reject $H_0^\dagger$ for the remaining $(1-\alpha)\left(J!\right)^I$ permutations of $\overrightarrow{\mathbf{Y}}$. The only choice you have is which of the $\alpha\left(J!\right)^I$ within-block permutations of $\overrightarrow{\mathbf{Y}}$ should lead to rejection of $H_0^\dagger$.

In brief, starting from the seemingly innocuous requirement (3.12) that the test rejects with probability α when the null hypothesis $H_0^\dagger$ is true, we conclude from (3.12)–(3.14) that the test *must* be a permutation test that rejects for $\alpha\left(J!\right)^I$ of the $\left(J!\right)^I$ permutations of the rows of $\overrightarrow{\mathbf{Y}}$. Stating the same conclusion in the converse: if your test correctly claims to have level α but is not a permutation test, then it must have restricted $\left\{F_1\left(\cdot\right), \ldots, F_I\left(\cdot\right)\right\}$ in some way; for instance, perhaps it restricted $F_i\left(y\right)$ to have the form $F_i\left(y\right) = \Phi\left\{\left(y - \beta_i\right)/\sigma\right\}$ where $\Phi\left(\cdot\right)$ is the standard Normal distribution and $\sigma > 0$ and β_i, $i = 1, \ldots, I$ are unknown block parameters.

Condition (3.12) leads to the conclusion that $\varpi\left(\mathbf{Y}\right)$ must be a permutation test if it is to have size α; however, not all such tests seem reasonable here. In particular, we want $\varpi\left(\mathbf{Y}\right)$ to distinguish the treated responses in column one from the control responses in columns $2, \ldots, J$, but under $H_0^\dagger$, there is nothing interesting about the ordering of control responses, $Y_{i2}, \ldots, Y_{iJ}$, so we want $\varpi\left(\mathbf{Y}\right)$ to be unchanged by reordering the control responses in any block. There are $(J-1)!$ ways to permute $Y_{i2}, \ldots, Y_{iJ}$, and $\varpi\left(\mathbf{Y}\right)$ should reject $H_0^\dagger$ for all of them or fail to reject $H_0^\dagger$ for all of them. The only relevant aspect of a within-block permutation is who gets picked for treatment, and there are J ways to decide that. That is, we want to restrict attention to a subset of the permutation tests, namely, those $\varpi\left(\mathbf{Y}\right)$ that take the same value for all

$\{(J-1)!\}^I$ ways to order the controls within the I rows. In other words, we want to split the $(J!)^I$ within-block permutations of $\overrightarrow{\mathbf{Y}}$ into J^I sets each of size $\{(J-1)!\}^I$, so that $\varpi(\mathbf{Y})$ is constant inside each set, and each set reflects the J^I ways to pick one treated person in each block. Thinking of each of the J^I sets as one $\mathbf{z} \in \mathcal{Z}$, the relevant permutation tests are those in Chap. 2, and their null distributions are given by Proposition 2.2.

Obviously, it would be a bit odd to say that there is a treatment effect if $H_0^\dagger$ is true. If $H_0^\dagger$ is true, then in every block i, the distribution of responses under treatment equals the distribution of responses under control, although that distribution may vary with i. And yet, every test of $H_0^\dagger$ that has size α is identical to a randomization test of Fisher's sharp null hypothesis, $H_0 : \boldsymbol{\delta} = \mathbf{0}$—the same observable data $(\mathbf{R}, \mathbf{Z})$ entail the same P-values testing $\tau = 0$, and the same confidence intervals and point estimates for τ obtained in the usual way by inverting the tests. This is all true even though $H_0^\dagger$ does not imply $H_0 : \boldsymbol{\delta} = \mathbf{0}$.

3.3 *Further Reading

Dawid's article [2] should be read by anyone interested in causal inference, and this is also true of the discussion of permutation and randomization tests in Lehmann and Romano [10, §5.8–§5.12]. Also interesting is an article by Lehmann and Stein [11].

Problems

3.1 Covariate Imbalance

In Table 3.1, use Bayes theorem to deduce $\Pr(\mathbf{X} = \mathbf{x} \mid Z = 1)$ and $\Pr(\mathbf{X} = \mathbf{x} \mid Z = 0)$ from $\Pr(\mathbf{X} = \mathbf{x})$ and $\Pr(Z = 1 \mid \mathbf{X} = \mathbf{x})$. That is: Derive the last two columns of Table 3.1 from the earlier columns.

3.2 Covariate Imbalance Given $\Pr(Z = 1 \mid \mathbf{X} = \mathbf{x})$

Use Table 3.1 to deduce Table 3.2.

3.3 t-tests and Gaussian Linear Models

Review the model in Problem 2.9. If you did not do Problem 2.9(ix), do it now; that is, give the linear model t-test of $H_0 : \tau = 0$ in the model in Problem 2.9.

3.4 $H_{\tau_0}^\dagger$ and Gaussian Linear Models

The null hypothesis $H_{\tau_0}^\dagger$ was defined in Sect. 3.2. In the Gaussian linear model in Problem 3.3, is $H_{\tau_0}^\dagger$ true if $\tau = \tau_0$?

3.5 Permutation tests and Gaussian Linear Models

Let α be a possible size for a permutation test in a blocked experiment with I blocks of size J; that is, $\alpha = k/I^J$ for some $k \in \{1, 2, \ldots, I^J - 1\}$. Under the Gaussian linear model in Problem 3.3, can a permutation test of $\tau = \tau_0$ based on (3.10) have exact size α?

3.6 Compatible Conclusions
Explain why your conclusions in Problems 3.3–3.5 are compatible with the conclusion from Lehmann and Romano [10, Ch. 5], as developed here in Sect. 3.2, that: "Only Permutation Tests Have Size α When Testing $H_0^{\dagger}$."

3.7 Nonparametric Linear Block Models
Change the model in Problem 3.3 in the following way: The IJ bivariate vectors $(\epsilon_{Tij}, \epsilon_{Cij})$ are independent, and in block i, the distribution of the J vectors $(\epsilon_{Tij}, \epsilon_{Cij})$ have the same exchangeable distribution whose common unknown marginal distribution, F_i, is continuous and may depend upon i, for $i = 1, \ldots, I$. Without further assumptions, does the t-test that you devised in Problem 3.3 still have size α when testing $\tau = \tau_0$ under this new model? Does a permutation test based on (3.10) in Problem 3.5 have exact size α when testing $\tau = \tau_0$?

References

1. Conover, W.J., Salsburg, D.S.: Locally most powerful tests for detecting treatment effects when only a subset of patients can be expected to "respond" to treatment. Biometrics **44**, 189–196 (1988)
2. Dawid, A.P.: Conditional independence in statistical theory. J. R. Stat. Soc. B **41**(1), 1–15 (1979)
3. Dawid, A.P.: Conditional independence for statistical operations. Ann. Stat. **8**(3), 598–617 (1980)
4. Fraser, D.A.S.: Completeness of order statistics. Can. J. Math. **6**, 42–45 (1954)
5. Fraser, D.A.S.: Nonparametric Methods in Statistics. Wiley, New York (1957)
6. Hodges, J., Lehmann, E.: Estimates of location based on rank tests. Ann. Math. Stat. **34**(2), 598–611 (1963)
7. Hollander, M., Wolfe, D.A., Chicken, E.: Nonparametric Statistical Methods, 3rd edn. Wiley, New York (2013)
8. Lehmann, E.L.: Nonparametrics. Holden-Day, San Francisco (1975)
9. Lehmann, E.L.: The Fisher, Neyman-Pearson theories of testing hypotheses: one theory or two? J. Am. Stat. Assoc. **88**(424), 1242–1249 (1993)
10. Lehmann, E.L., Romano, J.P.: Testing Statistical Hypotheses, 3rd edn. Springer, New York (2005)
11. Lehmann, E.L., Stein, C.: On the theory of some non-parametric hypotheses. Ann. Math. Stat. **20**(1), 28–45 (1949)
12. Little, R.J.A.: A note about models for selectivity bias. Econometrica **53**, 1469–1474 (1985)
13. Rosenbaum, P.R.: Hodges-Lehmann point estimates of treatment effect in observational studies. J. Am. Stat. Assoc. **88**(424), 1250–1253 (1993)
14. Rosenbaum, P.R.: Effects attributable to treatment: inference in experiments and observational studies with a discrete pivot. Biometrika **88**(1), 219–231 (2001)
15. Rosenbaum, P.R.: Confidence intervals for uncommon but dramatic responses to treatment. Biometrics **63**(4), 1164–1171 (2007)
16. Rosenbaum, P.R.: Causal Inference. MIT Press, New York (2023)

Part II
Adjustments for Observed Covariates

Chapter 4
Propensity Scores and Ignorable Treatment Assignment

Abstract Several key concepts are introduced: the propensity score, ignorable treatment assignment, and the principal unobserved covariate. The data in an observational study are from a population, and these concepts describe that population. The propensity score $e(\mathbf{x})$ is the conditional probability of treatment given the observed covariates, $e(\mathbf{x}) = \Pr(Z = 1 \mid \mathbf{X} = \mathbf{x})$, and it is determined by the distribution of observable quantities, $(R, Z, \mathbf{X})$; so, $e(\mathbf{x})$ can be estimated from the observable data. In contrast, the principal unobserved covariate is $\zeta = \zeta(r_T, r_C, \mathbf{X}) = \Pr(Z = 1 \mid r_T, r_C, \mathbf{X} = \mathbf{x})$, and it is not a function of observable quantities, $(R, Z, \mathbf{X})$, because (r_T, r_C) are never jointly observed. Treatment assignment is ignorable given the observed covariates $\mathbf{X}$ if $0 < e(\mathbf{x}) = \zeta(r_T, r_C, \mathbf{X}) < 1$, that is, if the propensity score equals the principal unobserved covariate and is never 0 or 1. If treatment assignment was ignorable given the observed covariates $\mathbf{X}$, then causal inference would be comparatively straightforward; so, the central problem in observational studies is the absence of grounds for believing, and the abundance of grounds for doubting, that treatment assignment is ignorable given $\mathbf{X}$. If $0 < \zeta < 1$, then treatment assignment is always ignorable given $(\mathbf{X}, \zeta)$; so, the central problem in observational studies can always be expressed in terms of one scalar unobserved covariate, ζ, where $0 \le \zeta \le 1$.

4.1 Notation and Identification

The concepts in this chapter refer to a population, to a probability distribution, not to data from that population. In that sense, these concepts, by themselves, are inadequate for inference from a sample to a population. In causal inference, the population itself may be inadequate for inference—even if you had all of the observable data from the population, even if you were handed an explicit form for the probability distributions of observable data, it might not be enough. Expressing the

© The Author(s), under exclusive license to Springer Nature Switzerland AG 2025
P. R. Rosenbaum, *An Introduction to the Theory of Observational Studies*, Springer Texts in Statistics, https://doi.org/10.1007/978-3-031-90494-3_4

same thought in a different way: Causal effects in the population may not be identified by the probability distribution of observable data—situations with different causal effects may have the same observable probability distribution [11,12]. The concepts in this chapter clarify certain problems, direct attention to certain considerations, justify certain goals in research design, and inspire certain data analyses, but that is all they do. Inference will have to wait to later chapters.

In the population, a person is treated, $Z = 1$, or not, $Z = 0$. If treated with $Z = 1$, the person exhibits response r_T; if the person is untreated with $Z = 0$—if the person is a control—then the observed response is r_C. The response we observe is $R = Z\, r_T + (1 - Z)\, r_C$; so, we observe (Z, R), but not the causal effect (r_T, r_C). The formal expression of causal effects as comparisons of potential outcomes under competing treatments is due to Jerzy Neyman [13] and Donald Rubin [28]. We observe also a covariate $\mathbf{X}$. A covariate is a quantity describing an individual prior to treatment and hence unaffected by the treatment the individual has not yet received. An outcome, (r_T, r_C), exists in two versions depending upon the treatment received, but a covariate is unaffected by a treatment not yet received, so a covariate, $\mathbf{X}$, exists in a single version. Mistaking an outcome for a covariate—i.e., adjusting for an outcome as if it were a covariate—can create a bias in causal inference that would not otherwise be present [16]. We are under no illusion that the covariate, $\mathbf{X}$, that we happened to measure comprises an adequate description of a person prior to treatment. We must entertain and address the possibility that $\mathbf{X}$ omits an important unmeasured covariate, u, that predicts both treatment received, Z, and outcome exhibited, R.

In this setting, many distributions are identified and many others are not. The distribution of responses to control, r_C, for people who happen to receive the control, $Z = 0$, is identified. How do we know this? Imagine that we could have a random sample from the population, a sample of any size we desired. The observable data from the population includes the joint distribution of (Z, R), so we can certainly estimate from our sample the conditional distribution $\Pr(R \mid Z = 0)$ by the empirical distribution of R for controls, that is, for people with $Z = 0$. However, when $Z = 0$, the observed response is $R = r_C$, so $\Pr(r_C \mid Z = 0) = \Pr(R \mid Z = 0)$. So, $\Pr(r_C \mid Z = 0)$ is identified.

Not identified is the distribution $\Pr(r_C)$ of responses r_C that would be observed if everyone in the population were assigned to control. How do we know this? From elementary properties of conditional distributions,

$$\Pr(r_C) = \Pr(r_C \mid Z = 0)\Pr(Z = 0) + \Pr(r_C \mid Z = 1)\Pr(Z = 1)\,, \qquad (4.1)$$

where $\Pr(r_C \mid Z = 0)$, $\Pr(Z = 0) = 1 - \Pr(Z = 1)$ are identified, but we never see r_C if $Z = 1$; so, $\Pr(r_C \mid Z = 1)$ is definitely a problem. We will make limited progress toward solving this problem by taking account of $\mathbf{X}$—in fact, that is what propensity scores do—but that progress is distinctly limited. For simplicity in the rest of this paragraph, suppose that we have no observed covariates $\mathbf{X}$, recognizing that observed covariates help only a bit when we have them. In this case, we would have no information at all about $\Pr(r_C \mid Z = 1)$; so, if

$\Pr(Z = 0) = \Pr(Z = 1) = \frac{1}{2}$, then lacking $\Pr(r_C \mid Z = 1)$ is lacking half of what we need to calculate $\Pr(r_C)$. As Charles Manski [11] emphasizes, if you fill in different distributions for $\Pr(r_C \mid Z = 1)$ in (4.1), then you will obtain very different distributions for $\Pr(r_C)$; moreover, nothing you will ever see in this population will ratify one form for $\Pr(r_C \mid Z = 1)$ or reject another, because there are no observable data about $\Pr(r_C \mid Z = 1)$. This is a problem with the population, with the probability distributions that yield the observed data, not a problem with inferring features of a population from a finite sample. If a fair coin is flipped to assign treatments, as in the toy randomized experiment in Sect. 3.1, then treatment Z is independent of r_C, or $Z \perp\!\!\!\perp r_C$; so $\Pr(r_C \mid Z = 0) = \Pr(r_C \mid Z = 1) = \Pr(r_C)$ and our estimate of $\Pr(r_C \mid Z = 0)$ based on the empirical distribution function is also an estimate of both $\Pr(r_C \mid Z = 1)$ and $\Pr(r_C)$. As in Chap. 2, random assignment to treatment or control makes a challenging problem into a straightforward one.

The propensity score [23, 27] is the conditional probability of treatment, $Z = 1$, given the observed covariates $\mathbf{X}$ or $\Pr(Z = 1 \mid \mathbf{X} = \mathbf{x})$. To emphasize that the propensity score is both a function of the observed covariates and a random variable, it is written either as the function $e(\mathbf{x}) = \Pr(Z = 1 \mid \mathbf{X} = \mathbf{x})$ or as the random variable $e(\mathbf{X})$. Because the population provides complete data on $(Z, \mathbf{X})$, the propensity score is identified by the observable data in the population. Is the propensity score useful?

4.2 Looking at Estimates of the Propensity Score

Returning to the binge drinking example in Sect. 1.5, two propensity scores will be separately estimated using $(Z, \mathbf{X})$, one for each type of control, those who never binged (N) and those who binged in the past but subsequently quit (P). Of course, the notation $Z = 0$ has a different meaning for N and P controls. Each estimate uses a linear logit model,

$$\log\left\{\frac{\Pr(Z = 1 \mid \mathbf{X} = \mathbf{x})}{\Pr(Z = 0 \mid \mathbf{X} = \mathbf{x})}\right\} = \log\left\{\frac{e(\mathbf{x})}{1 - e(\mathbf{x})}\right\} = \beta_0 + \beta_1 x_1 + \cdots + \beta_K x_K, \quad (4.2)$$

fitted in R by maximum likelihood [3]; see Problem 4.1. One could reasonably fit a more complex model, perhaps with an interaction between age and sex, or a quadratic or a spline for age. It is helpful to look at two propensity scores in this example, because they turn out to be quite different in relevant ways; however, the typical application of propensity scores has one control group and one propensity score.

Table 4.1 shows the usual summary output from R for each of two propensity scores for each of the two control groups. Table 4.1 contains the maximum likelihood estimates of the β_k in (4.2), their approximate standard errors, the deviates that are compared to the standard Normal distribution to test the hypothesis that $\beta_k = 0$, and the associated P-values.

Notably in Table 4.1, the two propensity scores are similar in some ways and different in others. For both control groups, the coefficient of age is negative: Current

Table 4.1 Logit regression results for two estimated propensity scores in the binge drinking data There is one propensity score for each control group, "N" and "P." For binary 1/0 covariates, 1 means "yes." For "smoke now," 1 means daily smoking, and 3 means nonsmoker.

Control Group	"N" or Never Controls				"P" or Past Binge Controls			
Covariate	Estimate	Std. Error	z value	P-value	Estimate	Std. Error	z value	P-value
Constant	0.17	1.11	0.16	0.876	2.95	1.38	2.13	0.033
Age	− 0.02	0.01	− 4.15	0.000	− 0.05	0.01	− 5.94	0.000
Female, 1/0	− 0.88	0.19	− 4.66	0.000	0.14	0.24	0.59	0.555
Education, 1-5	− 0.12	0.07	− 1.82	0.069	0.04	0.08	0.49	0.625
Smoke Now, 1-3	− 1.16	0.09	− 12.74	0.000	− 0.15	0.12	− 1.26	0.207
Smoked But Quit, 1/0	1.00	0.22	4.61	0.000	− 0.66	0.25	− 2.65	0.008
BP Meds, 1/0	0.18	0.20	0.93	0.351	0.05	0.22	0.23	0.815
BMI	− 0.01	0.01	− 0.80	0.422	− 0.02	0.01	− 1.64	0.101
Vigorous Activity, 1/0	0.45	0.16	2.80	0.005	0.10	0.19	0.50	0.617
Waist/Hip Ratio	1.72	1.30	1.33	0.185	− 0.44	1.55	− 0.29	0.775

binge drinkers are typically younger than both control groups, as was already visible in Fig. 1.6. Both control groups are more likely than current binge drinkers to have smoked regularly in the past but quit. There is no sign that the two measures of obesity—BMI and waist/hip ratio—predict binge drinking. In contrast, when compared to current binge drinkers, control group N is less likely to currently smoke, less likely to engage in vigorous activity, and more likely to be female; however, these patterns are not seen in comparison with control group P.

Several quantiles of the estimated propensity scores, $\widehat{e}(\mathbf{X})$, are shown in Table 4.2, specifically the median, quartiles, eights, and extremes. Here, $\widehat{e}(\mathbf{X})$ is obtained from the maximum likelihood estimate of model (4.2), plugging in each individual's $\mathbf{X}$ to produce an estimate $\widehat{e}(\mathbf{X})$ of $\Pr(Z = 1 \mid \mathbf{X})$. The estimated propensity scores are also depicted in Fig. 4.1. There are far fewer past-bingers (P) than never bingers (N); so, in a trivial way, the propensity scores $\widehat{e}(\mathbf{X})$ for the comparison with group N tend to be smaller than for the comparison with group P. For each propensity score, N or P, the distributions of $\widehat{e}(\mathbf{X})$ overlap for treated ($Z = 1$) and control ($Z = 0$) groups, but the distributions are nonetheless quite different, particularly for the N or never propensity scores. As one might expect given its construction in (4.2) using all of the covariates, the separation of treated and control groups is greater for the propensity score than for any individual covariate in Figs. 1.6 and 1.7.

Each panel of Fig. 4.1 contains three boxplots. The third boxplot shows the highest 206 estimated propensity scores for controls, for N controls in the left panel and for P controls in the right panel. Partly because there are many N controls to choose from, it is possible to select 206 N controls with estimated propensity scores as large or larger than the propensity scores for the binge group B. That is, pair matching can remove the large imbalance seen in the left panel of Fig. 4.1. In contrast, for P controls in the right panel of Fig. 4.1, even the largest 206 propensity scores for P controls have an upper quartile below the upper quartile for the 206 binge drinkers, B. Pair matching can equate the median propensity scores for P controls, but it cannot completely match the B distribution of propensity scores—there just are not enough P controls with large estimated propensity scores.

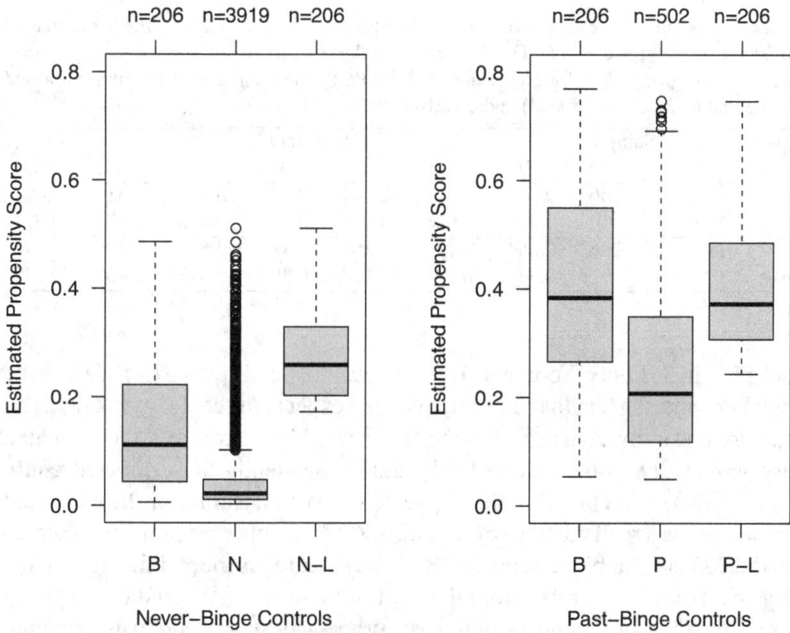

Fig. 4.1 Boxplots of two estimated propensity scores, $\widehat{e}(\mathbf{X})$, for two types of controls, N = never-binge and P = past-binge controls, compared to current binge drinkers (B). The plots N-L and P-L depict the $n = 206$ largest estimated propensity scores for groups N and P; so, they indicate whether a pair matching for the propensity score is feasible.

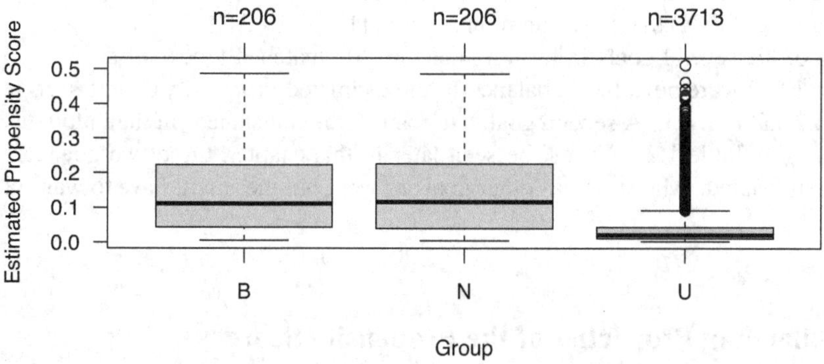

Fig. 4.2 The estimated propensity scores, $\widehat{e}(\mathbf{X})$, when matching binge drinkers (B) to never-binge controls (N). Group U consists of the unmatched individuals from group N

Table 4.2 Two estimated propensity scores in the binge data. The scores have the same treated group, the 206 current binge drinkers. For this one treated group, there are two propensity scores, one for each control group, "N" for Never and "P" for Past. The table shows the minimum and maximum, median (1/2), quartiles (1/4) and eighths (1/8)

Group	Sample				Quantile			
	Size	Min	1/8	1/4	1/2	3/4	7/8	Max
Binge, Z = 1	206	0.006	0.025	0.044	0.112	0.222	0.311	0.487
Never Binge, Z = 0	3919	0.003	0.008	0.011	0.022	0.048	0.083	0.511
Binge, Z = 1	206	0.054	0.171	0.267	0.384	0.550	0.635	0.770
Past Binge, Z = 0	502	0.049	0.085	0.118	0.207	0.348	0.455	0.747

Samuel Pimentel, Frank Yoon and Luke Keele [14] call $\{1 - e(\mathbf{X})\}/e(\mathbf{X})$ the "entire number" and suggest that, in principle, one expects to see $\{1 - e(\mathbf{X})\}/e(\mathbf{X})$ controls per treated individual at $\mathbf{X}$. For the N or never-binged controls, the estimated propensity scores $\widehat{e}(\mathbf{X})$ rarely exceed 0.5, and consequently the estimated entire number $\{1 - \widehat{e}(\mathbf{X})\}/\widehat{e}(\mathbf{X})$ rarely falls below 1; so, pair matching for the estimated propensity score has a realistic hope of finding 206 N controls with propensity scores similar to the 206 current binge drinkers (B). The situation is more difficult with the propensity scores for P controls: More than 1/4 of these scores exceed 0.5 in group B, so there is a deficit of P controls with large propensity scores, and pair matching cannot completely equate the empirical distributions of propensity scores for group B and control group P. Donald Rubin [29] observed that there is a maximum bias that can be removed by pair matching. Other, more flexible forms of matching can remove more bias than pair matching. For instance, "full matching" permits a treated individual to be matched to one or more controls, or a control to be matched to one or more treated individuals, and it can, in principle, remove all the bias in two distributions of $\widehat{e}(\mathbf{X})$ that have common support [1,7,8,19,31].

One of the several goals in forming the $I = 206$ matched blocks of size $J = 3$ in Sect. 1.5 is to remove the imbalance in the estimated propensity scores seen in Table 4.2 and Fig. 4.1. A second goal is to remove the imbalances in the individual covariates in Table 1.2. As will be seen later in this chapter, these two goals are intimately related. Matching has other goals as well, but these will have to wait for Chap. 5.

4.3 Balancing Properties of the Propensity Score

The Propensity Score Balances Observed Covariates

For each of the two control groups, the estimated propensity scores in Fig. 4.1 have very different distributions in the treated, $Z = 1$, and control groups, $Z = 0$, and this is not a small problem. That is, Fig. 4.1 suggests that $\Pr\{e(\mathbf{X}) \mid Z = 1\}$ is very different from $\Pr\{e(\mathbf{X}) \mid Z = 0\}$ for each control group, or equivalently that it is false that $e(\mathbf{X}) \perp\!\!\!\perp Z$. Of course, $e(\mathbf{X})$ is just one function of $\mathbf{X}$; so, it seems conceivable, at least at first, that there could be many other imbalances in **X** besides the imbalance in $e(\mathbf{X})$ in Fig. 4.1. There is a sense, however, that the entire problem of imbalances in observed covariates **X** is depicted in Fig. 4.1; that is, there is a sense in which, if the one problem in Fig. 4.1 was fixed, then all of the problems with the observed covariates **X** would be fixed as well, leaving us to face the important, untouched remaining problem with unmeasured covariates. The current section discusses a first aspect of that sense, namely, the balancing properties of the propensity score. Having examined *estimated* propensity scores in Sect. 4.2, this section returns to the *population* perspective from Sect. 4.1.

Proposition 4.1 states the basic balancing property of propensity scores (Rosenbaum and Rubin [23]). Essentially, Proposition 4.1 says that treated and control individuals with the same propensity score $e(\mathbf{X})$ have the same distribution of all of the observed covariates **X** that were used to define the score. Proposition 4.1 says nothing about covariates that were not measured and nothing about potential outcomes (r_T, r_C).

Proposition 4.1 *For any function* $\mathbf{f}(\mathbf{X})$*,*

$$\mathbf{X} \perp\!\!\!\perp Z \mid e(\mathbf{X}) \tag{4.3}$$

and

$$\mathbf{X} \perp\!\!\!\perp Z \mid \{e(\mathbf{X}), \mathbf{f}(\mathbf{X})\}. \tag{4.4}$$

Before proving Proposition 4.1, consider its implications. Here, (4.3) is the balancing property of the propensity score: It says that the observed covariates **X** are conditionally independent of the assigned treatment, Z, given the propensity score, $e(\mathbf{X})$, or equivalently that

$$\Pr\{\mathbf{X} \mid e(\mathbf{X}),\ Z = 1\} = \Pr\{\mathbf{X} \mid e(\mathbf{X}),\ Z = 0\};$$

so, at each value of the propensity score, $e(\mathbf{X})$, treated and control individuals have the same distribution of the observed covariates **X**. Now, (4.3) is equivalent to

$$\Pr\{Z = 1 \mid \mathbf{X},\ e(\mathbf{X})\} = \Pr\{Z = 1 \mid e(\mathbf{X})\}. \tag{4.5}$$

because of (3.4); that is, all of the information in **X** that is useful in predicting Z are captured by $e(\mathbf{X})$.

We often match for both the propensity score and certain other aspects of **X**; for instance, in both alcohol examples in Sects. 1.4 and 1.5, the blocks were matched for sex, say $\mathbf{f}(\mathbf{X})$. Then, (4.4) in Proposition 4.1 says that the balancing property of propensity scores is not lost by matching for both $e(\mathbf{X})$ and $\mathbf{f}(\mathbf{X})$.

Proof If (4.3) were true, then (4.4) would follow from Lemma 3.2(ii) with $A = \mathbf{X}$, $B = Z$, $C = e(\mathbf{X})$ and $D = \mathbf{f}(\mathbf{X})$; so, it suffices to prove (4.3). Expressions (4.3) and (4.5) are equivalent by (3.4), so it suffices to prove (4.5). Now,

$$\Pr(Z = 1 \mid \mathbf{X}) = \Pr\{Z = 1 \mid \mathbf{X},\ e(\mathbf{X})\}, \tag{4.6}$$

simply because $e(\mathbf{X})$ is a function of $\mathbf{X}$. By definition, $e(\mathbf{X}) = \Pr(Z = 1 \mid \mathbf{X})$. Generally, $\mathrm{E}(A \mid C) = \mathrm{E}\{\mathrm{E}(A \mid B, C) \mid C\}$, so taking $A = Z$, $B = \mathbf{X}$, and $C = e(\mathbf{X})$ yields

$$\begin{aligned}\Pr\{Z = 1 \mid e(\mathbf{X})\} &= \mathrm{E}\{Z \mid e(\mathbf{X})\} = \mathrm{E}[\mathrm{E}\{Z \mid \mathbf{X}, e(\mathbf{X})\} \mid e(\mathbf{X})] \\ &= \mathrm{E}[\Pr\{Z = 1 \mid \mathbf{X}, e(\mathbf{X})\} \mid e(\mathbf{X})] \\ &= \mathrm{E}[\Pr\{Z = 1 \mid \mathbf{X}\} \mid e(\mathbf{X})] \text{ by (4.6)} \\ &= \mathrm{E}[e(\mathbf{X}) \mid e(\mathbf{X})] \\ &= e(\mathbf{X}) = \Pr(Z = 1 \mid \mathbf{X}) = \Pr\{Z = 1 \mid \mathbf{X}, e(\mathbf{X})\}, \text{ by (4.6),}\end{aligned}$$

proving (4.5). □

Matching For $\widehat{e}(\mathbf{X})$ Alone in the Binge Drinking Data

To illustrate Proposition 4.1 using the binge drinking example from Sect. 1.5, consider matching the current binge drinkers (B) to never-binge controls (N) using the propensity score alone.[1] Figure 4.2 shows the estimated propensity scores, $\widehat{e}(\mathbf{X})$, for the $I = 206$ matched pairs B-N pairs and for the $3919 - 206 = 3713$ unmatched N controls. Figure 4.1 had suggested that the imbalance in $\widehat{e}(\mathbf{X})$ could be removed by pair matching for N controls, and this is confirmed by Fig. 4.2. Although there are 3713 unmatched controls in Fig. 4.2, many of them look nothing like binge drinkers in terms of $\mathbf{X}$.

Table 4.3 shows the covariate balance in $I = 206$ matched pairs. Notably, the match removed large imbalances in the covariates age, female, education, current smoking, vigorous activity, and blood pressure medication.

The covariate balance seen in Table 4.3 is important, and yet its importance can easily be overstated. It is important that, to the eye, the matched groups look comparable in terms of measured covariates, because many published comparisons compare groups that are nowhere near comparable, and the publication provides no indication that this is so. If nothing else, a balance table like Table 4.3 provides an indication. However, particularly in large samples, statistical methods make distinctions that are too subtle for the eye to see; so, those methods may be biased by incomparability that is too subtle for the eye to see in Table 4.3. Moreover, Table 4.3 is about covariate means, and covariate distributions can differ yet have similar means. The P-values in Table 4.3 are, at most, an informal benchmark, particularly for $\widehat{e}(\mathbf{X})$, which was built from the same data to separate groups B and N, and then controlled by a matching algorithm that tried to bring groups B and N together in terms of $\widehat{e}(\mathbf{X})$. Checking covariate balance is discussed at greater length in Chap. 6.

---

[1] The match used both a caliper on the estimated propensity score and a fine-balance constraint on the estimated propensity score. These techniques are described in Chap. 5.

Table 4.3 Covariate means for binge drinkers (B) matched to never-binge controls (N) using the estimated propensity score alone. Also shown are the means for the controls who were not included in the match (U) and the P-values from the usual two-sample t-test comparing the B-versus-N means. For binary covariates, 1 means "yes"

Covariate	Binge B	Control N	Unmatched U	P-value
Sample Size	206	206	3713	206-vs-206
Age	46.76	46.28	53.59	0.751
Female 1/0	0.29	0.33	0.60	0.340
Education, 1–5	3.27	3.37	3.60	0.368
BMI	29.27	29.61	30.21	0.634
Waist/Hip Ratio	0.95	0.95	0.93	0.952
Vigorous Activity 1/0	0.53	0.52	0.35	0.768
Smoke Now 1-3	2.02	2.04	2.83	0.879
Smoked but Quit 1/0	0.20	0.17	0.19	0.452
Blood pressure medications 1/0	0.26	0.25	0.34	0.735
$\widehat{e}(\mathbf{X})$	0.15	0.15	0.04	0.971

Although the covariate means in Table 4.3 look similar, matching for $\widehat{e}(\mathbf{X})$ makes no effort to pair individuals who are similar in terms of $\mathbf{X}$ itself. For instance, pair $i = 3$ of the $I = 206$ pairs consisted of a male binge drinker of age 30 with a BMI of 61.9 and a female never-binge control of age 21 with a BMI of 20.6. Table 4.3 shows that these differences within pairs tend to cancel out over all $I = 206$ pairs, as suggested by Proposition 4.1. Still, there are reasons to pair for both $\widehat{e}(\mathbf{X})$ and some aspects $f(\mathbf{X})$ of the rest of $\mathbf{X}$, so that paired individuals are closer in terms of $\mathbf{X}$, and ways to do this are discussed in Chap. 5.

The Limitations of Exact Matching

A first thought, natural yet mistaken, is that one can match for $\mathbf{X}$ by cutting each coordinate into categories and then match exactly for the categories. If each coordinate of $\mathbf{X}$ were split into just two categories at its median, then with a K-dimensional covariate $\mathbf{X}$ there would be 2^K categories or types of people, or about one type of person for each person on earth if $K = 33$, as $2^{33} \doteq 8.6$ billion. Even with so many categories, there are not enough categories: The median age for everyone in Table 4.3 is 55, but two categories of age, < 55 and ≥ 55, are not enough to represent age adequately.

Pair matching of binge drinkers (B) to never-binge controls (N) in Sect. 1.5 is not, in principle, very difficult. There are only $K = 9$ covariates, setting aside the estimated propensity score $\widehat{e}(\mathbf{X})$ that was built from those nine covariates. There are 206 binge drinkers and 3919 N controls to choose from. Most importantly, the left or N panel of Fig. 4.1 shows that there will be no problem correcting the imbalance in $\widehat{e}(\mathbf{X})$ using 206 controls with larger values of $\widehat{e}(\mathbf{X})$, and Proposition 4.1 suggests that consideration is the crucial one.

Suppose instead that we cut the three continuous coordinates of **X** each into four broad categories: (i) age as [20, 30), [30, 45), [45, 60), [60, ∞); (ii) BMI as [0, 25), [25, 30), [30, 35), [35, ∞); (iii) waist/hip ratio as [0, 0.8), [0.8, 0.9), [0.9, 1), [1, ∞). There are then $2^4 \times 3 \times 4^3 \times 5 = 15360$ categories.

Using these categories, of the 206 binge drinkers, only 104 binge drinkers can be matched exactly to N controls, even though 3919 N controls are available for matching. Of equal importance, 92 of the 206 binge drinkers are daily smokers ("Smoke Now" = 1), or about 45%. Among the 3919 potential N controls, 364 are daily smokers, or about 9%; so, because 364 > 92, by choosing the matched N controls carefully, we could have a matched sample in which 45% of N controls are daily smokers. However, there are only 48 N controls who are daily smokers and who match for the 15360 categories. In other words, we had 364 daily smokers in the N group, we needed 92 of 364 daily smokers to balance daily smoking, but the misguided attempt to match for 15360 coarse categories would lead us to discard 364 − 48 = 316 daily smokers from the N group.

The left or N panel of Table 4.1 clearly indicates that there are substantial imbalances in smoking behavior, age, sex, and vigorous activity, and the estimated propensity score $\widehat{e}(\mathbf{X})$ varies strongly with these covariates. By matching for $\widehat{e}(\mathbf{X})$—that is, by emphasizing smoking behavior, age, sex, and vigorous activity in $\widehat{e}(\mathbf{X})$—the match in Table 4.3 matched all 206 binge drinkers and balanced all nine covariates.

Again, the binge drinking example in Sect. 1.5 is a textbook example, with just a few covariates selected to permit concise exposition and easy replication by the reader using the `R` package `iTOS`. In scientific practice, there are often dozens or hundreds of covariates, as in the anesthesia example in Sect. 1.2. Matching exactly for covariates is rarely a practical option.

Balancing Scores

A function of the observed covariates, $\mathbf{b}(\mathbf{X})$, is said to be a balancing score [23, §2.2] if

$$\mathbf{X} \perp\!\!\!\perp Z \mid \mathbf{b}(\mathbf{X}). \tag{4.7}$$

As its name suggests, matching for a balancing score, $\mathbf{b}(\mathbf{X})$, balances observed covariates in treated and control groups; that is, (4.7) says

$$\Pr\{\mathbf{X} \mid Z = 1, \mathbf{b}(\mathbf{X})\} = \Pr\{\mathbf{X} \mid Z = 0, \mathbf{b}(\mathbf{X})\}.$$

Proposition 4.1 says that the propensity score, $e(\mathbf{X})$, is a balancing score, but so is $\mathbf{b}(\mathbf{X}) = \{e(\mathbf{X}), \mathbf{f}(\mathbf{X})\}$ for any function $\mathbf{f}(\mathbf{X})$. One might express this by saying that a score $\mathbf{b}(\mathbf{X})$ that makes distinctions at least as fine as those made by $e(\mathbf{X})$ is a balancing score.[2]

The converse is also true: $\mathbf{b}(\mathbf{X})$ cannot be a balancing score unless it makes distinctions as fine or finer than the propensity score. For suppose that a function $\mathbf{b}(\cdot)$ is not finer than the propensity score $e(\cdot)$, in the sense that there are $\mathbf{x}$ and $\mathbf{x}'$ such that $\mathbf{b}(\mathbf{x}) = \mathbf{b}(\mathbf{x}') = \overline{\mathbf{b}}$, say, but $e(\mathbf{x}) \neq e(\mathbf{x}')$. Then $\mathbf{b}(\mathbf{X})$ is not a balancing score because

$$\Pr\left\{Z = 1 \mid \mathbf{X} = \mathbf{x}, \mathbf{b}(\mathbf{X}) = \overline{\mathbf{b}}\right\} = \Pr\{Z = 1 \mid \mathbf{X} = \mathbf{x}\} = e(\mathbf{x})$$

$$\neq e(\mathbf{x}') = \Pr\left\{Z = 1 \mid \mathbf{X} = \mathbf{x}', \mathbf{b}(\mathbf{X}) = \overline{\mathbf{b}}\right\},$$

so (4.7) does not hold as a consequence of (3.4) with $A = \mathbf{X}$, $B = Z$, and $C = \mathbf{b}(\mathbf{X})$.

Lemma 4.1 is often useful, but similar to Proposition 4.1; so, the proof of Lemma 4.1 is Problem 4.2. (The solution to Problem 4.2 is at the end of the book.)

Lemma 4.1 *If* $\mathbf{b}(\mathbf{X}) = \{e(\mathbf{X}), \mathbf{f}(\mathbf{X})\}$, *then*

$$\Pr\{Z = 1 \mid \mathbf{b}(\mathbf{X})\} = \Pr(Z = 1 \mid \mathbf{X}) = e(\mathbf{X}).$$

4.4 Ignorable Treatment Assignment

Definition of Ignorable Treatment Assignment

Treatment assignment is said to be ignorable given covariates $\mathbf{V}$ if

$$Z \perp\!\!\!\perp (r_T, r_C) \mid \mathbf{V} \text{ and } 0 < \Pr(Z = 1 \mid \mathbf{V}) < 1. \tag{4.8}$$

In particular, as the propensity score is $e(\mathbf{X}) = \Pr(Z = 1 \mid \mathbf{X})$, treatment assignment is ignorable [23] given the observed covariates[3] $\mathbf{X}$ if

[2] Strictly speaking, one should say that $\mathbf{b}(\mathbf{X}) = \{e(\mathbf{X}), \mathbf{f}(\mathbf{X})\}$ is a balancing score for every measurable function, $\mathbf{f}(\mathbf{X})$, and that $\mathbf{b}(\mathbf{X})$ is a balancing score if the sigma-algebra generated by $\mathbf{b}(\mathbf{X})$ is finer (or includes) the sigma-algebra generated by $e(\mathbf{X})$.

[3] There are at least two definitions of ignorable treatment assignment, one for frequentist inference [23] and one for Bayesian inference [30]. The definition given here is the frequentist definition. The two definitions are similar in spirit but differ in detail. The frequentist version involves the factorization of probability distributions without reference to parameters. The Bayesian definition also refers to a factorization of a likelihood including factorization of its parameters. In the Bayesian version, viewing treatment assignment Z as fixed is the same as conditioning on Z if treatment assignment is ignorable; otherwise, the correct likelihood has a factor that cannot be ignored when conditioning on Z, so fixing Z and conditioning on Z are different things. In particular, randomized treatment assignment led to ignorable treatment assignment in the Bayesian sense, so Bayesians too benefited from randomized experiments [30]. The frequentist version is sometimes called strongly ignorable treatment assignment, but as only the frequentist version appears in this book, I will

$$Z \perp\!\!\!\perp (r_T, r_C) \mid \mathbf{X} \text{ and } 0 < e(\mathbf{X}) < 1, \tag{4.9}$$

or equivalently if

$$0 < \Pr(Z = 1 \mid \mathbf{X}) = \Pr(Z = 1 \mid \mathbf{X}, r_T, r_C) < 1. \tag{4.10}$$

The balancing properties of propensity scores in Proposition 4.1 are visible in data, because they refer to properties of the distribution of quantities $(Z, \mathbf{X})$ that are observed. In contrast, because we observe r_T only when $Z = 1$ and we observe r_C only when $Z = 0$, condition (4.9) or (4.10) refers to properties that cannot be checked by examining the observed distribution of $(R, Z, \mathbf{X})$. If treatments Z were assigned by independent flips of a fair coin, as in a randomized experiment, then (4.9) or (4.10) would be true based on properties of fair coins.

For example, in the binge drinking data in Sect. 1.5, we saw evidence consistent with (4.3) in Table 4.3, but there is nothing in the data on $(R, Z, \mathbf{X})$ alone that could tell us whether (4.9) or (4.10) are true or false.

Adjustments for X and Ignorable Treatment Assignment

In various senses, if treatment assignment is ignorable given the observed covariates $\mathbf{X}$, then appropriate adjustments for $\mathbf{X}$ can yield reasonable estimates of expected treatment effects. In various senses, if treatment assignment is *not* ignorable given the observed covariates, then adjustments for $\mathbf{X}$ may fail to deliver reasonable estimates of treatment effects. A simple formal translation of "reasonable" might be "consistent;" that is, estimates that converge to the truth as the sample size increases.

In particular, we can always estimate the two regressions

$$\mu_T(\mathbf{x}) = \mathrm{E}(R \mid Z = 1, \mathbf{X} = \mathbf{x}) = \mathrm{E}(r_T \mid Z = 1, \mathbf{X} = \mathbf{x})$$

and

$$\mu_C(\mathbf{x}) = \mathrm{E}(R \mid Z = 0, \mathbf{X} = \mathbf{x}) = \mathrm{E}(r_C \mid Z = 0, \mathbf{X} = \mathbf{x}),$$

because we have data from the distribution of $(R, Z, \mathbf{X})$, and $R = r_T$ when $Z = 1$ or $R = r_C$ when $Z = 0$. There are many methods that might be used to estimate $\mu_T(\mathbf{x})$ and $\mu_C(\mathbf{x})$, and different methods will have somewhat different properties, but there is nothing special about estimating $\mu_T(\mathbf{x})$ and $\mu_C(\mathbf{x})$, because the relevant quantities are all observed. For instance, with additional modeling assumptions, one might estimate $\mu_T(\mathbf{x})$ and $\mu_C(\mathbf{x})$ separately by fitting two linear models by least squares or by robust fitting using M-estimation.

The problem with $\mu_T(\mathbf{x})$ and $\mu_C(\mathbf{x})$ is that, in general, they do not tell us about

$$\rho_T(\mathbf{x}) = \mathrm{E}(r_T \mid \mathbf{X} = \mathbf{x}), \quad \rho_C(\mathbf{x}) = \mathrm{E}(r_C \mid \mathbf{X} = \mathbf{x})$$

---

simply call it ignorable treatment assignment. In both Bayesian and frequentist versions, the term "ignorable" is said in the tone of gentle reproach: You should only ignore the process that assigned treatments to individuals when it is ignorable, as it is in a randomized experiment.

and the expected causal effect at $\mathbf{X} = \mathbf{x}$, namely

$$\mathrm{E}\,(r_T - r_C \mid \mathbf{X} = \mathbf{x}) = \rho_T\,(\mathbf{x}) - \rho_C\,(\mathbf{x})\,.$$

If treatment assignment were ignorable given the observed covariates $\mathbf{X}$, then this problem would disappear, because (i) $Z \perp\!\!\!\perp (r_T, r_C) \mid \mathbf{X}$ implies $\rho_T\,(\mathbf{x}) = \mu_T\,(\mathbf{x})$ and $\rho_C\,(\mathbf{x}) = \mu_C\,(\mathbf{x})$ using (3.4), and (ii) $0 < e\,(\mathbf{X}) < 1$ means that some people receive treatment and others receive control at each value of $\mathbf{X}$. If treatment assignment was ignorable given $\mathbf{X}$, we could estimate $\mathrm{E}\,(r_T - r_C \mid \mathbf{X} = \mathbf{x})$ by estimating $\mu_T\,(\mathbf{x})$ and $\mu_C\,(\mathbf{x})$ and taking the difference of the two estimates.

To estimate the average treatment effect $\mathrm{E}\,(r_T - r_C)$ rather than $\mathrm{E}\,(r_T - r_C \mid \mathbf{X} = \mathbf{x})$, sample a value of $\mathbf{X}$ at random from the distribution $\Pr(\mathbf{X} = \mathbf{x})$, sample a treated individual, $Z = 1$, and a control individual, $Z = 0$, with this value of $\mathbf{X}$; then, the difference in their responses is unbiased for

$$\mathrm{E}\,[\mathrm{E}\,\{\mu_T\,(\mathbf{X}) - \mu_C\,(\mathbf{X}) \mid \mathbf{X}\}]\,,$$

and if treatment assignment is ignorable given $\mathbf{X}$, then this equals

$$\mathrm{E}\,[\mathrm{E}\,\{\rho_T\,(\mathbf{X}) - \rho_C\,(\mathbf{X}) \mid \mathbf{X}\}] = \mathrm{E}\,\{\mathrm{E}\,(r_T - r_C \mid \mathbf{X})\} = \mathrm{E}\,(r_T - r_C)\,.$$

To instead estimate the average effect, $\mathrm{E}\,(r_T - r_C \mid Z = 1)$, of the treatment on the treated population [25], sample a treated individual, $Z = 1$, at random, noting the value of $\mathbf{X}$ for this individual, and sample a control with the same value of $\mathbf{X}$. The difference of their responses is unbiased for

$$\mathrm{E}\,[\mathrm{E}\,\{\mu_T\,(\mathbf{X}) - \mu_C\,(\mathbf{X}) \mid \mathbf{X},\, Z = 1\}]\,,$$

and if treatment assignment is ignorable given $\mathbf{X}$, then this equals

$$\mathrm{E}\,\{\mathrm{E}\,(r_T - r_C \mid \mathbf{X},\, Z = 1) \mid Z = 1\} = \mathrm{E}\,(r_T - r_C \mid Z = 1)\,.$$

For instance, recall the data in Sect. 1.4 about light daily drinking and HDL cholesterol, in which each of the $I = 406$ light daily drinkers (D) was matched to a never-drinker (N) for a three-dimensional $\mathbf{X}$ composed of (age, female, education), yielding 406 matched pair differences in HDL cholesterol levels. These 406 pairs have the distribution of age, female, and education that is found in the treated group, $\Pr(\mathbf{X} \mid Z = 1)$, as seen in Table 1.1: 34% female, a mean age of about 57, and a mean education of "some college" or 4; so they are older, better educated, and disproportionately male compared to the N group before matching, $\Pr(\mathbf{X} \mid Z = 0)$. The average pair difference in HDL cholesterol levels is 13.1 with a standard error of 1.2. This average would estimate the average effect of light daily drinking on the type of person who engages in light daily drinking, namely, $\mathrm{E}\,(r_T - r_C \mid Z = 1)$, if treatment assignment was ignorable given $\mathbf{X}$.[4]

---

[4] Review Problem 1.4(e) to think about whether the expected pair difference, $\mathrm{E}\,(r_T - r_C \mid Z = 1)$, is the best way to characterize the typical difference in HDL cholesterol levels.

Speaking informally, if treatment assignment is ignorable given the observed covariates **X**, then adjustments for **X** suffice to draw inferences about treatment effects.

The Propensity Score and Ignorable Treatment Assignment

In Sect. 4.3, we saw that matching for every coordinate of **X** can be difficult when there are more than a few covariates, but with the same data, it may not be difficult to match for the scalar estimated propensity score, $\widehat{e}(\mathbf{X})$. Also, Proposition 4.1 said that, in the population, matching for $e(\mathbf{X})$ balances all of **X**. Is balancing **X** helpful in estimating treatment effects, such as $\mathrm{E}(r_T - r_C)$, $\mathrm{E}(r_T - r_C \mid Z = 1)$, and $\mathrm{E}(r_T - r_C \mid \mathbf{X} = \mathbf{x})$? Proposition 4.2 from [23, Thm. 3] says: If treatment assignment is ignorable given **X**, then it is ignorable given any balancing score $\mathbf{b}(\mathbf{X}) = \{e(\mathbf{X}), \mathbf{f}(\mathbf{X})\}$. In particular, $e(\mathbf{X})$ is always a balancing score, so Proposition 4.2 is true with $\mathbf{b}(\mathbf{X}) = e(\mathbf{X})$. Concisely, if it suffices to adjust for **X**, then it suffices to adjust for $e(\mathbf{X})$.

Proposition 4.2 *Let* $\mathbf{b}(\mathbf{X}) = \{e(\mathbf{X}), \mathbf{f}(\mathbf{X})\}$ *be a balancing score. If treatment assignment is ignorable given the observed covariates* **X***, then treatment assignment is ignorable given* $\mathbf{b}(\mathbf{X})$*; that is,*

$$0 < \Pr(Z = 1 \mid \mathbf{X}) = \Pr(Z = 1 \mid \mathbf{X}, r_T, r_C) < 1 \tag{4.11}$$

implies

$$0 < \Pr\{Z = 1 \mid \mathbf{b}(\mathbf{X})\} = \Pr\{Z = 1 \mid r_T, r_C, \mathbf{b}(\mathbf{X})\} < 1. \tag{4.12}$$

Proof Assume (4.11). Then

$$\Pr\{Z = 1 \mid r_T, r_C, \mathbf{b}(\mathbf{X})\} = \mathrm{E}[\Pr\{Z = 1 \mid r_T, r_C, \mathbf{X}\} \mid r_T, r_C, \mathbf{b}(\mathbf{X})]$$

$$= \mathrm{E}\{\Pr(Z = 1 \mid \mathbf{X}) \mid r_T, r_C, \mathbf{b}(\mathbf{X})\} \text{ using (4.11)}, \tag{4.13}$$

$$= \mathrm{E}[\Pr\{Z = 1 \mid \mathbf{b}(\mathbf{X})\} \mid r_T, r_C, \mathbf{b}(\mathbf{X})] \text{ by Lemma 4.1},$$
$$= \Pr\{Z = 1 \mid \mathbf{b}(\mathbf{X})\}, \text{ because } \Pr\{Z = 1 \mid \mathbf{b}(\mathbf{X})\} \text{ is a function of } \mathbf{b}(\mathbf{X}),$$

proving the equality in (4.12). Because $0 < \Pr(Z = 1 \mid \mathbf{X}) < 1$, it follows that $0 < \mathrm{E}\{\Pr(Z = 1 \mid \mathbf{X}) \mid r_T, r_C, \mathbf{b}(\mathbf{X})\} < 1$ in (4.13), proving the inequalities in (4.12). □

Proposition 4.2 says much less than we might hope. It does not say that it suffices to adjust for the propensity score $e(\mathbf{X})$ or a balancing score $\mathbf{b}(\mathbf{X}) = \{e(\mathbf{X}), \mathbf{f}(\mathbf{X})\}$. Proposition 4.2 says: If it suffices to adjust for the observed covariates **X**, then it suffices to adjust for either $e(\mathbf{X})$ or $\mathbf{b}(\mathbf{X}) = \{e(\mathbf{X}), \mathbf{f}(\mathbf{X})\}$; however, it provides no reason to believe the premise, namely, that it suffices to adjust for **X**.

4.5 The Principal Unobserved Covariate

What Is the Principal Unobserved Covariate?

Treatment assignment may not be and, except in randomized experiments, cannot safely be assumed to be, ignorable given the observed covariates $\mathbf{X}$. This is the central problem in observational studies. An aid to understanding and discussing this central problem is the principal unobserved covariate [21, 27]. The principal unobserved covariate is $\zeta = \Pr(Z = 1 \mid \mathbf{X}, r_T, r_C)$. The principal unobserved covariate ζ is a function of $(\mathbf{X}, r_T, r_C)$, and it is unobserved because the potential outcomes, (r_T, r_C), are not jointly observed. The observed response, $R = Z\, r_T + (1 - Z)\, r_C$, changes when the treatment assignment Z changes, but (r_T, r_C) does not change; so, Constantine Fragakis and Donald Rubin [6] refer to potential outcomes, (r_T, r_C), as principal strata, a type of covariate.

As ζ is a probability, it follows that $0 \le \zeta \le 1$. If $0 < \zeta < 1$, then by (4.10), treatment assignment is ignorable given the observed covariates $\mathbf{X}$ if the principal unobserved covariate, $\zeta = \Pr(Z = 1 \mid \mathbf{X}, r_T, r_C)$, equals the propensity score, $e(\mathbf{X}) = \Pr(Z = 1 \mid \mathbf{X})$.

The Key Property of the Principal Unobserved Covariate

In a sense, Proposition 4.3 says that there is only one scalar unobserved covariate u that matters in causal inference and that covariate is the principal unobserved covariate, $u = \zeta = \Pr(Z = 1 \mid \mathbf{X}, r_T, r_C)$, where $0 \le u \le 1$.

Proposition 4.3 *Let* $\zeta = \Pr(Z = 1 \mid \mathbf{X}, r_T, r_C)$ *be the principal unobserved covariate. If* $0 < \zeta < 1$, *then:*
(i) treatment assignment is ignorable given ζ,
(ii) treatment assignment is ignorable given $(\mathbf{X}, \zeta)$, *and*
(iii) for any function $\mathbf{f}(\mathbf{X})$, *treatment assignment is ignorable given* $\{\mathbf{f}(\mathbf{X}), \zeta\}$.

Proof Because the random variable $\zeta = \Pr(Z = 1 \mid \mathbf{X}, r_T, r_C)$ is a function of $(\mathbf{X}, r_T, r_C)$, it follows that

$$\Pr(Z = 1 \mid \mathbf{X}, r_T, r_C, \zeta) = \Pr(Z = 1 \mid \mathbf{X}, r_T, r_C) = \zeta. \tag{4.14}$$

Also,

$$\Pr(Z = 1 \mid \zeta) = \mathrm{E}\{\Pr(Z = 1 \mid \mathbf{X}, r_T, r_C, \zeta) \mid \zeta\} = \mathrm{E}(\zeta \mid \zeta) = \zeta. \tag{4.15}$$

Combining (4.14) and (4.15) yields

$$\Pr(Z = 1 \mid \mathbf{X}, r_T, r_C, \zeta) = \Pr(Z = 1 \mid \zeta)$$

or equivalently

$$Z \perp\!\!\!\perp (r_T, r_C, \mathbf{X}) \mid \zeta,$$

from which (i)–(iii) follow from (3.4) and Lemma 3.2. □

The proof of Proposition 4.3 also proves Corollary 4.1, omitting the premise that $0 < \zeta < 1$.

Corollary 4.1 *Let* $\zeta = \Pr(Z = 1 \mid \mathbf{X}, r_T, r_C)$ *be the principal unobserved covariate. Then*

$$Z \perp\!\!\!\perp (r_T, r_C, \mathbf{X}) \mid \zeta.$$

The Central Problem in Observational Studies and the Principal Unobserved Covariate

If a randomized experiment assigns treatments by independent flips of a fair coin, then treatment assignment is ignorable given the observed covariates $\mathbf{X}$, and $\mathrm{E}(r_T - r_C \mid \mathbf{X})$ is identified by the observable distribution of $(R, Z, \mathbf{X})$.

In an observational study, treatment assignment would be ignorable given $\mathbf{X}$ if the propensity score equaled the principal unobserved covariate with

$$0 < e(\mathbf{X}) = \Pr(Z = 1 \mid \mathbf{X}) = \Pr(Z = 1 \mid \mathbf{X}, r_T, r_C) = \zeta < 1; \tag{4.16}$$

however, the observable distribution of $(R, Z, \mathbf{X})$ provides no evidence that can justify (4.16). To believe (4.16) on the basis of $(R, Z, \mathbf{X})$ is, at best, wishful thinking; at worst, it is malfeasance.

Proposition 4.3 says that treatment assignment is always ignorable given $(\mathbf{X}, u)$ for $u = \zeta = \Pr(Z = 1 \mid \mathbf{X}, r_T, r_C)$, providing $0 < \zeta < 1$. So, the central problem in observational studies can always be expressed in terms of the single unobserved covariate ζ.

Departures from Ignorable Treatment Assignment: $e(\mathbf{X}) \neq \zeta$

A key way that (4.16) may fail to hold is that

$$e(\mathbf{X}) \neq \Pr(Z = 1 \mid \mathbf{X}) \neq \Pr(Z = 1 \mid \mathbf{X}, r_T, r_C) = \zeta. \tag{4.17}$$

In this case, the difference

$$\mu_T(\mathbf{x}) - \mu_C(\mathbf{x}) = \mathrm{E}(R \mid Z = 1, \mathbf{X} = \mathbf{x}) - \mathrm{E}(R \mid Z = 0, \mathbf{X} = \mathbf{x}) \tag{4.18}$$

of estimable quantities need not equal the expected treatment effect at $\mathbf{x}$, so that adjustments for $\mathbf{X}$ may be inadequate even for the basic task of estimating an average treatment effect $\mathrm{E}(r_T - r_C)$. Here, I say “may be inadequate” rather than “is inadequate” because failure of (4.16) blocks the reasoning that justifies various estimates of $\mathrm{E}(r_T - r_C)$. For instance, it is not logically impossible that mistaken values of $\mathrm{E}(r_T - r_C \mid \mathbf{X} = \mathbf{x})$ for each $\mathbf{x}$ aggregate to the correct value for $\mathrm{E}(r_T - r_C)$; however, without some tangible basis, cancelling biases would be something of a miracle, and inference cannot be hostage to miracles.

It is often unhelpful to think of (4.16) as a condition that either holds or fails to hold, and more helpful to think of the degree to which (4.16) fails to hold. In the case of smoking as a cause of lung cancer, it was found by Jerome Cornfield and colleagues [2] that only an enormous failure of (4.16) could explain the observed association as anything but an effect caused by smoking. It it is often helpful to make such evaluations.

It is useful to quantify the discrepancy between $e(\mathbf{X}) = \Pr(Z = 1 \mid \mathbf{X})$ and $\zeta = \Pr(Z = 1 \mid \mathbf{X}, r_T, r_C)$. Consider two people with the same $\mathbf{X}$, and hence the same propensity score $e(\mathbf{X})$, but different potential responses, (r_T, r_C) and $\left(r_T', r_C'\right)$, and so possibly different values of the principal unobserved covariates, $\zeta = \Pr(Z = 1 \mid \mathbf{X}, r_T, r_C)$ and $\zeta' = \Pr\left(Z = 1 \mid \mathbf{X}, r_T', r_C'\right)$. We say that the bias in treatment assignment is at most $\Gamma \geq 1$ if

$$\frac{1}{\Gamma} \leq \frac{\Pr(Z = 1 \mid \mathbf{X}, r_T, r_C) \times \Pr\left(Z = 0 \mid \mathbf{X}, r_T', r_C'\right)}{\Pr\left(Z = 1 \mid \mathbf{X}, r_T', r_C'\right) \times \Pr(Z = 0 \mid \mathbf{X}, r_T, r_C)} \tag{4.19}$$
$$= \frac{\zeta(1-\zeta')}{\zeta'(1-\zeta)} \leq \Gamma \text{ for all } \mathbf{X},\ (r_T, r_C) \text{ and } \left(r_T', r_C'\right).$$

If $\Gamma = 1$ in (4.19), then treatment assignment is ignorable given the observed covariates; that is, (4.16) holds. For sufficiently large Γ, any value $0 < \zeta = \Pr(Z = 1 \mid \mathbf{X}, r_T, r_C) < 1$ is possible; so, Γ is a yardstick measuring departures from ignorable treatment assignment [18]. The parameter Γ plays a role in Chap. 8.

Departures from Ignorable Assignment: Failure of $0 < \zeta < 1$

A simple way that (4.16) may fail to hold is that $e(\mathbf{X}) = \Pr(Z = 1 \mid \mathbf{X}) = \Pr(Z = 1 \mid \mathbf{X}, r_T, r_C) = \zeta$ but $e(\mathbf{x})$ equals zero or one for some values of $\mathbf{x}$. If $e(\mathbf{x}) = 0$, then r_T is never observed when $\mathbf{X} = \mathbf{x}$, preventing the identification of $\mathrm{E}(r_T - r_C \mid \mathbf{X} = \mathbf{x})$. In parallel, if $e(\mathbf{x}) = 1$, then r_C is never observed when $\mathbf{X} = \mathbf{x}$, preventing the identification of $\mathrm{E}(r_T - r_C \mid \mathbf{X} = \mathbf{x})$. In this simple case, if the population were restricted to $\mathcal{X} = \{\mathbf{x} : 0 < e(\mathbf{x}) < 1\}$, then $\mathrm{E}(r_T - r_C \mid \mathbf{X} = \mathbf{x})$ would be identified for $\mathbf{x} \in \mathcal{X}$, and $\mathrm{E}(r_T - r_C \mid \mathbf{X} \in \mathcal{X})$ would also be identified. Along these lines, practical strategies for dealing with limited covariate overlap are described by Fogarty et al. [4], Crump et al. [5] and Rosenbaum [20].

The situation is more complex if

$$e(\mathbf{X}) = \Pr(Z = 1 \mid \mathbf{X}) \neq \Pr(Z = 1 \mid \mathbf{X}, r_T, r_C) = \zeta.$$

In this case, it could be true that $0 < e(\mathbf{X}) < 1$, yet false that $0 < \zeta < 1$; see Problem 4.3. In this situation, some individuals may be destined for treatment with $\zeta = 1$, and others may be destined for control with $\zeta = 0$, but this may not be evident from the distributions of propensity scores, $e(\mathbf{X})$, in treated and control groups. One approach assumes that $\zeta = 1$ or $\zeta = 0$ is possible, but only for unspecified individuals in a fraction $0 < \eta < 1$ of the population, perhaps $\eta = 1\%$ or $\eta = 5\%$, while (4.19) holds in the remaining $1 - \eta$ fraction of the population [18, §4]. This will be discussed further in Sect. 8.5, and an alternative approach is discussed in Problems 8.4 and 8.5.

4.6 Ignorable Treatment Assignment and Randomization Inference

Suppose that treatment assignment is ignorable given observed covariates $\mathbf{X}$; that is, suppose (4.16) is true, and define $u = \zeta = \Pr(Z = 1 \mid \mathbf{X}, r_T, r_C)$. Then treatment assignment is also ignorable give any balancing score, $\mathbf{b}(\mathbf{X}) = \{e(\mathbf{X}), \mathbf{f}(\mathbf{X})\}$, by Proposition 4.2. Sample IJ individuals using $(Z, \mathbf{X})$ alone to form I blocks of size J, $i = 1, \ldots, I$, $j = 1, \ldots, J$, so that each block is homogeneous in the balancing score $\mathbf{b}(\mathbf{X}) = \{e(\mathbf{X}), \mathbf{f}(\mathbf{X})\}$, with $1 = \sum_{j=1}^{J} Z_{ij}$ for each i.[5] It then follows from (4.16) and Proposition 4.2 that the distribution of treatment assignments, $\Pr(\mathbf{Z} = \mathbf{z} \mid \mathcal{F}, \mathcal{Z})$ is the randomization distribution (2.4); so, all of the methods in Chap. 2 are applicable.

To repeat, saying that the methods in Chap. 2 would be applicable if treatment assignment was ignorable given $\mathbf{X}$ is not at all the same as saying the methods in Chap. 2 are applicable in an observational study. Rather, it says that the possibility that (4.16) is false, and the inability to provide evidence for (4.16) using the observable distribution of $(R, Z, \mathbf{X})$ are what separates a randomized experiment from an observational study. In a randomized block experiment, (2.4) is simply true by virtue of randomization, but nothing like that is available in an observational study.

[5] A more precise statement follows. Write $u = \zeta$. In an infinite population, sample independently I times a $\mathbf{b}(\mathbf{X})$, and each time sample $J - 1$ controls $(r_T, r_C, Z = 0, \mathbf{X}, u)$ from the conditional distribution given $\{Z = 0, \mathbf{b}(\mathbf{X})\}$, and sample one treated individual $(r_T, r_C, Z = 1, \mathbf{X}, u)$ from the conditional distribution given $\{Z = 1, \mathbf{b}(\mathbf{X})\}$. Use random numbers to make up noninformative subscripts $j = 1, \ldots, J$ for these J individuals in block i, so that only variables and not subscripts carry information about people. Create $\mathcal{F} = \{(r_{Tij}, r_{Cij}, \mathbf{X}_{ij}, u_{ij})\}$ and the $I \times J$ matrix $\mathbf{Z}$ containing the Z_{ij}. Note that the sampling ensures that event $\mathcal{Z}$ has occurred. One could alternatively sample $\mathbf{b}(\mathbf{X})$ from its conditional distribution given $Z = 1$, thereby weighting by the distribution of $\mathbf{b}(\mathbf{X})$ among treated individuals. The important point is that the conditional distribution $\Pr(\mathbf{Z} = \mathbf{z} \mid \mathcal{F}, \mathcal{Z})$ is given by (2.4) because of (4.16).

4.7 *Further Reading

This chapter is based on various articles that Donald Rubin and I wrote [15,17,18,21–27].

Problems

4.1 Estimating a Propensity Score Using a Logit Model
In the `iTOS` package in `R`, use the unmatched `binge` data to estimate a propensity score for the "N" or never controls; see Table 4.1. Specifically:

```
library(iTOS)
data(binge)
zN<-rep(NA,dim(binge)[1])
zN[binge$AlcGroup=="B"]<-1
zN[binge$AlcGroup=="N"]<-0
dN<-binge[!is.na(zN),]
zN<-zN[!is.na(zN)]
attach(dN)

propmodN<-glm(zN age+female+education+smokenow+smokeQuit+bpRX+
bmi+vigor+waisthip,family=binomial)

pN<-propmodN$fitted.values
detach(dN)
summary(propmodN)
```

4.2 Proof of Lemma 4.1
Prove Lemma 4.1.

4.3 Overlap for Observed and Unobserved Covariates
Show that $0 < \zeta < 1$ implies $0 < e(\mathbf{X}) < 1$, but the converse is untrue.

4.4 Boxplots of the Propensity Score
Imagine a pair of boxplots of the propensity score, $e(\mathbf{X})$, for treated and control groups, $Z = 1$ and $Z = 0$. Suppose that for some values of $\mathbf{X}$, the propensity score is $e(\mathbf{X}) = 0$ or $e(\mathbf{X}) = 1$. In large samples, will the two boxplots exhibit the same support? (Hint: $e(\mathbf{x}) = \Pr(Z = 1 | \mathbf{X} = \mathbf{x})$.)

4.5 Overlap in the Estimated Propensity Score
Suppose that you compare boxplots of the estimated propensity score, $\widehat{e}(\mathbf{x})$, for treated and control groups, $Z = 1$ and $Z = 0$. In particular, you pay close attention to whether these two boxplots have the same or similar supports. In light of Problem 4.3, what does such a pair of boxplots tell you, and what does it not tell you, about

the corresponding unobservable boxplots of the principal unobserved covariate, ζ? Consider separately two cases: (i) $\widehat{e}(\mathbf{x})$ is a good estimate of $e(\mathbf{x})$ and (ii) $\widehat{e}(\mathbf{x})$ has been over-fitted.

References

1. Austin, P.C., Stuart, E.A.: Optimal full matching for survival outcomes: a method that merits more widespread use. Stat. Med. **34**(30), 3949–3967 (2015)
2. Cornfield, J., Haenszel, W., Hammond, E.C., Lilienfeld, A.M., Shimkin, M.B., Wynder, E.L.: Smoking and lung cancer: recent evidence and a discussion of some questions. J. Natl. Cancer Inst. **22**(1), 173–203 (1959)
3. Cox, D.R.: The Analysis of Binary Data. Methuen, London (1970)
4. Crump, R.K., Hotz, V.J., Imbens, G.W., Mitnik, O.A.: Dealing with limited overlap in estimation of average treatment effects. Biometrika **96**(1), 187–199 (2009)
5. Fogarty, C.B., Mikkelsen, M.E., Gaieski, D.F., Small, D.S.: Discrete optimization for interpretable study populations and randomization inference in an observational study of severe sepsis mortality. J. Am. Stat. Assoc. **111**(514), 447–458 (2016)
6. Frangakis, C.E., Rubin, D.B.: Principal stratification in causal inference. Biometrics **58**(1), 21–29 (2002)
7. Hansen, B.B.: Full matching in an observational study of coaching for the sat. J. Am. Stat. Assoc. **99**(467), 609–618 (2004)
8. Hansen, B.B., Klopfer, S.O.: Optimal full matching and related designs via network flows. J. Comput. Graph. Stat. **15**(3), 609–627 (2006)
9. Haviland, A., Nagin, D.S., Rosenbaum, P.R.: Combining propensity score matching and group-based trajectory analysis in an observational study. Psychol. Methods **12**(3), 247–267 (2007)
10. Joffe, M.M., Rosenbaum, P.R.: Invited commentary: Propensity scores. Am. J. Epidemiol. **150**(4), 327–333 (1999)
11. Manski, C.F.: Identification Problems in the Social Sciences. Harvard University Press, Cambridge, MA (1995)
12. Manski, C.F.: Partial Identification of Probability Distributions. Springer, New York (2003)
13. Neyman, J.: On the application of probability theory to agricultural experiments. Stat. Sci. **5**, 465–472 (1923). Republication in English in 1990 of a paper published in Polish in 1923
14. Pimentel, S.D., Yoon, F., Keele, L.: Variable-ratio matching with fine balance in a study of the peer health exchange. Stat. Med. **34**(30), 4070–4082 (2015)
15. Rosenbaum, P.R.: Conditional permutation tests and the propensity score in observational studies. J. Am. Stat. Assoc. **79**(387), 565–574 (1984)
16. Rosenbaum, P.R.: The consequences of adjustment for a concomitant variable that has been affected by the treatment. J. R. Stat. Soc. A **147**(5), 656–666 (1984)
17. Rosenbaum, P.R.: Model-based direct adjustment. J. Am. Stat. Assoc. **82**(398), 387–394 (1987)
18. Rosenbaum, P.R.: Sensitivity analysis for certain permutation inferences in matched observational studies. Biometrika **74**(1), 13–26 (1987)
19. Rosenbaum, P.R.: A characterization of optimal designs for observational studies. J. R. Stat. Soc. Ser. B Methodol. **53**(3), 597–610 (1991)
20. Rosenbaum, P.R.: Optimal matching of an optimally chosen subset in observational studies. J. Comput. Graph. Stat. **21**(1), 57–71 (2012)
21. Rosenbaum, P.R.: Modern algorithms for matching in observational studies. Annu. Rev. Stat. Appl. **7**, 143–176 (2020)
22. Rosenbaum, P.R., Rubin, D.B.: Assessing sensitivity to an unobserved binary covariate in an observational study with binary outcome. J. R. Stat. Soc. Ser. B Methodol. **45**(2), 212–218 (1983)

23. Rosenbaum, P.R., Rubin, D.B.: The central role of the propensity score in observational studies for causal effects. Biometrika **70**(1), 41–55 (1983)
24. Rosenbaum, P.R., Rubin, D.B.: Reducing bias in observational studies using subclassification on the propensity score. J. Am. Stat. Assoc. **79**(387), 516–524 (1984)
25. Rosenbaum, P.R., Rubin, D.B.: The bias due to incomplete matching. Biometrics **41**, 103–116 (1985)
26. Rosenbaum, P.R., Rubin, D.B.: Constructing a control group using multivariate matched sampling methods that incorporate the propensity score. Am. Stat. **39**(1), 33–38 (1985)
27. Rosenbaum, P.R., Rubin, D.B.: Propensity scores in the design of observational studies for causal effects. Biometrika **110**, 1–13 (2023)
28. Rubin, D.B.: Estimating causal effects of treatments in randomized and nonrandomized studies. J. Educ. Psychol. **66**(5), 688 (1974)
29. Rubin, D.B.: Multivariate matching methods that are equal percent bias reducing, II: Maximums on bias reduction for fixed sample sizes. Biometrics **32**, 121–132 (1976)
30. Rubin, D.B.: Bayesian inference for causal effects: the role of randomization. Ann. Stat. **6**, 34–58 (1978)
31. Stuart, E.A., Green, K.M.: Using full matching to estimate causal effects in nonexperimental studies: examining the relationship between adolescent marijuana use and adult outcomes. Dev. Psychol. **44**(2), 395 (2008)

Chapter 5
Algorithms for Matching

Abstract Concepts of matching are introduced by building three matched samples for the binge drinking example. Each matched sample is a solution to an optimization problem, and each is implemented by finding a minimum cost flow in a network. The third matched sample is judged the best of these three: It pairs closely for important covariates and balances other covariates.

5.1 Matching as Balancing, Matching as Pairing

Beyond Balancing Covariates

Chapter 4 suggested that matching for one covariate, the propensity score, might balance many observed covariates without closely pairing for those covariates. Covariates are balanced if the distribution of covariates after matching is similar in treated and control groups. Close pairing for a covariate is different: It means that in each pair, or in most pairs, the two paired individuals are similar in terms of that covariate. As discussed in Sect. 4.3, it is not possible to pair closely for many covariates, but it is possible to balance low-dimensional summaries of many covariates [58, §3.3].

In addition to balancing many covariates, there are often reasons to pair closely for a few important observed covariates [57]. Pairing closely for a few aspects of $\mathbf{x}_{ij}$ that predict $\left(r_{Tij}, r_{Cij}\right)$ can make a treatment effect stand out more clearly in comparison to background noise, thereby increasing insensitivity to unmeasured biases in treatment assignment [52, 74]. If the magnitude of a treatment effect varies with a covariate—if there is effect modification—then pairing closely for that covariate permits intact pairs with different levels of the covariate to be examined separately, that is, it permits subgroup analyses with intact pairs. If the treatment effect is larger in a subgroup defined by observed covariates, then firmer conclusions

© The Author(s), under exclusive license to Springer Nature Switzerland AG 2025
P. R. Rosenbaum, *An Introduction to the Theory of Observational Studies*,
Springer Texts in Statistics, https://doi.org/10.1007/978-3-031-90494-3_5

may be possible in that subgroup (or, more precisely, the causal inference may be insensitive to larger unmeasured biases in that subgroup [25]). So, covariate balance for many covariates is important, but so is close pairing for a few key covariates.

Quite a bit has been written in recent decades about matching algorithms. The current chapter merely illustrates a few ideas and methods using three examples.

Algorithms for Matching: Three Examples

This chapter compares three matched samples built by optimization algorithms that implement the concepts in Chap. 4. For the binge drinking example in Sect. 1.5, each of the examples pairs the 206 binge drinkers (B) to 206 never-binge controls (N). The first two matched samples control the propensity score and nothing else, but even in this case, the first matched sample is much worse than the second. The third matched sample combines an effort to balance covariates with an effort to form close pairs.

Before explaining how the methods work and how they differ, consider their performance at the first task of balancing covariates. Table 5.1 shows the covariates and their means in the treated group of 206 binge drinkers (B) and in three different matched control groups comprised of 206 never-binge controls (N).[1] You have seen two of these matched samples in earlier chapters. The N controls in Table 1.2 are the "two-criteria" controls in Table 5.1. As seen in Table 1.2, there were substantial imbalances in covariates before matching, but there are only small imbalances after matching. For instance, the binge drinkers (B) were 29% female, the N controls were 59% female before matching, and the N controls were 29% female after matching. The controls in Table 4.3 are the "caliper/fine" controls in Table 5.1, and in terms of covariate balance, they look similar to the "two-criteria" controls.

The match labeled "quintile" in Table 5.1 cuts the propensity score into five groups at its quintiles, each quintile containing 20% of the combined B+N group before matching, and paired people who were in the same quintile. The N controls from the "quintile" match are much closer to group B than was the control group before matching, but the "quintile" match was less successful than the other matches at balancing the propensity score and current smoking.

Table 5.2 shows the counts for current smoking. Notably, the B and N counts are the same for the "two-criteria" match, but are quite different for the "quintile" match where the control group has an excess of nonsmokers.

For the treated group B and the three matched control groups, Fig. 5.1 depicts the distribution of estimated propensity scores. All three matches substantially reduced the difference in the propensity scores. For each of the three matches, the upper quartile of the propensity score among unmatched controls is below the lower quartile of propensity scores in the treated group; so, most of the unmatched N controls are nothing like the binge drinkers (B). Nonetheless, the quintile match did not eliminate

---

[1] The variable labels in Table 5.1, such as age and female, are also used in later tables and are found in the `binge` data in the `iTOS` package in R.

Table 5.1 Comparison of covariate means in three matched samples comparing 206 binge drinkers (B) to 206 controls (N) matched by three different methods, "Quintile," "Caliper/Fine," and "Two Criteria." An asterisk indicates a two-sided P-value from the two-sample t-test less than 0.005, while the absence of an asterisk indicates a P-value above 0.15. Notably, current smoking and the estimated propensity score are out of balance in the "Quintile" match. For "Smoke Now," 1 is "everyday," 2 is "some days," 3 is "not at all"

		Treated	Three Matched Control Groups		
			Quintile	Caliper/Fine	Two Criteria
Covariate	Label	B	N	N	N
Age, years	age	46.8	47.5	46.3	47.2
Female, 1/0	female	0.29	0.27	0.33	0.29
Education, 1–5	educ	3.27	3.35	3.37	3.28
Body-Mass Index, BMI	bmi	29.3	29.8	29.6	29.5
Waist/Hip Ratio	waisthip	0.95	0.96	0.95	0.96
Vigorous Activity, 1/0	vigor	0.53	0.54	0.52	0.53
Smoke Now, 1–3	smokenow	2.02	2.30*	2.04	2.02
Smoked But Quit 1/0	smokeQuit	0.20	0.26	0.17	0.20
Blood Pressure Medication, 1/0	bpRX	0.26	0.29	0.25	0.26
Propensity Score	p	0.15	0.11*	0.15	0.15

Table 5.2 Counts of current smokers in the treated group (B) and the three matched control groups (N). Smoking is poorly balanced in the quintile match and perfectly balanced in the two-criteria match

	Treated	Three Matched Control Groups		
		Quintile	Caliper/Fine	Two Criteria
Covariate	B	N	N	N
Every day	92	66	95	92
Some days	17	12	8	17
Not at all	97	128	103	97
Total	206	206	206	206

the imbalance in the propensity score. The tick marks on the right vertical axis of the plot for the quintile match show the quintiles of the estimated propensity score before matching. Because the top quintile extends from 0.064 to 0.511 and contains 135 of the 206 binge drinkers, the top quintile is too broad to secure adequate control for the propensity score.

*Are t-Tests Useful in Judging Covariate Balance?

The asterisks in Table 5.1 note the P-values from the familiar two-sample t-test for the equality of two means. Two of these P-values are below 0.005, and the rest are above 0.15. The two small P-values are for current smoking and the propensity score in the quintile match. A few comments are needed.

Aside from familiarity, the t-test does not have much to recommend it in this context. Strictly speaking, the usual t-test is not a randomization test, so it is imperfect even as an informal benchmark comparing the imbalance in a covariate to the imbalance expected in a covariate in a randomized experiment.[2] A better approach to benchmarking is discussed in Chap. 6. Also, the t-test can perform poorly relative to other tests when the covariate is not Gaussian [26], and neither the propensity score nor current smoking resembles a Gaussian random variable. Even in a completely randomized experiment, we expect 1-in-20 covariates to exhibit a P-value of 0.05 or less for imbalance when tested using a randomization test; so, the 0.05 standard cannot be quite right for many covariates. Finally, the estimated propensity score was built using the data at hand to distinguish treated and control groups, $Z = 1$ and $Z = 0$, and therefore embodies some degree of over-fitting; so, asking whether the mean age is different for $Z = 1$ and $Z = 0$ is not the same as asking whether the *estimated* propensity score is different for $Z = 1$ and $Z = 0$.

A natural thought—but in my view a mistaken thought—is that a paired test, such as the paired t-test, should be used for covariate balance in matched pairs, not a two-sample test. The difficulty with this is that pairing affects the standard deviation of the pair differences, which may or may not become smaller as the difference in means becomes smaller. It is as if the yardstick is changing length as you measure different things. In Table 5.1, the treated and control means of the propensity score are close for the caliper/fine match (0.15 versus 0.15) but are not close for the quintile match (0.15 versus 0.11). However, in making the means closer, the caliper/fine match also made the standard deviation of the pair differences in the propensity score much smaller, 0.0088 for the caliper/fine match, compared with 0.1210 for the quintile match; so, the caliper/fine match is being held to a standard that is 0.1210/0.0088 = 13.7 times more stringent. The standard deviation of the pair differences for the propensity score in the two-criteria match is in between at 0.0257, even though the means are still close (0.15 versus 0.15). The paired t-test might prefer a match in which the treated-control means are further apart to a match in which they are closer, just because the standard deviation of the pair differences has changed. In principle, covariate balance does not refer to the pairing but rather to the comparability of the marginal distributions of the covariate. Two matched samples with the same imbalance in the marginal distributions of a covariate but different pairing (as in [52,74]) should be judged equivalent in terms of covariate balance, but different in terms of pairing. As will be seen, the pairing for ten covariates is much better in the two-criteria matched sample than in the caliper/fine match even though the standard deviation of the pair difference in the propensity score is larger, 0.0257 versus 0.0088. Indeed, it is better *because* it is larger. The two-criteria matched sample provided excellent balance for the propensity score, as seen in Fig. 5.1, but it worked harder at pairing for individual covariates than did the caliper/fine match, which devoted all of its attention to the propensity score alone. In brief, paired tests fail to distinguish balanced marginal distributions from close individual pairs, so they can send you in the wrong direction when appraising the qualities of a matched sample.

[2] The two sample t-tests were performed by the `t.test` function in the `stats` package in R, which uses the separate variance estimates in the two groups.

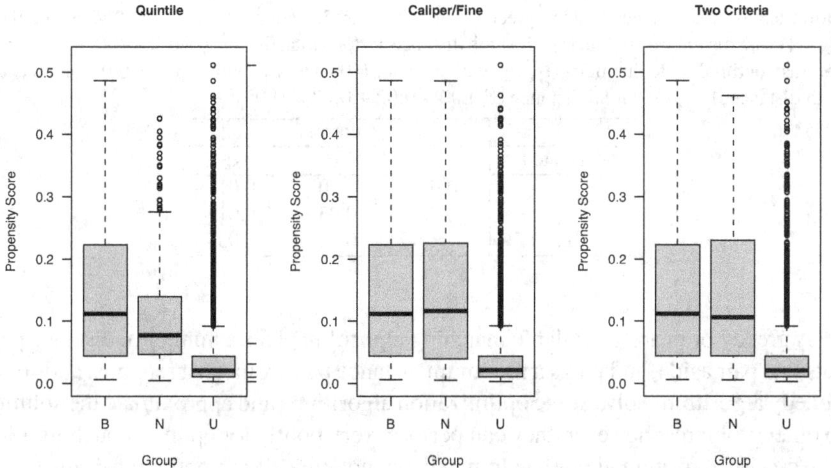

Fig. 5.1 The distribution of estimated propensity scores among binge drinkers (B), matched never-bingers (N), and unmatched never-bingers (U), when matching in three different ways. The tick marks on the right vertical axis of the "Quintile" plot indicate the quintiles of the estimated propensity score for the combined group, B ∪ N ∪ U, before matching. Unlike the other methods, the quintile method has provided inadequate control for the propensity score, largely because most of group B is in the top quintile, which extends from 0.064 to 0.511

5.2 Optimal Pair Matching

What Is Optimal Pair Matching?

In pair matching, the L treated individuals are paired with L distinct controls selected from a reservoir of $M \geq L$ potential controls. In optimal pair matching, there is an $L \times M$ distance matrix, where in row ℓ and column m is a nonnegative number indicating the degree to which treated individual ℓ and potential control m differ in terms of measured covariates.

The distances need not be—and often are not—distances in the topological sense of satisfying the triangle inequality. Infinite distances may be used to forbid certain pairings. Asymmetric distances may be used to oppose the natural direction of the bias: A control 5 years younger than the treated individual may be given a smaller distance than a control 5 years older than the treated individual if the control reservoir tends to be older than the treated group [66].

An optimal pair matching selects L distinct controls, so that the sum of the L within-pair distances is minimized [50]. This optimization problem is standard [5, 6, 30, 31, 44], but not trivial as it calls for the selection of *distinct* controls: You cannot solve it by selecting the minimum distance column in each row, because the same column or control might be selected more than once. There are $M!/(M-L)!$ possible pair matchings, typically an enormous number. Of these $M!/(M-L)!$ pairs, the goal is to find one with minimum total distance.

Table 5.3 In this distance matrix, greedy matching pairs in sequence (t_1, c_2) with distance 0.00, (t_2, c_3) with distance 0.01, and (t_3, c_1) with distance ∞, for a total distance of $0.00+0.01+\infty = \infty$. In contrast, optimal matching pairs (t_1, c_2) with distance 0.00, (t_2, c_1) with distance 0.02, and (t_3, c_3) with distance 0.03, for a total distance of $0.00 + 0.02 + 0.03 = 0.05$

	Controls		
Treated	c_1	c_2	c_3
t_1	0.03	0.00	0.01
t_2	0.02	0.03	0.01
t_3	∞	0.02	0.03

A greedy or nearest-available matching algorithm picks a minimum distance pair, sets that pair aside, and picks a minimum distance pair from what remains, and so on. Greedy algorithms solve some optimization algorithms and approximate the solution to other problems; however, they can perform very poorly for optimal matching [30]. The greedy algorithm yields a pair match, but not typically an optimal pair match. In Table 5.3, the greedy match has an infinite total distance, and the optimal match has a small distance. When there is competition for the same control, the greedy algorithm starts strong with many small initial distances, but it paints itself into a corner, and it must accept large distances later on. Often, there are treated individuals with high propensity scores who lack close controls, and a greedy algorithm may match them last, after all the controls with high propensity scores are taken [59, Figure 4.1].

In the binge drinking example, there are $L = 206$ binge drinkers (B) and $M = 3919$ never-binge controls (N). The distance matrix is 206×3919 with 807,314 distances. There are $M!/(M - L)! = 3919!/(3919 - 206)!$ possible matched samples, an unthinkably large number. It is, however, possible to find almost instantaneously one minimum distance pairing from the $3919!/(3919 - 206)!$ possible pairings by finding a minimum cost flow in a network.[3]

An Optimal Pair Match for the Binge Drinking Example

The quintile match in Table 5.1 and Fig. 5.1 is a simple example of optimal pair matching. Table 5.4 is a 2×6 piece of the 206×3919 distance matrix. In this distance matrix, a zero distance indicates a treated individual and a control who are in the same quintile of the propensity score, as is true for t_1 and c_2. A distance of 1000 indicates a treated individual and a control who are in adjacent quintiles of the propensity score, as is true for t_1 and c_4; that is, 1000 signifies a one-quintile separation. In parallel, distances of 2000, 3000, or 4000 indicate a 2, 3, or 4 quintile

[3] This can be done using Ben Hansen's `optmatch` package in R, which calls the RELAX IV code of Dimitri Bertsekas and Paul Tseng [5, 7]. The RELAX IV code finds a minimum cost flow in a network [6], and is directly available in R using the `callrelax` function in Samuel Pimentel's `rcbalance` package. In the `iTOS` package associated with this book, an optimal pair match is produced by the `makematch` function by setting the right cost matrix to zero, and setting the left cost matrix to the distance matrix.

Table 5.4 A 2×6 portion of the 206×3919 distance matrix between 206 binge drinkers and 3919 never-bingers in the "Quintile" match. A zero distance indicates the same quintile of the estimated propensity score, a 1000 distance indicates adjacent categories, etc. The "Quintile" match paired (t_1, c_6) and (t_2, c_5) contributing $0 + 0 = 0$ to the total within-pair distance

		c_1	c_2	c_3	c_4	c_5	c_6
SEQN		119571	122215	122760	124417	124723	124818
109315	t_1	2000	0	2000	1000	2000	0
109365	t_2	0	2000	0	3000	0	2000

Table 5.5 The first two matched pairs in the quintile match. Here, mset is the matched set indicator, $1, 2, \ldots, 206$. As expected, the pairs are somewhat close on p, but not on individual covariates

SEQN			mset	p	age	female	educ	BMI	waisthip	vigor	smokenow	bpRX	smokeQuit
109315	t_1	B	1	0.02	30	1	4	32	0.92	1	3	0	0
124818	c_6	N	1	0.03	40	0	5	38	0.97	0	3	0	0
109365	t_2	B	2	0.10	49	1	4	32	0.99	0	1	0	0
124723	c_5	N	2	0.07	27	0	2	22	0.87	1	3	0	0

separation.[4] Given that we have already viewed Fig. 5.1, we know that this distance and matching method produces inferior balance for the propensity score than do other methods, but we know this because we have already tried other methods.

Having built an optimal pair match using the method described in the next subsection, Table 5.5 shows the first 2 of 206 matched pairs.[5] These two pairs happen to be from the small portion of the 206×3919 distance matrix that is displayed in Table 5.4: Specifically, t_1 was paired with c_6 for a distance of 0 and t_2 was paired with c_5 for a distance of 0. In fact, every 1 of the 206 pairs had a distance of zero, so the total distance was zero.[6]

The two pairs in Table 5.5 are fairly close on the estimated propensity score (p), but in several other respects, they are quite different. Again, a close pairing for the true propensity score is expected to balance covariates in the matched sample as a whole but not yield a close pairing for individual covariates. For instance, in both pairs, a female binge drinker (B) was paired with a male never-binger (N), even though there are plenty of female never-bingers available to use as controls. Both pairs are mismatched for education and vigorous exercise, and the second pair is mismatched for smoking. In the second pair in Table 5.5, a heavy, middle-aged female smoker who does not exercise vigorously is paired with a light, younger male

[4] In the `iTOS` package in R, the function `addquantile` creates a distance matrix of this form and adds it to an existing distance matrix. The `startcost` function creates an initial distance matrix of zeros.

[5] In Table 5.5 and elsewhere, SEQN is the NHANES identification number for a person. You can use SEQN to locate the eight people in Table 5.5 in the `binge` data in the `iTOS` package in R.

[6] A total distance of zero is not a success given that the propensity score is not balanced in Fig. 5.1. The zero distance tells us that we asked for too little, that the match is optimal for an unambitious objective, and that we should have had a more ambitious objective. In several respects, the "two criteria" match in Fig. 5.1 is a much better match, even though its total distance is larger than zero. The "two criteria" match had a different distance: It imperfectly achieved a much more ambitious objective.

Table 5.6 Counts in propensity score quintiles in the pair match of 206 binge drinkers (B) and 206 never-binge controls (N). The quintile boundaries refer to 206 + 3919 = 4125 individuals before matching. The quintiles exhibit perfect balance, with the same counts in each quintile; that is, the marginal distributions are the same. That is, there is "fine balance." Not seen in this table: Each B-N pair consists of two individuals from the same quintile; that is, individuals are exactly paired for the quintile. Reflecting the nature of the treated or B group, most people are in the top quintile, which extends from 0.0641 to 1.000; so, paired individuals in that top quintile may have very different values of the propensity score

	Quintiles of the Propensity Score Before Matching				
	(0.000, 0.0101]	(0.0101, 0.0179]	(0.0179, 0.0311]	(0.0311, 0.0641]	(0.0641, 1.000]
B	6	8	20	37	135
N	6	8	20	37	135

nonsmoker who does exercise vigorously. Again, all of this might balance out over many pairs, but the individual pairs are not close on several covariates.

Tables 5.1, 5.2, and 5.6 are implicitly critical of the optimal "quintile" match that we have constructed. Indeed, the limitations of this match are evident in Table 5.6 even without comparing this match to the two better matches in Fig. 5.1. Table 5.6 shows that we have indeed perfectly balanced the quintiles of the propensity score. However, the top quintile contains the majority of the B group, 135/206 = 65.5%, in a category that is very broad. The distance matrix regarded everyone with an estimated propensity score above 0.0641 as the same. This explains why this match failed even to balance the propensity score.

Matching should be completed before outcomes are examined [60]. Delaying examination of outcomes means that we may compare several matched designs, as in Table 5.1, and pick the best design, as we would in designing an experiment. Indeed, comparing several designs for an observational study, *before* examining outcomes, is an important step in the design of an observational study. In the illustration in this chapter, we will ultimately prefer the "two-criteria" match in Table 5.1, but it is common to make many small improvements in a matched design rather than taking the two large steps in Table 5.1. For instance, in the "quintile" match, we might fix (i) the problem with the propensity score in Fig. 5.1 by rejecting quintile categories and (ii) the imbalance in smoking in Table 5.2 by including smoking in the distance; then, we would reexamine covariate balance to determine what additional repairs are needed.

The optimal "quintile" match could be fixed in a variety of ways, but to fix something you must first notice that it is broken, know the tools available for repair, and then take action. A better distance matrix would help quite a bit. Even in the first article on propensity score matching [57], Donald Rubin and I compared three distances, concluding that a distance should prioritize fairly close pairing for the propensity score, but should also seek a close pairing for a few key covariates, when possible, using a lower priority distance. The optimal "quintile" match has done neither of these things: The propensity score quintiles are too wide in the treated group, and other covariates are not represented in the distance matrix. In addition to a better distance matrix, modern methods provide additional tools, as discussed in Sect. 5.3 and Sect. 5.4.[7]

Finding an Optimal Pair Matching Using Network Optimization

Figure 5.2 depicts a network used in optimal pair matching. This network has ten nodes, $\mathcal{N} = \{S, s, t_1, t_2, c_1, c_2, c_3, c_4, c_5, c_6\}$, where S is the source, s is the sink, t_1 and t_2 are the treated individuals in Table 5.4, and $c_1, \ldots, c_6$ are the controls in Table 5.4. The actual network used to produce the optimal "quintiles" match has $4127 = 1 + 1 + 206 + 3919$ nodes for the source, sink, 206 treated individuals, and 3919 potential controls.

A directed edge is an ordered pair of nodes, such as (S, t_2), (t_1, c_2), or (c_4, s), all of which are directed edges of Fig. 5.2. If (a, b) is a directed edge, we say it is from a to b. We might draw a directed edge (a, b) as an arrow with its tail at a and its head at b, but I have drawn the edges in Fig. 5.2 as line segments to minimize clutter, with the understanding that every directed edge has its tail on the left and its head on the right, so every edge points to the right. Everything flows from left to right. As undirected edges do not appear in this book, I will speak of an edge rather than a directed edge. In brief, the set of edges $\mathcal{E}$ of a network is a subset of all the ordered pairs of nodes in $\mathcal{N}$, that is, $\mathcal{E} \subseteq \mathcal{N} \times \mathcal{N}$.

The network for pair matching in this chapter has L treated nodes, $t_1, \ldots, t_L$, and M control nodes $c_1, \ldots, c_M$, where $L = 2$ and $M = 6$ in Fig. 5.2. The network also has additional nodes. Figure 5.2 has a source S and a sink s, such that no edge points to S, and s points to no edge; that is, $\mathcal{E}$ contains no edge of the form (a, S) and no edge of the form (s, b). Everything starts at the source S and ends at the sink s.

Finding an optimal match is finding a minimum cost flow, an idea that will now be defined. An edge $e = (a, b) \in \mathcal{E}$ has a capacity κ_e to carry flow, which is a nonnegative integer. In Fig. 5.2, every edge has capacity one, $\kappa_e = 1$ for every $e = (a, b) \in \mathcal{E}$. A flow assigns to each edge $e = (a, b) \in \mathcal{E}$ a nonnegative integer $f_e \geq 0$ subject to several requirements. First, the flow attached to an edge must not exceed the capacity of the edge to carry flow, $f_e \leq \kappa_e$ for all $e = (a, b) \in \mathcal{E}$. In Fig. 5.2, f_e is an integer with $0 \leq f_e \leq 1 = \kappa_e$; so, a flow attaches either a zero flow, $f_e = 0$, or a one flow, $f_e = 1$, to each edge $e \in \mathcal{E}$. We often speak of the total flow

---

[7] Specifically, in 1985 Rubin and I [57] suggested matching using a symmetric caliper on the propensity score together with a Mahalanobis distance computed from a few key covariates. That is a better distance than the quintile distance in Table 5.4. As one would expect, there have been substantial advances in matching since 1985, including the introduction of balance constraints in Sect. 5.3 and Sect. 5.4. However, a very simple but highly effective method for improving a distance matrix is due to Ruoqi Yu [66]. She shows that more bias is removed using a distance with asymmetrical caliper penalties that work against the direction of the bias. Propensity scores are higher and smoking is more common among binge drinkers (B). An asymmetric caliper might then assign a smaller distance to mismatching a nonsmoking B to a smoking N and a larger distance to mismatching a smoking B to a nonsmoking N, knowing that the former are rare and the latter are common.

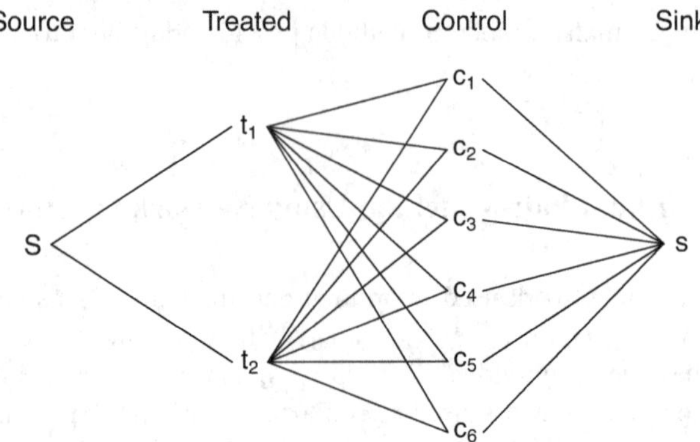

Fig. 5.2 A network for minimum cost pair matching of two treated individuals, t_1 and t_2, to two of six potential controls, $c_1, \ldots, c_6$. Each edge or line segment can carry either 0 or 1 unit of flow, with the source, S, issuing two units of flow, and the sink, s, collecting two units of flow. The edge (t_j, c_k) connecting nodes t_j and c_k has cost given in the distance matrix, and other edges have cost zero. A minimum cost flow picks two edges (t_j, c_k) with distinct nodes to form two matched pairs

into a node $d \in \mathcal{N}$, meaning the total of $f_{(a,d)}$ over all $(a, d) \in \mathcal{E}$, or the total flow out from d, meaning the total of $f_{(d,b)}$ over all $(d, b) \in \mathcal{E}$; here, a or b is varying, but d is fixed. The source S issues L units of flow, meaning the total flow from S to other nodes over edges (S, b) is L, or in symbols $L = \sum_{e\in\mathcal{E}:e=(S,b)} f_e$. In Fig. 5.2, this equality $L = \sum_{e\in\mathcal{E}:e=(S,b)} f_e$ is simply $L = f_{(S,t_1)} + f_{(S,t_2)}$. The sink collects L units of flow, meaning the total flow into s from other nodes over edges (a, s) is L, or in symbols $L = \sum_{e\in\mathcal{E}:e=(a,s)} f_e$. In Fig. 5.2, this equality $L = \sum_{e\in\mathcal{E}:e=(a,s)} f_e$ is simply $L = f_{(c_1,s)} + \cdots + f_{(c_M,s)}$. Aside from the source S and the sink s, a node passes along whatever flow it receives from other edges—the flow is conserved—meaning that, for each node $d \in \mathcal{N} - \{S, s\}$, the total flow into d equals the total flow out from d, or in symbols $\sum_{e\in\mathcal{E}:e=(a,d)} f_e = \sum_{e\in\mathcal{E}:e=(d,b)} f_e$. For instance, in Fig. 5.2, taking $d = c_3$, the flow into c_3 is $f_{(t_1,c_3)} + f_{(t_2,c_3)}$, and the flow out from c_3 is $f_{(c_3,s)}$, so conservation of flow at node c_3 means $f_{(t_1,c_3)} + f_{(t_2,c_3)} = f_{(c_3,s)}$. Notice that all of the requirements in this paragraph that define a flow are of three kinds: linear equality constraints like the conservation of flow constraint, linear inequality constraints like $0 \leq f_e \leq \kappa_e$, and the so-called "integrality" constraints that require each f_e be a nonnegative integer, $f_e \in \{0, 1, 2, \ldots\}$.

Each edge $e \in \mathcal{E}$ has a nonnegative cost per unit of flow, $w_e \geq 0$. In Fig. 5.2, the cost $w_e = w_{(t_\ell,c_m)}$ of the edge $e = (t_\ell, c_m)$ connecting treated individual t_ℓ to control c_m is given by the distance matrix in Table 5.4, and the other edges have $w_e = 0$. The total cost of a flow is $\sum_{e\in\mathcal{E}} f_e\, w_e$. A minimum cost flow f_e, $e \in \mathcal{E}$, meets the requirements (or constraints) in the previous paragraph and, subject to doing that, minimizes the total cost, $\sum_{e\in\mathcal{E}} f_e\, w_e$.

What is the connection between a minimum cost flow and optimal pair matching? Look again at Fig. 5.2 and also at Fig. 5.3. The source S issues L units of flow that must pass over L edges (S, t_ℓ), $\ell = 1, \ldots, L$, each of which has capacity $\kappa_{(S,\,t_\ell)} = 1$ to carry flow; so, every edge (S, t_ℓ) must carry one unit of flow. In Fig. 5.3, the

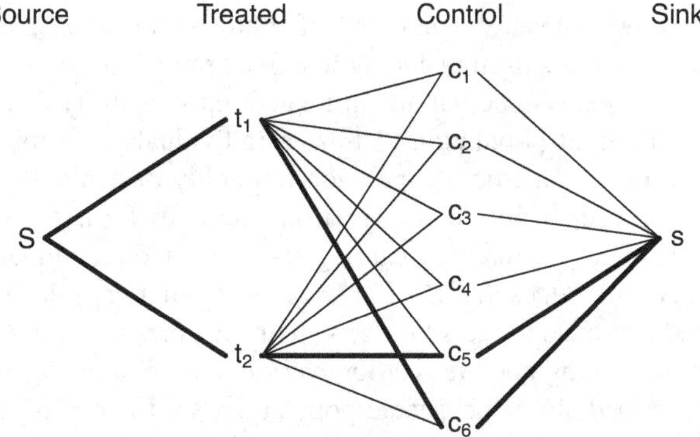

Fig. 5.3 A network for minimum cost pair matching of two treated individuals, t_1 and t_2, to two of six potential controls, $c_{1]}, \ldots, c_6$. The thick lines show a minimum cost flow for the distances in Table 5.4, resulting in the pairing $(t_1,\ c_6)$ and $(t_2,\ c_5)$ with a total cost of $0 = 0 + 0$. In this network, there are $6 \times 5 = 30$ possible pair matches

$L = 2$ edges leaving the source S are both heavy, as they both carry a unit of flow. Because $f_{(t_\ell, c_m)} = 0$ or $f_{(t_\ell, c_m)} = 1$ for every $(t_\ell, c_m) \in \mathcal{E}$, each treated unit t_ℓ must send one unit of flow to one control and zero units of flow to the remaining $M - 1$ controls. In Fig. 5.3, the edges (t_1, c_6) and (t_2, c_5) are heavy, signifying that they carry a unit of flow, $f_{(t_1, c_6)} = 1$ and $f_{(t_2, c_5)} = 1$. Now, control c_m must send all of the flow it receives from treated individuals to the sink s along the edge $(c_m,\ s)$, which has capacity $\kappa_{(c_m,\ s)} = 1$; so, $f_{(c_m,\ s)} = 0$ or $f_{(c_m,\ s)} = 1$, with the consequence that c_m can receive either one or zero units of flow from treated individuals. In Fig. 5.3, $f_{(c_5,\ s)} = 1$ and $f_{(c_6,\ s)} = 1$. Consequently, every one of the L treated individuals t_ℓ is paired with a different control c_m, and we recognize this pairing from the fact that $f_{(t_\ell, c_m)} = 1$ rather than $f_{(t_\ell, c_m)} = 0$. In Fig. 5.3, (t_1, c_6) and (t_2, c_5) are the two matched pairs. Finally, because edges connected to the source or the sink have zero cost, the total cost of the flow, $\sum_{e \in \mathcal{E}} f_e w_e$, is the total of the L within-pair distances. In brief, a minimum cost flow is a minimum distance pairing.

*Obtaining Other Designs by Altering the Network

Small adjustments to the network in Fig. 5.2 provide new options for study design. To obtain a minimum distance match with two controls matched to each treated individual [50, §3.1]: (i) increase the capacity of edges $(S,\ t_\ell)$, $\ell = 1, \ldots, L$ from $\kappa_{(S,\ t_\ell)} = 1$ to $\kappa_{(S,\ t_\ell)} = 2$; (ii) increase the flow issued by the source from L to $2L$; and (iii) increase the flow absorbed by the sink from L to $2L$. To optimally form L_1 matched pairs and L_2 1-to-2 matched sets [50, §3.3], where $L = L_1 + L_2$: (i) Add a second source that issues L_2 units of flow; (ii) connect the new source to each treated individual with an edge of capacity one; and (iii) increase the flow absorbed by the sink from L to $L + L_2 = L_1 + 2L_2$. Problems 5.2 and 5.3 ask you to extend this method to matching with variable numbers of controls and to consider how variable numbers of controls differ from matching in a fixed ratio [39, 50].

Subset matching pairs some but not all treated individuals, typically with a view to describing a different population of treated individuals who might easily have been controls instead. This new population implicitly or explicitly avoids treated individuals whose propensity scores are near one. To form $L^* < L$ minimum distance matched pairs, optimally discarding $L - L^*$ treated individuals [53]: (i) Add a bypass node B with edges (t_ℓ, B), $\ell = 1, \ldots, L$ having capacity $\kappa_{(t_\ell, B)} = 1$ and cost zero; (ii) add an edge to the sink (B, s) with capacity $\kappa_{(B, s)} = L - L^*$ and cost zero; and (iii) increase by one the cost for every treated-control edge (t_ℓ, c_m). The method just described alters the treated population, so it alters the expected effect of the treatment on the treated population [56]. There are several other methods of matching some but not all treated individuals [14, 16], and each method has certain attractive features not shared by the others, although certain methods may be used in combination [45, §6.4.4].

5.3 Optimal Pair Matching with Fine Balance

An Example of Matching with Fine Balance

Section 5.2 tried to accomplish two tasks with one tool, namely, to balance covariates and pair closely for covariates by minimizing a distance between treated individuals and their matched controls. In Sect. 5.3 and Sect. 5.4, these same two tasks employ two tools rather than one. Part of the network is devoted to balancing covariates, ignoring who is paired with whom. Another part of the network is focused on who is paired with whom. This allows us to balance less important covariates while pairing closely for more important covariates. It also allows us to tell the matching algorithm: "balancing a covariate is more important than pairing for it; if you cannot do both, then accept a larger within-pair distance instead of tolerating a substantial imbalance in a covariate." Section 5.3 focuses on fine-balance constraints, while Sect. 5.4 discusses a substantial generalization of fine-balance constraints.

A fine-balance constraint [50, §3.2] forces perfect balance for the marginal distribution of a nominal covariate, perhaps a nominal covariate with many levels. Table 5.6 exhibits fine balance for the quintiles of the propensity score, but this was achieved by pairing exactly for these quintiles.

The current section continues to match solely for the estimated propensity score but makes three improvements in how this is done: (i) better cutpoints for the propensity score; (ii) a fine-balance constraint using those better cutpoints; and (iii) a distance using a caliper on the propensity score. These improvements define the "caliper/fine" match. As already seen in Tables 5.1 and 5.2 and in Fig. 5.1, these three improvements produce a much better match for the propensity score, but also a much better match for current smoking.

Instead of cutting at the quintiles of the propensity score in the B∪N group before matching, the five categories of the propensity are defined by higher cuts that better divide the treated group (B). The four cuts that define the five groups are 0.05, 0.10, 0.15, and 0.20. Table 5.7 shows that the "caliper/fine" match is finely balanced for these five categories. In Table 5.7, 60 binge drinkers (B) and 60 matched controls (N) are in category 5, which comprises 29.1% of the B group. Notably, 42.2% = 29.1% + 13.1% of the treated individuals are in categories 4 or 5, but only 6.3% = 4.0% + 2.3% of the control group was in categories 4 or 5 before matching. Table 5.8 shows that the marginal frequencies in the five categories agree perfectly, but the paired individuals need not come from the same category. The fine-balance constraint paid no attention at all to whether paired individuals came from the same category; that tendency in Table 5.8 was produced solely by the caliper portion of the "caliper/fine" match.

Table 5.7 Categories of the estimated propensity score in the "caliper/fine" match for frequent binge drinkers (B) and never-binge controls (N). The categories are: 1 for [.00, .05], 2 for (.05, .10], 3 for (.10, .15], 4 for (.15, .20], and 5 for (.20, 1.00]

	Counts						Percents					
Group	1	2	3	4	5	Total	1	2	3	4	5	Total
B	58	37	24	27	60	206	28.2	18.0	11.7	13.1	29.1	100.0
Matched N	58	37	24	27	60	206	28.2	18.0	11.7	13.1	29.1	100.0
All N	2990	528	154	89	158	3919	76.3	13.5	3.9	2.3	4.0	100.0

The standard deviation of the estimated propensity score was 0.0718 among all 4125 = 3919 + 206 B or N individuals before matching. The caliper was set at 20% of this standard deviation [57], or 0.0144 = 0.0718 × 0.2. If a treated individual and a control had estimated propensity scores that differ in absolute value by less than 0.0144, then the distance between them is zero. If the absolute difference in propensity scores is at least 0.0144 but below 2 × 0.0144, then the distance is 10; however, if it is greater than 2 × 0.0144, then the distance is 20; see Table 5.9.[8] The "caliper/fine" match *required* perfect marginal balance for the five categories of the propensity score in Table 5.7, and subject to that marginal constraint it *minimized* the total caliper violation using the distances like those in Table 5.9. Balance for the propensity score categories was prioritized as a constraint, but much closer pairing for the propensity score was attempted subject to that constraint.

[8] The two-step caliper is an improvement upon a single-step caliper. If there is no way to avoid violating the narrower caliper, a two-step caliper tries to pick a control who is just a little further away. Multiplying distances by a positive constant yields the same minimum cost flow and the same optimal match; so, distances of 0, 1, and 2 are the same as 0, 10, and 20. Later on, in Sect. 5.4, the magnitude of a distance is used to prioritize several goals. Even in this very simple case, we could have changed the distances to express certain priorities. Had we changed the costs from 0, 10, 20 to 0, 10, 1000, and if violations of the narrow caliper were unavoidable, then the revised distances would have emphasized minimizing the number of violations of the wide caliper while seeking to respect the narrow caliper when possible.

Table 5.8 Tabulation of 206 pairs showing the joint behavior of the propensity score category for the treated individual and the matched control. Notably, the marginal totals are perfectly balanced, as in Table 5.7, but individuals in the same pair may come from different categories

Treated B	Controls N					
	1	2	3	4	5	Total
1	54	4	0	0	0	58
2	4	31	2	0	0	37
3	0	2	22	0	0	24
4	0	0	0	25	2	27
5	0	0	0	2	58	60
Total	58	37	24	27	60	206

Table 5.9 A 2×6 portion of the 206×3919 distance matrix between 206 binge drinkers and 3919 never-bingers in the "caliper/fine" match. The distance refers to the magnitude of the violation of the 0.0144 caliper. The "caliper/fine" match paired (t_1, c_4) and (t_2, c_3), contributing $0 + 0 = 0$ to the within-pair distance. The sinks indicate the category to which a control belongs, and only two of the five categories are represented in this 2×6 portion of the distance matrix

		c_1	c_2	c_3	c_4	c_5	c_6
SEQN		119571	122215	122760	124417	124723	124818
109315	t_1	20	0	20	0	20	0
109365	t_2	0	20	0	20	10	20
sink		s_2	s_1	s_2	s_1	s_2	s_1

Table 5.10 shows the first two pairs in the "caliper/fine" match. They are close on the propensity score. In fact, all 206 pairs were matched inside the caliper, and marginal balance was achieved in Table 5.7; that is, the total within-pair distance was zero, and the marginal distributions in the five categories were identical. As the caliper/fine match gave us everything we asked of it, perhaps we are still not asking for enough.

Often, fine-balance and related constraints are applied with more than five categories; for instance, Samuel Pimentel and colleagues [47] balance 2.9 million categories.

Table 5.10 The first two matched pairs in the "caliper/fine" match. As expected, the pairs are not close on individual covariates, but the propensity score, p, is closer here than in Table 5.5

SEQN		Group	mset	p	age	female	educ	bmi	waisthip	vigor	smokenow	bpRX	smokeQuit
109315	t_1	B	1	0.02	30	1	4	32	0.92	1	3	0	0
124417	c_4	N	1	0.01	25	1	5	26	0.78	0	3	0	0
109365	t_1	B	2	0.10	49	1	4	32	0.99	0	1	0	0
122760	c_3	N	2	0.09	48	0	4	31	0.98	0	2	1	0

Table 5.11 Tabulation of 206 pairs showing the joint behavior of the propensity score category for the treated individual and the matched control, when matching using a propensity score caliper alone, unaided by a fine-balance constraint

Treated B	Controls N					
	1	2	3	4	5	Total
1	58	0	0	0	0	58
2	7	30	0	0	0	37
3	0	3	20	1	0	24
4	0	0	6	20	1	27
5	0	0	0	6	54	60
Total	65	33	26	27	55	206

How Does Fine Balance Improve a Caliper Match?

Does fine balance for propensity categories actually improve the match given that there is a fairly narrow caliper on the propensity score? It is a reasonable question, and the answer is not evident in Table 5.10. Fine balance is a property of marginal distributions, so it is not evident in two pairs.

To see the contribution of fine balance, the match was repeated using the caliper alone. Removing the fine-balance constraint does not increase the minimum total distance—removing a constraint never increases the minimum achieved in a minimization problem—so, the caliper match also matches all 206 individuals within the 0.0144 caliper. Table 5.11 is analogous to Table 5.8, except that Table 5.11 refers to the balance achieved by a caliper match unaided by a fine-balance constraint.

Table 5.11 has two undesirable properties, both of which are avoided in Table 5.8. First, fine-balance is not achieved using the caliper alone: (i) There are 65 controls in the lowest propensity score category, but only 58 treated individuals; and (ii) there are 55 controls in the highest propensity score category, fewer than the 60 treated individuals. By construction, the estimated propensity score tends to be higher in the treated group, as was seen in Fig. 4.1, and the marginal distributions in Table 5.11 show that this tendency has not been completely removed by the caliper alone. In different ways, Fig. 4.1, Fig. 5.1 and Table 5.11 all show that removing the imbalance in the estimated propensity score is possible for the N controls; so, the use of the caliper alone has failed to achieve what can easily be achieved.

The second undesirable property does not refer to the marginal distributions in Table 5.11 but rather to the joint distribution. There are 24 pairs that contain individuals from different propensity score categories, and in 22 of those 24 pairs, the propensity score is higher for the treated individual. The chance that a fair coin would produce either 22 or more heads or 22 or more tails in 24 flips is 0.000036; so, this pattern is not an accident and reflects a degree of residual bias in the propensity score. When pairs are mismatched, the mismatch is almost always in the same direction; more precisely, in $22/24 = 92\%$ of mismatched pairs, the imbalance is in the same direction. This property of the joint distribution was not implied by the marginal distributions in Table 5.11. These 24 pairs could have the mismatch pattern seen in Table 5.11, with all the remaining $182 = 206 - 24$ pairs also mismatched in ways that balance out, so that the marginal distributions are as in Table 5.11. Then, instead of $22/24 = 92\%$ of mismatched treated individuals having higher propensity scores, it would have been $(22 + 182/2)/206 = 55\%$, not far from 50%. For comparison, imbalances cancel exactly in Table 5.8: In 16 pairs, treated individuals and controls belong to different propensity score categories, but in $8/16 = 50\%$, the category is higher for the treated individual.

Fine balance is even more helpful when we are concerned with pairing for other covariates besides the propensity score. The caliper/fine match applied a belt plus suspenders to the propensity score alone, ignoring individual covariates. Sometimes we want to use the belt to ensure close pairing for some covariates and the suspenders to balance all covariates. For instance, we might balance the distribution of the propensity score with between four and ten categories of the propensity score, but not pair for the propensity score, instead pairing closely for a few key covariates thought to predict the outcome or to exhibit effect modification. This could be implemented by replacing the caliper on the propensity score by a different distance.

Minimum Distance Fine Balance by Network Optimization

Figure 5.4 is a network for minimum distance matching with a fine-balance constraint in the case of two fine balance categories [50, §3.2]. In Fig. 5.4, there are two sinks rather than one sink, as in Fig. 5.2. In general, there is one sink for each fine-balance category, or five sinks for the five propensity score categories in the "caliper/fine" match. A control c_ℓ has an edge to the one sink that represents the category to which c_ℓ belongs; see Table 5.9. Where the one sink in Fig. 5.2 collects all $L = 206$ units of flow, the five sinks together collect all $L = 206$ units of flow. Each sink collects flow equal to the number of treated individuals in that category; so, Table 5.7 indicates that sink s_1 collects 58 units of flow, sink s_2 collects 37 units, and so on. This structure constrains the flow to select controls c_ℓ from category k in proportion to the frequency of treated individuals in category k, and subject to doing that, it minimizes the total within-pair distance for matched individuals.

The heavy lines in Fig. 5.4 represent a flow for the individuals in Tables 5.9 and 5.10. As it turns out, c_4 is in propensity category [.00, .05] represented by s_1 in Fig. 5.7, while c_3 is in propensity score category (.05, .10] represented by s_2. In Table 5.10, t_2 has a propensity score that rounds to 0.10, but the pairing in the match would be indifferent to whether t_2 had a propensity score of 0.10001 or 0.99999, because the category boundaries have no direct effect on the pairing.[9]

[9] The construction of the caliper/fine match is reproduced in the documentation for the `binge` data in the `R` package `iTOS`.

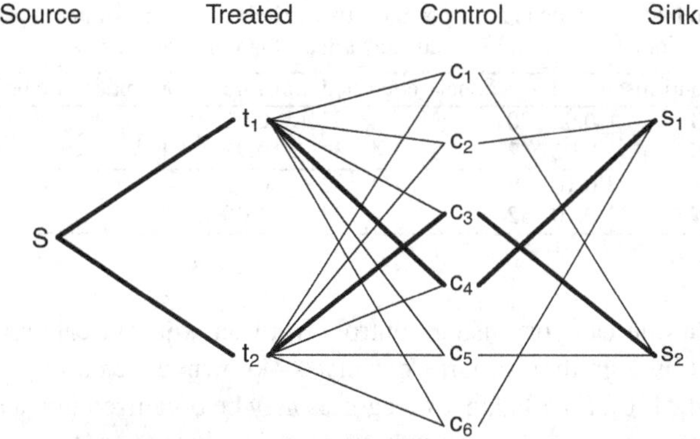

Fig. 5.4 A network for minimum cost pair matching with fine balance. As in Figure 5.2, the source, S, issues two units of flow, but now there are two sinks, s_1 and s_2, that each collect one unit of flow, forcing exactly one matched control to be connected to each sink. The sinks are two fine-balance categories of the propensity score. The heavy edges carry a unit of flow; so, (t_1, c_4) is one matched pair and (t_2, c_3) is another, where c_4 is from fine-balance category s_1 and c_3 is from fine-balance category s_2

5.4 Two-Criteria Matching

Two Distance Matrices, One for Pairing, One for Balance

Two-criteria matching was proposed by Bo Zhang and colleagues [70] as a generalization of both minimum distance matching and matching with fine balance. Unlike minimum distance matching, in two-criteria matching there are two $L \times M$ distance matrices indicating the distance between the L treated individuals $t_1, \ldots, t_L$ and the M potential controls $c_1, \ldots, c_M$. The first distance matrix indicates how we prefer to pair treated individuals t_ℓ and controls c_m. The second distance matrix indicates how we wish to select controls, c_m, ignoring who will be paired to these selected controls. Obviously, the controls we select must be the controls we pair, so selection and pairing are not unrelated, but having selected L of M controls, there are still $L!$ possible pairings.

If the second distance matrix is an $L \times M$ matrix of zeros then, in effect, there is no second criterion, and the result is a minimum distance pair match, as in Fig. 5.2. If the second distance matrix has an infinite distance between a treated individual t_ℓ and a control c_m who belong to different fine-balance categories, then the result is minimum distance match subject to a fine-balance constraint, as in Fig. 5.4. There are many useful variations on this theme, and a few are now briefly mentioned. Sometimes a fine-balance category has more treated individuals than potential controls, so the fine balance constraint has no feasible solution. If the infinite distance is replaced by a large but finite distance, the result exhibits balance that is said to be near-fine, meaning that the constraint is violated to the smallest feasible extent [63]. Fine balance was feasible in Table 5.7, but if it had been infeasible, it is desirable to make

Table 5.12 The first two matched pairs in the "Two Criteria" match. Although paired individuals do differ, they are much closer on individual covariates than in Table 5.10

SEQN		Group	mset	p	age	female	educ	bmi	waisthip	vigor	smokenow	bpRX	smokeQuit
109315	t_1	B	1	0.02	30	1	4	32	0.92	1	3	0	0
122215	c_2	N	1	0.02	42	1	4	30	0.93	1	3	0	0
109365	t_2	B	2	0.10	49	1	4	32	0.99	0	1	0	0
119571	c_1	N	2	0.10	52	1	4	38	1.06	0	1	0	0

up a deficit in one category using controls from an adjacent category, and this is accomplished by a grading of large distances—known as penalties—in the second distance matrix [70]. Fine-balance categories may be organized into a tree structure, so that balance near the root is more important than balance at the leaves [47], and this too can be represented in a second distance matrix. Fine-balance categories may have a nominal factorial structure, and near-fine balance may be imposed by a Hamming distance between factorial categories in the second distance matrix, so agreement on all factors is a distance of zero, disagreement on one factor is a distance of 1000, disagreement on two factors is a distance of 2000, and so on [70]. By using a mixture of large and small penalties, several goals may be pursued at the same time, with larger penalties enforcing priorities.

A Two-Criteria Match of Binge Drinkers and Controls

For quite some time, you have been looking at a two-criteria match of binge drinkers (B) and never-binge controls (N), and sometimes also past binge controls (P); see again Tables 1.2, 5.1, and 5.2 and Figs. 1.6, 1.7, and 5.1. Only in Table 5.2 for smoking did the two-criteria match look better than the caliper/fine match for the propensity score. We are about to look more closely at the two-criteria match, and we will see that it improves upon the caliper/fine match in several ways.

Table 5.12 shows the first two pairs from the two-criteria match. Compare Tables 5.10 and 5.12. In Table 5.10, we see that the caliper/fine mismatched one pair for each of female, education, vigorous exercise, current smoking, and taking blood pressure medication. In Table 5.10, these covariates were matched exactly for both pairs. Of course, these are 2 of 206 matched pairs.

In Table 5.1, both the caliper/fine match and the two-criteria match balanced the mean age, and indeed all of the observed covariates. Table 5.13 compares the caliper/fine match and the two-criteria match in terms of pairing for age in four broad categories. In the caliper/fine match, only 62 of 206 pairs were matched for the age category, but all 206 pairs in the 2-criteria match were matched for the age category. In the caliper/fine match, 6 binge drinkers over 60 years old were matched to controls who were at most 30 years old. Table 5.14 displays the number of exactly matched pairs for several covariates. Throughout Table 5.14, two-criteria matching produced more exactly matched pairs. This is not surprising, because the caliper/fine

Table 5.13 Comparison of the caliper/fine match and the two-criteria match in terms of four age categories. Only 62 = 7 + 21 + 20 + 14 of 206 caliper/fine controls are matched exactly for the age category, while all 206 = 29 + 61 + 67 + 49 2-criteria controls were matched exactly for the age category

	Caliper/Fine Controls N				Two-criteria Controls N			
Treated (B)	(0,30]	(30,45]	(45,60]	(60,∞)	(0,30]	(30,45]	(45,60]	(60,∞)
(0,30]	7	10	7	5	29	0	0	0
(30,45]	14	21	13	13	0	61	0	0
(45,60]	9	19	20	19	0	0	67	0
(60,∞)	6	15	14	14	0	0	0	49

Table 5.14 Number of pairs matched exactly for several nominal covariates in the caliper/fine match and the two-criteria match. Each match has 206 pairs

Match	age4	female	educ	vigor	smokenow	bpRX
Two-criteria	206	206	145	206	206	206
Caliper/fine	62	143	55	109	160	129

Table 5.15 The first (or left or pairing) distance matrix for the two-criteria match. The two-criteria match paired (t_1, c_2) and (t_2, c_1), contributing 0.53 + 0.74 = 1.27 to the total within-pair left distance

		c_1	c_2	c_3	c_4	c_5	c_6
SEQN		119571	122215	122760	124417	124723	124818
109315	t_1	141.03	0.53	20132.25	117.56	10111.08	10019.77
109365	t_2	0.74	137.78	20019.66	232.90	10254.59	10131.10

Table 5.16 The second (or right or balancing) distance matrix for the two-criteria match. Although the left and right parts of the two-criteria match must use the same control group of 206 of 3919 controls, this right distance matrix affects which 206 controls are selected into the match, but not their pairing with the 206 treated individuals

		c_1	c_2	c_3	c_4	c_5	c_6
SEQN		119571	122215	122760	124417	124723	124818
109315	t_1	2006.83	0.38	1004.37	11.54	23.01	14.60
109365	t_2	0.03	2026.51	1005.58	2043.75	2029.29	2045.14

match aimed only for covariate balance, while two-criteria matching aimed both for covariate balance and close pairs.

Tables 5.15 and 5.16 are 2×6 portions of the two 206×3919 distance matrices. Table 5.15 is the first distance matrix, or the left distance matrix, or the matrix used for pairing. It is the sum of several distance matrices with different objectives. The left distance matrix strongly emphasized pairing for female, current smoking, bpRX, and the four age categories, with some attention to vigor and smokenow. In Table 5.14, the pairing is exact for these covariates. Continuous covariates, like age, bmi, and waisthip, also appeared with limited emphasis as continuous variables in a robust Mahalanobis distance [54, §9.3] along with other covariates.[10]

[10] All details of the construction of the two-criteria match for the `binge` data are in the example in the documentation for the `makematch` function in the `iTOS` package in R.

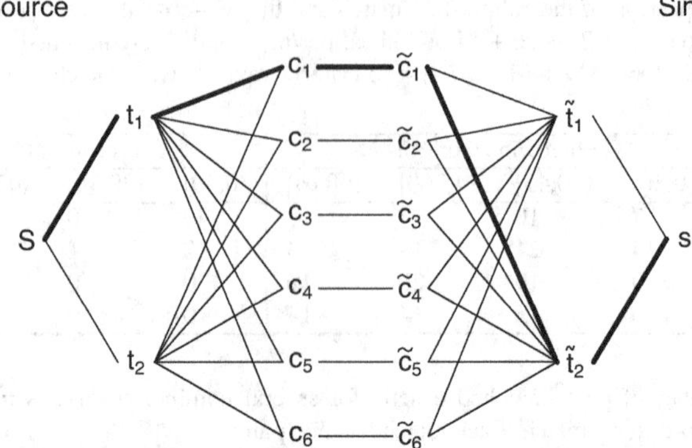

Fig. 5.5 A network for minimum cost pair matching with two-criteria matching. Each treated individual and each control appear twice in this network, with a connection between each control and its copy. All edges can carry 0 or 1 unit of flow. The pairing is defined by a unit of flow connecting t_i and c_j, but c_j must pass that unit of flow to $\widetilde{c}_j$, who must pass it to a $\widetilde{t}_k$ who must pass it to the sink. The heavy lines show the path taken by one unit of flow

In contrast, the right distance matrix affects the selection of controls but ignores who is paired with whom. The mechanics of this are explained in the next subsection, but the method is similar to matching with fine balance. As with the left distance matrix, the right distance matrix was the sum of several distance matrices with different objectives. The right distance matrix had a different emphasis: It strongly emphasized current smoking and emphasized the propensity score, education, and having quit smoking. An asymmetrical caliper tolerated pairing controls with much higher propensity scores than treated individuals but penalized the selection of controls with much lower propensity scores than treated individuals. A robust Mahalanobis distance included just three covariates: the propensity score, age, and sex. Notice that, by using this pair of distance matrices, the propensity score and education influenced which controls were selected into the matched sample, but they had only indirect effects on who was paired with whom.

Two-Criteria Matching as a Minimum Cost Flow

The network for two-criteria matching [70] is depicted in Fig. 5.5. Each control c_m is duplicated as $\widetilde{c}_m$ and an edge $(c_m, \widetilde{c}_m)$ connects each control to its duplicate. The balance categories in Fig. 5.4 are removed and replaced by a second copy of the treated individuals, $\widetilde{t}_1, \ldots, \widetilde{t}_L$, as in Fig. 5.5. The second copies of treated individuals are connected to the sink, s. Every edge $e \in \mathcal{E}$ has capacity one, $\kappa_e = 1$.

A total of L units of flow are emitted by the source S and collected by the sink s, and for all other nodes, flow is conserved. The costs w_e for edges $e = (t_\ell, c_m)$ are given by the left distance matrix, and the costs w_e for edges $e = (\widetilde{c}_m, \widetilde{t}_\ell)$ are given by the right distance matrix. Other edges have cost $w_e = 0$. So, the total cost of the flow is $\sum_{e=(t_\ell, c_m)} w_e + \sum_{e=(\widetilde{c}_m, \widetilde{t}_\ell)} w_e$.

Because there are L treated individuals and L treated duplicates, every edge $e = (S, t_\ell)$ and every edge $e = (\widetilde{t}_\ell, s)$ has flow $f_e = 1$. Because every f_e is 0 or 1, if $f_{(t_\ell, c_m)} = 1$ then $f_{(c_m, \widetilde{c}_m)} = 1$ and there is some $\widetilde{t}_{\ell'}$ such that $f_{(\widetilde{c}_m, \widetilde{t}_{\ell'})} = 1$. Typically $\ell \neq \ell'$; that is, pairing and balancing are separated, with pairing on the left and balancing on the right. The edges (t_ℓ, c_m) with $f_{(t_\ell, c_m)} = 1$ define the matched pairs. The edges $(\widetilde{c}_m, \widetilde{t}_{\ell'})$ with $f_{(\widetilde{c}_m, \widetilde{t}_{\ell'})} = 1$ affect the total cost of the flow and consequently affect the choice of L controls with $f_{(c_m, \widetilde{c}_m)} = 1$; however, the pairing implied by $f_{(\widetilde{c}_m, \widetilde{t}_{\ell'})} = 1$ is ignored when forming matched pairs.

In the binge drinking example, education strongly affected the balancing cost, $\sum_{e=(\widetilde{c}_m, \widetilde{t}_\ell)} w_e$, while the four age categories strongly affected the pairing cost, $\sum_{e=(t_\ell, c_m)} w_e$. This explains why age and education are both balanced for the two-criteria match in Table 5.1, while the pairing for age categories is perfect in Table 5.14 but the pairing for education is imperfect.

Small modifications in the network can accommodate: (i) matching each treated individual to a fixed number of controls, say 2 controls, or (ii) matching an optimally chosen subset of the treated individuals. The modifications are similar to those in Sect. 5.2.

5.5 *Further Reading

Literature Reviews: Several recent reviews of the literature on matching are available [20, 43, 54, 55, 62, 77].

Fine Balance: A compromise between fine balance of a nominal covariate and pairing for that covariate is to seek exact equality in the margins of a table like Table 5.8 while also trying to maximize the total count along its diagonal; that is, off-diagonal counts are minimally tolerated but must perfectly counterbalance one another [75]. Ruoqi Yu [64] examines the increased cost of imposing a fine-balance constraint on an optimal match, concluding that the increase in distance is often small. With some care, it is possible to combine matching with fine balance and matching with a variable matching ratio [49]. Fine balance need not be a hard constraint: if imposed by a distance penalty, it can be gradually relaxed in an effort to also accomplish other goals [46], as briefly illustrated in Sect. 5.4.

Block designs: So far, block designs with multiple control groups, as in Sect. 1.4 and Sect. 1.5, have been built by pairing each control group separately to the treated group. An alternative approach builds treated-first-control pairs for the first control group, then pairs individuals in the second control group to these existing treated-first-control pairs [27, 41]. This topic is related to approximation algorithms for the three-dimensional assignment problem [13]. There are advantages to each approach. The two treated-control differences in covariates are expected to be smaller in the first approach, but the three covariate differences, including the control-control difference, are expected to be smaller in the second approach.

Matching structure: This chapter has emphasized 1-to-1 pair matching, and it has [21] mentioned that 1-to-2 or 1-to-3 matching involves little more than increasing the flow out of the source from L to $2L$ or $3L$. Matching in variable ratio [39,40], such as a mixture of 1-to-1 pairs and 1-to-2 triples, is slightly more complex only because the meaning of fine balance becomes more complex [49]. Another option is full matching in which a matched set may have either one treated individual and one or more controls, or one control and one or more treated individuals [1,17,22,23,51]. Katherine Brumberg and colleagues [11] proposed "triplet matching," in which every matched set contains three individuals, either one treated and two controls, or two treated and one control. Unlike full matching, in triplet matching, there are no pairs. They demonstrate that triplet matching can remove more bias and use more controls than pair matching while also increasing design sensitivity in the sense of Sect. 10.2.

Nonbipartite matching: Matching need not begin with a treated group and a control group. Instead, it can begin with a single group that is optimally subdivided into pairs to minimize the total distance within pairs [19,30,32,35,44]. This method has been used to strengthen an instrument [2–4,15,28,42], to match with doses of treatment [38,69], to form an incomplete block design with three treatments [37], or in risk-set matching [33,34,36]. It is also used in randomized experiments to match before randomization [18].

Integer programming: The minimum cost flow problem is a type of integer program that can be solved quickly. Other forms of integer programming add new options for matching [9,10,12,71,72,74,76]. Bijan Niknam and José Zubizarreta [43] provide an introduction to this large and important topic.

Multilevel matching: If individuals are nested within clusters—for example, if students attend different schools, or patients are treated at different hospitals—multilevel matching pairs similar clusters and similar individuals within those clusters [29,48,72]. Sometimes, a treatment is given to whole clusters, not to individuals [8,24,61]. At other times, a treatment is common in some clusters and rare in others [73].

Matching in large data sets. A matching network for T treated individuals and C controls can have $O(T \times C)$ edges, and that can make optimal matching difficult when

T and C are quite large. Many of these edges represent possible pairs that are quickly seen to be unattractive. Several strategies for optimal matching with fine balance in large data sets try to reduce the number of edges from $O(T \times C)$ to $O(T + C)$ without making the optimization problem infeasible [47, 65, 67, 68].

Problems

5.1 Apply Two-Criteria Matching to the Binge Data
(i) In the `iTOS` package in `R`, run the examples in the documentation for the `makematch` function, thereby creating the `bingeM` matched data in Sect. 1.5 from the unmatched `binge` data.
(ii) Having run the examples, examine the code in these examples. Notice that you build two distance matrices, one for pairing, `left`, and the other for balancing, `right`. For instance, in the code, `left<-startcost(z)` creates a distance matrix of zeros. Also,

```
left<-addNearExact(left,z,female,penalty = 10000)
```

adds a penalty of 10000 to the current distance matrix between any treated individual and any control of different sexes. This penalty will strongly encourage men to be matched to men, and women to be matched to women. Try removing the above "near-exact" penalty and rerunning the match. Notice that `female` also appears in the Mahalanobis distance on both the left and the right.
(iii) Conceptually, in two-criteria matching, what is the difference between:

```
left<-addNearExact(left,z,female,penalty = 10000)
```

and

```
right<-addNearExact(right,z,female,penalty = 10000)?
```

5.2 Minimum distance matching with between 1 and 3 controls
The final subsection of Sect. 5.2 explained how to use a minimum cost flow algorithm to match L_1 treated individuals to one control, and L_2 treated individuals to two controls, where $L = L_1 + L_2$. Suppose that you wanted to match each treated individual to between 1 and 3 controls, in such a way that $L' > L$ controls are included in the match. How should you adjust the network in Fig. 5.2 to obtain a match of this form that minimizes the sum of the within-set treated-control covariate distances?

5.3 Smaller total distances by matching with variable controls
In problem 5.2, suppose $L' = 2L$. In this case, we could match every treated individual to two controls or match with between one and three controls. Consider (a) a minimum distance match in which each treated individual is matched to two controls and (b) a minimum distance match in which each treated individual is matched to between one and three controls.
(i) Why is the total distance in case (b) never larger than in case (a)?
(ii) Suppose that high estimated propensity scores are common in the treated group

and rare in the control group before matching. In case (b), would you expect 1-1 pairs to have high or low propensity scores compared to 1-3 matched sets?

References

1. Austin, P.C., Stuart, E.A.: Optimal full matching for survival outcomes: a method that merits more widespread use. Stat. Med. **34**(30), 3949–3967 (2015)
2. Baiocchi, M., Kang, H.: Matching with instrumental variables. In: Zubizarreta, J.R., Stuart, E.A., Small, D.S., Rosenbaum, P.R. (eds.) Handbook of Matching and Weighting Adjustments for Causal Inference, pp. 135–152. Chapman and Hall/CRC, Boca Raton (2023)
3. Baiocchi, M., Small, D.S., Lorch, S., Rosenbaum, P.R.: Building a stronger instrument in an observational study of perinatal care for premature infants. J. Am. Stat. Assoc. **105**(492), 1285–1296 (2010)
4. Baiocchi, M., Small, D.S., Yang, L., Polsky, D., Groeneveld, P.W.: Near/far matching: a study design approach to instrumental variables. Health Services Outcomes Res. Methodol. **12**, 237–253 (2012)
5. Bertsekas, D.P.: A new algorithm for the assignment problem. Math. Program. **21**(1), 152–171 (1981)
6. Bertsekas, D.P.: Linear Network Optimization. MIT Press, Cambridge (1991)
7. Bertsekas, D.P., Tseng, P.: The relax codes for linear minimum cost network flow problems. Ann. Oper. Res. **13**(1), 125–190 (1988)
8. Bruce, M.L., Ten Have, T.R., Reynolds III, C.F., Katz, I.I., Schulberg, H.C., Mulsant, B.H., Brown, G.K., McAvay, G.J., Pearson, J.L., Alexopoulos, G.S.: Reducing suicidal ideation and depressive symptoms in depressed older primary care patients: a randomized controlled trial. J. Am. Med. Assoc. **291**(9), 1081–1091 (2004)
9. Brumberg, K., Ellis, D.E., Small, D.S., Hennessy, S., Rosenbaum, P.R.: Using natural strata when examining unmeasured biases in an observational study of neurological side effects of antibiotics. J. Roy. Stat. Soc. C (Applied Statistics) **72**(2), 314–329 (2023)
10. Brumberg, K., Small, D.S., Rosenbaum, P.R.: Using randomized rounding of linear programs to obtain unweighted natural strata that balance many covariates. J. Roy. Stat. Soc. A **185**(4), 1931–1951 (2022)
11. Brumberg, K., Small, D.S., Rosenbaum, P.R.: A new design for observational studies applied to the study of the effects of high school football on cognition late in life. Ann. Appl. Stat. **18**, 3507–3527 (2024)
12. Brumberg, K., Small, D.S., Rosenbaum, P.R.: Optimal refinement of strata to balance covariates. Biometrics **80**(3) (2024). https://doi.org/10.1093/biomtc/ujae061
13. Crama, Y., Spieksma, F.C.: Approximation algorithms for three-dimensional assignment problems with triangle inequalities. Eur. J. Oper. Res. **60**(3), 273–279 (1992)
14. Crump, R.K., Hotz, V.J., Imbens, G.W., Mitnik, O.A.: Dealing with limited overlap in estimation of average treatment effects. Biometrika **96**(1), 187–199 (2009)
15. Ertefaie, A., Small, D.S., Rosenbaum, P.R.: Quantitative evaluation of the trade-off of strengthened instruments and sample size in observational studies. J. Am. Stat. Assoc. **113**(523), 1122–1134 (2018)
16. Fogarty, C.B., Mikkelsen, M.E., Gaieski, D.F., Small, D.S.: Discrete optimization for interpretable study populations and randomization inference in an observational study of severe sepsis mortality. J. Am. Stat. Assoc. **111**(514), 447–458 (2016)
17. Fredrickson, M.M., Hansen, B.B.: Optimal full matching. In: Zubizarreta, J.R., Stuart, E.A., Small, D.S., Rosenbaum, P.R. (eds.) Handbook of Matching and Weighting Adjustments for Causal Inference, pp. 87–104. Chapman and Hall/CRC, Boca Raton (2023)
18. Greevy, R., Lu, B., Silber, J.H., Rosenbaum, P.: Optimal multivariate matching before randomization. Biostatistics **5**(2), 263–275 (2004)

19. Greevy, R.A., Lu, B.: Optimal nonbipartite matching. In: Zubizarreta, J.R., Stuart, E.A., Small, D.S., Rosenbaum, P.R. (eds.) Handbook of Matching and Weighting Adjustments for Causal Inference, pp. 227–238. Chapman and Hall/CRC, Boca Raton (2023)
20. Greifer, N., Stuart, E.A.: Matching methods for confounder adjustment: an addition to the epidemiologist's toolbox. Epidemiol. Rev. **43**(1), 118–129 (2021)
21. Gu, X.S., Rosenbaum, P.R.: Comparison of multivariate matching methods: Structures, distances, and algorithms. J. Comput. Graph. Stat. **2**(4), 405–420 (1993)
22. Hansen, B.B.: Full matching in an observational study of coaching for the sat. J. Am. Stat. Assoc. **99**(467), 609–618 (2004)
23. Hansen, B.B., Klopfer, S.O.: Optimal full matching and related designs via network flows. J. Comput. Graph. Stat. **15**(3), 609–627 (2006)
24. Hansen, B.B., Rosenbaum, P.R., Small, D.S.: Clustered treatment assignments and sensitivity to unmeasured biases in observational studies. J. Am. Stat. Assoc. **109**(505), 133–144 (2014)
25. Hsu, J., Small, D., Rosenbaum, P.R.: Effect modification and design sensitivity in observational studies. J. Am. Stat. Assoc. **108**(501), 135–148 (2013)
26. Jones, D.H., Sethuraman, J.: Bahadur efficiencies of the student's t-tests. Annals of Statistics, pp. 559–566 (1978)
27. Karmakar, B., Small, D.S., Rosenbaum, P.R.: Using approximation algorithms to build evidence factors and related designs for observational studies. J. Comput. Graph. Stat. **28**(3), 698–709 (2019)
28. Keele, L., Harris, S., Pimentel, S.D., Grieve, R.: Stronger instruments and refined covariate balance in an observational study of the effectiveness of prompt admission to intensive care units. J. Roy. Stat. Soc. Ser. A **183**(4), 1501–1521 (2020)
29. Keele, L., Pimentel, S.D.: Matching with multilevel data. In: Zubizarreta, J.R., Stuart, E.A., Small, D.S., Rosenbaum, P.R. (eds.) Handbook of Matching and Weighting Adjustments for Causal Inference, pp. 185–204. Chapman and Hall/CRC, Boca Raton (2023)
30. Korte, B.H., Vygen, J.: Combinatorial Optimization, 5th edn. Springer, Berlin (2012)
31. Kuhn, H.W.: The Hungarian method for the assignment problem. Naval Res. Logist. Q. **2**(1-2), 83–97 (1955)
32. Lawler, E.L.: Combinatorial Optimization: Networks and Matroids. Dover, Mineola (2001)
33. Li, Y.P., Propert, K.J., Rosenbaum, P.R.: Balanced risk set matching. J. Am. Stat. Assoc. **96**(455), 870–882 (2001)
34. Lu, B.: Propensity score matching with time-dependent covariates. Biometrics **61**(3), 721–728 (2005)
35. Lu, B., Greevy, R., Xu, X., Beck, C.: Optimal nonbipartite matching and its statistical applications. Am. Stat. **65**(1), 21–30 (2011)
36. Lu, B., Greevy, R.A.: Risk set matching. In: Zubizarreta, J.R., Stuart, E.A., Small, D.S., Rosenbaum, P.R. (eds.) Handbook of Matching and Weighting Adjustments for Causal Inference, pp. 169–184. Chapman and Hall/CRC, Boca Raton (2023)
37. Lu, B., Rosenbaum, P.R.: Optimal pair matching with two control groups. J. Comput. Graph. Stat. **13**(2), 422–434 (2004)
38. Lu, B., Zanutto, E., Hornik, R., Rosenbaum, P.R.: Matching with doses in an observational study of a media campaign against drug abuse. J. Am. Stat. Assoc. **96**(456), 1245–1253 (2001)
39. Ming, K., Rosenbaum, P.R.: Substantial gains in bias reduction from matching with a variable number of controls. Biometrics **56**(1), 118–124 (2000)
40. Ming, K., Rosenbaum, P.R.: A note on optimal matching with variable controls using the assignment algorithm. J. Comput. Graph. Stat. **10**(3), 455–463 (2001)
41. Nattino, G., Lu, B., Shi, J., Lemeshow, S., Xiang, H.: Triplet matching for estimating causal effects with three treatment arms: a comparative study of mortality by trauma center level. J. Am. Stat. Assoc. **116**(533), 44–53 (2021)
42. Neuman, M.D., Rosenbaum, P.R., Ludwig, J.M., Zubizarreta, J.R., Silber, J.H.: Anesthesia technique, mortality, and length of stay after hip fracture surgery. J. Am. Med. Assoc. **311**(24), 2508–2517 (2014)
43. Niknam, B.A., Zubizarreta, J.R.: Using cardinality matching to design balanced and representative samples for observational studies. J. Am. Med. Assoc. **327**(2), 173–174 (2022)

44. Papadimitriou, C.H., Steiglitz, K.: Combinatorial Optimization: Algorithms and Complexity. Prentice Hall, Englewood Cliffs (1982)
45. Pimentel, S.D.: Fine balance and its variations in modern optimal matching. In: Zubizarreta, J.R., Stuart, E.A., Small, D.S., Rosenbaum, P.R. (eds.) Handbook of Matching and Weighting Adjustments for Causal Inference, pp. 105–134. Chapman and Hall/CRC, Boca Raton (2023)
46. Pimentel, S.D., Kelz, R.R.: Optimal tradeoffs in matched designs comparing US-trained and internationally-trained surgeons. J. Am. Stat. Assoc. **115**(532), 1675–1688 (2020)
47. Pimentel, S.D., Kelz, R.R., Silber, J.H., Rosenbaum, P.R.: Large, sparse optimal matching with refined covariate balance in an observational study of the health outcomes produced by new surgeons. J. Am. Stat. Assoc. **110**(510), 515–527 (2015)
48. Pimentel, S.D., Page, L.C., Lenard, M., Keele, L.: Optimal multilevel matching using network flows: an application to a summer reading intervention. Ann. Appl. Stat. **12**(3), 1479–1505 (2018)
49. Pimentel, S.D., Yoon, F., Keele, L.: Variable-ratio matching with fine balance in a study of the peer health exchange. Stat. Med. **34**(30), 4070–4082 (2015)
50. Rosenbaum, P.R.: Optimal matching for observational studies. J. Am. Stat. Assoc. **84**(408), 1024–1032 (1989)
51. Rosenbaum, P.R.: A characterization of optimal designs for observational studies. J. Roy. Stat. Soc. Ser. B (Methodological) **53**(3), 597–610 (1991)
52. Rosenbaum, P.R.: Heterogeneity and causality: Unit heterogeneity and design sensitivity in observational studies. Am. Stat. **59**(2), 147–152 (2005)
53. Rosenbaum, P.R.: Optimal matching of an optimally chosen subset in observational studies. J. Comput. Graph. Stat. **21**(1), 57–71 (2012)
54. Rosenbaum, P.R.: Design of Observational Studies, 2nd edn. Springer, New York (2020)
55. Rosenbaum, P.R.: Modern algorithms for matching in observational studies. Ann. Rev. Stat. Appl. **7**, 143–176 (2020)
56. Rosenbaum, P.R., Rubin, D.B.: The bias due to incomplete matching. Biometrics **41**, 103–116 (1985)
57. Rosenbaum, P.R., Rubin, D.B.: Constructing a control group using multivariate matched sampling methods that incorporate the propensity score. Am. Stat. **39**(1), 33–38 (1985)
58. Rosenbaum, P.R., Rubin, D.B.: Propensity scores in the design of observational studies for causal effects. Biometrika **110**, 1–13 (2023)
59. Rosenbaum, P.R., Zubizarreta, J.R.: Optimization techniques in multivariate matching. In: Zubizarreta, J.R., Stuart, E.A., Small, D.S., Rosenbaum, P.R. (eds.) Handbook of Matching and Weighting Adjustments for Causal Inference, pp. 63–86. Chapman and Hall/CRC, Boca Raton (2023)
60. Rubin, D.B.: The design versus the analysis of observational studies for causal effects: parallels with the design of randomized trials. Stat. Med. **26**(1), 20–36 (2007)
61. Small, D.S., Ten Have, T.R., Rosenbaum, P.R.: Randomization inference in a group–randomized trial of treatments for depression: covariate adjustment, noncompliance, and quantile effects. J. Am. Stat. Assoc. **103**(481), 271–279 (2008)
62. Stuart, E.A.: Matching methods for causal inference: A review and a look forward. Stat. Sci. **25**(1), 1 (2010)
63. Yang, D., Small, D.S., Silber, J.H., Rosenbaum, P.R.: Optimal matching with minimal deviation from fine balance in a study of obesity and surgical outcomes. Biometrics **68**(2), 628–636 (2012)
64. Yu, R.: How well can fine balance work for covariate balancing? Biometrics **79**, 2346–2356 (2023)
65. Yu, R.: Matching methods for large observational studies. In: Zubizarreta, J.R., Stuart, E.A., Small, D.S., Rosenbaum, P.R. (eds.) Handbook of Matching and Weighting Adjustments for Causal Inference, pp. 239–260. Chapman and Hall/CRC, Boca Raton (2023)
66. Yu, R., Rosenbaum, P.R.: Directional penalties for optimal matching in observational studies. Biometrics **75**(4), 1380–1390 (2019)
67. Yu, R., Rosenbaum, P.R.: Graded matching for large observational studies. J. Comput. Graph. Stat. **31**(4), 1406–1415 (2022)

68. Yu, R., Silber, J.H., Rosenbaum, P.R.: Matching methods for observational studies derived from large administrative databases (with Discussion). Stat. Sci. **35**(3), 338–355 (2020)
69. Zhang, B., Mackay, E.J., Baiocchi, M.: Statistical matching and subclassification with a continuous dose: characterization, algorithm, and application to a health outcomes study. Ann. Appl. Stat. **17**(1), 454–475 (2023)
70. Zhang, B., Small, D.S., Lasater, K.B., McHugh, M., Silber, J.H., Rosenbaum, P.R.: Matching one sample according to two criteria in observational studies. J. Am. Stat. Assoc. **118**, 1140–1151 (2022)
71. Zubizarreta, J.R.: Using mixed integer programming for matching in an observational study of kidney failure after surgery. J. Am. Stat. Assoc. **107**(500), 1360–1371 (2012)
72. Zubizarreta, J.R., Keele, L.: Optimal multilevel matching in clustered observational studies: a case study of the effectiveness of private schools under a large-scale voucher system. J. Am. Stat. Assoc. **112**(518), 547–560 (2017)
73. Zubizarreta, J.R., Neuman, M., Silber, J.H., Rosenbaum, P.R.: Contrasting evidence within and between institutions that provide treatment in an observational study of alternate forms of anesthesia. J. Am. Stat. Assoc. **107**(499), 901–915 (2012)
74. Zubizarreta, J.R., Paredes, R.D., Rosenbaum, P.R.: Matching for balance, pairing for heterogeneity in an observational study of the effectiveness of for-profit and not-for-profit high schools in Chile. Ann. Appl. Stat. **8**(1), 204–231 (2014)
75. Zubizarreta, J.R., Reinke, C.E., Kelz, R.R., Silber, J.H., Rosenbaum, P.R.: Matching for several sparse nominal variables in a case-control study of readmission following surgery. Am. Stat. **65**(4), 229–238 (2011)
76. Zubizarreta, J.R., Small, D.S., Goyal, N.K., Lorch, S., Rosenbaum, P.R.: Stronger instruments via integer programming in an observational study of late preterm birth outcomes. Ann. Appl. Stat. **7**, 25–50 (2013)
77. Zubizarreta, J.R., Stuart, E.A., Small, D.S., Rosenbaum, P.R.: Handbook of Matching and Weighting Adjustments for Causal Inference. Chapman and Hall/CRC Press (2023)

Chapter 6
Evaluating the Balance of Observed Covariates

Abstract Several recent articles by Brumberg et al. (Biometrics 80(3) 2024), Hansen and Bowers (Stat Sci 23:219–236, 2008), Pimentel et al. (J Am Stat Assoc 110(510):515–527, 2015), and Yu (Biometrics 77(4)L1276–1288, 2021) have suggested comparing the covariate balance in a pair-matched or 1-to-K matched sample to the covariate balance in simulated completely randomized experiments built from the same covariate data. This technique is illustrated and discussed.

6.1 A Benchmark for Covariate Balance

What Benchmarks Can and Cannot Do

A benchmark does not tell you what to do; rather, it provides you with something to consider as you decide what to do.

Suppose that you are trying to decide between two options. You could spend the next 4 years training for the 100-meter dash at the Olympics. Or, you can spend the next 4 years working toward a BA degree in computer science. You would, of course, think about how fast you can run and about whether you enjoy computer programming. However, one of several useful benchmarks is that Usain Bolt ran the 100-meter dash at the 2012 Olympics in 9.65 seconds [2]. That is something to consider as you decide.

An important decision in designing a matched sample is when to stop trying to improve covariate balance. It is almost always the case that you are dissatisfied with your initial attempt to construct a matched sample, and that small changes in the match quickly produce meaningful improvements. After a while, an improvement here is offset by a degradation there. When do you stop?

We know that it is impossible to match exactly for many covariates; so, whether or not you have matched exactly for many covariates is not a useful benchmark.

© The Author(s), under exclusive license to Springer Nature Switzerland AG 2025
P. R. Rosenbaum, *An Introduction to the Theory of Observational Studies*,
Springer Texts in Statistics, https://doi.org/10.1007/978-3-031-90494-3_6

Matching is often implemented by optimizing some criterion or other. We know that we can always optimize a criterion; so, successfully optimizing a criterion is not a useful benchmark either. What you can never do, and what you can always do, are not useful benchmarks. If you are trying to decide whether you have what it takes for an Olympic 100-meter dash, it is not useful to focus on your inability to run 100 meters in half a second, nor on your commitment to running as fast as you can.

So, at the least, a useful benchmark is neither impossible nor tautological. Also, it is a consideration worthy of your attention as you make your decision. That decision will often weigh several incommensurate considerations that are all worthy of your attention.

Optimal Procedures and Situations as Benchmarks

In modern statistical theory, optimal statistical procedures and research designs serve as benchmarks. Given n independent observations from a Normal distribution with expectation μ and variance σ^2, the sample mean is the optimal estimator of the center of symmetry of the distribution of those observations, and it has variance σ^2/n. As you consider other estimators of the center of symmetry of the distribution of those observations, the variance of the mean, σ^2/n, is a useful benchmark: It is possible to achieve it, but most estimators neither achieve it nor come close.

If the mean is optimal, then why consider other estimators? The mean is optimal if the data are from a Normal distribution, but you can never be certain the data are from a Normal distribution. The mean is not robust to small departures from the Normal distribution [1]. A benchmark might help you evaluate a robust estimator of the center of symmetry of a symmetric unimodal distribution. For example, you might usefully compare this estimator's variance when applied to Normal data to the optimal benchmark in this situation, namely, σ^2/n. For instance, the Hodges-Lehmann [9, 15] estimator is robust, yet it is almost as efficient as the mean for Normal data.

One Benchmark for Covariate Balance

We have been considering observational block designs with I blocks of size J, with one treated individual and $J-1$ controls. From Chap. 2, you know that a completely randomized experiment, had it been feasible, would have been better as a study design than using matching to form blocks in an effort to fix imbalances in covariates in the absence of randomization. Balance for observed covariates is only a small part of this "better," but nonetheless large randomized trials are quite remarkable at balancing many observed covariates [21, §3.3]. This suggests one benchmark.

Complete randomization produces a degree of balance in observed covariates. Suppose that we took IJ people and picked I people at random, calling them group

$G = 1$, and defined group $G = 0$ to be the remaining $I(J - 1)$ people. That would produce a degree of imbalance in the observed covariates $\mathbf{x}_{ij}$. We could use those same IJ people but pick another I people at random, creating another complementary group of $I(J - 1)$ people. We could do that many times. Each time, we would see one realization of the imbalance in observed covariates that is produced by complete randomization. So that is a fixed benchmark, like an Olympic record. How does the imbalance in observed covariates in the observational block design compare with the imbalance that randomization would have produced had the same IJ people been in a completely randomized experiment?

Why is this a reasonable benchmark? First, it is not tautological. We may have optimized a criterion to produce a matched sample, but that alone tells us nothing about how the observational block design compares with complete randomization. To know how the covariate balance in the observational study compares with the benchmark, you have to look at the observational study and at the benchmark.

Second, this benchmark does not ask for a kind of covariate balance that is simply impossible. The covariate imbalance produced by complete randomization of IJ people is possible, because randomization does produce it. This benchmark is unlike the impossible goal of matching exactly for many covariates.

Third, the benchmark is not theoretical, not about what would happen with multivariate Normal covariates or whatever. The benchmark is about the covariate balance that is possible with the IJ people under study, and with their covariates, $\mathbf{x}_{ij}$.

Fourth, by definition, covariate balance refers to the distribution of covariates in treated and control groups, not to who is paired with whom. This benchmark also refers to the distribution of covariates in treated and control groups, not to who is paired with whom. A benchmark that is affected by who is paired with whom may be a benchmark for something, but it is not a benchmark for covariate balance.[1]

Assessing covariate balance by comparing a match to repeated randomizations has been proposed, in various forms, by Katherine Brumberg and colleagues [5], Ben Hansen and Jake Bowers, [8] Samuel Pimentel and colleagues [18], and Ruoqi Yu [24]. The current chapter is a brief illustration of their ideas.

The covariate balance produced by randomization is a useful, objective benchmark, nothing more. The use of this benchmark is not unlike the use of regression diagnostics [7] to check whether a linear model is adequate, and, if not, to improve it. In Chap. 5, the quintile match proved inadequate but was substantially improved by the two-criteria match, and an objective, empirical benchmark is helpful in making such comparisons.

There is no guarantee that adequate pair matching is achievable at all, by any method [22, 23]; see the discussion of Fig. 4.1 in Sect. 4.2. Conversely, even randomization produces small imbalances in observed covariates.

[1] Of course, one might also want to evaluate the quality of the pairing, but for that other benchmarks are needed. Pairing serves several purposes unrelated to covariate balance, including aiding the study of effect modification [10, 13, 14], and decreasing heterogeneity of responses as a way to increase insensitivity to unmeasured biases [20, 27].

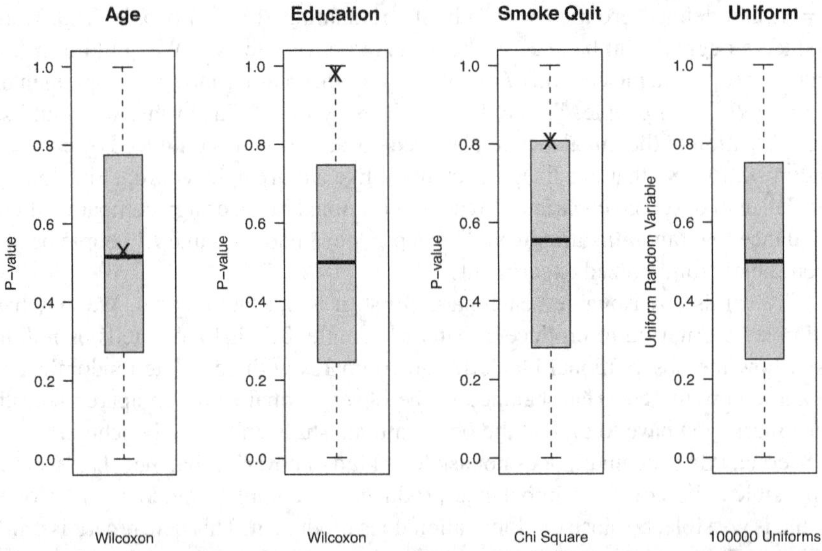

Fig. 6.1 Balance in the matched sample (X) compared with 1000 randomized experiments. For age in years and the five integer values of education, the Wilcoxon rank sum test is used to evaluate balance, but for the binary variable `smokeQuit`, the chi square test is used. The final boxplot shows 100000 uniform random variables

6.2 Covariate Balance in the Binge Drinking Match

Many Randomized Experiments with the Observed Covariates

Covariate balance will be evaluated for the two-criteria match in Sect. 5.4 of the binge drinking data. As an illustration, the binge drinking group will be compared to the combination of the never binge group and the past binge group; so, $J = 3$ in this example.[2]

The $IJ = 206 \times 3 = 618$ matched individuals are randomly split into a group of $I = 206$ individuals with $G = 1$ and a group of $I(J-1) = 412$ individuals with $G = 0$. This random split ignores both the 206 blocks and the identity of the treated individual in each block. This random split might have defined the treated and control groups in a completely randomized experiment with 206 treated individuals and 412 controls.

Ignoring the block structure, the marginal covariate balance produced in the actual matched sample is compared to the 1000 randomized experiments.

[2] The calculations are replicated for the example in the documentation for the `evalBal` function in the iTOS package, except you must increase the `reps` parameter from its default to 1000. That example also checks the balance for one control group, namely, past binge drinkers.

Looking at Covariates One at a Time

For age recorded in years, the two-sample Wilcoxon rank sum test is computed 1001 times, once for the matched block design ignoring the blocks, and then from the 1000 randomized experiments. The usual two-sided P-value is computed and plotted in the first boxplot in Fig. 6.1, where X indicates the value for the actual matched block design, and the boxplot indicates the 1000 values for the 1000 randomized experiments. As the Wilcoxon rank sum test is a randomization test, it is not surprising that the boxplot of P-values resembles the uniform distribution in the fourth boxplot in Fig. 6.1. The X is close to the median P-value for the 1000 randomized experiments; so, the imbalance in age resembles that expected from complete randomization.

Figure 6.1 also shows P-values from the Wilcoxon test for the heavily tied one-to-five categories of education, and P-values from the chi-square test for a 2×2 table for the binary covariate "used to smoke but quit"or `smokeQuit`. In both cases, the P-value from the matched data is higher than typical, suggesting somewhat better balance than expected by complete randomization.

The Minimum P-value For Several Covariates

Each of the nine covariates in Table 5.1, excluding the estimated propensity score, has a P-value for balance in the actual study and 1000 associated P-values produced by complete randomization. The minimum of the nine P-values is not, itself, a P-value; rather, we expect the distribution of the minimum P-value to be stochastically smaller than the uniform distribution, even in a randomized experiment. However, the minimum P-value is a statistic, and we can compare its behavior in the matched sample to its behavior in the 1000 randomized experiments. This comparison is suggested by Ruoqi Yu [24]. Because the empirical distribution of the minimum P-value is used for comparison, no assumption is required about the dependence among nine covariates.

Figure 6.2 compares the minimum of nine P-values in the actual match (marked by an X) and in 1000 completely randomized experiments. The minimum P-value in the actual match is 0.53, and only 4/1000 randomized experiments produced a larger minimum P-value. So, the actual imbalance in the most imbalanced of 9 covariates—which happens to be age with P-value 0.53—is a small imbalance compared to the most imbalanced of 9 covariates in 1000 randomized experiments. Of course, in the 1000 randomized experiments, the minimum of nine P-values tends to be smaller than the uniform distribution that is expected for any one of those nine P-values.

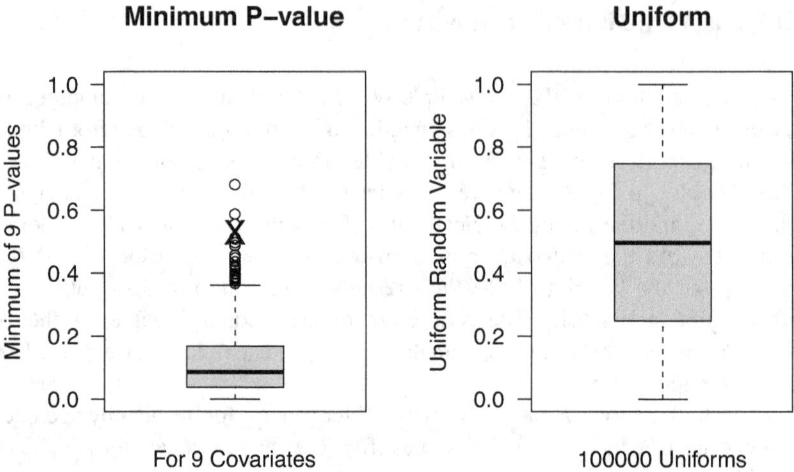

Fig. 6.2 The minimum P-value for nine covariates. Balance in the matched sample (the X in the boxplot) is compared with 1000 randomized experiments. Only 4 of 1000 randomized experiments had a larger minimum P-value than the actual matched sample. The second boxplot shows 100000 uniform random variables, and it serves as a reminder that the smallest of 9 P-values has a distribution that is much smaller than a uniform distribution even in a randomized experiment

The Truncated Product of P-values for Several Covariates

Zaykin and colleagues [26] suggest combining independent P-values by taking the product of those P-values that are less than or equal to a threshold, conventionally 0.2, or perhaps 0.1. The product is defined to be one if all P-values are above the threshold. They determine the distribution of the truncated product of independent uniform P-values. If instead the threshold is set to 1, then their method reduces to Fisher's method of combining P-values [3].

The P-values for the nine covariates are not independent, because the covariates themselves are not independent. However, independence of covariates is not needed to compare an observed truncated product to the *empirical* distribution of the 1000 truncated products from the 1000 randomized experiments.

Figure 6.3 compares the actual match and 1000 randomized experiments in terms of the truncated product of nine P-values with truncation points 0.2 and 1.0, the latter being the product of all nine P-values or Fisher's method. By either standard, the actual match exhibits better covariate balance than most of the 1000 randomized experiments. Truncated at 0.2, the product for the matched sample is 1.0, because all P-values exceed 0.2, but this is true also in 198/1000 randomized experiments.

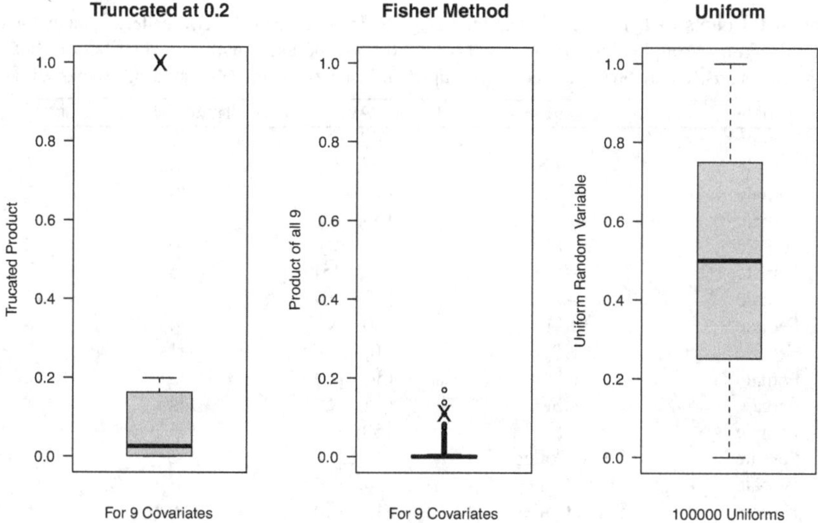

Fig. 6.3 The truncated product of P-values for nine covariates, with truncation 0.2 or 1.0 (i.e., no truncation or Fisher's method). Balance in the matched sample (X) is compared with 1000 randomized experiments. Truncating at 0.2, the match has a truncated product of 1, but so do 198/1000 randomized experiments. The actual product of all 9 P-values is 0.1109 and only 2/1000 randomized experiments yield a larger product. The third boxplot shows 100000 uniform random variables, and it serves as a reminder that a truncated product of 9 P-values has a distribution that is much smaller than a uniform distribution even in a randomized experiment

The product of all nine P-values is 0.1109 in the matched sample, and it is larger for only 2/1000 randomized experiments.

Are Interactions Among Covariates Balanced?

Table 6.1 shows the joint distribution of treatment and a factor variable, FEA, for female (F), five education categories (E), and four age categories (A), for the two-criteria match of binge drinkers compared to both types of controls. In a completely randomized experiment, treatment would be independent of the $40 = 2 \times 5 \times 4$ covariate categories of FEA. Four such three-factor variables will be examined, FEA, FES, FAS and EAS, where S is current smoking with three levels.

Many of the counts in Table 6.1 are too low to trust the large-sample chi-square null distribution in a test of independence of treatment and category. However, we may follow Samuel Pimentel and colleagues [18, Table 1] by comparing the chi-square statistic for the matched sample to its distribution in 1000 randomized

Table 6.1 Counts of Female × Education × Age × Treatment in the two-criteria match for the binge drinking example. The counts are too low to trust the chi-square null distribution, but the chi-square statistic may be compared to its empirical distribution in 1000 randomized experiments

Female	Education	Age	Treated	Control
Female	< 9th	(0, 30)	0	1
Female	< 9th	[30, 45)	0	1
Female	< 9th	[45, 60)	0	1
Female	< 9th	[60, ∞)	0	0
Female	9–11	(0, 30)	0	2
Female	9–11	[30, 45)	5	7
Female	9–11	[45, 60)	6	11
Female	9–11	[60, ∞)	4	8
Female	HS	(0, 30)	1	2
Female	HS	[30, 45)	3	12
Female	HS	[45, 60)	4	8
Female	HS	[60, ∞)	3	6
Female	Some College	(0, 30)	2	3
Female	Some College	[30, 45)	7	13
Female	Some College	[45, 60)	9	16
Female	Some College	[60, ∞)	4	8
Female	≥ BA	(0, 30)	1	4
Female	≥ BA	[30, 45)	5	7
Female	≥ BA	[45, 60)	4	6
Female	≥ BA	[60, ∞)	2	4
Male	< 9th	(0, 30)	0	1
Male	< 9th	[30, 45)	2	8
Male	< 9th	[45, 60)	4	5
Male	< 9th	[60, ∞)	3	4
Male	9–11	(0, 30)	5	9
Male	9–11	[30, 45)	9	17
Male	9–11	[45, 60)	8	15
Male	9–11	[60, ∞)	8	18
Male	HS	(0, 30)	9	10
Male	HS	[30, 45)	14	25
Male	HS	[45, 60)	8	30
Male	HS	[60, ∞)	13	18
Male	Some College	(0, 30)	9	14
Male	Some College	[30, 45)	13	33
Male	Some College	[45, 60)	21	33
Male	Some College	[60, ∞)	10	27
Male	≥ BA	(0, 30)	2	2
Male	≥ BA	[30, 45)	3	10
Male	≥ BA	[45, 60)	3	8
Male	≥ BA	[60, ∞)	2	5
		Total	206	412

experiments. A row with a zero row total, like row 4 in Table 6.1, does not contribute to the test.

Figure 6.4 shows the chi-square statistics for 1000 randomized experiments and for the matched sample (X). For all four 3-factor variables, the chi-square statistic is smaller in the matched sample than in most of the 1000 randomized experiments. In

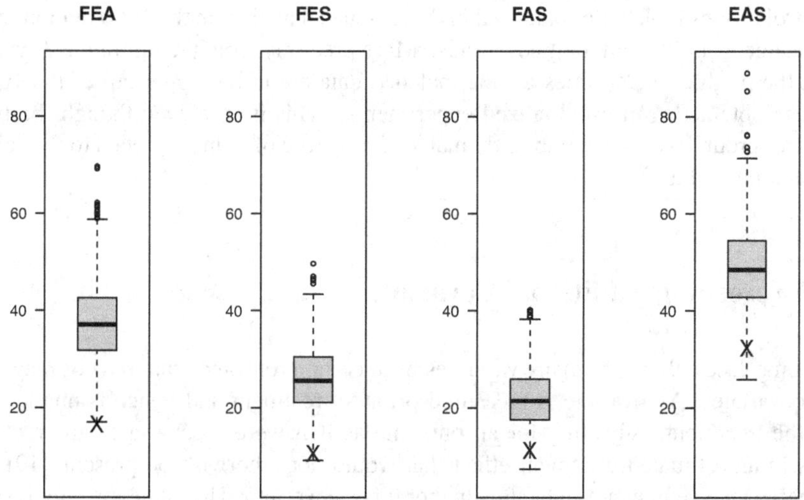

Fig. 6.4 Checking imbalances in four three-factor interactions among covariates F = female (2 levels), E = education (5 levels), A = age (4 categories), S = current smoking (three categories). Here, FEA denotes the 2 × 5 × 4 for female × education × age, as in Table 6.1. Plotted values are chi-square statistics testing independence of treatment and a 3-way factor in 1000 randomized experiments and in the actual matched sample (X)

the randomized experiments, treatment is actually independent of these four three-factor covariates. In brief, Fig. 6.4 says these four three-factor covariates are better balanced than in most of the 1000 randomized experiments.

Comparing Multiple Control Groups

Of course, the treated group, the binge drinkers (B), could be checked separately for covariate balance compared to each of the two control groups, never binge (N) and past binge (P). Implicitly, the two control groups, N and P, are matched to each other by virtue of being matched to the same current binge drinker (B), that is, by virtue of being in the same block i. So, the two control groups can be checked for covariate balance with each other.

If the covariates in the two control groups are compared to each other using the Wilcoxon rank sum test or chi-square test for a 2×2 table, then the smallest of the nine P-values for the nine covariates in Table 5.1 is 0.431 for age. Of 1000 randomized experiments, 566 had a larger P-value for age, and, more importantly, 11/1000 had a larger minimum P-value. Fisher's product of the nine P-values was 0.0608, and 9/1000 randomized experiments had a larger product of P-values. Considering all nine covariates in terms of the minimum P or the product of P-values, the two control groups look better balanced in the matched data than in the 1000 randomized experiments built from their covariates. More precisely, both the minimum P-value and the product of P-values for the matched data are in the upper tail of the 1000 values obtained from randomized experiments. This is true even though the two control groups were only implicitly matched by virtue of being matched to the same treated individual.[3]

6.3 Screening Additional Covariates

In some cases, there are many variables of uncertain relevance that may or may not be covariates. A covariate is measured prior to treatment and hence is unaffected by the treatment. Adjusting for an outcome as if it were a covariate can create a bias in an estimated treatment effect that would not otherwise be present [19]. A variable's name may not indicate whether it is a covariate: The name may not reveal when it was measured. A variable whose name suggests it describes the past may nonetheless have been assessed after treatment, so the assessed value of the variable is an outcome, possibly affected by the treatment. Substantial errors of this sort have been documented [17]. To avoid such errors, an investigator should adjust for a variable only after due thought and consideration. What should be done with a list of doubtful additional variables that is too long for due thought and consideration?

Cochran [6, §3.1] evaluated a simple screening procedure that was updated by Ruoqi Yu and colleagues [25, §3.1]. In its updated form, a preliminary matched sample is constructed, matching for covariates thought to be relevant. The study's intended outcomes are set aside; they play no role in the screening procedure. The screening procedure is a diagnostic check of a tentatively matched sample. In this tentatively matched sample, each entry on a long list of doubtful candidates is checked, one at a time, for residual imbalance in the matched treated and control groups. Due thought and consideration are given to variables that exhibit a residual imbalance, usually a much shorter list. In her example, a study of the effect of hormone replacement therapy on survival, Yu et al. [25, Fig. 3] found one variable on a list of 45 variables that showed an extremely large residual imbalance, with a t-statistic of 35, a difference in means in units of the standard deviation of 0.4, and a large Kullback-Leibler divergence [12]. Due thought and consideration given to that one variable established its unambiguous status as a covariate and as a covariate that a priori considerations suggest is likely to be relevant to survival.

This process suggests a few additional variables for thoughtful consideration and does this prior to the examination of outcomes.

[3] Some matching methods pair controls explicitly, taking account of control-control covariate distances [11, 16].

6.4 *Further Reading

The references for this chapter are Branson [4], Brumberg and colleagues [5], Hansen and Bowers [8], Pimentel and colleagues [18], Yu [24], and Yu and colleagues [25].

Problems

6.1 Check covariate balance for control group P
Run the annotated example in the documentation for the `evalBal` function in the R package `iTOS` to check for covariate balance in the binge data comparing the treated group (B) to the past-binge controls (P). If you are not in an enormous hurry, set reps=1000, rather than reps=100 as in the documentation. As the procedure uses random numbers, you must set the seed if you want to be able to reproduce exactly the same analysis at a later date.

6.2 Check covariate balance for control group N
Repeat Problem 6.1 for control group N. The documentation for `evalBal` does not do this, but the steps are similar to those in Problem 6.1.

6.3 Balance and pairing
Using the matched data in `bingeM` in the `iTOS` package, make four comparisons of age in treated group B and control group P. Do two unpaired tests of 206 ages in group B and 206 ages in group P using the Wilcoxon rank sum test and the unpaired t-test. Do two paired tests on the 206 B-P matched pair differences in age using the Wilcoxon signed rank test and the t-test. Plot the data in various ways. In all cases, produce a point estimate and confidence interval for the typical difference in ages, in addition to a P-value. (This is produced automatically by the `t.test` function in the `stats` package in R, but for the Wilcoxon tests, you must set `conf.int=TRUE` in the `wilcox.test` function in the `stats` package in R.) First, what is the estimated difference in typical ages by these four methods? Is it a large difference in age? What are the four P-values for the four tests? What is the usual (i.e., Pearson) correlation between the paired ages in groups B and P? What would this correlation be if you had matched exactly for age in groups B and P, so a 50-year-old is always paired with a 50-year-old, and a 20-year-old is always paired with a 20-year-old? What would this correlation be if you had always mismatched by 2ϵ for very small $\epsilon > 0$, always matching a 50+ϵ B to a 50-ϵ P, and a 20+ϵ B to a 20-ϵ P? What would the values of the paired and unpaired t-statistics be if you mismatched by 2ϵ in this way? I have argued that balance checks should examine covariate balance without reference to who is paired with whom, but not everyone agrees, and you should form your own opinion. The calculations you have just done for the `bingeM` data provide one view of the issues that are involved.

6.4 Should you check the imbalance in the estimated propensity score?
There is a propensity score for each control group, N and P; see Table 4.2. So, if

you are going to check covariate balance for the propensity score, then you must do it separately for the two control groups. You have already checked the imbalance in the covariates that were used to estimate the propensity score. Should you also check the imbalance in the estimated propensity score itself? Unlike a true covariate, the estimated propensity score was fitted to the observed treatment assignments, Z; so, due to over-fitting, it would tend to be out of balance even if fitted in a randomized experiment in which the true propensity score is 1/2 for all $2I$ individuals. Here are two possibilities. (i) You estimate the propensity score in the matched data, forget that you estimated it, and treat it like age or BMI for purposes of balance checking, comparing its imbalance to 1000 randomized experiments. (ii) In each randomized experiment, you estimate a propensity score from the data for that experiment. You then compare the imbalance in the estimated propensity score in the matched sample to the imbalance in these 1000 other estimated propensity scores from 1000 randomized experiments. Discuss and compare the advantages and disadvantages of methods (i) and (ii).

References

1. Andrews, D.F., Hampel, F.R., Bickel, P.J., Huber, P.J., Rogers, W.H., Tukey, J.W.: Robust Estimates of Location: Survey and Advances. Princeton University Press, Princeton (1972)
2. BBC: Usain Bolt wins Olympics 100m gold in London. BBC Sport (2012). https://www.bbc.com/sport/olympics/19137390
3. Berk, R.H., Cohen, A.: Asymptotically optimal methods of combining tests. Journal of the American Statistical Association **74**(368), 812–814 (1979)
4. Branson, Z.: Randomization tests to assess covariate balance when designing and analyzing matched datasets. Observ. Stud. **7**(2), 1–36 (2021)
5. Brumberg, K., Small, D.S., Rosenbaum, P.R.: Optimal refinement of strata to balance covariates. Biometrics **80**(3) (2024). https://doi.org/10.1093/biomtc/ujae061
6. Cochran, W.G.: The planning of observational studies of human populations (with Discussion). J. Roy. Stat. Soc. A **128**(2), 234–266 (1965)
7. Cook, R.D., Weisberg, S.: Residuals and Influence in Regression. Chapman & Hall/CRC, Boca Raton (1980)
8. Hansen, B.B., Bowers, J.: Covariate balance in simple, stratified and clustered comparative studies. Stat. Sci. **23**, 219–236 (2008)
9. Hodges, J., Lehmann, E.: Estimates of location based on rank tests. Ann. Math. Stat. **34**(2), 598–611 (1963)
10. Hsu, J., Zubizarreta, J.R., Small, D., Rosenbaum, P.R.: Strong control of the familywise error rate in observational studies that discover effect modification by exploratory methods. Biometrika **102**(4), 767–782 (2015)
11. Karmakar, B., Small, D.S., Rosenbaum, P.R.: Using approximation algorithms to build evidence factors and related designs for observational studies. J. Comput. Graph. Stat. **28**(3), 698–709 (2019)
12. Kullback, S., Leibler, R.A.: Information and sufficiency. Ann. Math. Stat. **22**(1), 79–86 (1951)
13. Lee, K., Small, D.S., Hsu, J.Y., Silber, J.H., Rosenbaum, P.R.: Discovering effect modification in an observational study of surgical mortality at hospitals with superior nursing. J. Roy. Stat. Soc. Ser. A: Stat. Soc. **181**(2), 535–546 (2018)
14. Lee, K., Small, D.S., Rosenbaum, P.R.: A powerful approach to the study of moderate effect modification in observational studies. Biometrics **74**(4), 1161–1170 (2018)

15. Lehmann, E.L.: Nonparametrics. Holden-Day, San Francisco (1975)
16. Nattino, G., Lu, B., Shi, J., Lemeshow, S., Xiang, H.: Triplet matching for estimating causal effects with three treatment arms: a comparative study of mortality by trauma center level. J. Am. Stat. Assoc. **116**(533), 44–53 (2021)
17. Niknam, B.A., Arriaga, A.F., Rosenbaum, P.R., Hill, A.S., Ross, R.N., Even-Shoshan, O., Romano, P.S., Silber, J.H.: Adjustment for atherosclerosis diagnosis distorts the effects of percutaneous coronary intervention and the ranking of hospital performance. J. Am. Heart Assoc. **7**(11), e008366 (2018)
18. Pimentel, S.D., Kelz, R.R., Silber, J.H., Rosenbaum, P.R.: Large, sparse optimal matching with refined covariate balance in an observational study of the health outcomes produced by new surgeons. J. Am. Stat. Assoc. **110**(510), 515–527 (2015)
19. Rosenbaum, P.R.: The consequences of adjustment for a concomitant variable that has been affected by the treatment. J. Roy. Stat. Soc. A **147**(5), 656–666 (1984)
20. Rosenbaum, P.R.: Heterogeneity and causality: unit heterogeneity and design sensitivity in observational studies. Am. Stat. **59**(2), 147–152 (2005)
21. Rosenbaum, P.R., Rubin, D.B.: Propensity scores in the design of observational studies for causal effects. Biometrika **110**, 1–13 (2023)
22. Rubin, D.B.: Matching to remove bias in observational studies. Biometrics **29**, 159–183 (1973)
23. Rubin, D.B.: Multivariate matching methods that are equal percent bias reducing, II: maximums on bias reduction for fixed sample sizes. Biometrics **32**, 121–132 (1976)
24. Yu, R.: Evaluating and improving a matched comparison of antidepressants and bone density. Biometrics **77**(4), 1276–1288 (2021)
25. Yu, R., Small, D.S., Rosenbaum, P.R.: The information in covariate imbalance in studies of hormone replacement therapy. Ann. Appl. Stat. **15**(4), 2023–2042 (2021)
26. Zaykin, D.V., Zhivotovsky, L.A., Westfall, P.H., Weir, B.S.: Truncated product method for combining p-values. Genetic Epidemiol. **22**(2), 170–185 (2002)
27. Zubizarreta, J.R., Paredes, R.D., Rosenbaum, P.R.: Matching for balance, pairing for heterogeneity in an observational study of the effectiveness of for-profit and not-for-profit high schools in Chile. Ann. Appl. Stat. **8**(1), 204–231 (2014)

Chapter 7
Covariance Adjustment

Abstract Covariance adjustment and other model-based adjustments are used, for different tasks, in both randomized experiments and observational studies. We ask less of model-based adjustments in randomized experiments; so, we have greater reason to expect success in this smaller task. In an observational study, the distribution of observed covariates $\mathbf{x}$ may be different in treated and control groups, so in certain regions of $\mathbf{x}$, there may be few observed r_T's, and in other regions of $\mathbf{x}$, there may be few observed r_C's. It can be difficult to recognize that a model does not accurately predict r_T in a region of $\mathbf{x}$ where there are few r_T's. Of course, the same is true for r_C. One of Donald Rubin's examples is recalled to illustrate this issue.

7.1 What Is Covariance Adjustment?

In 1957, William Cochran [2] wrote "Analysis of covariance: Its nature and uses," which reviewed the literature on covariance adjustment over the previous quarter century. The article was "intended as an introduction to the subsequent papers" of a special issue of *Biometrics* devoted to covariance adjustment. Cochran [2, pp. 262–263] describes the "principal uses" of the analysis of covariance, listing first "to increase precision in randomized experiments," describing this as "probably the most frequent application," first illustrated by Fisher in 1932:

> The variate x was the yield of tea per plot in the period preceding the start of the experiment, while y was the tea yield at the end of a period of application of treatments ... Adjustment of the responses y for their regression on x removes the effects of variations in initial yields from the experimental errors, insofar as these effects are measured by the linear regression. ... In this use, the function of covariance is the same as that of local control (pairing or blocking). It removes the effects of an environmental source of variation that would otherwise inflate experimental error.

In this quotation, it is important that x was determined prior to treatment and hence unaffected by treatment, that y was determined after the application of treatment and

© The Author(s), under exclusive license to Springer Nature Switzerland AG 2025
P. R. Rosenbaum, *An Introduction to the Theory of Observational Studies*,
Springer Texts in Statistics, https://doi.org/10.1007/978-3-031-90494-3_7

so might be affected by treatment, and that adjustment for x is intended to reduce experimental error, not to model or predict future y's. Here, randomization alone had provided an unbiased estimate of the causal effect of the treatment, and covariance adjustment sought to remove that part of the randomized variation in y that could be anticipated from randomized variation in x. In contrast, blocking for x prior to randomization, if feasible, prevents randomized variation in x; therefore, blocking provides greater precision than covariance adjustment for accidental imbalances in x [4, expression (1)].

Cochran's [2, pp. 264–265] second principal use of covariance adjustment is:

> To remove the effects of disturbing variables in observational studies ... Unfortunately, observational studies are subject to difficulties of interpretation from which randomized experiments are free. Although matching and covariance have been skillfully applied, we can never be sure that bias may not be present from some disturbing variable that was overlooked. In randomized experiments, the effects of this variable are distributed among the groups by the randomization in a way that is taken into account in the standard tests of significance. There is no such safeguard in the absence of randomization. Secondly, when the x-distributions show real differences—the case in which adjustment is needed most—covariance adjustments involve a greater or less degree of extrapolation. ... When the groups differ widely in x, these difficulties imply that the interpretation of an adjusted analysis is speculative rather than soundly based.

To what extent do the "x-distributions show real differences [... so that ...] covariance adjustments involve a greater or less degree of extrapolation?" Some insight is gleaned from examining boxplots of the propensity score, as in Fig. 4.1.

7.2 Covariance Adjustment Without Matching

Rubin's Comparisons

In the 1970s, Donald Rubin [11, 12] did several large simulations to compare methods of adjustment for measured covariates in observational studies when there is no bias from unmeasured covariates. He compared matching alone, covariance adjustment alone, and various combinations of matching and covariance adjustment. He concluded [11, p. 185] "the combination of regression adjustment in matched samples generally produces the least biased estimate."

Rubin also compared several alternative methods of performing least-squares regression adjustment on matched samples. These methods included (a) regression applied to a matched sample ignoring who is matched to whom and (b) an alternative method in which the fitted model takes account of the pairing. For paired data, Rubin's version implemented the alternative method (b) by regressing matched-pair differences in outcomes on matched-pair differences in covariates. This is almost the same as fitting one pair parameter for each matched pair, and this alternative implementation is applicable also to matched blocks, with one block parameter for each block. The discussion of method (b) in this book refers to models with pair or block parameters. When the linear model that is used for analysis is also the model that actually generated the data, then methods (a) and (b) both yield unbiased estimates of an additive treatment effect. If the model used for analysis is misspecified—if the model used for analysis differs from the model that generated the data—then Rubin [11, p. 201] judged method (b) "may often be superior" to method (a).

Rubin's simulations involve quite a bit of detail, too much detail to present here. Instead, I will present a single example similar to one of his simulated cases to illustrate some of the issues.

A Simple Theoretical Illustration

Figure 7.1 depicts one simple case of the type considered by Rubin [11]. There is a single observed covariate X, and there is no bias in treatment assignment from unobserved covariates; that is, treatment assignment is ignorable given a single covariate X. In the treated group, X is Normally distributed with expectation 1/2 and variance 1/2, while in the control group X is Normally distributed with expectation $-1/2$ and variance 4; so, X has a standard deviation in the control group that is $\sqrt{4/(1/2)} = \sqrt{8} = 2.83$ times larger than in the treated group. Figure 7.1 includes at least 99% of both of these Normal distributions. The covariate means are not far apart, as seen in the two short vertical line segments on the x-axis in Panel (i) of Fig. 7.1. The propensity score is not monotone in X in Panel (i) of Fig. 7.1: Both the smallest and largest X's tend to be controls. In this example, the number of treated individuals equals the number of potential controls.

There is zero expected treatment effect, $\mathrm{E}(r_T - r_C \mid X) = 0$, in this illustration, so $\mathrm{E}(R \mid X, Z) = \mathrm{E}(r_T \mid X) = \mathrm{E}(r_C \mid X) = \upsilon(X)$, say. The usual covariance adjustment fits the linear model, $\mathrm{E}(R \mid X, Z) = \beta_0 + \beta_1 X + \tau Z$ and takes the least the least-squares estimate of τ as the estimate of the treatment effect. In this example, $\mathrm{E}(R \mid X, Z) = \upsilon(X) = \exp(X/2)$, so the model $\mathrm{E}(R \mid X, Z) = \beta_0 + \beta_1 X + \tau Z$ is misspecified in the sense that $\exp(X/2) \neq \beta_0 + \beta_1 X + \tau Z$ for every value of (β_0, β_1, τ).

Panel (ii) of Fig. 7.1 depicts $\upsilon(X) = \exp(X/2)$ as a solid curve. Although $\upsilon(X)$ is dramatically convex, looking back at Panel (i) reminds us that X's in the control group are only occasionally in the region of dramatic curvature of $\upsilon(X)$, and X's in the treated group are almost never in that dramatic portion of $\upsilon(X)$. Fitting the incorrect model $\beta_0 + \beta_1 X + \tau Z$ to $\upsilon(X)$ yields the parallel lines in Panel (ii) of Fig. 7.1, where the line for the control group is above the line for the treated group, incorrectly suggesting that there is a negative treatment effect, when in fact there is no treatment effect. The greater dispersion of X in the control group, together with the marked convexity of $\upsilon(X)$, has pulled up the line for the control group. In Fig. 7.1(ii), the true curve $\upsilon(X)$ is close to the lower line near the expected value $\mathrm{E}(X \mid Z = 1) = 1/2$ of X in the treated group. At $X = -2$ and $X = 2$, there are few treated individuals, but controls are common. The true curve $\upsilon(X)$ crosses the upper line near $X = \pm 2$ in Fig. 7.1(ii).

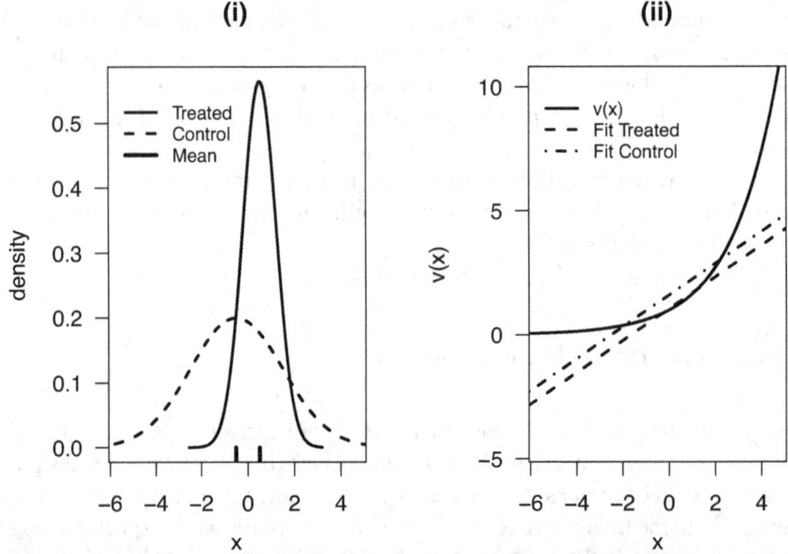

Fig. 7.1 Simulated example of covariance adjustment with a single covariate X and a misspecified model adapted from Rubin [11]. Panel (i) shows the distribution of X in treated and control groups: X is $N(1/2, 1/2)$ in the treated group and X is $N(-1/2, 4)$ in the control group, so the propensity score is not monotone in X, and the standard deviation of X is 2.83 = $\sqrt{8}$ times larger in the control group. Panel (ii) shows the response surface under treatment and control, $\mathrm{E}(r_T \mid X) = \mathrm{E}(r_C \mid X) = \exp(X/2) = v(X)$, say, so there is no expected treatment effect. The dashed lines in Panel (ii) fit a linear covariance adjustment model to $v(X)$ as a linear combination of Z and X, where the difference between the two parallel lines is the (nonzero) expectation of the estimate of the treatment effect

If we computed the means of R in treated and control groups ignoring X, then the difference in means would estimate

$$\begin{aligned} &\mathrm{E}\{\mathrm{E}(R \mid X) \mid Z = 1\} - \mathrm{E}\{\mathrm{E}(R \mid X) \mid Z = 0\} \\ &= \mathrm{E}\{v(X) \mid Z = 1\} - \mathrm{E}\{v(X) \mid Z = 0\} = 0.083; \end{aligned}$$

so, that would be a positively biased estimate of the true average treatment effect of zero,[1] namely,

$$\mathrm{E}\{\mathrm{E}(r_T - r_C \mid X)\} = \mathrm{E}\{\mathrm{E}(r_T \mid X)\} - \mathrm{E}\{\mathrm{E}(r_C \mid X)\} = \mathrm{E}\{v(X) - v(X)\} = 0.$$

In contrast, the incorrect parallel model $\beta_0 + \beta_1 X + \tau Z$ depicted in Fig. 7.1(ii) estimates the average treatment effect with a negative bias of − 0.564. So, in this

[1] Numerical values are based on treated and control samples each of size fifty million. Figure 7.1 is based on samples each of size 50,000.

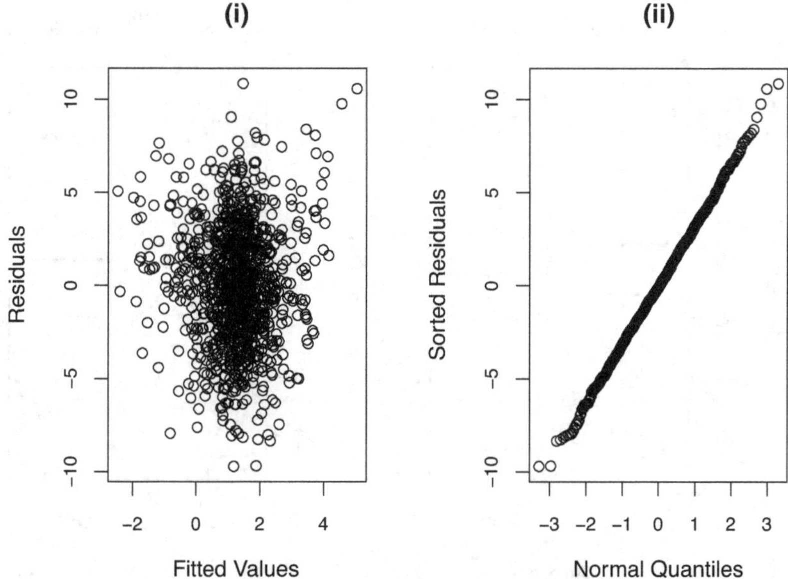

Fig. 7.2 Diagnostic plots for the linear covariance adjustment model fitted to the situation in Fig. 7.1 after adding Normal errors with mean 0 and standard deviation 3. There are 500 observations in the treated group and 500 observations in the control group

illustration, covariance adjustment has changed the sign of the bias while also increasing its absolute magnitude by more than sixfold.

Would a data analyst detect that $\upsilon(X)$ is misspecified by a model of the form $\beta_0 + \beta_1 X + \tau Z$? Figure 7.1 depicts probability distributions and conditional expectations, not data; so, the problem in Fig. 7.1 looks much clearer than it would look in noisy data. So far, we have been talking about and looking at expectations, not data. To simulate data, we add noise to expectations. Suppose the data were $R = \upsilon(X) + \varepsilon$ where X and ε are independent, and ε's are independently sampled from a Normal distribution with expectation 0 and standard deviation 3. With treated and control samples each of size 500, we might fit the incorrect model $\beta_0 + \beta_1 X + \tau Z$ and look for model misspecification using various regression diagnostics. Figure 7.2 shows the two most common diagnostic plots: a plot of residuals against fitted values in Panel (i) and a Normal plot of residuals in Panel (ii). Neither plot reveals much. The Shapiro-Wilk [13] test applied to the residuals yields a P-value of 0.94, leaving the same impression as the Normal plot. A careless data analyst might be satisfied with the model $\beta_0 + \beta_1 X + \tau Z$, reporting a least-squares estimate effect of $\widehat{\tau} = -0.499$,

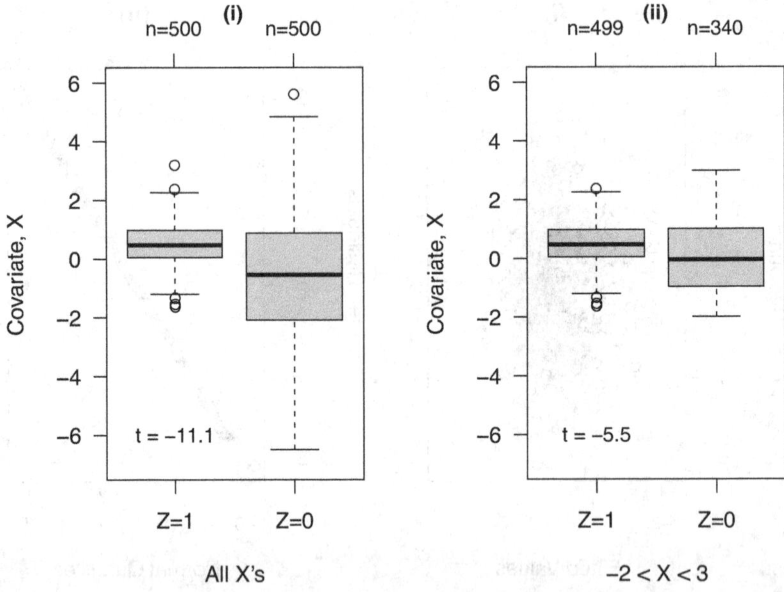

Fig. 7.3 Boxplots of the covariate X by treatment group Z. Panel (i) shows all 1000 individuals. Panel (ii) restricts attention to $-2 < X < 3$. The two-sample separate-variance t-statistic is inside the plot, and the sample sizes are at the top of the plot. One treated individual has $X = 3.19$

a P-value testing $H_0 : \tau = 0$ of 0.021 and a 95% confidence interval for τ of $[-0.922, -0.076]$.[2]

How would things be different if we tried to match for X before fitting the misspecified covariance adjustment model, $\beta_0 + \beta_1 X + \tau Z$? As in Chap. 1, the first task is to understand how the distribution of observed covariates differs in treated and control groups prior to matching. With just one observed covariate, X, that task should not be too difficult. Panel (i) of Fig. 7.3 shows the distribution of X for treated ($Z = 1$) and control ($Z = 0$) groups. The groups are very different. There seems to be no hope of estimating $\mathrm{E}(r_T \mid X)$ at $X = \pm 4$, because there are no treated individuals anywhere near $X = \pm 4$, and hence r_T has never been seen near $X = \pm 4$. We cannot estimate $\mathrm{E}\{\mathrm{E}(r_T - r_C \mid X)\} = \mathrm{E}\{\mathrm{E}(r_T \mid X)\} - \mathrm{E}\{\mathrm{E}(r_C \mid X)\}$ averaging over the full range of X if we have no data about r_T for much of the range of X. Perhaps we can redefine the study population [3], and then estimate the expected effect for individuals with $-2 < X < 3$, that is, $\mathrm{E}\{\mathrm{E}(r_T - r_C \mid X) \mid -2 < X < 3\}$. Even if we restrict attention to individuals with $-2 < X < 3$, the distributions of X still look very different in Panel (ii) of Fig. 7.3.

[2] A careful data analyst might add Cleveland's [1] lowess curve to the plot of residuals against fitted values, and this does show curvature. Instead, a careful analyst might test for curvature by adding a quadratic in X to the model, and this too does show curvature. In truth, a careful data analyst would not be trying to estimate $\mathrm{E}(r_T - r_C)$ from these data.

What happens if we fit the model, $\beta_0+\beta_1 X+\tau Z$, only on an interval of X's where we have seen both r_T's and r_C's? What happens if we fit the incorrect covariate adjustment model, $\beta_0+\beta_1 X+\tau Z$, but restrict attention to individuals in Fig. 7.3(ii) with X's in the interval $-2 < X < 3$? It is helpful to reexamine Fig. 7.1, confining attention to $-2 < X < 3$: There, we have both r_T's and r_C's, and the degree of convexity of $\upsilon(X)$ is not extreme. The regression is fit to $499+340 = 839$ of the 1000 individuals, and we can only interpret the model as an estimate of $\mathrm{E}(r_T - r_C \mid X)$ for X in $-2 < X < 3$. Doing this, the least-squares estimate of effect τ is $\widehat{\tau} = -0.088$, the P-value testing $H_0 : \tau = 0$ is 0.695 and the 95% confidence interval for τ is $[-0.529, 0.353]$. The model gives no indication that $\mathrm{E}(r_T \mid X) - \mathrm{E}(r_C \mid X)$ is nonzero on $-2 < X < 3$, and that is more tolerable given $\upsilon(X) - \upsilon(X) = \mathrm{E}(r_T \mid X) - \mathrm{E}(r_C \mid X)$ is truly zero. Essentially, the only evidence we have that says $0 \neq \mathrm{E}(r_T \mid X) - \mathrm{E}(r_C \mid X)$ comes from $X \notin (-2, 3.2)$ where we have never observed an r_T, and, of course, that is no evidence at all. Sometimes you hear it said: If you don't use all of the data that you have to estimate $\mathrm{E}(r_T \mid X) - \mathrm{E}(r_C \mid X)$, then you are "throwing away part of the data." It is more accurate to say: If you estimate $\mathrm{E}(r_T \mid X) - \mathrm{E}(r_C \mid X)$ in an interval of X's that contains no treated individuals, and hence no r_T's, then you are "hallucinating part of the data that you need but do not have."

7.3 Covariance Adjustment in Randomized Experiments

Testing a Simple Null Hypothesis About Treatment Effects

Recall that Sect. 2.8 tested a simple null hypothesis that specified IJ treatment effects, $H_0 : \boldsymbol{\delta} = \boldsymbol{\delta}_0$ in a randomized block experiment (2.4). A test statistic, $T^{\delta_0} = t\left(\mathbf{Z}, \mathbf{R}^{\delta_0}\right)$, was computed, where $\mathbf{R}^{\delta_0}$ is the $I \times J$ matrix of observed responses adjusted for the hypothesized treatment effect, $R_{ij}^{\delta_0} = R_{ij} - Z_{ij}\,\delta_{0ij}$. If $H_0 : \boldsymbol{\delta} = \boldsymbol{\delta}_0$ were true, then $R_{ij}^{\delta_0} = r_{Cij}$ and $\mathbf{R}^{\delta_0} = \mathbf{r}_C$, and these are part of $\mathcal{F}$, so they are fixed by conditioning on $\mathcal{F}$ in (2.4) and Proposition 2.2. So, the P-value for testing $H_0 : \boldsymbol{\delta} = \boldsymbol{\delta}_0$ in a randomized block design entails in (2.12) counting the number of $\mathbf{z} \in \mathcal{Z}$ such that $t(\mathbf{z}, \mathbf{r}_C) \geq k$ when k is set to the observed value of T^{δ_0}. That P-value is the chance that a blocked randomization $\mathbf{Z}$ would produce a value of T^{δ_0} as large or larger than the observed value if $H_0 : \boldsymbol{\delta} = \boldsymbol{\delta}_0$ were true.

Does this approach work with covariance adjustment? Indeed, it does [8]. Let $T^{\delta_0} = t_{\mathbf{X}}\left(\mathbf{Z}, \mathbf{R}^{\delta_0}\right)$ be a test statistic that also depends upon the observed covariates $\mathbf{X}$. As $\mathbf{X}$ is also part of $\mathcal{F}$, it too is fixed by conditioning on $\mathcal{F}$ in (2.4) and Proposition 2.2. So, the same argument applies to any test statistic that depends upon $t_{\mathbf{X}}\left(\mathbf{Z}, \mathbf{R}^{\delta_0}\right)$. This argument depends upon randomized treatment assignment (2.4) and not on a model linking r_{Cij} and $\mathbf{x}_{ij}$.

A simple version computes $R_{ij}^{\delta_0} = R_{ij} - Z_{ij}\,\delta_{0ij}$ from $H_0 : \boldsymbol{\delta} = \boldsymbol{\delta}_0$ and the observed responses, R_{ij}; then, regresses $R_{ij}^{\delta_0}$ on $\mathbf{x}_{ij}$ using some form of regression to obtain residuals, $v_{ij}^{\delta_0}$ and $\mathbf{V}^{\delta_0}$, where $\mathbf{V}^{\delta_0}$ is the $I \times J$ matrix of $v_{ij}^{\delta_0}$. If $H_0 : \boldsymbol{\delta} = \boldsymbol{\delta}_0$ were true, then $\mathbf{V}^{\delta_0}$ is a function of $\mathbf{R}^{\delta_0} = \mathbf{r}_C$ and $\mathbf{X}$, which are fixed by conditioning upon $\mathcal{F}$. The test statistic $t_{\mathbf{X}}\left(\mathbf{Z}, \mathbf{R}^{\delta_0}\right)$ is then taken as a conventional test statistic, such as one of those in Sect. 2.6-Sect. 2.7, applied with $\mathbf{V}^{\delta_0}$ in place of $\mathbf{R}^{\delta_0}$; that is, $t_{\mathbf{X}}\left(\mathbf{Z}, \mathbf{R}^{\delta_0}\right) = t\left(\mathbf{Z}, \mathbf{V}^{\delta_0}\right)$. Then, Proposition 2.2 gives the randomization distribution (2.12) of $t\left(\mathbf{Z}, \mathbf{V}^{\delta_0}\right)$ when $H_0 : \boldsymbol{\delta} = \boldsymbol{\delta}_0$ is true in a randomized block experiment (2.4).

*Technical Comments: Residuals, Multiple Testing, Block Parameters

A few technical comments follow. The argument above is not restricted to tests based on residuals—that is, $t_{\mathbf{X}}\left(\mathbf{Z}, \mathbf{R}^{\delta_0}\right)$ need not have the form $t\left(\mathbf{Z}, \mathbf{V}^{\delta_0}\right)$—but that form is convenient when comparing analyses with and without covariance adjustment. It is also convenient when comparing analyses with different covariance adjustment methods or models. If the hypothesis $H_0 : \boldsymbol{\delta} = \boldsymbol{\delta}_0$ is tested more than once, say with and without covariance adjustment, or with alternative covariance adjustment models, then it is best to plan the study, so that one of these analyses is the "primary analysis," with the rest as supporting analyses. To emphasize, the primary analysis is chosen during planning, before any R_{ij} is examined. The primary analysis is reported, come what may, as the main analysis, with the supporting analyses reported as checks on the primary analysis. Without a single primary analysis, repeated tests of $H_0 : \boldsymbol{\delta} = \boldsymbol{\delta}_0$ require corrections for multiple testing, such as the use of the Bonferroni inequality. Given that one is committed to the primary analysis before seeing the R_{ij}, the primary analysis should be a robust analysis.

The regression that produces residuals $v_{ij}^{\delta_0}$ may or may not include I additive block parameters, one for each of the I blocks, or $I - 1$ block parameters if the model includes a constant term. The method of fitting the linear model and the specific form that the model takes do not affect the validity of the null distribution (2.12) in a randomized experiment, but they may affect (i) the power of the test and (ii) the robustness of the test in the face of outliers, and other matters. As in Cochran's first use of covariance adjustment in Sect. 7.1, the hope in a randomized experiment is that the residuals v_{ij} have removed some of the variability in $R_{ij}^{\delta_0}$ that can be predicted from $\mathbf{x}_{ij}$; however, the validity of the randomization test of $H_0 : \boldsymbol{\delta} = \boldsymbol{\delta}_0$ depends upon randomization (2.4), not on having a model that generated the data. Conversely, the tests described in this chapter may not be valid if (2.4) does not hold, even if one fits the model that did generate the data.

Table 7.1 Randomization based, one-sided hypothesis tests and 95% confidence limits for the effect τ of binge drinking on systolic blood pressure. There are two covariance adjustment models, one without block parameters, the other with $I - 1 = 205$ block parameters

Covariance adjustment	$H_0 : \tau = 0$	$H_0 : \tau = 5$	95% CI
None	0.000	0.037	$\tau \geq 5.33$
Without Block Parameters	0.000	0.044	$\tau \geq 5.14$
With Block Parameters	0.000	0.009	$\tau \geq 5.83$

Table 7.2 Robust regression results used in testing $H_0 : \tau = 0$ in models without and with block parameters. Residuals from these regressions form the basis for the tests. Age is represented by a quadratic orthogonal polynomial and is not scaled in years. The model with block parameters omits female and bpRX, which were exactly matched, and adds $I - 1 = 205$ block parameters that are not shown here

	Without Block Parameters			With Block Parameters		
	Coefficient	Std. Error	t value	Coefficient	Std. Error	t value
(Intercept)	123.72	11.38	10.87	102.00	22.88	4.46
age	124.09	20.71	5.99	60.19	57.17	1.05
age^2	13.95	17.63	0.79	-42.63	34.66	-1.23
education	-1.11	0.65	-1.71	-0.72	1.23	-0.59
bmi	0.12	0.12	0.98	-0.08	0.19	-0.40
waisthip	2.31	12.51	0.18	10.75	20.92	0.51
vigor	1.81	1.47	1.23	7.80	5.80	1.34
smokenow	-0.81	0.89	-0.90	0.59	2.67	0.22
smokeQuit	-0.74	2.04	-0.36	-0.77	3.69	-0.21
female	-6.74	1.80	-3.74	—	—	—
bpRX	7.62	1.76	4.32	—	—	—

Covariance Adjustment in the Binge Drinking Example

Ignoring for a moment the absence of randomization in the binge drinking example, consider applying covariance adjustment to the matched comparison for systolic blood pressure in Fig. 1.8, which is based on the two-criteria match in Chap. 5. The covariance model does not distinguish the two control groups, N and P. The covariates are those in Table 5.1, including linear and quadratic terms for age;[3] however, the propensity score is not included as it is a function of the other covariates. The linear model is fitted by a method of robust regression that limits the influence of a few extreme blood pressure measurements; specifically, Huber's [6, 7] M-estimates are used.[4]

The covariate means in treated and control groups are quite close in the matched sample, as seen in part in Table 5.1. Perhaps for that reason, covariance adjustment

---

[3] More precisely, age is represented by orthogonal linear and quadratic terms produced by the `poly` function in the `stats` package in R. Age is scaled by this function, so the coefficient of age does not multiply age in years.

[4] More precisely, the model is fit using the `rlm` function in the `MASS` package in R with the default settings. The default settings use M-estimation with Huber's weight function, whose influence function resembles that of a trimmed mean.

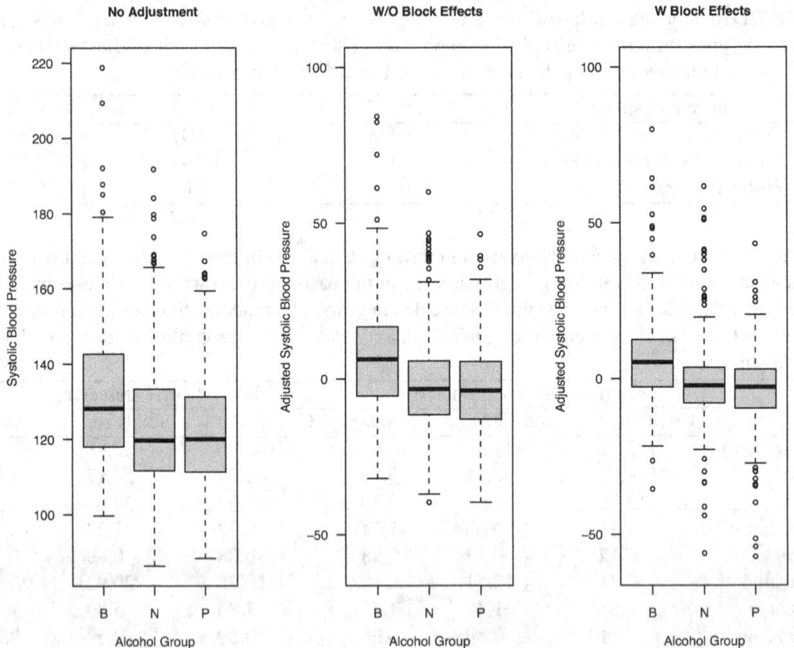

Fig. 7.4 Systolic blood pressure before and after robust covariance adjustment in linear models without (W/O) or with (W) the $I - 1 = 205$ block parameters. B = binge drinker, N = never, P = binge drinker in the past

may not greatly alter our sense of what is happening with systolic blood pressure but let us do the calculation and see what happens.

The confidence interval will be obtained from tests of the hypothesis $H_0 : \boldsymbol{\delta} = \tau_0 \mathbf{1}$, where $\mathbf{1}$ is an $I \times J$ matrix of ones and τ_0 is a scalar. For each hypothesized value of τ_0, we compute adjusted systolic blood pressures, $R_{ij}^{\tau_0 \mathbf{1}} = R_{ij} - Z_{ij}\,\tau_0$, regress these on covariates to obtain residuals $v_{ij}^{\tau_0 \mathbf{1}}$, and compare a test statistic, $t\left(\mathbf{Z}, \mathbf{V}^{\tau_0 \mathbf{1}}\right)$, to its randomization distribution (2.12), and this would be a valid test of $H_0 : \boldsymbol{\delta} = \tau_0 \mathbf{1}$ in a blocked randomized experiment (2.4). Note carefully that the linear model must be refit for each new hypothesized value τ_0. There is no assumption that the linear model generated the responses, but condition (2.4) is a very strong assumption in the absence of randomized treatment assignment. For this illustration, Quade's statistic $t(\cdot, \cdot)$ in Sect. 2.6 is used.[5]

Table 7.1 tests two values of τ_0 against the one-sided alternative $\tau > \tau_0$, namely, $\tau_0 = 0$ and $\tau_0 = 5$, and reports a one-sided 95% confidence interval as the smallest τ_0 not rejected by the test. This table reports three analyses, the unadjusted analysis without covariance adjustment, and two versions of covariance adjustment. All three

[5] One could pair covariance adjustment by M-estimation with an M-statistic as the basis for the test [9, 10], or one could pair a rank-based fit of a linear model [5] with a rank-based test, such as Quade's test; however, there is no need to do this.

analyses use Quade's statistic, but one analysis applies it to $R_{ij}^{\tau_0 \mathbf{1}} = R_{ij} - Z_{ij}\,\tau_0$ without covariance adjustment, and two analyses apply it to residuals, $v_{ij}^{\tau_0 \mathbf{1}}$ computed from a linear model regressing $R_{ij}^{\tau_0 \mathbf{1}}$ on covariates. One linear model includes only the covariates as predictors, and it is analogous to Rubin's method [11, 12] of applying covariance adjustment to a matched sample, ignoring who is paired with whom. The second linear model includes covariates and $I - 1 = 205$ block parameters; it is analogous to Rubin's method of applying covariance adjustment to matched-pair differences. Block parameters depend upon the $J = 3$ individuals in each of I blocks, so block parameters are not precisely estimated; however, they are commonly included in least-squares covariance adjustments in block designs. The blocks were matched for the covariates, so most of the information in the covariates is also in the blocks, albeit in a different form.

In Table 7.1, the inferences from the three methods are similar. The 95% confidences intervals differ by less than one point of systolic blood pressure, and they all suggest an effect larger than five points. Again, these inferences would be appropriate had treatments been randomly assigned within blocks, but of course that did not happen.

Table 7.2 compares the regression coefficients in the two linear models fit by M-estimation. Notably, several of the covariates have large t-statistics in the model without block parameters, but none have large t-statistics in the model with block parameters. In part, this is because the blocks and the covariates both represent the same information in different forms. In Table 7.1, the smallest P-values and the shortest confidence interval came from the model with block parameters.

Figure 7.4 depicts the responses, $R_{ij}^{\tau_0 \mathbf{1}}$, or residuals, $v_{ij}^{\tau_0 \mathbf{1}}$, used to test $H_0 : \boldsymbol{\delta} = \tau_0 \mathbf{1}$ for $\tau_0 = 0$ in Table 7.1. The binge drinkers in group B have the highest $R_{ij}^{\tau_0 \mathbf{1}}$ or $v_{ij}^{\tau_0 \mathbf{1}}$ in all three panels of Fig. 7.4. Quade's test always takes account of the block structure, but only the third panel of Fig. 7.4 removes the variability that can be predicted from the block structure.

7.4 Covariance Adjustment in Observational Studies

A simple common use of covariance adjustment in observational studies is as a check on the adequacy of matching or blocking. In Table 7.1, the addition of covariance adjustment barely alters the blocked comparison; so, perhaps our work with the observed covariates is done, and attention can turn to addressing potential biases from covariates that were not measured.

The randomization-based covariance adjustment described in Sect. 7.3 lends itself to analyses in later chapters that focus on ways (2.4) may fail to hold in observational studies. For example, we may ask how these randomization inferences using covariance adjustment would be altered by departures from (2.4) measured in terms of the principal unobserved covariate and Γ in (4.19). The methods in Chap. 8 may be applied with covariance adjustment for measured covariates by replacing adjusted responses $R_{ij}^{\delta_0}$ by adjusted residuals $v_{ij}^{\delta_0}$ from the covariance adjustment model [8].

As will be discussed in Sect. 10.4, a treatment effect of fixed size will be insensitive to larger unmeasured biases if the effect stands out more clearly in comparison with background noise. If covariance adjustment leaves the treatment effect unaltered but reduces background noise, it may affect sensitivity to unmeasured biases.

7.5 *Further Reading

Cochran's article [2] reminds us about the perspective that covariance adjustment is not part of predictive modeling but rather part of experimental design. Rubin's articles from the 1970s on matching and covariance adjustment continue to be worth reading. Sections 7.3 and 7.4 are based on my article [8], which also discusses the use of covariance adjustment with instruments.

References

1. Cleveland, W.S.: Robust locally weighted regression and smoothing scatterplots. J. Am. Stat. Assoc. **74**(368), 829–836 (1979)
2. Cochran, W.G.: Analysis of covariance: its nature and uses. Biometrics **13**(3), 261–281 (1957)
3. Fogarty, C.B., Mikkelsen, M.E., Gaieski, D.F., Small, D.S.: Discrete optimization for interpretable study populations and randomization inference in an observational study of severe sepsis mortality. J. Am. Stat. Assoc. **111**(514), 447–458 (2016)
4. Greevy, R., Lu, B., Silber, J.H., Rosenbaum, P.: Optimal multivariate matching before randomization. Biostatistics **5**(2), 263–275 (2004)
5. Hettmansperger, T.P., McKean, J.W.: Robust Nonparametric Statistical Methods. Chapman & Hall/CRC Press, Boca Raton (2010)
6. Huber, P.J.: Robust regression: Asymptotics, conjectures and Monte Carlo. Ann. Stat. **1**(5), 799–821 (1973)
7. Huber, P.J.: Robust Statistics. John Wiley & Sons, London (1981)
8. Rosenbaum, P.R.: Covariance adjustment in randomized experiments and observational studies. Stat. Sci. **17**(3), 286–327 (2002)
9. Rosenbaum, P.R.: Sensitivity analysis for M-estimates, tests, and confidence intervals in matched observational studies. Biometrics **63**(2), 456–464 (2007)
10. Rosenbaum, P.R.: Weighted M-statistics with superior design sensitivity in matched observational studies with multiple controls. J. Am. Stat. Assoc. **109**(507), 1145–1158 (2014)
11. Rubin, D.B.: The use of matched sampling and regression adjustment to remove bias in observational studies. Biometrics **29**, 185–203 (1973)
12. Rubin, D.B.: Using multivariate matched sampling and regression adjustment to control bias in observational studies. J. Am. Stat. Assoc. **74**(366a), 318–328 (1979)
13. Shapiro, S.S., Wilk, M.B.: An analysis of variance test for normality. Biometrika **52**(3/4), 591–611 (1965)

Part III
Sensitivity of Inferences to Covariates That Were Not Observed

People who reason badly may sometimes accept bad principles of inference; but normally what they do is better thought of as, in some way or other, misapplying good principles.

Paul Grice
Aspects of Reason

It is not always obvious at first that a position is obviously inadequate.

Robert J. Fogelin
Pyrrhonian Reflections on Knowledge and Justification

Chapter 8
Sensitivity of Causal Inferences to Unmeasured Biases in Treatment Assignment

Abstract A sensitivity analysis considers departures from randomized treatment assignment of various magnitudes. In an $I \times J$ block design, this means that the probability θ_{ij} that individual j receives treatment in block i may depart from $\overline{\theta}_{ij} = 1/J$. The sensitivity analysis determines the degree to which an inference about causal effects could change in the presence of departures from randomization, $\theta_{ij} \neq 1/J$ of various magnitudes, thereby placing bounds on inference quantities, such as P-values, point estimates, and endpoints of confidence intervals. A sensitivity analysis replaces the true but useless statement "association does not imply causation," by the equally true but far more useful statement "to explain the association actually seen in data, the bias in treatment assignment must exceed a particular magnitude."

8.1 Structural Elements

Recap: The Central Problem in Observational Studies

Our situation in a randomized experiment in Chap. 2 was good: not perfect, but good. We could not see an individual causal effect, $\delta_{ij} = r_{Tij} - r_{Cij}$; so, we could not see the IJ-dimensional vector $\boldsymbol{\delta}$ of causal effects. That inability to see causal effects is the central problem in causal inference, and randomized experimentation came close to solving it. If treatment assignments Z_{ij} are determined by a truly random device (2.4) in a blocked experiment, then it follows from Lemma 2.1 that $\Pr\left(Z_{ij} = 1 \,\middle|\, \mathcal{F}, \mathcal{Z}\right) = 1/J$ for each ij, with $1 = \sum_{j=1}^{J} Z_{ij}$ for each i and with treatment assignments $\mathbf{Z}_i = (Z_{i1}, \ldots, Z_{iJ})$ being independent in distinct blocks i. Using these properties of randomized treatment assignment and Proposition 2.2, we may find the null distribution of any test statistic $T = t\left(\mathbf{Z}, \mathbf{R}^{\delta_0}\right)$ under any simple null hypothesis $H_0 : \boldsymbol{\delta} = \boldsymbol{\delta}_0$ about the causal effects $\boldsymbol{\delta}$. This immediately leads to (i)

© The Author(s), under exclusive license to Springer Nature Switzerland AG 2025
P. R. Rosenbaum, *An Introduction to the Theory of Observational Studies*, Springer Texts in Statistics, https://doi.org/10.1007/978-3-031-90494-3_8

tests in Sect. 2.9 of composite null hypotheses, $H_0 : \delta \in \Delta_0$, for a set Δ_0 of δ_0's, and (ii) confidence intervals and point estimates in Sect. 2.10 and Sect. 2.11.

The situation in observational studies is much more difficult. Chapter 4 defined the propensity score, $e(\mathbf{X}) = \Pr(Z = 1 \mid \mathbf{X})$, in Sect. 4.3, and the principal unobserved covariate, $\zeta = \zeta(\mathbf{X}, r_T, r_C) = \Pr(Z = 1 \mid \mathbf{X}, r_T, r_C)$, in Sect. 4.5. The principal unobserved covariate is not observed because we do not see (r_T, r_C) jointly; so, we cannot calculate $\Pr(Z = 1 \mid \mathbf{X}, r_T, r_C)$ from the observed data, $(R, Z, \mathbf{X})$. Treatment assignment is ignorable (or unconfounded) given the observed covariates $\mathbf{X}$ if two conditions hold: (i) $0 < e(\mathbf{X}) < 1$, and (ii) the propensity score and the principal unobserved covariate are equal; that is, (i) and (ii) hold if

$$0 < \zeta = \Pr(Z = 1 \mid \mathbf{X}, r_T, r_C) = \Pr(Z = 1 \mid \mathbf{X}) = e(\mathbf{X}) < 1. \tag{8.1}$$

Chapter 4 showed that various methods of analysis would permit inference about causal effects if treatment assignments were ignorable given the observed covariates $\mathbf{X}$; however, these methods may otherwise fail. The central problem in observational studies is that (8.1) may be false. If $0 < \zeta < 1$, then treatment assignment is always ignorable given $(\mathbf{X}, \zeta)$, or even given $\{\mathbf{h}(\mathbf{X}), \zeta\}$ for any function $\mathbf{h}(\cdot)$, but this is of limited help because ζ is not observed. Addressing this central problem is the topic of the remainder of this book.

Positivity or Common Support

Condition (i) in the definition of ignorable treatment assignment, namely, $0 < e(\mathbf{X}) < 1$, is a claim about the distribution of the observable data $(R, Z, \mathbf{X})$; so, relevant information is contained in the observable data. One informal diagnostic technique entails plotting the distribution of estimated propensity scores, $\widehat{e}(\mathbf{X})$, in treated and control groups, as in Figs. 4.1 and 4.2. This informal plot creates concern if it is clear that there are regions of $\widehat{e}(\mathbf{X})$ with no treated individual or no control. If $\widehat{e}(\mathbf{X})$ is estimated by a logit model and if there are regions of $\widehat{e}(\mathbf{X})$ with no treated individual or no control, then there are regions of $\mathbf{X}$ with no treated individual or no control.

When condition (i) appears to be false, the issue is usually addressed by redefining the study population to consist of individuals who have some reasonable prospect of receiving both treatments [13,21,71]. The method of Colin Fogarty and colleagues [21] is particularly attractive, because it finds a new study population that is intelligible and recognizable in which condition (i) does hold. Specifically, in their method, an optimization algorithm tries to find a rectangle defined by a few coordinates of $\mathbf{X}$, such that inside this rectangle condition (i) does hold. A randomized clinical trial is typically confined to a specific population of patients; that is, it is restricted to such a covariate rectangle—to patients aged 40 to 70 with stage 2 or stage 3 colon cancer, say. The algorithm of Fogarty et al. [21] asks of observational data whether there is any definition of such a substantial rectangle such that condition (i) holds on that rectangle. Although this task requires some thought and care, it is not intrinsically a difficult task, because decisions are based on observable data $(Z, \mathbf{X})$.

Observational Block Designs and the Principal Unobserved Covariate

Suppose that N individuals are independently sampled from a population, and $(Z, \mathbf{x})$ is observed for these individuals. A function $\mathbf{h}(\cdot)$ is defined, and $\mathbf{h}(\mathbf{x})$ is computed for each individual. Using $\{Z, \mathbf{h}(\mathbf{x})\}$ alone, $IJ \leq N$ of these individuals are selected and arranged into I blocks of size J, in such a way that

$$\mathbf{h}(\mathbf{x}_{i1}) = \mathbf{h}(\mathbf{x}_{i2}) = \cdots = \mathbf{h}(\mathbf{x}_{iJ}) \text{ and } 1 = \sum_{j=1}^{J} Z_{ij} \text{ for } i = 1, \ldots, I. \tag{8.2}$$

Then $R = Z\,r_T + (1 - Z)\,r_C$ is observed for these IJ individuals. In (8.2), the subscript j carries no information and does not identify the one treated individual with $Z_{ij} = 1$.[1] Define $\mathcal{F}$ and $\mathcal{Z}$ as in Sect. 2.1 for these IJ individuals, where the unobserved covariate u_{ij} in $\mathcal{F}$ either is the principal unobserved covariate, $u_{ij} = \zeta_{ij} = \zeta(\mathbf{x}_{ij}, r_{Tij}, r_{Cij})$, or includes the principal unobserved covariate.[2]

This is a simplified description of the construction of an observational block design. Here, matching is described as sampling and then conditioning on the values of certain random variables, followed by rearrangement of the data set using these quantities that have been fixed by conditioning. It is an approximate but reasonable description of the study of light alcohol consumption and HDL cholesterol in Chap. 1, where there were three covariates, sex, age in years, and education in five categories.[3] If we had coarsened age, say into ten-year age categories, then (8.2) might very closely describe the resulting match, but it is usually better to have a tighter match for age and allow (8.2) to be an approximate description of that tighter match. In contrast, recall the process that built the match in Chap. 5 for the study of binge drinking and blood pressure. That process is more complex than (8.2), but it is also

[1] For instance, after forming blocks so that (8.2) holds, random numbers are used to assign the subscript j to individuals in block i, independently in distinct blocks, and random numbers are used to assign the subscript i to blocks. This just says that information about people is in random variables, observed or not; that is, no information about a person is hidden in a subscript.

[2] To say that u_{ij}, which might be a vector, includes ζ_{ij} is to say that ζ_{ij} is a function of u_{ij}. It is sometimes useful to talk about a specific covariate, say a genetic variant, rather than insist that every conversation about an unobserved covariate must refer solely to the principal unobserved covariate. It is convenient to allow the notation to cover both cases. Strictly speaking, the principal unobserved covariate, $\zeta_{ij} = \zeta(\mathbf{x}_{ij}, r_{Tij}, r_{Cij})$, is a function of $(\mathbf{x}_{ij}, r_{Tij}, r_{Cij})$, which is part of $\mathcal{F}$; so, any reference to u_{ij} is already somewhat redundant. If we were willing to restrict discussion of unobserved covariates to the principal unobserved covariate, the notation could omit any reference to u_{ij}. It is important that conditioning on $\mathcal{F}$ partitions the sample space by the IJ vectors $(\mathbf{x}_{ij}, r_{Tij}, r_{Cij})$; however, the rest is merely a manner of speaking. Both $\mathcal{F}$ and $\zeta_{ij} = \zeta(\mathbf{x}_{ij}, r_{Tij}, r_{Cij})$ involve (r_{Tij}, r_{Cij}), which are not jointly observed; so, neither $\mathcal{F}$ nor $\zeta_{ij} = \zeta(\mathbf{x}_{ij}, r_{Tij}, r_{Cij})$ is observed.

[3] An alternative and reasonable mathematical formulation takes all of the treated individuals in some population and matches them to a sample of controls with a similar distribution of the observed covariates $\mathbf{X}$, thereby attempting to estimate the average effect of the treatment on treated individuals [82]; see Sect. 4.4. Although this distinction is important for some purposes, the same sensitivity analyses apply in this case, except that the matched design is understood to refer to a population with a different distribution of observed covariates, $\mathbf{X}$.

a better match than could be produced by adhering exactly to the structure (8.2). My own preference is to have an approximate description of an excellent study design, rather than an exact description of a poor study design; however, I acknowledge that tastes vary, and my preference is not everyone's preference.

8.2 Departures from Randomization in Block Designs

Biased Treatment Assignment in Observational Block Designs

For the J individuals in block i, the chance that j is treated with $Z_{ij} = 1$ and the remaining $J-1$ individuals are controls with $Z_{ik} = 0$ is $\zeta_{ij} \prod_{k \neq j} (1 - \zeta_{ik})$. We want the conditional probability, say θ_{ij}, that $Z_{ij} = 1$ given $1 = \sum_{\ell=1}^{J} Z_{i\ell}$. First, observe the trivial but useful identity:

$$\zeta_{ij} \prod_{k \neq j} (1 - \zeta_{ik}) = \frac{\zeta_{ij}}{1 - \zeta_{ij}} \prod_{j=1}^{J} (1 - \zeta_{ik}) . \tag{8.3}$$

Hence, conditioning on $1 = \sum_{j=1}^{J} Z_{ij}$ or on $\mathcal{Z}$ yields

$$\Pr\left(Z_{ij} = 1 \,\middle|\, \mathcal{F}, 1 = \sum\nolimits_{j=1}^{J} Z_{ij} \right) = \Pr\left(Z_{ij} = 1 \,\middle|\, \mathcal{F}, \mathcal{Z} \right)$$
$$= \frac{\zeta_{ij} \prod_{k \neq j} (1 - \zeta_{ik})}{\sum_{\ell=1}^{J} \zeta_{i\ell} \prod_{k \neq \ell} (1 - \zeta_{ik})} = \frac{\zeta_{ij} / (1 - \zeta_{ij})}{\sum_{\ell=1}^{J} \zeta_{i\ell} / (1 - \zeta_{i\ell})} = \theta_{ij}, \tag{8.4}$$

using (8.3). Let us pause for a moment to connect (8.4) with ideas from earlier chapters.

(i) Randomized experiments: In a blocked randomized experiment (2.4), $\theta_{ij} = 1/J$ for all ij as a consequence of the use of a truly random device to assign treatments. This led to all of the inferences in Chap. 2 and to randomization-based covariance adjustment in Sect. 7.3.

(ii) Ignorable treatment assignment: In an observational study, if treatment assignments were ignorable given the observed covariates $\mathbf{x}$ in the sense of (8.1) and if the propensity score $e(\mathbf{x})$ were included in $\mathbf{h}(\mathbf{x})$, in the sense that people who have the same $\mathbf{h}(\mathbf{x})$ have the same $e(\mathbf{x})$, then $\zeta_{ij} = e(\mathbf{x}_{ij})$ by (8.1), and $e(\mathbf{x}_{i1}) = \cdots = e(\mathbf{x}_{iJ})$ for each i by (8.2), so once again $\theta_{ij} = 1/J$ for all ij, as in Sect. 4.6 and Sect. 7.4. In earlier chapters, various analyses acted as if the two observational studies of alcohol were randomized experiments. Those analyses would be reasonable if treatment assignments were ignorable given $\mathbf{x}_{ij}$ and if $\mathbf{h}(\mathbf{x})$ included $e(\mathbf{x})$.

(iii) Departures from ignorable assignment: Ignorable treatment assignment in (8.1) fails to hold if $\zeta = \Pr(Z = 1 \mid \mathbf{X}, r_T, r_C) \neq \Pr(Z = 1 \mid \mathbf{X}) = e(\mathbf{X})$, that is, if two individuals with the same $\mathbf{X}$ or the propensity score $\Pr(Z = 1 \mid \mathbf{X})$, have different values of the principal unobserved covariate, $\zeta = \Pr(Z = 1 \mid \mathbf{X}, r_T, r_C)$. So, it is natural to measure the degree of departure from ignorable assignment as the degree to which $\zeta = \Pr(Z = 1 \mid \mathbf{X}, r_T, r_C)$ may vary within blocks that satisfy (8.2). In (4.19), the magnitude of departure from ignorable assignment was at most $\Gamma \geq 1$ if

$$\Gamma \geq \frac{\zeta_{ij}\left(1-\zeta_{ij'}\right)}{\zeta_{ij'}\left(1-\zeta_{ij}\right)} \geq \frac{1}{\Gamma} \text{ for all } i, j, j'. \tag{8.5}$$

Combining (8.4) and (8.5) yields

$$\Gamma \geq \frac{\theta_{ij}}{\theta_{ij'}} = \frac{\frac{\zeta_{ij}/(1-\zeta_{ij})}{\sum_{\ell=1}^{J}\zeta_{i\ell}/(1-\zeta_{i\ell})}}{\frac{\zeta_{ij'}/(1-\zeta_{ij'})}{\sum_{\ell=1}^{J}\zeta_{i\ell}/(1-\zeta_{i\ell})}} = \frac{\zeta_{ij}\left(1-\zeta_{ij'}\right)}{\zeta_{ij'}\left(1-\zeta_{ij}\right)} \geq \frac{1}{\Gamma} \text{ for all } i, j, j'; \tag{8.6}$$

so an odds ratio in the principal unobserved covariate ζ_{ij} in (8.5) becomes a ratio of conditional probabilities, $\theta_{ij}/\theta_{ij'}$, in (8.6).

(iv) Imprecise matching for observed covariates: Conditions (8.5) and (8.6) are usually understood to refer to bias in treatment assignment Z from unmeasured covariates u, or from (r_T, r_C), but these conditions may be understood more broadly. At various points we have noticed that blocking has produced treatment groups that look comparable in terms of the distribution of the observed covariates, $\mathbf{x}$, but the blocks were not perfectly homogeneous in terms of $\mathbf{x}$. Conditions may be understood to refer to the degree to which the principal unobserved covariate, $\zeta = \Pr(Z = 1 \mid \mathbf{X}, r_T, r_C)$, varies within blocks, regardless of whether that variation is due to (r_T, r_C) or $\mathbf{X}$ or a combination of the two.

The Sensitivity Model in Terms of Linear Constraints

At various times, it is convenient to think of the sensitivity analysis model (8.6) as defined in terms of linear equality and inequality constraints. Write

$$\boldsymbol{\theta} = \begin{bmatrix} \theta_{11} & \theta_{12} & \cdots & \theta_{1J} \\ \vdots & \vdots & & \vdots \\ \theta_{I1} & \theta_{I2} & \cdots & \theta_{IJ} \end{bmatrix} \tag{8.7}$$

for the $I \times J$ matrix of θ_{ij} in (8.4). Then (8.6) is equivalently defined by

$$1 = \sum_{j=1}^{J} \theta_{ij} \text{ for } i = 1, \ldots, I, \tag{8.8}$$

$$\theta_{ij} \leq \Gamma\theta_{ij'} \text{ for all } i, j, j', \tag{8.9}$$

$$\frac{1}{1+(J-1)\,\Gamma} \le \theta_{ij} \le \frac{\Gamma}{\Gamma+(J-1)} \quad \text{for all } i, j. \tag{8.10}$$

Of course, (8.8) follows from (8.4). Rearranging $\Gamma \ge \theta_{ij}/\theta_{ij'} \ge 1/\Gamma$ in (8.6) yields (8.9). Then, $0 \le \theta_{ij} \le 1$ combines with (8.8) and (8.9) to yield (8.10). For instance, θ_{i1} could be as small as $1/\{1+(J-1)\,\Gamma\}$ if $\theta_{i2} = \cdots = \theta_{iJ} = \Gamma/\{1+(J-1)\,\Gamma\}$ where (8.8)–(8.10) hold, or θ_{i1} could be as large as $\Gamma/\{\Gamma+(J-1)\}$ if $\theta_{i2} = \cdots = \theta_{iJ} = 1/\{\Gamma+(J-1)\}$ where (8.8)–(8.10) still hold.

Because (8.10) can be deduced from $0 \le \theta_{ij} \le 1$, (8.8) and (8.9), constraint (8.10) could be replaced by $0 \le \theta_{ij} \le 1$ for all ij. However, the sharper bound (8.10) provides more insight, and it may accelerate computations, as an optimization algorithm does not need to entertain as a possible solution a $\boldsymbol{\theta}$ that violates (8.10) but satisfies $0 \le \theta_{ij} \le 1$ for all ij.

Write B_Γ for the set of $I \times J$-dimensional arrays $\boldsymbol{\theta}$ in (8.7) such that (8.8)–(8.10) hold. Although each $\boldsymbol{\theta}$ is a point of dimension IJ, the set B_Γ resides in an $I \times (J-1)$-dimensional flat, because of (8.8). The set B_Γ is closed and bounded and hence compact. Also, B_Γ is convex. Finally, the sets are nested in the sense that $B_\Gamma \subset B_{\Gamma'}$ for $\Gamma < \Gamma'$.

If $\Gamma = 1$, then $\theta_{ij} = 1/J$ for all i, j; so, $\Gamma = 1$ entails ignorable treatment assignment given the matched covariates, $\mathbf{h}(\mathbf{X})$, resulting in randomization inferences. Equivalently, if $\Gamma = 1$, then $B_\Gamma = B_1$ contains a single point, $B_1 = \left\{\overline{\boldsymbol{\theta}}\right\}$, where

$$\overline{\boldsymbol{\theta}} = \begin{bmatrix} 1/J & 1/J & \cdots & 1/J \\ \vdots & \vdots & & \vdots \\ 1/J & 1/J & \cdots & 1/J \end{bmatrix}$$

for the randomization distribution in Chap. 2. Using (8.8)–(8.10), it is evident that $\overline{\boldsymbol{\theta}} \in B_\Gamma$ for all $\Gamma \ge 1$.

If $\Gamma = 1.01$, then $B_\Gamma = B_{1.01}$ contains infinitely many $\boldsymbol{\theta}$s, all of which closely resemble $\overline{\boldsymbol{\theta}}$. Indeed, for blocks of size $J = 3$, using (8.10) we have $1/(1+2\times 1.01) = 0.3311 \le \theta_{ij} \le 0.3355 = 1.01/(1.01+2)$ for all ij and for all $\boldsymbol{\theta} \in B_{1.01}$, as opposed to $\overline{\theta}_{ij} = 1/J = 1/3$ in a randomized block experiment.

If $\boldsymbol{\theta}$ is any $I \times J$ matrix satisfying (8.8) and $0 < \theta_{ij} < 1$ for all ij, then there exists some $\Gamma \ge 1$ such that $\boldsymbol{\theta} \in B_\Gamma$.[4] In this sense, to assume either that $\boldsymbol{\theta} = \overline{\boldsymbol{\theta}} \in B_1$ or that $\boldsymbol{\theta} = \overline{\boldsymbol{\theta}} \in B_{1.01}$ is to assume a great deal about unmeasured biases in treatment assignment, whereas to assume $\boldsymbol{\theta} \in B_3$ is to assume much less. An assumption that $\boldsymbol{\theta} \in B_2$ is a statement about the world: it is true or false, and data may reveal it to be false or implausible; see, for instance, Chap. 12. In contrast, to assume that there exists some unspecified $\Gamma \ge 1$ such that $\boldsymbol{\theta} \in B_\Gamma$ is barely to assume anything at all; in fact, it is to assume only that $0 < \theta_{ij} < 1$ for all ij. The collection of sets $\{B_\Gamma : \Gamma \in [1, \infty)\}$ is not a model, but rather a yardstick for measuring how far

[4] We can say a bit more. Let $\mathcal{T}$ be the set of all $I \times J$ matrices that satisfy (8.8) and $0 < \theta_{ij} < 1$ for all ij. Then, for any $\boldsymbol{\theta} \in \mathcal{T}$ there exists a unique $\Gamma \ge 1$ such that every open neighborhood of $\boldsymbol{\theta}$ has a nonempty intersection with both B_Γ and its complement in $\mathcal{T}$, namely, $\mathcal{T} - B_\Gamma$. In other words, for every $\boldsymbol{\theta} \in \mathcal{T}$ there exists a smallest $\Gamma \ge 1$ such that $\boldsymbol{\theta} \in B_\Gamma$.

treatment assignment probabilities $\boldsymbol{\theta}$ depart from randomized assignment, $\overline{\boldsymbol{\theta}}$. There are other yardsticks, and Sect. 8.5 discusses a different yardstick that permits limited violations of positivity or common support; that is, it permits some $\theta_{ij} = 0$ or $\theta_{ij} = 1$.

For each $\boldsymbol{\theta} \in B_\Gamma$, there is a distribution of treatment assignments given $(\mathcal{F}, \mathcal{Z})$, namely,

$$\Pr(\mathbf{Z} = \mathbf{z} \mid \mathcal{F}, \mathcal{Z}) = \prod_{i=1}^{I} \prod_{j=1}^{J} \theta_{ij}^{z_{ij}} \text{ for } \mathbf{z} \in \mathcal{Z}, \tag{8.11}$$

which reduces to (2.4) for $\boldsymbol{\theta} = \overline{\boldsymbol{\theta}} \in B_\Gamma$.

8.3 Sensitivity of Causal Inferences to Biased Treatment Assignment

Sensitivity of Tests of Hypotheses About Treatment Effects

In Sect. 2.8, a simple hypothesis, $H_0 : \boldsymbol{\delta} = \boldsymbol{\delta}_0$, about causal effects, $\delta_{ij} = r_{Tij} - r_{Cij}$ was tested in a randomized block experiment by (i) using the observed responses, R_{ij}, to compute adjusted responses, $R_{ij}^{\delta_0} = R_{ij} - Z_{ij}\,\delta_{0ij}$, where $R_{ij}^{\delta_0} = r_{Cij}$ if H_0 is true; (ii) selecting a test statistic, $T^{\delta_0} = t\left(\mathbf{Z}, \mathbf{R}^{\delta_0}\right)$, which rejects H_0 when T^{δ_0} is large, (iii) momentarily presuming H_0 to be true in order to determine the distribution of T^{δ_0} under H_0; and (iv) realizing that this null distribution $\Pr(T \geq a \mid \mathcal{F}, \mathcal{Z})$ of T under H_0 is (2.12). Then, an α-level test rejects H_0 if this null distribution attaches probability at most α to values of $T^{\delta_0} = t\left(\mathbf{Z}, \mathbf{R}^{\delta_0}\right)$ as large or larger than the observed value, that is, if $\Pr\left(T^{\delta_0} \geq a \,\middle|\, \mathcal{F}, \mathcal{Z}\right) \leq \alpha$ under H_0 with $a = t\left(\mathbf{Z}, \mathbf{R}^{\delta_0}\right)$. The P-value is the smallest α that leads to rejection of H_0.

Proposition 8.1 generalizes Proposition 2.2 to any one specific $\boldsymbol{\theta} \in B_\Gamma$; that is, Proposition 2.2 is the special case of Proposition 8.1 with $\boldsymbol{\theta} = \overline{\boldsymbol{\theta}}$.

Proposition 8.1 *If $H_0 : \boldsymbol{\delta} = \boldsymbol{\delta}_0$ is true and treatment assignments $\mathbf{Z}$ have the distribution (8.11), then (i) $\mathbf{r}_C = \mathbf{R}^{\delta_0}$, and (ii) given $\mathcal{F}$ and $\mathcal{Z}$, the distribution of $T^{\delta_0} = t\left(\mathbf{Z}, \mathbf{R}^{\delta_0}\right)$ is*

$$\Pr\left\{t\left(\mathbf{Z}, \mathbf{r}_C\right) \geq a \mid \mathcal{F}, \mathcal{Z}\right\} = \sum_{\mathbf{z} \in \mathcal{Z}: t(\mathbf{z}, \mathbf{r}_C) \geq a} \prod_{i=1}^{I} \prod_{j=1}^{J} \theta_{ij}^{z_{ij}}. \tag{8.12}$$

Proof Assume H_0 is true for the purpose of testing it; then, $\mathbf{R}^{\delta_0} = \mathbf{r}_C$, as in Proposition 2.2, where $\mathbf{r}_C$ is part of $\mathcal{F}$ and is fixed by conditioning on $\mathcal{F}$. The set $\{\mathbf{z} \in \mathcal{Z} : t(\mathbf{z}, \mathbf{r}_C) \geq a\}$ contains the possible values $\mathbf{z}$ of $\mathbf{Z}$ such that $t(\mathbf{Z}, \mathbf{r}_C) \geq a$. The event $\mathbf{Z} = \mathbf{z}$ has probability (8.11), yielding (8.12). □

Proposition 8.1 provides an α-level test of $H_0 : \boldsymbol{\delta} = \boldsymbol{\delta}_0$ for a specific $\boldsymbol{\theta} \in B_\Gamma$, formed by calculating the probability (8.12) for $a = t\left(\mathbf{Z}, \mathbf{R}^{\delta_0}\right)$ and rejecting H_0 if $\Pr\left\{t\left(\mathbf{Z}, \mathbf{r}_C\right) \geq a \mid \mathcal{F}, \mathcal{Z}\right\} \leq \alpha$. As yet, that calculation is not useful, because we do not know the principal unobserved covariate ζ_{ij}, so we cannot derive the true θ_{ij} from it. In brief, $\boldsymbol{\theta}$ is unknown.

Suppose that we repeated this calculation with $a = t\left(\mathbf{Z}, \mathbf{R}^{\delta_0}\right)$ for every $\boldsymbol{\theta} \in B_\Gamma$, and suppose that $\Pr\{t(\mathbf{Z}, \mathbf{r}_C) \geq a \mid \mathcal{F}, \mathcal{Z}\} \leq \alpha$ for all $\boldsymbol{\theta} \in B_\Gamma$; that is, suppose

$$\max_{\boldsymbol{\theta} \in B_\Gamma} \sum_{\mathbf{z} \in \mathcal{Z}: t(\mathbf{z}, \mathbf{r}_C) \geq a} \prod_{i=1}^{I} \prod_{j=1}^{J} \theta_{ij}^{z_{ij}} \leq \alpha. \tag{8.13}$$

If (8.13) were true, then we could correctly say several things. First, because $\overline{\boldsymbol{\theta}} \in B_\Gamma$, the hypothesis $H_0 : \boldsymbol{\delta} = \boldsymbol{\delta}_0$ would have been rejected at level α by the randomization test in Proposition 2.2. Moreover, if treatment assignments were ignorable given $\mathbf{X}$ and if the blocking had been controlled for either $\mathbf{X}$ or the true propensity score $e(\mathbf{X})$, then this same test would have rejected $H_0 : \boldsymbol{\delta} = \boldsymbol{\delta}_0$ at level α. More importantly, the deviations $\boldsymbol{\theta} \in B_\Gamma$ from randomization or ignorable assignment are too small to alter this conclusion; that is, the bias in treatment assignment would have to be larger than Γ to alter the conclusion that $H_0 : \boldsymbol{\delta} = \boldsymbol{\delta}_0$ is rejected at level α. In this case, we say that rejection of $H_0 : \boldsymbol{\delta} = \boldsymbol{\delta}_0$ at level α is insensitive to a bias in treatment assignment of magnitude Γ. The smallest α leading to rejection of $H_0 : \boldsymbol{\delta} = \boldsymbol{\delta}_0$ for all $\boldsymbol{\theta} \in B_\Gamma$ is the upper bound on the P-value.

In Chap. 2, inferences of all kinds were built from tests of simple hypotheses, including (i) tests of composite hypotheses, $H_0 : \boldsymbol{\delta} \in \Delta_0$, (ii) $1 - \alpha$ confidence sets and intervals, (iii) point estimates, and (iv) "standard errors" understood in terms of 2/3 confidence intervals. Although there are still some technical details to be worked out, Proposition 8.1 and (8.13) will yield sensitivity analyses for inferences (i)–(iv) with almost no additional effort once we can determine whether the inequality in (8.13) holds.

Example: Alcohol and HDL Cholesterol

In the study of light daily alcohol consumption and HDL cholesterol levels in Sect. 1.4 and Fig. 1.3, daily drinkers (D) were compared to never drinkers (N), rare drinkers (R), and people who used to engage in regular binge drinking in the past but quit (B). There were $I = 406$ blocks, matched for age, sex, and education, with one individual from each group, and somewhat higher HDL levels were observed for the daily drinkers. Consider a one-sided, α-level test of Fisher's simple hypothesis of no treatment effect $H_0 : \boldsymbol{\delta} = \mathbf{0}$ against positive effects in the presence of a bias in treatment assignment of at most Γ, for various values of $\Gamma \geq 1$. As in Sect. 2.9, rejection of Fisher's hypothesis, $H_0 : \boldsymbol{\delta} = \mathbf{0}$, will also imply rejection of the composite null hypothesis $H_0 : \boldsymbol{\delta} \in \Delta_0$ where Δ_0 is the set of all $I \times J$ matrices $\boldsymbol{\delta}$ with $\delta_{ij} \leq 0$ for all i and j.

Table 8.1 displays the upper bound on the P-value for several values of $\Gamma \geq 1$ and for four test statistics. Two of the test statistics were discussed in Sect. 2.6. The blocked Wilcoxon statistic ranks the observed responses R_{ij} from 1 to $J = 4$

Table 8.1 Upper bounds on the one-sided P-value testing the null hypothesis of no treatment effect in the study of alcohol and HDL cholesterol. Results for four weighted rank statistics are compared: the blocked Wilcoxon rank sum statistic, Quade's statistic, and the default statistic, U868, in the `weightedRank` package in R, plus U878. In each column, a P-value close to 0.05 is in **bold**. The P-value bounds are rounded to four digits

	Four test statistics			
Γ	Wilcoxon	Quade	U868	U878
1	0.0000	0.0000	0.0000	0.0000
2	0.0000	0.0000	0.0000	0.0000
3.5	**0.0603**	0.0002	0.0000	0.0000
4	0.3478	0.0052	0.0003	0.0001
4.5	0.7401	**0.0447**	0.0028	0.0010
5	0.9429	0.1775	0.0154	0.0050
5.5	0.9926	0.4123	**0.0537**	0.0174
6	0.9994	0.6642	0.1340	**0.0456**

within each block i and sums the $I = 406$ ranks q^*_{ij} for the 406 treated individuals (D) with $Z_{ij} = 1$. It gives equal weight to the $I = 406$ blocks. Quade's statistic emphasizes blocks i in which the within-block ranges, w_i in (2.11), are larger. Specifically, Quade's ranks are formed by multiplying Wilcoxon's ranks, q^*_{ij}, by a number proportional to the ranks b_i of the block ranges, w_i, ranking the ranges from 1 to I. Quade's statistic equals Wilcoxon's other statistic, his signed rank statistic, when $J = 2$ for matched pairs. In Quade's statistic, the block with the largest range, w_i, has a weight that is about I times larger than the block with the smallest range.

The third statistic, U868, is the default option in the `wgtRank` function in the `weightedRank` package in R. The statistics U868 and U878 are also weighted rank statistics, but they pay very little attention to the blocks with the smallest within-block ranges [69, 72, 79]. All of the statistics in Table 8.1 are weighted rank statistics, as discussed in Sect. 2.6, in the sense that they have the form $T = t(\mathbf{Z}, \mathbf{R}) = \sum_{i=1}^{I} \sum_{j=1}^{J} Z_{ij}\, q_{ij}$ with $q_{ij} = \phi\left(q^*_{ij}\right) \varphi\left\{b_i/(I+1)\right\}$, where $\phi(\cdot)$ and $\varphi(\cdot)$ are two nonnegative, monotone increasing functions. The $\varphi(\cdot)$ functions for the four statistics are depicted in Fig. 8.1. Properties of U868 and U878 are discussed in Chaps. 9 and 11. Notably, the blocked Wilcoxon rank sum statistic gives the most weight to blocks with small ranges, w_i, and U878 gives them the least weight.

Recall that $\Gamma = 1$ yields the randomization distribution (2.4) or ignorable treatment assignment or "no unmeasured confounders." For $\Gamma = 1$ the P-values in Table 8.1 are all very small. If the HDL cholesterol data had come from a randomized block experiment, then there would have been very strong evidence against the hypothesis of no effect, $H_0 : \boldsymbol{\delta} = \mathbf{0}$, and also against any pattern of nonpositive effects, $H_0 : \boldsymbol{\delta} \in \Delta_0$. Moreover, this conclusion is insensitive to substantial biases in treatment assignment. At $\Gamma = 3.4$, even the blocked Wilcoxon rank sum statistic has a maximum P-value of 0.0357, moving to 0.0603 at $\Gamma = 3.5$.

A bias in treatment assignment of $\Gamma = 3.5$ is a substantial departure from a blocked randomized experiment (2.4). With blocks of size $J = 4$, a randomized experiment has $\theta_{ij} = 1/J = 0.25$ for all i and j, but from the upper bound in

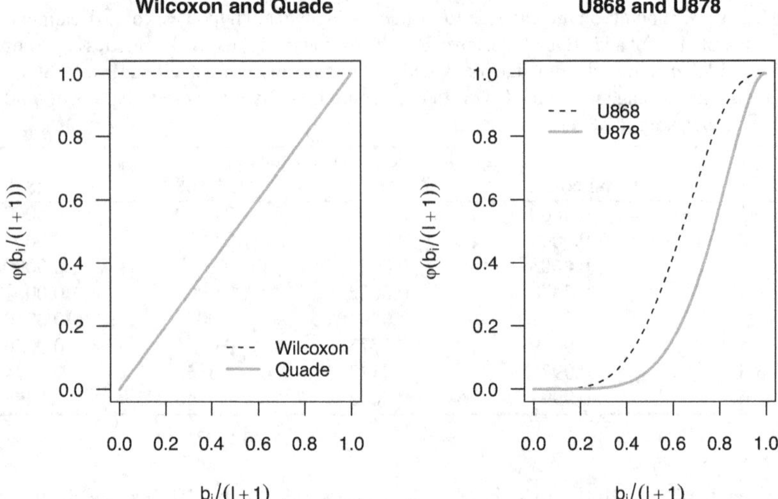

Fig. 8.1 The $\varphi(\cdot)$ functions for the four weighted rank statistics in Table 8.1. In a weighted rank statistic, the $\varphi(\cdot)$ function weights block i by $\varphi(b_i/(I+1))$, where b_i is the rank of the within-block range of the R_{ij}'s in block i

(8.10), an observational study with $\Gamma = 3.5$ might have $\theta_{ij} = \Gamma/\{\Gamma + (J-1)\} = 3.5/(3.5+3) = 0.538$ for one j and $\theta_{ij} = 1/\{\Gamma + (J-1)\} = 1/(3.5+3) = 0.154$ for the remaining three js. Here,

$$\frac{0.538}{0.154} = \frac{\frac{\Gamma}{\Gamma+(J-1)}}{\frac{1}{\Gamma+(J-1)}} = \Gamma = 3.5 \text{ and } 1 = \frac{\Gamma}{\Gamma+(J-1)} + (J-1) \times \frac{1}{\Gamma+(J-1)}.$$

An interesting aspect of Table 8.1 is that different test statistics report very different degrees of sensitivity to unmeasured biases. In one sense, this is not surprising: different test statistics differ in performance even in randomized experiments, so why should that not happen also in observational studies? The blocked Wilcoxon rank sum statistic reported sensitivity to an unmeasured bias of $\Gamma = 3.5$, in the sense that a bias of that size could barely push its P-value above $\alpha = 0.05$ when H_0 is true. Quade's statistic passes from a maximum P-value of 0.0447 at $\Gamma = 4.5$ to a maximum P-value of 0.0621 at $\Gamma = 4.6$. The statistic U868 passes from a maximum P-value of 0.0431 at $\Gamma = 5.4$ to a maximum P-value of 0.0537 at $\Gamma = 5.5$. As discussed in the previous paragraph, at $\Gamma = 3.5$ one θ_{ij} might be as large as 0.538 rather than 0.25, and the rest of the θ_{ij}'s in block i might be as small as 0.154; however, at $\Gamma = 5.5$ one θ_{ij} might be as large as $5.5/(5.5+3) = 0.647$ with the other three θ_{ij}'s as small as $1/(5.5+3) = 0.118$. Clearly, we will need some theoretical guidance about which statistics to use and which to avoid when examining sensitivity to unmeasured bias. Chapters 9 and 11 address this need. The statistic U868 and other statistics are discussed in Chaps. 9 and 11. Also, we will need some theoretical guidance about how decisions made when designing a study affect its sensitivity to unmeasured biases, and Chap. 10 addresses this need. Section 8.7 discusses an additional way to interpret the magnitude of Γ.

To anchor the discussion of Table 8.1, in Hammond's [33] study, a bias of $\Gamma = 6$ could explain away, as biased treatment assignment, the effect of heavy smoking on lung cancer [66, Table 4.1]; however, a bias of $\Gamma = 3.5$, though large, could not begin to explain Hammond's findings. So, $\Gamma = 6$ is a very large departure from a randomized experiment.

The same reasoning applies to confidence intervals. Instead of testing $H_0 : \boldsymbol{\delta} = \mathbf{0}$, we may test $H_0 : \boldsymbol{\delta} = \tau_0 \times \mathbf{1}$ for every real τ_0, where $\mathbf{1}$ is an $I \times J$ matrix of ones. Retaining those τ_0 that are not rejected at level α for a specific Γ yields a $1 - \alpha$ confidence interval for an additive effect τ in the presence of a bias of at most Γ. As in Sect. 2.9, rejection of the simple hypothesis $H_0 : \boldsymbol{\delta} = \tau_0 \times \mathbf{1}$ entails also rejecting every hypothesis $\boldsymbol{\delta} = \boldsymbol{\delta}_0$ with $\delta_{0ij} \le \tau_0$ for all i and j.

Set $\Gamma = 2$, and consider the four 95% confidence intervals for the four test statistics in Table 8.1. All four tests have rejected $\tau_0 = 0$ at $\Gamma = 2$, so their intervals will be strictly positive. The one-sided 95% confidence intervals at $\Gamma = 2$ are $\tau \ge 5$ for the blocked Wilcoxon statistic, $\tau \ge 6.5$ for Quade's statistic, and $\tau \ge 7$ for both the U868 and U878 statistics. As always, a test that tends to reject more null hypotheses tends to produce shorter confidence intervals, simply because the confidence interval is a record of the null hypotheses that the test did not reject.

8.4 Null Expectation and Variance of a Test Statistic

Simple Formulas for the Expectation and Variance

Under the distribution (8.12), consider testing $H_0 : \boldsymbol{\delta} = \boldsymbol{\delta}_0$ using a test statistic of the form $T^{\boldsymbol{\delta}_0} = t\left(\mathbf{Z}, \mathbf{R}^{\boldsymbol{\delta}_0}\right) = \sum_{i=1}^{I} \sum_{j=1}^{J} Z_{ij}\, q_{ij}$, where q_{ij} is a function of $\mathbf{R}^{\boldsymbol{\delta}_0}$; see Sect. 2.6–Sect. 2.7 for many such statistics, including the blocked Wilcoxon rank sum statistic and Quade's statistic. Here, q_{ij} depends upon $\boldsymbol{\delta}_0$, but the notation does not indicate this explicitly. If $H_0 : \boldsymbol{\delta} = \boldsymbol{\delta}_0$ were true, then $\mathbf{R}^{\boldsymbol{\delta}_0} = \mathbf{r}_C$ is fixed by conditioning on $\mathcal{F}$ in (8.12), so the null distribution of $T^{\boldsymbol{\delta}_0} = \sum_{i=1}^{I} \sum_{j=1}^{J} Z_{ij}\, q_{ij}$ is the distribution of the sum of I independent random variables, where the ith random variable, $A_i = \sum_{j=1}^{J} Z_{ij}\, q_{ij}$, is one of the scores $q_{i1}, \ldots, q_{iJ}$, picked with probabilities $\theta_{i1}, \ldots, \theta_{iJ}$. Proposition 8.2 is parallel to Proposition 2.3, but with different treatment assignment probabilities, θ_{ij}, rather than $1/J$. Aside from using (8.12) in place of (2.4) and θ_{ij} in place of $1/J$, the proof of Proposition 8.2 is the same as the proof of Proposition 2.3.

Proposition 8.2 *If $H_0 : \boldsymbol{\delta} = \boldsymbol{\delta}_0$ is true and treatment assignments are governed by (8.12), then conditionally given $\mathcal{F}$, $\mathcal{Z}$: (i) the statistic $T^{\boldsymbol{\delta}_0} = \sum_{i=1}^{I} \sum_{j=1}^{J} Z_{ij}\, q_{ij}$*

is the sum of I independent random variables; (ii) the ith of these I independent random variables, $A_i = \sum_{j=1}^{J} Z_{ij}\, q_{ij}$*, is one of the J fixed scores,* $q_{i1}, \ldots, q_{iJ}$*, picked with probability* $\theta_{i1}, \ldots, \theta_{iJ}$*; and (iii) the expectation and variance of* $T^{\delta_0} = \sum_{i=1}^{I} \sum_{j=1}^{J} Z_{ij}\, q_{ij}$ *are*

$$\mathrm{E}\left(T^{\delta_0} \mid \mathcal{F}, \mathcal{Z}\right) = \sum_{i=1}^{I} \mu_{\theta i}, \text{ where } \mu_{\theta i} = \sum_{j=1}^{J} \theta_{ij}\, q_{ij} = \mathrm{E}(A_i \mid \mathcal{F}, \mathcal{Z}), \tag{8.14}$$

and

$$\mathrm{var}\left(T^{\delta_0} \mid \mathcal{F}, \mathcal{Z}\right) = \sum_{i=1}^{I} \sigma_{\theta i}^2, \text{ where } \sigma_{\theta i}^2 = \sum_{j=1}^{J} \theta_{ij}\, \left(q_{ij} - \mu_{\theta i}\right)^2 = \mathrm{var}(A_i \mid \mathcal{F}, \mathcal{Z}). \tag{8.15}$$

Sensitivity Analysis for Point Estimates of Treatment Effects

In a randomized experiment in Sect. 2.10, a Hodges-Lehmann point estimate $\widehat{\tau}$ of an additive effect, $\boldsymbol{\delta} = \tau\times\mathbf{1}$, was found by solving the equation $\mathrm{E}\left(T^{\tau_0\times\mathbf{1}} \mid \mathcal{F}, \mathcal{Z}\right) = T^{\tau_0\times\mathbf{1}}$ for τ_0. For a given $\Gamma \geq 1$, there is an interval of possible values for $\mathrm{E}\left(T^{\tau_0\times\mathbf{1}} \mid \mathcal{F}, \mathcal{Z}\right)$ in (8.14) for $\boldsymbol{\theta} \in B_\Gamma$ and a corresponding interval of Hodges-Lehmann point estimates [60]. For a weighted rank statistic in Sect. 2.6, this interval of possible values for $\mathrm{E}\left(T^{\tau_0\times\mathbf{1}} \mid \mathcal{F}, \mathcal{Z}\right)$ does not change as τ_0 increases, but $T^{\tau_0\times\mathbf{1}}$ is monotone decreasing as τ_0 increases; see Proposition 2.4. Consequently, an interval of values of $\mathrm{E}\left(T^{\tau_0\times\mathbf{1}} \mid \mathcal{F}, \mathcal{Z}\right)$ for $\boldsymbol{\theta} \in B_\Gamma$ gives an interval of solutions $\left[\widehat{\tau}_{\text{low}}, \widehat{\tau}_{\text{high}}\right]$ to the equation $\mathrm{E}\left(T^{\tau_0\times\mathbf{1}} \mid \mathcal{F}, \mathcal{Z}\right) = T^{\tau_0\times\mathbf{1}}$.[5]

The interval $\left[\widehat{\tau}_{\text{low}}, \widehat{\tau}_{\text{high}}\right]$ is an interval of point estimates, not a confidence interval. As with point estimates generally, $\left[\widehat{\tau}_{\text{low}}, \widehat{\tau}_{\text{high}}\right]$ makes no allowance for sampling uncertainty; rather, it allows for a bias in treatment assignment of magnitude at most Γ. At $\Gamma = 1$ for randomization or ignorable treatment assignment, $\widehat{\tau}_{\text{low}} = \widehat{\tau}_{\text{high}}$ is a Hodges-Lehmann estimate for a randomization distribution, and it is a single point. As Γ increases, the interval $\left[\widehat{\tau}_{\text{low}}, \widehat{\tau}_{\text{high}}\right]$ becomes longer.

Continuing the sensitivity analysis for alcohol and HDL cholesterol in Table 8.1, at $\Gamma = 2$, the interval of point estimates is $\left[\widehat{\tau}_{\text{low}}, \widehat{\tau}_{\text{high}}\right] = [6, 20]$ using the blocked Wilcoxon statistic, [8, 18] using Quade's statistic, and [9, 17.5] using the statistic U868.

---

[5] A similar approach works with statistics that are not rank statistics, such as M-estimates [68]. The situation is only slightly more complex, because now both $\mathrm{E}\left(T^{\tau_0\times\mathbf{1}} \mid \mathcal{F}, \mathcal{Z}\right)$ and $T^{\tau_0\times\mathbf{1}}$ change with τ_0, so for $\boldsymbol{\theta} \in B_\Gamma$ one determines the set of solutions τ_0 to the equation $0 = \mathrm{E}\left(T^{\tau_0\times\mathbf{1}} \mid \mathcal{F}, \mathcal{Z}\right) - T^{\tau_0\times\mathbf{1}}$.

8.5 Several Views of the Mathematics of Sensitivity Analysis

Introduction: Four Views of Sensitivity Analysis

For any one hypothesis, $H_0 : \delta = \delta_0$, the sensitivity analysis asks: Is (8.13) true? In other words: Would we reject at level α the simple null hypothesis $H_0 : \delta = \delta_0$ if the bias in treatment assignments were of magnitude at most Γ? That is the question at the atomic level, and once we can answer it we can use the atomic answer to build the larger molecules of inference. We answer the atomic question repeatedly for different hypotheses and different levels α, thereby producing confidence intervals, point estimates, and P-values, as in Chap. 2. Also, as in Chap. 2, knowing the answer about a simple null hypothesis often settles the answer about a composite null hypothesis. So, in Sect. 8.5, we ask: Is (8.13) true?

There are several ways to view this question. One lens, the lens used in the current subsection, sees the answer as a simple type of optimization problem. A second lens, the lens sketched in the next subsection, sees the answer as a problem in applied probability. The third lens is a general exact solution that is difficult to compute if there are many blocks or strata. The fourth lens, the most general and adequate lens, is bifocal: it alternates between the perspectives of optimization and probability, and it is sketched in the final subsection of Sect. 8.5.

For most conceptual and data analytic purposes, it is sufficient to view sensitivity analysis through the lens of optimization, with the computer as a black box that solves the optimization problem. The second lens is helpful when proving theorems about how sensitivity analyses are likely to turn out under various research designs, analyzed using various test statistics, under various sampling models. You can simulate the answers to such questions using the first lens—repeatedly simulate a sample and give it to the black box—but to substitute proof for simulation, the second lens is helpful. The third lens is directly useful for some problems, but is mostly a stepping stone to the fourth lens. The fourth lens yields general statements about broad classes of test statistics and study designs and fast algorithms that are easy to program even for large problems, such as the example in Sect. 1.2 with $I = 54{,}996$ blocks.

An Optimization Lens: A Convex Quadratic Program

Suppose throughout this subsection that $H_0 : \delta = \delta_0$ is true and treatment assignment is governed by (8.12). Suppose further that $T^{\delta_0} = \sum_{i=1}^{I}\sum_{j=1}^{J} Z_{ij}\, q_{ij}$ satisfies a central limit theorem as $I \to \infty$ with $\mathrm{E}\left(T^{\delta_0} \mid \mathcal{F}, \mathcal{Z}\right)$ and $\mathrm{var}\left(T^{\delta_0} \mid \mathcal{F}, \mathcal{Z}\right)$ given in Proposition 8.2. One such central limit theorem is given in Appendix Sect. 8.10. For any one fixed $\boldsymbol{\theta} \in B_\Gamma$, an approximate two-sided α-level test of $H_0 : \delta = \delta_0$ rejects H_0 if

$$\frac{\left|T^{\delta_0} - \mathrm{E}\left(T^{\delta_0} \mid \mathcal{F}, \mathcal{Z}\right)\right|}{\sqrt{\mathrm{var}\left(T^{\delta_0} \mid \mathcal{F}, \mathcal{Z}\right)}} \geq \Phi^{-1}(1-\alpha/2), \tag{8.16}$$

where $\Phi(\cdot)$ is the standard normal cumulative distribution. For instance, $\Phi^{-1}(1-\alpha/2) \doteq 1.96$ for $\alpha = 0.05$. Write $\varsigma_{\alpha/2} = \Phi^{-1}(1-\alpha/2)^2$, so $\varsigma_{0.05} \doteq 1.96^2 = 3.84$, and write

$$f_{\alpha/2}(\boldsymbol{\theta}) = \left(T^{\delta_0} - \sum_{i=1}^{I}\sum_{j=1}^{J} \theta_{ij}\, q_{ij}\right)^2 - \varsigma_{\alpha/2} \sum_{i=1}^{I} \left\{ \left(\sum_{j=1}^{J} \theta_{ij}\, q_{ij}^2\right) - \left(\sum_{j=1}^{J} \theta_{ij}\, q_{ij}\right)^2 \right\}. \tag{8.17}$$

Proposition 8.3 *For one fixed $\boldsymbol{\theta} \in B_\Gamma$, condition (8.16) holds if and only if*

$$f_{\alpha/2}(\boldsymbol{\theta}) \geq 0.$$

Proof Squaring (8.16) and rearranging gives the equivalent condition:

$$\left\{T^{\delta_0} - \mathrm{E}\left(T^{\delta_0} \mid \mathcal{F}, \mathcal{Z}\right)\right\}^2 \geq \varsigma_{\alpha/2}\, \mathrm{var}\left(T^{\delta_0} \mid \mathcal{F}, \mathcal{Z}\right).$$

Substitution using Proposition 8.2 gives another equivalent condition, namely,

$$\left(T^{\delta_0} - \sum_{i=1}^{I}\sum_{j=1}^{J} \theta_{ij}\, q_{ij}\right)^2 - \varsigma_{\alpha/2} \sum_{i=1}^{I}\sum_{j=1}^{J} \theta_{ij}\left(q_{ij} - \mu_{\boldsymbol{\theta} i}\right)^2 \geq 0.$$

Using $\mu_{\boldsymbol{\theta} i} = \sum_{j=1}^{J} \theta_{ij}\, q_{ij}$, it follows that

$$\sum_{j=1}^{J} \theta_{ij}\left(q_{ij} - \mu_{\boldsymbol{\theta} i}\right)^2 = \sum_{j=1}^{J} \theta_{ij}\left(q_{ij}^2 - 2\mu_{\boldsymbol{\theta} i} q_{ij} + \mu_{\boldsymbol{\theta} i}^2\right)$$

$$= \left(\sum_{j=1}^{J} \theta_{ij}\, q_{ij}^2\right) - \mu_{\boldsymbol{\theta} i}^2 = \left(\sum_{j=1}^{J} \theta_{ij}\, q_{ij}^2\right) - \left(\sum_{j=1}^{J} \theta_{ij}\, q_{ij}\right)^2,$$

proving the proposition. □

Although $f_{\alpha/2}(\boldsymbol{\theta})$ in (8.17) is a nonlinear function, it is the nicest kind of nonlinear function, as indicated by Proposition 8.4.

Proposition 8.4 *The function $f_{\alpha/2}(\boldsymbol{\theta})$ is a convex quadratic function of $\boldsymbol{\theta}$.*

The proof of Proposition 8.4 is in Appendix Sect. 8.9. The proof consists of routine checking and is not difficult, but it is placed in an appendix because it is a bit long. Remark 8.1 in Sect. 8.9 notes that, in general, $f_{\alpha/2}(\boldsymbol{\theta})$ is not strictly convex, for instance, if there is a within-block tie, $q_{ij} = q_{ij'}$ for $j \neq j'$.[6]

Recall that B_Γ is the set of $\boldsymbol{\theta}$ that satisfy the linear equalities and inequalities (8.8)–(8.10). Define

$$F_{\Gamma,\alpha/2} = \min_{\boldsymbol{\theta} \in B_\Gamma} f_{\alpha/2}(\boldsymbol{\theta}).$$

In light of Proposition 8.4, one can calculate $F_{\Gamma,\alpha/2}$ by finding the minimum of a convex quadratic function subject to linear equality and inequality constraints. That is easy to do using a solver such as `gurobi` for a problem with $I = 406$ blocks of size $J = 4$, as in Sect. 1.4, where $\boldsymbol{\theta}$ is of dimension $IJ = 1624$.

Here is the important point. If $F_{\Gamma,\alpha/2} \geq 0$, then Proposition 8.3 says that $H_0 : \boldsymbol{\delta} = \boldsymbol{\delta}_0$ is rejected at level α for every $\boldsymbol{\theta} \in B_\Gamma$; that is, rejection of H_0 is insensitive to all biased treatment assignments $\boldsymbol{\theta}$ that deviate from random assignment by a magnitude of at most Γ. More precisely, the approximate two-sided α-level test in (8.16) is insensitive to a bias of magnitude at most Γ if $F_{\Gamma,\alpha/2} \geq 0$. In this sense, a two-sided sensitivity analysis entails finding the minimum of a convex quadratic function (8.17) of $\boldsymbol{\theta}$, subject to linear equality and inequality constraints (8.8)–(8.10).

The one-sided test in (8.12) and (8.13) requires a small change. Pick an $\alpha < 1/2$, commonly $\alpha = 0.05$. For a fixed $\boldsymbol{\theta}$, the approximate one-sided α-level test of $H_0 : \boldsymbol{\delta} = \boldsymbol{\delta}_0$ rejects H_0 if

$$\frac{T^{\boldsymbol{\delta}_0} - \mathrm{E}\left(T^{\boldsymbol{\delta}_0} \mid \mathcal{F}, \mathcal{Z}\right)}{\sqrt{\mathrm{var}\left(T^{\boldsymbol{\delta}_0} \mid \mathcal{F}, \mathcal{Z}\right)}} \geq \Phi^{-1}(1-\alpha). \tag{8.18}$$

Note the change from $\alpha/2$ in the two-sided test in (8.16) to α in (8.18). We can no longer determine whether (8.18) holds by examining its square, as we did in Proposition 8.3, because squaring discards the sign of $T^{\boldsymbol{\delta}_0} - \mathrm{E}\left(T^{\boldsymbol{\delta}_0} \mid \mathcal{F}, \mathcal{Z}\right) = T^{\boldsymbol{\delta}_0} - \sum_{i=1}^{I} \sum_{j=1}^{J} \theta_{ij}\, q_{ij} = g(\boldsymbol{\theta})$, say. In other words, it is possible that $f_\alpha(\boldsymbol{\theta}) \geq 0$ because $T^{\boldsymbol{\delta}_0}$ is far below $\mathrm{E}\left(T^{\boldsymbol{\delta}_0} \mid \mathcal{F}, \mathcal{Z}\right)$, but this would not lead to rejection of H_0 in the one-sided test in (8.18), because $g(\boldsymbol{\theta}) \leq 0$.

The method for one-sided sensitivity analyses is simple, although it takes a moment to understand why this simple method works. Recall that $\overline{\boldsymbol{\theta}}$ comprises the probabilities in randomization inference, $\theta_{ij} = 1/J$ for all i and j. The method says (8.18) holds for all $\boldsymbol{\theta} \in B_\Gamma$ if and only if $g\left(\overline{\boldsymbol{\theta}}\right) > 0$ and $f_\alpha(\boldsymbol{\theta}) \geq 0$ for all $\boldsymbol{\theta} \in B_\Gamma$. In other words, solve the quadratic program for the two-sided test, and if $\min_{\boldsymbol{\theta} \in B_\Gamma} f_\alpha(\boldsymbol{\theta}) \geq 0$, then check that you are in the upper tail by verifying that

[6] In what senses is $f_{\alpha/2}(\boldsymbol{\theta})$ a nice function in light of Proposition 8.4? Here are a few answers. Let $C \subseteq B_\Gamma$ be a closed and convex subset of B_Γ; most commonly $C = B_\Gamma$. Because B_Γ is bounded, C is also bounded and hence compact. Because $f_{\alpha/2}(\boldsymbol{\theta})$ is quadratic, it is continuous, and so it achieves a minimum on C. Because $f_{\alpha/2}(\boldsymbol{\theta})$ is convex: (i) any local minimum of $f_{\alpha/2}(\boldsymbol{\theta})$ on C is a global minimum on that C, and (ii) the set of global minima of $f_{\alpha/2}(\boldsymbol{\theta})$ on C is a convex set. Because $f_{\alpha/2}(\boldsymbol{\theta})$ is quadratic, its $IJ \times IJ$ second derivative matrix does not change with $\boldsymbol{\theta}$, and because of the special form of $f_{\alpha/2}(\boldsymbol{\theta})$, the second derivative matrix can be represented in terms of IJ numbers rather than $(IJ)^2$ numbers; see (8.32).

$g\left(\overline{\theta}\right) > 0$. Briefly, it is the same method, with α in place of $\alpha/2$, with one check at the end that $g\left(\overline{\theta}\right) > 0$ to make sure that you are rejecting because T^{δ_0} is too large, not too small. Why does this work? Proposition 8.5 says that a sensitivity analysis is like an ordinary hypothesis test: you can reject in the upper tail because T^{δ_0} is high or in the lower tail because T^{δ_0} is low, but you do not reject in the upper tail for some $\boldsymbol{\theta} \in B_\Gamma$ and in the lower tail for some other $\boldsymbol{\theta} \in B_\Gamma$.

Let us say the q_{ij} are *not constant within blocks* if, for at least one block i, it is not true that $q_{i1} = \cdots = q_{iJ}$.

Proposition 8.5 *Assume the q_{ij} are not constant within blocks. Suppose that (i) $g\left(\overline{\theta}\right) > 0$ and (ii) $f_\alpha(\boldsymbol{\theta}) \geq 0$ for all $\boldsymbol{\theta} \in B_\Gamma$. Then $g(\boldsymbol{\theta}) > 0$ for all $\boldsymbol{\theta} \in B_\Gamma$.*

Proof To obtain a contradiction, suppose that $f_\alpha(\boldsymbol{\theta}) \geq 0$ for all $\boldsymbol{\theta} \in B_\Gamma$ and $g\left(\overline{\theta}\right) > 0$, but there is a $\boldsymbol{\theta}^* \in B_\Gamma$ such that $g(\boldsymbol{\theta}^*) \leq 0$. As B_Γ is convex, for each $\lambda \in [0, 1]$, the convex combination $\lambda\overline{\boldsymbol{\theta}} + (1-\lambda)\boldsymbol{\theta}^*$ is also in B_Γ. Now $h(\lambda) = g\left\{\lambda\overline{\boldsymbol{\theta}} + (1-\lambda)\boldsymbol{\theta}^*\right\}$ is a continuous function of $\lambda \in [0,1]$, where $h(1) = g\left(\overline{\theta}\right) > 0 \geq g(\boldsymbol{\theta}^*) = h(0)$; so, by the intermediate value theorem, there is a $\lambda^\ddagger \in [0, 1]$ such that $0 = h\left(\lambda^\ddagger\right)$. Define $\boldsymbol{\theta}^\ddagger = \lambda^\ddagger\,\overline{\boldsymbol{\theta}} + \left(1-\lambda^\ddagger\right)\boldsymbol{\theta}^*$, so $\boldsymbol{\theta}^\ddagger \in B_\Gamma$ and $g\left(\boldsymbol{\theta}^\ddagger\right) = 0$. Using (8.17), if the q_{ij} are not constant within blocks, then $\{g(\boldsymbol{\theta})\}^2 > f_\alpha(\boldsymbol{\theta})$ for all $\boldsymbol{\theta} \in B_\Gamma$, for all $\Gamma \geq 1$, and for all $\alpha \in (0, 1/2)$. However, $0 = \left\{g\left(\boldsymbol{\theta}^\ddagger\right)\right\}^2 > f_\alpha\left(\boldsymbol{\theta}^\ddagger\right)$ contradicting the premise that $f_\alpha(\boldsymbol{\theta}) \geq 0$ for all $\boldsymbol{\theta} \in B_\Gamma$. □

In summary, sensitivity analyses can be reduced to solving a convex quadratic program. This can be conceptually attractive: one can view the optimization problem as separate from the statistical problem, leaving the optimization problem to the computer to solve, as statisticians commonly do when finding, say, maximum likelihood estimates.

There are good reasons to look a bit further into some of the details of sensitivity analyses, and some of these reasons are sketched in the remainder of Sect. 8.5. However, for data analysis and for a general understanding of most of the rest of this book, you could think of sensitivity analysis as finding the minimum of a convex quadratic function (8.17), and you could regard that optimization problem as a problem for the computer, not for you.

A Probability Lens: Stochastic Order

For certain problems, it is possible to determine the $\boldsymbol{\theta} \in B_\Gamma$ that maximizes the upper tail probability in (8.13), namely,

$$\max_{\boldsymbol{\theta} \in B_\Gamma} \sum_{\mathbf{z} \in \mathcal{Z}:\, t(\mathbf{z}, \mathbf{r}_C) \geq a} \prod_{i=1}^{I} \prod_{j=1}^{J} \theta_{ij}^{z_{ij}}, \tag{8.19}$$

without numerical optimization, simply by thinking about the problem in the right way. Obviously, this can speed computations. More importantly, an explicit form for the bound (8.19) is an aid to theoretical study of the way sensitivity analyses perform as statistical methods and how they behave in different research designs. Perhaps some methods are better than others when used in sensitivity analyses, as is suggested by Table 8.1. Perhaps some research designs are better than others, reliably yielding inferences that are less sensitive to unmeasured biases. An explicit form for the sensitivity bound is helpful in proving, rather than simulating, results along these lines.

Consider the simplest case in which we can find, without numerical optimization, a $\boldsymbol{\theta} \in B_\Gamma$ that yields the maximum in (8.19). This is the case of matched pairs—that is, blocks of size $J = 2$—in which $T^{\delta_0} = \sum_{i=1}^{I} \sum_{j=1}^{2} Z_{ij}\, q_{ij}$ for scores q_{ij} that are functions of $\mathbf{R}^{\delta_0} = \mathbf{r}_C$ when $H_0 : \boldsymbol{\delta} = \boldsymbol{\delta}_0$ is true. For example, this simplest case includes Wilcoxon's signed rank test, which is equivalent to Quade's test for $J = 2$. It also includes all signed-rank statistics, the mean pair difference, and Maritz's [52] version of Huber's M-estimate. In this case, block i has two probabilities, θ_{i1} and θ_{i2}. As is so often true, the correct solution in this case is intuitively obvious, and the effort does not go into *finding* the obvious solution, but rather into *clarifying* the sense in which the intuitively obvious solution is a solution at all. So, let me state the obvious solution, and then we can ponder why this solution is a solution, and how we can generalize it to cases that are no longer obvious. For $i = 1, \ldots, I$, the obvious solution sets

$$\begin{aligned} \theta_{i1} &= \frac{\Gamma}{1+\Gamma} \text{ and } \theta_{i2} = \frac{1}{1+\Gamma} \text{ if } q_{i1} \geq q_{i2} \\ \theta_{i1} &= \frac{1}{1+\Gamma} \text{ and } \theta_{i2} = \frac{\Gamma}{1+\Gamma} \text{ if } q_{i1} < q_{i2}. \end{aligned} \tag{8.20}$$

Notice first that the $2I$-dimensional $\boldsymbol{\theta}$ defined by (8.20) is in B_Γ and satisfies (8.8)–(8.10); so, this $\boldsymbol{\theta}$ is a feasible solution of the optimization problem. Notice second that, for each block i, an inequality in (8.10) holds as equality; that is, the constraints (8.10) are active at the $\boldsymbol{\theta}$ defined by (8.20). In practical terms, if $q_{i1} < q_{i2}$ and we made θ_{i1} smaller than in (8.20), then $\boldsymbol{\theta}$ would exit B_Γ. In parallel, if $q_{i1} > q_{i2}$ and we made θ_{i1} larger than in (8.20), then $\boldsymbol{\theta}$ would exit B_Γ. Stated informally, $\boldsymbol{\theta}$ in (8.20) has hit the wall or the boundary of B_Γ; go any further, and you are outside. Notice second that the solution in (8.20) is separable, in the sense that the solution for block i depends on q_{i1} and q_{i2}, but not on any information from other blocks.

It is intuitive that (8.20) makes $T^{\delta_0} = \sum_{i=1}^{I} \sum_{j=1}^{2} Z_{ij}\, q_{ij}$ as large as possible, because in each block i, the $\boldsymbol{\theta}$ in (8.20) attaches the highest possible probability to the larger of q_{i1} and q_{i2}. Although intuition is correct here, it takes a moment to understand what it means for a random variable to be "as large as possible." What is it, precisely, that is intuitively obvious?

Assume $H_0 : \boldsymbol{\delta} = \boldsymbol{\delta}_0$ is true for the purpose of testing it, so that $\mathbf{R}^{\delta_0} = \mathbf{r}_C$. For each $\boldsymbol{\theta} \in B_\Gamma$, there is a distribution of $\mathbf{Z}$ given by (8.11). Each distribution of $\mathbf{Z}$ given by (8.11) for a specific $\boldsymbol{\theta}$ yields a corresponding null probability distribution, say $W_{\boldsymbol{\theta}}(a \mid \mathcal{F}, \mathcal{Z}) = \Pr_{\boldsymbol{\theta}}\left(T^{\delta_0} \geq a \,\middle|\, \mathcal{F}, \mathcal{Z}\right)$, for the statistic $T^{\delta_0} = t(\mathbf{Z}, \mathbf{r}_C)$. Note that, because we reject H_0 when T^{δ_0} is large, $W_{\boldsymbol{\theta}}(a \mid \mathcal{F}, \mathcal{Z})$ is defined to give upper tail probabilities, as opposed to the lower tail probabilities given by cumulative distributions. It would be very convenient if there was one $\boldsymbol{\theta}^{\dagger} \in B_{\Gamma}$ that gave the bound in (8.19) for all a, so that

$$W_{\boldsymbol{\theta}^{\dagger}}(a \mid \mathcal{F}, \mathcal{Z}) = \sum_{\mathbf{z} \in \mathcal{Z}: t(\mathbf{z}, \mathbf{r}_C) \geq a} \prod_{i=1}^{I} \prod_{j=1}^{J} \left(\theta_{ij}^{\dagger}\right)^{z_{ij}} \tag{8.21}$$

$$= \max_{\boldsymbol{\theta} \in B_{\Gamma}} \sum_{\mathbf{z} \in \mathcal{Z}: t(\mathbf{z}, \mathbf{r}_C) \geq a} \prod_{i=1}^{I} \prod_{j=1}^{J} \theta_{ij}^{z_{ij}},$$

but alas (8.21) is not true in general. If (8.21) were true, then we could work explicitly with a single probability distribution $W_{\boldsymbol{\theta}^{\dagger}}(a \mid \mathcal{F}, \mathcal{Z})$, rather than making implicit reference to a $\boldsymbol{\theta}$ that is produced by an optimization algorithm. More importantly, as a varies in (8.19), the result is not a probability distribution, because the optimizing $\boldsymbol{\theta}$ may change as a changes. That is, (8.19) is a bound on a tail probability for a specific a, not a bounding probability distribution. Is there ever a "largest" probability distribution?

Let us state the same thought in a different way, using the concept of stochastic order. One probability distribution, say $W_{\boldsymbol{\theta}'}(\cdot \mid \mathcal{F}, \mathcal{Z})$, is said to be larger in stochastic order than another, say $W_{\boldsymbol{\theta}''}(\cdot \mid \mathcal{F}, \mathcal{Z})$, if $W_{\boldsymbol{\theta}'}(a \mid \mathcal{F}, \mathcal{Z}) \geq W_{\boldsymbol{\theta}''}(a \mid \mathcal{F}, \mathcal{Z})$ for all a.[7] In other words, no matter where you place the winning line, a, you are at least as likely to win with $\boldsymbol{\theta}'$ than with $\boldsymbol{\theta}''$. For example, a normal distribution with expectation 1 and variance 1 is larger in stochastic order than a normal distribution with expectation 0 and variance 1. Many pairs of probability distributions are not ordered in this way. For example, in terms of stochastic order, a normal distribution with expectation 0 and variance 1 is neither larger nor smaller than a normal distribution with expectation 0 and variance 2.

Now, we can state precisely what is intuitively obvious in (8.20): the distribution of T^{δ_0} is stochastically larger at the $\boldsymbol{\theta}$ in (8.20) than at any other $\boldsymbol{\theta} \in B_{\Gamma}$. Alas, now that we have stated precisely what is intuitively obvious, it is no longer so obvious that it is true. There are two parts. First, for each i, because $\sum_{j=1}^{2} Z_{ij}\, q_{ij}$ takes just two values, increasing the probability of $\max(q_{i1}, q_{i2})$ and decreasing the probability of $\min(q_{i1}, q_{i2})$ increases the distribution of $\sum_{j=1}^{2} Z_{ij}\, q_{ij}$ in the sense of stochastic order—that is immediate from the definition of stochastic order. Second, because the I blocks are independent, $T^{\delta_0} = \sum_{i=1}^{I} \sum_{j=1}^{2} Z_{ij}\, q_{ij}$ is made stochastically larger by making each of its I components, $\sum_{j=1}^{2} Z_{ij}\, q_{ij}$ for $i = 1, \ldots, I$, larger. The second part takes a small amount of effort to prove and holds more generally than I have stated it.[8]

There are many situations in which a little thought determines a $\boldsymbol{\theta}^{\dagger} \in B_{\Gamma}$, analogous to the $\boldsymbol{\theta}^{\dagger}$ in (8.20), such that $T^{\delta_0} = t(\mathbf{Z}, \mathbf{r}_C)$ is stochastically largest at this

---

[7] Notice the way this definition handles the case in which two distributions are the same. If $W_{\boldsymbol{\theta}'}(a \mid \mathcal{F}, \mathcal{Z}) = W_{\boldsymbol{\theta}''}(a \mid \mathcal{F}, \mathcal{Z})$ for all a, then $W_{\boldsymbol{\theta}'}(a \mid \mathcal{F}, \mathcal{Z})$ is larger than $W_{\boldsymbol{\theta}''}(a \mid \mathcal{F}, \mathcal{Z})$ and also $W_{\boldsymbol{\theta}''}(a \mid \mathcal{F}, \mathcal{Z})$ is larger than $W_{\boldsymbol{\theta}'}(a \mid \mathcal{F}, \mathcal{Z})$ in terms of stochastic order.

[8] If you are interested in a proof, I recommend the leisurely and pleasant discussion given by Shaked and Shanthikumar [89, §6.B, Theorem 6.B.16]. If you would like a short proof that is free online from `projecteuclid`, then see Ahmed et al. [1, Lemma 3.3]. For a very general version, see [46].

$\boldsymbol{\theta}^{\dagger}$. Again, this accelerates computation, but usually the insight provided by such a $\boldsymbol{\theta}^{\dagger}$ is more important than faster computation. A few examples follow [66, Ch. 4]. A stochastically largest distribution for $T^{\delta_0} = t(\mathbf{Z}, \mathbf{r}_C)$ is available: (i) for matched pairs using statistics $t(\mathbf{Z}, \mathbf{r}_C)$ that may not be of the form $\sum_{i=1}^{I} \sum_{j=1}^{2} Z_{ij}\, q_{ij}$, but that have the property of being a "decreasing reflection function" [16, 57]; (ii) for any application of the Mantel-Haenszel-Birch [5] statistic, $T^{\delta_0} = \sum_{i,j} Z_{ij}\, r_{Cij}$ with binary r_{Cij} in any $Z \times r_C \times I$ contingency table [61, §5.2]; and (iii) for certain statistics involving quantiles [61, 62]. For some statistics, not only is there a $\boldsymbol{\theta}^{\dagger} \in B_{\Gamma}$ that provides the stochastically largest null distribution, but in addition the exact null distribution of T^{δ_0} at $\boldsymbol{\theta}^{\dagger}$ is tractable and useful for small and moderate I. For instance, this is true of (i) Wilcoxon's signed rank statistic [75, Ch. 3, Appendix], (ii) the exact version of the Mantel-Haenszel-Birch statistic for a $2 \times 2 \times I$ table [61, Proposition 2], and even (iii) certain methods that adaptively select the best of several test statistics [70, 76, 85].

I have been saying that an explicit solution, $\boldsymbol{\theta}$, can supply insight, but I have not provided an example of such insight. Here is an example that can be stated briefly. As in (8.20), the example refers to matched pairs, so $J = 2$ and $\theta_{i2} = 1 - \theta_{i1}$. The requirement $\boldsymbol{\theta} \in B_{\Gamma}$ precludes the possibility that $\theta_{ij} = 0$ or $\theta_{ij} = 1$ for some i and j; that is, it precludes violations of positivity or common support in Sect. 8.1. What if there are limited violations? What if $\theta_{ij} = 0$ or $\theta_{ij} = 1$ for a limited number of individuals ij who cannot be identified? Perhaps, unknown to us, a few of the people in the two alcohol studies have some medical condition or some gene such that alcohol consumption makes them violently ill. People like that cannot be in the treated group; their θ_{ij} equals zero. We cannot exclude these people because we do not know who they are. Suppose that (8.6) holds except for m blocks where θ_{ij} is not constrained. Equivalently, suppose (8.9) and (8.10) hold for all but m of the I blocks. Let $B_{\Gamma m}$ be the corresponding set of $\boldsymbol{\theta}$s, noting that $B_{\Gamma m}$ is no longer a convex set for $1 \le m < I$. Does causal inference collapse completely from small violations of positivity or common support? Obviously, the conclusions are sensitive at a smaller Γ because $B_{\Gamma} \subset B_{\Gamma m}$, so $\min_{\boldsymbol{\theta} \in B_{\Gamma}} f_{\alpha/2}(\boldsymbol{\theta}) \ge \min_{\boldsymbol{\theta} \in B_{\Gamma m}} f_{\alpha/2}(\boldsymbol{\theta})$. Do we fall off a cliff for $m \ge 1$ or do we descend a gradual slope? A $\boldsymbol{\theta} \in B_{\Gamma m}$ that provides the upper bound null distribution for $T^{\delta_0} = \sum_{i=1}^{I} \sum_{j=1}^{2} Z_{ij}\, q_{ij}$ has the form (8.6) for the $I - m$ pairs i with the smallest $|q_{i1} - q_{i2}|$, and for the m remaining pairs has $\theta_{i1} = 1$ if $q_{i1} - q_{i2} > 0$ and $\theta_{i1} = 0$ if $q_{i1} - q_{i2} < 0$. In effect, the $I - m$ pairs with the largest $|q_{i1} - q_{i2}|$ are fixed in the null distribution, thereby failing to contribute to rejecting the null hypothesis [57, §4]. For Wilcoxon's signed rank statistic, the m pairs with the largest ranks are fixed. For small m, violations of positivity or common support have limited consequences if robust statistics are used.[9] [10]

---

[9] Certain rank statistics [8, 53, 55] for matched pairs sharply limit the influence of pairs with large pair differences, $|r_{Ci1} - r_{Ci2}|$. Some versions of these statistics exhibit good performance when used in a sensitivity analysis [73]. Fixing m of the pairs with large $|r_{Ci1} - r_{Ci2}|$ has particularly limited consequences for these statistics.

[10] Arguably, it is not reasonable to compare B_{Γ} and $B_{\Gamma m}$, because $B_{\Gamma} \subset B_{\Gamma m}$, so it is a foregone conclusion that $B_{\Gamma m}$ will report greater sensitivity to unmeasured biases. Arguably, it would be more reasonable to compare B_{Γ} and $B_{\Gamma' m}$, with $\Gamma' < \Gamma$, so that, in some aggregate sense, the

Particular cases aside, in general there is no $\boldsymbol{\theta} \in B_\Gamma$ that provides a null distribution stochastically larger than all other $\boldsymbol{\theta}$'s in B_Γ. That is, in general, changing a will change the $\boldsymbol{\theta} \in B_\Gamma$ that yields the maximum in (8.19). In principle, this can happen even for the stratified Wilcoxon rank sum statistic [26, Table 2]. This is not a problem in data analysis. The two sections that follow provide some insight into the general problem.

The Third Lens: A Partial But Exact Solution

As it turns out, under quite general conditions, the infinite set B_Γ contains a finite number of candidates $\boldsymbol{\theta} \in B_\Gamma$ for the bound in (8.19), and (at least) one of these candidates must yield the maximum in (8.19). Conceptually, one could just run through this finite list of $\boldsymbol{\theta}$s to find the maximum, and that does work for some important problems, but alas the list is sometimes a bit long. So far, this book has focused on $I \times J$ block designs with $1 = \sum_{j=1}^{J} Z_{ij}$ for each i, with test statistic $T^{\delta_0} = \sum_{i=1}^{I} \sum_{j=1}^{J} Z_{ij}\, q_{ij}$. So, let us consider this case first and in detail. In the final paragraph of this subsection, the general case is mentioned with references to the literature.

For notational convenience, use q_{ij} to sort the J people in block i into increasing order within block i, $q_{i1} \leq \cdots \leq q_{iJ}$. Of course, when we sort people, we move intact people into a new order, bringing their Z_{ij} and θ_{ij} to their new positions. Nothing we compute depends upon the ordering of people within blocks, so nothing but notation changes when we sort them by q_{ij}.

In block i, there are $J - 1$ candidates, $m = 1, \ldots, J - 1$, for the optimizing $(\theta_{i1}, \ldots, \theta_{iJ})$. Candidate m for $(\theta_{i1}, \ldots, \theta_{iJ})$ is

$$\frac{1}{m + (J-m)\,\Gamma}, \ldots, \frac{1}{m + (J-m)\,\Gamma}, \frac{\Gamma}{m + (J-m)\,\Gamma}, \ldots, \frac{\Gamma}{m + (J-m)\,\Gamma}, \tag{8.22}$$

where (8.22) has m terms $1/\{m + (J - m)\,\Gamma\}$ and $J - m$ terms $\Gamma/\{m + (J - m)\,\Gamma\}$. Because $q_{i1} \leq \cdots \leq q_{iJ}$, (8.22) gives the largest probabilities to the $J - m$ largest q_{ij} and the smallest probabilities to the m smallest q_{ij}. The constraints (8.8)–(8.10) are satisfied by each of these m candidates. Indeed, the constraints are just barely satisfied: the constraints would be violated by increasing any $\Gamma/\{m + (J - m)\,\Gamma\}$ or decreasing any $1/\{m + (J - m)\,\Gamma\}$.

For the blocked Wilcoxon rank sum statistic, the ranks are $q_{i1} = 1$, $q_{i2} = 2, \ldots,$ $q_{iJ} = J$. For $J = 4$, Table 8.2 shows the probabilities (8.22) that $\sum_{j=1}^{J} Z_{ij}\, q_{ij}$ equals

---

biases in B_Γ and $B_{\Gamma' m}$ are of similar magnitude. In a special case, Wang and Krieger [96] examine this issue. In effect, they argue in a special case that if you constrain the standard deviation of an unobserved covariate, then biases that affect every matched pair in the same way do more harm than biases that have a big effect on some pairs and smaller effects on others. In a sense, their technical argument is similar to Hoeffding [38] and Gleser [28], who compare a binomial distribution to the sum of Bernoulli trials with unequal probabilities of success. See Problems 8.4 and 8.5.

Table 8.2 Extreme probabilities in (8.22) for the contribution from block i to the blocked Wilcoxon rank sum statistic, for $J = 4$, $m = 1, 2, 3$, and for $\Gamma = 1, 2, 3$. Also given are expectation and variance computed using these probabilities

m	$q_{i1} = 1$	$q_{i2} = 2$	$q_{i3} = 3$	$q_{i4} = 4$	Total	Expectation	Variance
		$\Gamma = 1$					
1	0.250	0.250	0.250	0.250	1.000	2.500	1.250
2	0.250	0.250	0.250	0.250	1.000	2.500	1.250
3	0.250	0.250	0.250	0.250	1.000	2.500	1.250
		$\Gamma = 2$					
1	0.143	0.286	0.286	0.286	1.000	2.714	1.061
2	0.167	0.167	0.333	0.333	1.000	2.833	1.139
3	0.200	0.200	0.200	0.400	1.000	2.800	1.360
		$\Gamma = 3$					
1	0.100	0.300	0.300	0.300	1.000	2.800	0.960
2	0.125	0.125	0.375	0.375	1.000	3.000	1.000
3	0.167	0.167	0.167	0.500	1.000	3.000	1.333

j, together with the expectation and variance of $\sum_{j=1}^{J} Z_{ij}\, q_{ij}$, for $\Gamma = 1, 2, 3$. As $J = 4$, there are $J - 1 = 3$ candidates for $(\theta_{i1}, \ldots, \theta_{iJ})$, for $m = 1, 2, 3$. Of course, for $\Gamma = 1$, Table 8.2 reports the randomization distribution.

For fixed $\Gamma > 1$ in Table 8.2, no one candidate (8.22) is larger in stochastic order than another. For example, for $\Gamma = 2$, the chance that $\sum_{j=1}^{J} Z_{ij}\, q_{ij} \geq 2$ is $0.858 = 0.286 + 0.286 + 0.286$ for $m = 1$, 0.833 for $m = 2$, and 0.800 for $m = 3$, so the probability is highest for $m = 1$. At the same time, for $\Gamma = 2$, the chance that $\sum_{j=1}^{J} Z_{ij}\, q_{ij} \geq 3$ is 0.571 for $m = 1$, 0.667 for $m = 2$, and 0.600 for $m = 3$, so the probability is highest for $m = 2$. Of course, for $\Gamma > 1$, the highest probability that $\sum_{j=1}^{J} Z_{ij}\, q_{ij} \geq 4$ is for $m = 3$. In other words, there is no single distribution $\boldsymbol{\theta} \in B_\Gamma$ that is larger in stochastic order than all others, unlike (8.20) for $J = 2$.

Look also at the expectations and variances of $\sum_{j=1}^{J} Z_{ij}\, q_{ij}$ in Table 8.2. Suppose you are given two distributions with finite expectations, where the first distribution is larger in stochastic order than the second distribution; then, the first distribution has an expectation that is at least as large as the second distribution.[11] For fixed $\Gamma > 1$ in Table 8.2, no distribution is larger than another in stochastic order, even though the expectations do vary. For $\Gamma = 3$, the distributions for $m = 2$ and $m = 3$ have the same expectations but $m = 3$ has larger variance. For $\Gamma = 3$, the distribution for $m = 3$ attaches a larger probability to both $\sum_{j=1}^{J} Z_{ij}\, q_{ij} = 1$ and $\sum_{j=1}^{J} Z_{ij}\, q_{ij} = 4$ than does the distribution for $m = 2$. In a sense made precise in the next subsection, for $\Gamma = 3$, the distribution with $m = 3$ does more to increase the probability that $T^{\delta_0} = \sum_{i=1}^{I} \sum_{j=1}^{J} Z_{ij}\, q_{ij}$ is high in its upper tail than does the distribution with $m = 2$, even though they make the same contribution to the expectation of $T^{\delta_0} = \sum_{i=1}^{I} \sum_{j=1}^{J} Z_{ij}\, q_{ij}$.

A $\boldsymbol{\theta} \in B_\Gamma$ is on the finite list of candidates that may achieve the maximum of the exact probability (8.19) if the ith row of $\boldsymbol{\theta}$ is one of the $J - 1$ candidates in

[11] Indeed, if the first distribution is larger than the second in stochastic order and their expectations are the same, then the distributions are the same [89, Thm. 1.A.8].

(8.22) for $(\theta_{i1}, \ldots, \theta_{iJ})$ for $i = 1, \ldots, I$. Write $\mathfrak{B}_\Gamma$ for the finite set containing the candidates $\boldsymbol{\theta}$ on this list, so $\mathfrak{B}_\Gamma \subset B_\Gamma$. So, there are $(J-1)^I$ candidates $\boldsymbol{\theta}$ in $\mathfrak{B}_\Gamma$, or $(4-1)^{406} = 5.14 \times 10^{193}$ candidates for the alcohol and HDL cholesterol example in Sect. 1.4. I believe I did mention that the list, $\mathfrak{B}_\Gamma$, though finite, could be a bit long. A calculus argument ([66, §4.7.3] or [80, §3]) demonstrates that the search for an optimizing $\boldsymbol{\theta}$ can be confined to $\mathfrak{B}_\Gamma$; that is,

$$\max_{\boldsymbol{\theta} \in B_\Gamma} \sum_{\mathbf{z} \in \mathcal{Z}:\, t(\mathbf{z}, \mathbf{r}_C) \geq a} \prod_{i=1}^{I} \prod_{j=1}^{J} \theta_{ij}^{z_{ij}} = \max_{\boldsymbol{\theta} \in \mathfrak{B}_\Gamma} \sum_{\mathbf{z} \in \mathcal{Z}:\, t(\mathbf{z}, \mathbf{r}_C) \geq a} \prod_{i=1}^{I} \prod_{j=1}^{J} \theta_{ij}^{z_{ij}}. \tag{8.23}$$

For matched pairs, $J = 2$, there is just $1 = J - 1$ distribution in (8.22), namely, the distribution with $m = 1$. Consequently, for $J = 2$, the list of candidates $\mathfrak{B}_\Gamma$ contains a single $\boldsymbol{\theta}$, namely, (8.20). For block designs with $J > 2$ and large I, direct calculation in (8.23) is impractical, but (8.23) is a stepping stone to the practical methods in the next subsection.

The result (8.23) is not confined to statistics of the form $T^{\delta_0} = \sum_{i=1}^{I} \sum_{j=1}^{J} Z_{ij}\, q_{ij}$ and is not confined to balanced block designs [80]. In particular, (8.23) is a practical method when comparing n_1 treated individuals to n_2 controls without blocks, as $\mathfrak{B}_\Gamma$ contains only $n_1 + n_2 - 1$ candidates.[12] Also, (8.23) is a practical method with a few strata, say women and men.

A Bifocal Lens: Asymptotic Separability

With blocks larger than pairs, $J > 2$, as the number of blocks, I, increases, the finite set $\mathfrak{B}_\Gamma$ of candidate maximizers of (8.23) grows in size at an exponential rate; specifically, $\mathfrak{B}_\Gamma$ contains $(J-1)^I$ candidate $\boldsymbol{\theta}$s. That does not look promising for a discrete optimization problem, at least until you remember that some good things do happen as $I \longrightarrow \infty$.

As throughout this chapter, assume $H_0: \delta = \delta_0$ is true for the purpose of testing it, so that $\mathbf{R}^{\delta_0} = \mathbf{r}_C$, and let the q_{ij} be functions of $\mathbf{R}^{\delta_0} = \mathbf{r}_C$, so the q_{ij} are fixed by conditioning on $\mathcal{F}$. The test statistic is

$$t(\mathbf{Z}, \mathbf{r}_C) = T^{\delta_0} = \sum_{i=1}^{I} \sum_{j=1}^{J} Z_{ij}\, q_{ij} = \sum_{i=1}^{I} A_i \text{ where } A_i = \sum_{j=1}^{J} Z_{ij}\, q_{ij},$$

whose exact upper tail probability $\Pr\left(T^{\delta_0} \geq a \,\middle|\, \mathcal{F}, \mathcal{Z}\right)$ is given by (8.12) for each $\boldsymbol{\theta} \in B_\Gamma$, where $\mathrm{E}(A_i \mid \mathcal{F}, \mathcal{Z}) = \mu_{\boldsymbol{\theta} i}$, $\mathrm{var}(A_i \mid \mathcal{F}, \mathcal{Z}) = \sigma^2_{\boldsymbol{\theta} i}$, and the A_i are independent. As $I \rightarrow \infty$, Appendix Sect. 8.10 discusses a central limit theorem for T^{δ_0} for each $\boldsymbol{\theta} \in B_\Gamma$. For any one $\boldsymbol{\theta} \in B_\Gamma$, the central limit theorem suggests approximating the exact probability:

[12] This method is implemented in the `sen2sample` function of the `senstrat` package in R.

$$\Pr\left(T^{\delta_0} \geq a \mid \mathcal{F}, \mathcal{Z}\right) = \sum_{\mathbf{z}\in\mathcal{Z}:\, t(\mathbf{z}, \mathbf{r}_C)\geq a} \prod_{i=1}^{I} \prod_{j=1}^{J} \theta_{ij}^{z_{ij}} \tag{8.24}$$

in (8.12) as

$$\Pr\left(T^{\delta_0} \geq a \mid \mathcal{F}, \mathcal{Z}\right) \doteq 1 - \Phi\left(\frac{a - \sum_{i=1}^{I} \mu_{\theta i}}{\sqrt{\sum_{i=1}^{I} \sigma_{\theta i}^2}}\right). \tag{8.25}$$

This in turn suggests approximating the exact sensitivity bound (8.19) by the maximum of (8.25) over either $\boldsymbol{\theta} \in \mathfrak{B}_\Gamma$ or $\boldsymbol{\theta} \in B_\Gamma$, and of course this is very close to where we began, namely, the convex quadratic optimization problem in Propositions 8.3 and 8.4. Suppose, however, that we want to avoid solving the convex quadratic optimization problem, perhaps because I is large, as in Sect. 1.2 where $I = 54{,}996$. Sometimes, also, we want to say something about how the sensitivity analysis behaves as $I \to \infty$, and direct use of Propositions 8.3 and 8.4 is not practical for that either.

The convex quadratic optimization problem is not separable—you cannot solve it by finding an optimum in each block i separately and stitching together the I separate solutions. However, the problem of maximizing (8.25) is asymptotically separable, that is, almost separable for large I. The issues involved will be briefly sketched in a few steps, with references to the literature for technical details. In the first step, the separable approximation is stated; it is just a few steps of arithmetic in each block i, easily performed with $I = 54{,}996$ blocks. Second, the separable approximation is seen to fail to optimize (8.25) for some small I, in particular for $I = 1$. Third, a few ad hoc comparisons hint that the approximation is often adequate for $I = 10$ or $I = 15$, tiny sample sizes for an observational study. Fourth, intuition is offered suggesting that the separable approximation might work for large I. Fifth, in the technical literature, the intuition becomes a theorem in either of two ways [26, 74] that are briefly described.[13]

Definition 8.1 The separable approximation to (8.19) calculates $\mu_{\theta i}$ and $\sigma_{\theta i}^2$ at each of the $J - 1$ values of $(\theta_{i1}, \ldots, \theta_{iJ})$ in (8.22). It sets $\overline{\mu}_i$ equal to the maximum of these $J - 1$ values of $\mu_{\theta i}$. Let $\mathcal{B}_i$ be the subset of the $J - 1$ values $(\theta_{i1}, \ldots, \theta_{iJ})$ in (8.22) that produce this maximum, i.e., that have $\mu_{\theta i} = \overline{\mu}_i$. Let $\overline{\sigma}_i^2$ be the maximum of $\sigma_{\theta i}^2$ over $(\theta_{i1}, \ldots, \theta_{iJ}) \in \mathcal{B}_i$. The separable approximation to (8.19) is

$$1 - \Phi\left(\frac{a - \sum_{i=1}^{I} \overline{\mu}_i}{\sqrt{\sum_{i=1}^{I} \overline{\sigma}_i^2}}\right) \tag{8.26}$$

if $a > \sum_{i=1}^{I} \overline{\mu}_i$, and otherwise, this P-value bound is unambiguously above 1/2 and is therefore uninteresting.

---

13 A quite general implementation, not restricted to balanced block designs, is available in the `senstrat` package in R.

In Table 8.2, for $\Gamma = 2$, $\overline{\mu}_i = 2.833$ and $\overline{\sigma}_i^2 = 1.139$ as $\mathcal{B}_i$ contains only one $(\theta_{i1}, \ldots, \theta_{iJ})$. In contrast, for $\Gamma = 3$ in Table 8.2, $\mathcal{B}_i$ contains two $(\theta_{i1}, \ldots, \theta_{iJ})$, because solutions $m = 2$ and $m = 3$ both have $\mu_{\theta i} = \overline{\mu}_i = 3.000$; so, $\overline{\sigma}_i^2 = 1.333 > 1.000$.

Stated concisely, the separable approximation has maximized $\sum_{i=1}^{I} \overline{\mu}_i$ over $\boldsymbol{\theta} \in \mathfrak{B}_\Gamma$, and among all $\boldsymbol{\theta} \in \mathfrak{B}_\Gamma$ that maximize $\sum_{i=1}^{I} \overline{\mu}_i$, the separable approximation has maximized $\sum_{i=1}^{I} \overline{\sigma}_i^2$. Briefly, the separable approximation prioritizes maximizing the expectation of T^{δ_0}, but when there is a tie in that prioritized task, it breaks the tie by maximizing the variance of T^{δ_0}.

The separable approximation can fail to maximize $\Pr\left(T^{\delta_0} \geq a \,\middle|\, \mathcal{F}, \mathcal{Z}\right)$ for small I. It does fail in Table 8.2 in the case of a single block, $I = 1$, with $\Gamma = 3$ at $a = 3$. The maximum of $\Pr\left(T^{\delta_0} \geq 3 \,\middle|\, \mathcal{F}, \mathcal{Z}\right)$ is $0.375 + 0.375 = 0.750$ for $m = 2$ and is $0.167 + 0.500 = 0.667$ for $m = 3$, so the separable approximation picked the wrong m for a study comprised of a single block, $I = 1$.

Gastwirth et al. [26, Table 2] consider eight cases, with $I = 10$ or $I = 15$, with $J = 3$ or $J = 5$, with $\Gamma = 2$ or $\Gamma = 4$. In seven of the eight cases, the separable approximation, namely, $\left(T^{\delta_0} - \sum_{i=1}^{I} \overline{\mu}_i\right) / \sqrt{\sum_{i=1}^{I} \overline{\sigma}_i^2}$, was the minimum standardized deviate, and in the final case it was close to the minimum.

The intuition behind the separable approximation is as follows. Suppose you are given a bag containing a finite or infinite collection of normal distributions with different expectations and variances. These are the approximate null distributions for T^{δ_0} for a given Γ. You want to identify the one distribution in this bag that maximizes the probability that $T^{\delta_0} \geq a$. Clearly, a large expectation would help, but so would a large variance. Typically in sensitivity analyses in observational studies, a bias in treatment assignment that pushes up the expectation of T^{δ_0} also reduces its variance, so you do not have the option of picking from the bag a distribution that combines the largest expectation with the largest variance. The distributions in the bag are partially ordered, but not totally ordered, by their expectations and variances, so that maximizing the probability that $T^{\delta_0} \geq a$ involves working directly with the probability. Imagine instead a sequence of bags of normal distributions indexed by I, where the expectations of the distributions in bag I are tending to various nonzero limits as their variances are tending to zero. These are the limiting distributions of T^{δ_0} after a suitable rescaling by a sequence of constants, K_I, so T^{δ_0} is replaced by T^{δ_0}/K_I. For the blocked Wilcoxon rank sum statistic, $K_I = I$, making T^{δ_0} into a mean over I blocks rather than a sum over I blocks. In this case, as $I \to \infty$, increasing the limiting expectation, even just a little, trumps increasing the variance, and this motivates the separable approximation. The limiting distributions in the sequence of bags are tending to spikes located at their expectations; so, expectations are ultimately more important than variances.

As $I \to \infty$, the separable approximation makes negligible errors. There are two proofs of this, a probabilistic proof [26, Proposition 1] and an analytic proof [74, Proposition 1 and Remarks 4 and 5]. The probabilistic proof resembles the intuition given above and it has some regularity conditions. The analytic proof essentially tinkers with the negative of the convex function in Propositions 8.3 and 8.4 and the finite set $\mathfrak{B}_\Gamma$. A rough description of the analytic result follows. The separable approximation evaluates (8.25) at one $\boldsymbol{\theta} \in \mathfrak{B}_\Gamma$, say $\boldsymbol{\theta}_s$; so, it either maximizes (8.25) over $\boldsymbol{\theta} \in \mathfrak{B}_\Gamma$ or is too low. Using a concave function and its derivative at $\boldsymbol{\theta}_s$ provides an easily computed upper bound [74, Proposition 1] on the increase that could be attained by moving from $\boldsymbol{\theta}_s$ to a different $\boldsymbol{\theta} \in \mathfrak{B}_\Gamma$. For large enough I, the bound says no increase is possible by moving from $\boldsymbol{\theta}_s$ to a different $\boldsymbol{\theta} \in \mathfrak{B}_\Gamma$ [74, Remarks 4 and 5]. This is important for theoretical calculations about the limit as $I \to \infty$, because for large enough I the separable approximation equals the maximum of (8.25) over $\boldsymbol{\theta} \in \mathfrak{B}_\Gamma$, rather than merely approximating the maximum. Even when an increase is possible for finite I, it is often too tiny to be of concern, perhaps affecting just a few blocks i. Even if the increase is not tiny, the upper bound gives a directly useful conservative statement about the bounding P-value. In actual observational studies, I have not yet seen a case in which the separable approximation and the conservative bound differ by enough that it would matter which number was reported in a scientific journal.[14]

To illustrate, consider the examples in Sect. 1.4 and Sect. 1.5. The `wgtRank` function in the `weightedRank` package in `R` uses the separable approximation for weighted rank statistics, and its default statistic, U868, is used in the examples that follow. It is compared to the `senstrat` function in the `senstrat` package in `R`, adjusted to use the same test statistic, where `senstrat` computes both the separable approximation and also the upper bound. In the HDL cholesterol example in Sect. 1.4, with $I = 406$ blocks, at $\Gamma = 5.467$, both the separable approximation and the upper bound exactly agree, yielding the same P-value bound of $\alpha = 0.05003$. In the binge drinking example in Sect. 1.5, for systolic blood pressure with $I = 207$, at $\Gamma = 2.434$, both the separable approximation and the upper bound exactly agree, yielding a P-value bound of $\alpha = 0.05005$.

8.6 Sensitivity Value $\Gamma^{\bullet}$ and Associated Sets of Biases

The Sensitivity Value $\Gamma^{\bullet}$ as a Summary of a Sensitivity Analysis

Qingyuan Zhao [101] gives the name "sensitivity value," or $\Gamma^{\bullet}$, to the largest value of Γ that just barely leads to rejection of the null hypothesis at $\alpha = 0.05$. Any other fixed α could be used instead, but let us be tangible and conventional and fix $\alpha = 0.05$. The sensitivity value is not well defined if the randomization test, $\Gamma = 1$, fails to reject the null hypothesis at level $\alpha = 0.05$; so, define $\Gamma^{\bullet} = -\infty$ in this case. Consider the study of HDL cholesterol and light daily consumption of alcohol in

---

[14] The `senstrat` function in the `senstrat` package in `R` optionally computes both the separable approximation and the conservative bound.

Sect. 1.4. Using Quade's statistic, we find $\Gamma^{\bullet} = 4.5331$ because the left side of (8.13) exceeds $\alpha = 0.05$ for $\Gamma > 4.5331$.[15]

Unlike the parameter Γ and like a P-value, the sensitivity value $\Gamma^{\bullet}$ is a random variable: neither the P-value nor $\Gamma^{\bullet}$ are fixed in advance, and both are computed from the data, making them random variables. The sensitivity value $\Gamma^{\bullet}$ is related to the sensitivity parameter Γ in a way that is analogous to the relationship between a P-value and the level α of a test. The usual P-value is a random variable: it is the smallest level α that leads to rejection of the null hypothesis at level α using the current data. The sensitivity value $\Gamma^{\bullet}$ is also a random variable. The sensitivity value $\Gamma^{\bullet}$ is the largest Γ such that rejection of H_0 at a fixed level α is insensitive to a bias of magnitude Γ using the current data. The P-value and the sensitivity value $\Gamma^{\bullet}$ are both random variables because they depend upon the data. In contrast, the level α of a test and the sensitivity parameter Γ are fixed features of a procedure that issues a "reject" or "accept" decision. Rather than report "reject" or "accept" for one α and Γ, both the sensitivity value $\Gamma^{\bullet}$ and the P-value describe when the testing procedure data tips from reject to accept.

The distinction between the level, α, and the P-value, or between the sensitivity parameter, Γ, and the sensitivity value, $\Gamma^{\bullet}$, becomes very clear if you think about running a simulation to determine the power of a test against a specific alternative hypothesis. A probability model is specified that generates data under the alternative hypothesis, and many data sets are generated under this model, say many $I \times J$ blocked studies. To simulate the power of a conventional 0.05-level test, report the proportion of simulated data sets in which the test rejects the null hypothesis at level $\alpha = 0.05$. Instead of calculating power, closely related information is obtained by computing the P-value in each simulated data set and reporting some summary of the resulting simulated distribution of P-values. For example, Brian Joiner [45] suggests reporting the median P-value to estimate the level, say $\alpha_{0.5}$, at which the test has 50% power.[16] In parallel, the power of a 0.05-level sensitivity analysis in the presence of a bias of fixed size Γ is simulated as the proportion of rejections in (8.13) at $\alpha = 0.05$ for the fixed Γ. Instead, closely related information is obtained by computing the sensitivity value, $\Gamma^{\bullet}$, in each simulated data set and reporting a summary or a boxplot of the distribution of sensitivity values, $\Gamma^{\bullet}$. Based on such a simulation against a specific alternative, we might prefer Quade's statistic to the blocked Wilcoxon rank sum statistic either because Quade's statistic has greater power in a sensitivity analysis or because the distribution of sensitivity values $\Gamma^{\bullet}$ from Quade's statistic is stochastically larger than the distribution of sensitivity

[15] Actually, the calculation is an approximation based on the central limit theorem. The normal approximation (8.18) to (8.13) holds as an equality at $\Gamma^{\bullet} = 4.5331$. The issues are the same for (8.13), (8.18), and (8.16), so this section focuses on (8.13).

[16] Of course, 50% power is problematic, but that is why it is interesting. If we compared several statistical tests all of which had power near 1, or power near 0, then it would barely matter which test we use. In contrast, if power is in the vicinity of 50%, then it may matter a great deal which test we use. As you would expect, in conventional problems, $\alpha_{0.5}$ tends to zero as $I \to \infty$, but it does so at different rates for different test statistics. We would like $\alpha_{0.5}$ to go to zero as fast as possible as $I \to \infty$. For this reason, Raj Bahadur [2, 3] measured the efficiency of tests and estimates in terms of the rate at which $\alpha_{0.5}$ tends to zero as $I \to \infty$. We will return to this topic in Chap. 11.

values $\Gamma^\bullet$ from Wilcoxon's rank sum statistic. These tests did exhibit very different performance in the example in Table 8.1, and a simulation would let us determine whether Table 8.1 is some kind of fluke or else something we should expect in general. Questions of this sort are taken up in Chaps. 9 and 11.

The Insensitive Set $B_{\Gamma^\bullet}$ of Treatment Assignments $\boldsymbol{\theta}$

Recall that a sensitivity analysis at a particular Γ rejects $H_0 : \delta = \delta_0$ if and only if it rejects H_0 for each $\boldsymbol{\theta} \in B_\Gamma$, and $B_1 = \{\overline{\boldsymbol{\theta}}\} \subset B_\Gamma$ for all $\Gamma > 1$. Our convention defined $\Gamma^\bullet = -\infty$ if H_0 is not rejected in a randomization test with $\boldsymbol{\theta} = \overline{\boldsymbol{\theta}}$. In that way, $\Gamma^\bullet = 1$ if H_0 is rejected only for $\boldsymbol{\theta} = \overline{\boldsymbol{\theta}}$, and not for any $\boldsymbol{\theta} \neq \overline{\boldsymbol{\theta}}$, but $\Gamma^\bullet = -\infty$ if H_0 is not rejected for any $\boldsymbol{\theta}$, not even for $\boldsymbol{\theta} = \overline{\boldsymbol{\theta}}$.

As a yardstick measuring the magnitude of departure from randomized treatment assignment, $\overline{\boldsymbol{\theta}}$, the sensitivity analysis used the nested sets $\left\{\overline{\boldsymbol{\theta}}\right\} = B_1 \subset B_\Gamma \subset B_{\Gamma'}$ for $1 < \Gamma < \Gamma'$ defined by (8.8)–(8.10). It is convenient to lengthen this ordered collection by adding one more set, namely, the empty set $\emptyset$ at the beginning, so the revised collection is $B_{-\infty} = \emptyset \subset \left\{\overline{\boldsymbol{\theta}}\right\} = B_1 \subset B_\Gamma$. Associated with the sensitivity value $\Gamma^\bullet$ is one of these nested sets, the set denoted $B_{\Gamma^\bullet}$, where $H_0 : \delta = \delta_0$ is rejected at level $\alpha = 0.05$ for all $\boldsymbol{\theta} \in B_{\Gamma^\bullet}$ but not for some $\boldsymbol{\theta} \in B_\Gamma$ for every $\Gamma > \Gamma^\bullet$. In harmony with this, if $\Gamma^\bullet = -\infty$ because H_0 is not rejected even in a randomization test with treatment assignment probabilities $\overline{\boldsymbol{\theta}}$, then of course $B_{\Gamma^\bullet} = B_{-\infty} = \emptyset$ is the empty set, because there is no $\Gamma \geq 1$ that leads to rejection of H_0.

*The Troubling Set $\mathcal{J}$ of Barely Insensitive Biases $\boldsymbol{\theta}$

The current section has an asterisk, so it may be skipped, although it will be mentioned in a couple of sentences in Chap. 12; however, those sentences may also be skipped. The goal is to say that a certain set $\mathcal{J}$ containing specific biased treatment assignments $\boldsymbol{\theta} \in B_{\Gamma^\bullet}$ are especially interesting or troubling, because the study is just barely insensitive to $\boldsymbol{\theta}$, and the tiniest increase in Γ would make the study sensitive to a $\boldsymbol{\theta}'$ outside B_Γ but very near $\boldsymbol{\theta}$. If all such $\boldsymbol{\theta}$ could be shown to be implausible based on observable data, then we would increase the study's insensitivity to plausible biases [77, 78]. That is what makes $\mathcal{J}$ both interesting and troubling: perhaps we can make progress if we can render implausible these troublesome $\boldsymbol{\theta} \in \mathcal{J}$. The current section gives a little geometric structure to this conversation.

For each $\Gamma \geq 1$, the set B_Γ is a compact and convex set. Moreover, (8.12) is a continuous function on each B_Γ, so the maximum in (8.19) is achieved at some point $\boldsymbol{\theta} \in B_\Gamma$, although that point need not be unique. Write $\mathcal{M}_\Gamma$ for the set of $\boldsymbol{\theta} \in B_\Gamma$ that achieve the maximum in (8.19). We have just convinced ourselves that $\mathcal{M}_\Gamma$ is not empty, but we want to understand more about $\mathcal{M}_\Gamma$ than that. Let us continue to focus on statistics of the form $T^{\delta_0} = \sum_{i=1}^{I} \sum_{j=1}^{J} Z_{ij}\, q_{ij}$ where q_{ij} is a function of $\mathbf{R}^{\delta_0}$, where $\mathbf{R}^{\delta_0} = \mathbf{r}_C$ if $H_0 : \boldsymbol{\delta} = \boldsymbol{\delta}_0$ is true.[17] Also, add the nearly trivial assumption that (8.12) is not constant as a function of $\boldsymbol{\theta} \in B_\Gamma$ for $\Gamma > 1$.[18]

We know, for example, that in the case of matched pairs, $J = 2$, the set $\mathcal{M}_\Gamma$ contains the point $\boldsymbol{\theta}$ given by (8.20). However, it is clear in (8.20) that if $q_{i1} = q_{i2}$, then the value of $\theta_{i1} = 1 - \theta_{i2}$ does not matter; that is, it does not matter what probability you attach to picking q_{i1} rather than q_{i2} if $q_{i1} = q_{i2}$. So, ties in the scores q_{ij} can populate $\mathcal{M}_\Gamma$ with infinitely many optimizing $\boldsymbol{\theta}$'s.[19]

The geometric structure of $\mathcal{M}_\Gamma$ is simple in an important way, but it takes a moment to understand this simplicity. Write $\mathcal{L} = \left\{\boldsymbol{\theta} : 1 = \sum_{j=1}^{J} \theta_{ij},\ i = 1, \ldots, I\right\}$, noting that $B_\Gamma \subset \mathcal{L}$ for each Γ, but many elements of $\mathcal{L}$ are not vectors of treatment assignment probabilities, because θ_{ij} need not be in $[0, 1]$.[20] In other words, $\mathcal{L}$ is an $I(J-1)$-dimensional flat satisfying (8.8) but not (8.9) and (8.10); so, $\mathcal{L} - \overline{\boldsymbol{\theta}}$ is an $I(J-1)$-dimensional subspace which translates randomized treatment assignment $\overline{\boldsymbol{\theta}} \in \mathcal{L}$ to the origin, $\mathbf{0}$, in $\mathcal{L} - \overline{\boldsymbol{\theta}}$. Think of $\mathcal{L} - \overline{\boldsymbol{\theta}}$ as a vector space with the usual Euclidean norm, so that familiar ideas like an "open set" refer to an open set in $\mathcal{L}$, not in $\Re^{IJ}$. By definition, the boundary of the compact set B_Γ consists of points $\boldsymbol{\theta} \in B_\Gamma$ such that every open neighborhood of $\boldsymbol{\theta}$ in $\mathcal{L}$ contains points of $\mathcal{L}$ that are not in B_Γ. Informally, the boundary of B_Γ is the "skin" of the set B_Γ viewed as an inhabitant of $\mathcal{L}$. Formally, $\boldsymbol{\theta} \in B_\Gamma$ is a boundary point of B_Γ in $\mathcal{L}$ if at least one of the inequalities (8.9) holds as an equality, that is, if there is at least one $i, j \neq j'$ such that $\theta_{ij} = \Gamma\theta_{ij'}$. If this θ_{ij} were increased by even the tiniest amount while $\theta_{ij'}$ stays the same or decreases, then constraint (8.9) would be violated, and we would exit B_Γ. For example, in (8.20), for every pair i, either $\theta_{i1} = \Gamma\theta_{i2}$ or $\theta_{i2} = \Gamma\theta_{i1}$. If $\boldsymbol{\theta}$, $\boldsymbol{\theta}' \in B_\Gamma$ and if both $\theta_{ij} = \Gamma\theta_{ij'}$ and $\theta'_{ij} = \Gamma\theta'_{ij'}$, then every point on the line segment from $\boldsymbol{\theta}$ to $\boldsymbol{\theta}'$—every $\lambda\boldsymbol{\theta} + (1-\lambda)\,\boldsymbol{\theta}'$ for $\lambda \in [0, 1]$—is also a boundary point because $\lambda\theta_{ij} + (1-\lambda)\,\theta'_{ij} = \Gamma\left\{\lambda\theta_{ij'} + (1-\lambda)\,\theta'_{ij'}\right\}$.

A calculus argument applied after transforming $\boldsymbol{\theta}$ to the logit scale shows that every $\boldsymbol{\theta} \in \mathcal{M}_\Gamma$ is a boundary point [80, Proposition 2]. For $\Gamma < \Gamma'$, a boundary point of $B_{\Gamma'}$ cannot be a boundary point of B_Γ, because $\theta_{ij} \leq \Gamma\theta_{ij'} < \Gamma'\theta_{ij'}$ for every $\boldsymbol{\theta} \in B_\Gamma$; so, if $\boldsymbol{\theta} \in \mathcal{M}_{\Gamma'}$ then $\boldsymbol{\theta} \notin \mathcal{M}_\Gamma$.

---

[17] The properties to be discussed are true ([66, §4.7] or [80]) for a much larger class of statistics studied by Hollander, Proschan, and Sethuraman [39] called "functions decreasing in transposition" or "arrangement increasing functions" and the extension of this class to "decreasing reflection functions" that accommodate blocks, pairs, or strata [10, 16, 59].

[18] For example, (8.12) would be constant as a function of $\boldsymbol{\theta}$ if $q_{i1} = q_{i2} = \cdots = q_{iJ}$ for all $i = 1, \ldots, I$, and this case is excluded.

[19] Ties in the q_{ij} may occur when there are ties in the r_{Cij}, but they are not the same idea. Some useful statistics create heavily tied q_{ij} from completely untied r_{Cij}, e.g., [8, 53, 55]. For many weighted rank statistics, ties occur with probability zero when the data are from continuous distributions, like the normal distribution. In many contexts, including (8.20), the absence of within-block ties in the q_{ij} leads $\mathcal{M}_\Gamma$ to contain just a single $\boldsymbol{\theta}$.

[20] The set $\mathcal{L}$ is commonly called the affine hull of B_Γ for any $\Gamma > 1$; however, we will not need this common terminology.

Define the random set $\mathcal{J}$ of troubling biases $\boldsymbol{\theta}$ as $\mathcal{J} = \mathcal{M}_{\Gamma^\bullet} \subseteq \mathcal{B}_{\Gamma^\bullet}$. If $\Gamma^\bullet \geq 1$, then H_0 is rejected at level $\alpha = 0.05$ for every $\boldsymbol{\theta} \in \mathcal{J}$, but in every open neighborhood in $\mathcal{L}$ of each $\boldsymbol{\theta} \in \mathcal{J}$ there is a $\boldsymbol{\theta}'$ such that H_0 is not rejected. If $\Gamma^\bullet = -\infty$, then $\mathcal{J} = \emptyset$ because $\mathcal{B}_{\Gamma^\bullet} = \emptyset$; that is, in a trivial way, we do not have to worry about falsely rejecting H_0 due to biased treatment assignment if H_0 is not rejected for every $\Gamma \geq 1$.

In the simplest case, the paired case with $J = 2$, if $q_{i1} \neq q_{i2}$ for $i = 1, \ldots, I$, the set $\mathcal{J}$ contains a single point $\boldsymbol{\theta}^\bullet$—i.e., $\mathcal{J} = \{\boldsymbol{\theta}^\bullet\}$—given by (8.20) with $\Gamma = \Gamma^\bullet$. If there are some within-pair ties in the paired case, then $\mathcal{J}$ contains infinitely many $\boldsymbol{\theta}^\bullet \in \mathcal{B}_{\Gamma^\bullet}$, where untied pairs with $q_{i1} \neq q_{i2}$ have $\theta^\bullet_{ij}$ given by (8.20) with $\Gamma = \Gamma^\bullet$, and tied pairs have $\theta^\bullet_{i1} = 1 - \theta^\bullet_{i2}$ as any value between $1/(1+\Gamma^\bullet) \leq \theta^\bullet_{i1} \leq \Gamma^\bullet/(1+\Gamma^\bullet)$.

If we want to say more about unmeasured biases than can be said by a sensitivity analysis, then one natural focus of concern is with the biased treatment assignments $\boldsymbol{\theta} \in \mathcal{J}$. At a $\boldsymbol{\theta} \in \mathcal{J}$, the sensitivity analysis is about to give up. Is it ever possible to say, "Don't worry about biased treatment assignment probabilities $\boldsymbol{\theta} \in \mathcal{J}$, because they aren't actually plausible?" This issue is discussed further in Chap. 12.

8.7 Alternative Interpretations of Γ

It is convenient to use a scalar parameter Γ to measure the magnitude of departure of treatment assignment probabilities $\boldsymbol{\theta}$ from random assignment within blocks, $\overline{\boldsymbol{\theta}}$, where $\overline{\theta}_{ij} = 1/J$ for all ij. As discussed in Sect. 8.2, this parameter speaks directly about the principal unobserved covariate $\zeta = \Pr(Z = 1 \mid r_T, r_C, \mathbf{x})$, which is always the unobserved covariate responsible for unmeasured confounding.

At times, the conversation turns from ζ to a specific unobserved covariate, say u, for which no adjustments were made. One investigator says to another, "my study measured u and adjusted for $(\mathbf{x}, u)$, while your study adjusted for $\mathbf{x}$ but did not measure, adjust, or properly account for u, and that explains why your study reached an incorrect conclusion about the effects caused by the treatment." For instance, a study in 1981 suggested coffee as a cause of pancreatic cancer [51]. This association was subsequently claimed by critics to be due to an excess of patients with gastrointestinal disorders in the comparison group, that is, individuals who had been advised to reduce their consumption of coffee [92,95,97]. The point here is that a specific u is under discussion, so the conversation may be informed or constrained by scientific information about that specific u.

Suppose that R and Z are associated after adjustment for $\mathbf{x}$ because of the failure to adjust for u, and that R and Z would be conditionally independent given $(\mathbf{x}, u)$. Can a value of Γ be interpreted in terms of separate unobserved relationships between u and R, and between u and Z, that are jointly responsible for the spurious but observed relationship between R and Z? To say that the association is spurious is to say that there is no treatment effect, $R = r_T = r_C$; otherwise, the relationship between R and Z is not entirely spurious. I will speak about the association between r_C and u, rather than between R and u, although they are the same when there is no treatment effect. The advantage of speaking about r_C rather than R is that the discussion can then refer to a general hypothesis about causal effects, $H_0 : \boldsymbol{\delta} = \boldsymbol{\delta}_0$, tested using $\mathbf{R}^{\boldsymbol{\delta}_0}$, rather than restricting attention to $H_0 : \boldsymbol{\delta} = \mathbf{0}$.

A method will now be presented for interpreting Γ in this context [83]. A single matched pair, $J = 2$, is a useful benchmark. In a matched pair, $Z_{i1} - Z_{i2} = 1$ if individual $j = 1$ is treated, or $Z_{i1} - Z_{i2} = -1$ if individual $j = 2$ is treated. In that matched pair, $r_{Ci1} - r_{Ci2}$ is the difference in potential responses under control, and it equals $(R_{i1} - \delta_{0i1}) - (R_{i2} - \delta_{0i2})$ when $H_0 : \boldsymbol{\delta} = \boldsymbol{\delta}_0$ is true. Assuming matching has made $\mathbf{x}_{i1} = \mathbf{x}_{i2}$, suppose that (u_{i1}, u_{i2}) could at most increase the odds of $Z_{i1} - Z_{i2} = 1$ rather than $Z_{i1} - Z_{i2} = -1$ by a factor of $\Lambda \geq 1$; so,

$$\frac{1}{\Lambda} \leq \frac{\Pr(Z_{i1} - Z_{i2} = 1 \mid \mathbf{x}_{i1}, \mathbf{x}_{i2}, u_{i1}, u_{i2})}{\Pr(Z_{i1} - Z_{i2} = -1 \mid \mathbf{x}_{i1}, \mathbf{x}_{i2}, u_{i1}, u_{i2})} \leq \Lambda,$$

or equivalently

$$\frac{1}{1+\Lambda} \leq \Pr(Z_{i1} - Z_{i2} = 1 \mid \mathbf{x}_{i1}, \mathbf{x}_{i2}, u_{i1}, u_{i2}) \leq \frac{\Lambda}{1+\Lambda}. \tag{8.27}$$

The situation for $r_{Ci1} - r_{Ci2}$ is slightly different, because r_{Cij} may not be binary. So, consider the probability that $r_{Ci1} - r_{Ci2} > 0$ given the value of $|r_{Ci1} - r_{Ci2}|$. In a randomized experiment, this probability is $1/2$ if $|r_{Ci1} - r_{Ci2}| \neq 0$ and is 0 if $|r_{Ci1} - r_{Ci2}| = 0$, so that $r_{Ci1} - r_{Ci2}$ is symmetrically distributed about zero. Motivated by Douglas Wolfe's [98] semiparametric family of deformations of distributions symmetric about zero, the method introduces a parameter $\Psi \geq 1$ and assumes

$$\frac{1}{\Psi} \leq \frac{\Pr(r_{Ci1} - r_{Ci2} > 0 \mid \mathbf{x}_{i1}, \mathbf{x}_{i2}, u_{i1}, u_{i2}, |r_{Ci1} - r_{Ci2}|)}{\Pr(r_{Ci1} - r_{Ci2} < 0 \mid \mathbf{x}_{i1}, \mathbf{x}_{i2}, u_{i1}, u_{i2}, |r_{Ci1} - r_{Ci2}|)} \leq \Psi,$$

or equivalently

$$\frac{1}{1+\Psi} \leq \Pr(r_{Ci1} - r_{Ci2} > 0 \mid \mathbf{x}_{i1}, \mathbf{x}_{i2}, u_{i1}, u_{i2}, |r_{Ci1} - r_{Ci2}|) \leq \frac{\Psi}{1+\Psi}, \tag{8.28}$$

when $|r_{Ci1} - r_{Ci2}| \neq 0$, where of course

$$\Pr(r_{Ci1} - r_{Ci2} > 0 \mid \mathbf{x}_{i1}, \mathbf{x}_{i2}, u_{i1}, u_{i2}, |r_{Ci1} - r_{Ci2}|) = 0 \text{ if } |r_{Ci1} - r_{Ci2}| = 0.$$

It turns out that a matched pair sensitivity analysis using Γ is identical to a matched pair sensitivity analysis using (Λ, Ψ) whenever

$$\Gamma = \frac{\Lambda\Psi + 1}{\Lambda + \Psi}. \tag{8.29}$$

A careful statement and proof of this claim takes a few steps that are not presented here [83]. The careful statement says that two different sampling models give exactly the same paired sensitivity analyses. Most of this chapter has conditioned on $\mathcal{F}$, which includes (r_{Ci1}, r_{Ci2}), but (8.27) and (8.28) do not condition on (r_{Ci1}, r_{Ci2}), and that is the difference between the two sampling models.

For example, taking $(\Lambda, \Psi) = (2, 2)$ in (8.29) yields $(\Lambda\Psi + 1)/(\Lambda + \Psi) = 5/4 = 1.25 = \Gamma$. So, in a matched pair, $\Gamma = 1.25$ is equivalent to an unobserved covariate u that at most doubles the odds of treatment, $Z_{i1} - Z_{i2} = 1$, and at most doubles the odds of a positive pair difference in control responses, $r_{Ci1} - r_{Ci2} > 0$. It is, therefore, reasonable to regard $\Gamma = 1.25$ as a bias that is not enormous, but not small either.

The description in the previous paragraph is appropriate when testing the general hypothesis, $H_0 : \boldsymbol{\delta} = \boldsymbol{\delta}_0$ using $\mathbf{R}^{\boldsymbol{\delta}_0}$. If we are discussing the sensitivity of rejection of $H_0 : \boldsymbol{\delta} = \mathbf{0}$, then the description may be restated in a simpler way, because if $H_0 : \boldsymbol{\delta} = \mathbf{0}$ were true, then $r_{Cij} = R_{ij}$. In this special case: in a matched pair, $\Gamma = 1.25$ is equivalent to an unobserved covariate u that doubles the odds of treatment and at most doubles the odds of a positive difference in responses, $R_{i1} - R_{i2} > 0$.

Taking $(\Lambda, \Psi) = (3, 5)$ or $(\Lambda, \Psi) = (5, 3)$ in (8.29) yields $(\Lambda\Psi + 1)/(\Lambda + \Psi) = 16/8 = 2 = \Gamma$. So, in a matched pair, $\Gamma = 2$ is equivalent to an unobserved covariate u that triples the odds of treatment and increases by 5-fold the odds of a positive pair difference in control responses, $r_{Ci1} - r_{Ci2} > 0$. However, $\Gamma = 2$ is also equivalent to an unobserved covariate u that triples the odds of a positive pair difference in control responses and increases by 5-fold the odds of treatment.

In Table 8.1, rejection of the hypothesis of no effect of alcohol on HDL cholesterol levels using statistic U878 became sensitive to unmeasured bias at about $\Gamma = 6$. In a matched pair, $\Gamma = 6$ is equivalent to an unobserved covariate that increases the odds of light daily drinking by $\Lambda = 11$ fold and the odds of a higher HDL cholesterol level by $\Psi = 13$ fold, as $(\Lambda, \Psi) = (11, 13)$ in (8.29) yields $(\Lambda\Psi + 1)/(\Lambda + \Psi) = 144/24 = 6 = \Gamma$. Again, that is about what it would take to explain away the effect of smoking on lung cancer in Hammond's [33] study [66, Table 4.1].

A block design with $J > 2$ contains $I(J - 1)$ treated-control pairs; in particular, it contains a paired design with $J = 2$. For $J > 2$, one such paired design can be produced from a block design by selecting one of the $J - 1$ controls at random in each block. For any block design, it is reasonable to interpret a bias of magnitude Γ in terms of its impact on a single matched pair using (8.29), because the block design contains many such pairs, and each pair is an atom of the block design—i.e., it is the smallest component of the design that provides an estimate of the treatment effect. A unit of measure, here Γ, is often defined by referring to a simple situation, here a single matched pair; for instance, a gram is the mass of a milliliter of water at 4° Celsius. The interpretation (8.29) is simply an aid to conversations that wish to express Γ in terms of a specific unmeasured covariate u, as in the example of coffee and pancreatic cancer; it plays no formal role in calculations or theory.

Because (8.29) converts a single Γ into a two-dimension curve of (Λ, Ψ), expression (8.29) is called an amplification [83]. The entire curve (Λ, Ψ) converts to the same Γ and hence the same inference. An investigator may interpret Γ in terms of any one point on the curve, or as the entire curve.

Figure 8.2 depicts the amplification curves (Λ, Ψ) for $\Gamma = 1.25$ and $\Gamma = 2$. On the curve for $\Gamma = 1.25$, the point $(\Lambda, \Psi) = (2, 2)$ is indicated. On the curve for

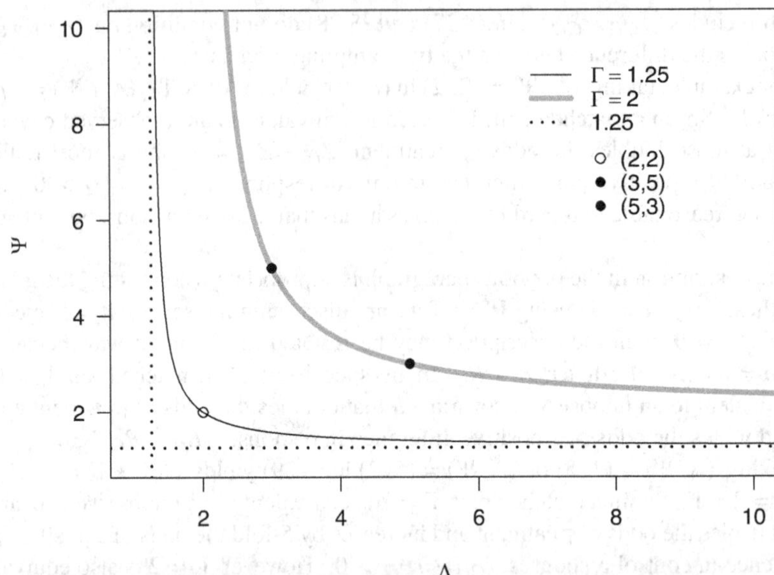

Fig. 8.2 The amplification of Γ into the curve (Λ, Ψ) using (8.29) for Γ = 1.25 and Γ = 2. Points (Λ, Ψ) = (2, 2) for Γ = 1.25 and (Λ, Ψ) = (3, 5) and (Λ, Ψ) = (5, 3) for Γ = 2 are distinguished. The asymptotes for the curve Γ = 1.25 are shown as vertical and horizontal lines at Λ = 1.25 and Ψ = 1.25

Γ = 2, the points (Λ, Ψ) = (3, 5) and (5, 3) are indicated. As is evident from (8.29), if $\Psi \to \infty$ with Γ fixed, then $\Lambda \to \Gamma$. Similarly, if $\Lambda \to \infty$ with Γ fixed, then $\Psi \to \Gamma$. This is visible in Fig. 8.2 by comparing the curve (Λ, Ψ) for Γ = 1.25 to the dotted horizontal and vertical lines at 1.25.

Reconsider the equivalence of (Λ, Ψ) = (3, 5) and Γ = 2 in (8.29). In (8.20), the probability that the treated individual in pair i has the larger rank score is $\Gamma/(1+\Gamma) = 2/(1+2) = 2/3$ for Γ = 2. In contrast, using (8.27) and (8.28), $r_{Ci1} - r_{Ci2}$ and $Z_{i1} - Z_{i2}$ can have the same sign in two ways: both $r_{Ci1} - r_{Ci2}$ and $Z_{i1} - Z_{i2}$ can be positive, or both $r_{Ci1} - r_{Ci2}$ and $Z_{i1} - Z_{i2}$ can be negative. In both of these two cases, the treated-minus-control difference, $(r_{Ci1} - r_{Ci2})(Z_{i1} - Z_{i2})$, is positive. The chance that $r_{Ci1} - r_{Ci2}$ and $Z_{i1} - Z_{i2}$ have the same sign is at most

$$\frac{\Lambda}{1+\Lambda}\frac{\Psi}{1+\Psi} + \frac{1}{1+\Lambda}\frac{1}{1+\Psi} = \frac{3}{1+3}\frac{5}{1+5} + \frac{1}{1+3}\frac{1}{1+5}$$
$$= \frac{15}{24} + \frac{1}{24} = \frac{16}{24} = \frac{2}{3};$$

so, the two formulations agree in this case, and indeed they agree in general [83].

8.8 *Further Reading

The first sensitivity analysis: The first sensitivity analysis in an observational study appeared in an article in 1959 by Cornfield et al. [11, 12] that reviewed the evidence available at that time concerning smoking and lung cancer. The article was an important conceptual advance. It said that association does not imply causation in an observational study, but it added a quantitative dimension [11, p. 193]:

> Cigarette smokers have a nine-fold greater risk of developing lung cancer than nonsmokers, while over-two-pack-a-day smokers have at least a 60-fold greater risk. Any characteristic proposed as a measure of the postulated cause common to both smoking status and lung-cancer risk must therefore be at least nine-fold more prevalent among cigarette smokers than among nonsmokers and at least 60-fold more prevalent among two-pack-a-day smokers.

The method of Cornfield et al. has been further developed and discussed [12, 14, 24, 27, 29, 99]. A variety of similar methods have been proposed [7, 81, 87, 94]. Though of fundamental importance as a conceptual advance, the method of Cornfield et al. [11] is limited in several ways. It ignores the difference between estimates and population parameters, so it can mistakenly suggest that a small observational study is insensitive to large biases simply because its point estimate is unstable. In part because it does not distinguish estimates and population parameters, it does not take account of the fact that as $\boldsymbol{\theta}$ departs from $\overline{\boldsymbol{\theta}}$, the sampling distribution changes. The method is for binary outcomes without adjustments for observed covariates. The method does not provide sensitivity analyses for inference quantities, such as P-values, point estimates, and confidence intervals. Most modern methods of sensitivity analysis address some or all of these issues.

Scope of the methods in this chapter: Although the chapter has emphasized the use of weighted rank statistics in block designs, the methods in this chapter apply to (i) other statistics, including M-estimates [68, 72], means [18, 19], attributable effects [63, 64], and quantiles [61, 62]; (ii) other designs [74, 80], including case-control studies [58], clustered treatment assignments [34], interference between units [67, §6], and attempts to demonstrate equivalence of effects [84]; (iii) use of covariance adjustment [65], instruments [43] [4, 17, 20, 35, 91], and multiple comparisons [22, 84]; and (iv) methods that attempt to discover effect modification, in which the magnitude of a treatment effect varies with measured covariates [40, 41, 47, 48].

Other approaches to sensitivity analysis: There are many approaches to sensitivity analysis in observational studies [6, 18, 19, 25, 56, 81]. These include Bayesian methods [54], conformal methods [44], inverse probability weighting methods [15, 102], logit regression methods [37, 50], semiparametric methods [36, 56, 86], and trend tests [100].

Amplification: The amplification [83] in Sect. 8.7 builds upon an earlier approach of Gastwirth et al. [25]. One difference between these two approaches is that, in the method in Sect. 8.7, the relationship between Γ and (Λ, Ψ) does not depend upon the test statistic.

Issues besides unmeasured confounding: Sensitivity analyses are often used to address causal issues besides unmeasured confounding [42,49,88,90].

8.9 *Appendix: Proof of Proposition 8.4

This appendix demonstrates the convexity of $f_{\alpha/2}(\boldsymbol{\theta})$ in (8.17); that is, it proves Proposition 8.4. Remark 8.1 observes that, in general, $f_{\alpha/2}(\boldsymbol{\theta})$ is not strictly convex, noting in particular the case of a within-block tie, $q_{ij} = q_{ij'}$ for $j \neq j'$.

Proof Alas, this is a proof for your wrist rather than for your head. First, we need to rearrange $f_{\alpha/2}(\boldsymbol{\theta})$ to distinguish terms that involve θ_{ij} alone from those that involve $\theta_{ij}\,\theta_{i'j'}$. In (8.17),

$$\left(T^{\delta_0} - \sum_{i=1}^{I}\sum_{j=1}^{J}\theta_{ij}\,q_{ij}\right)^2 = \left(T^{\delta_0}\right)^2 - 2T^{\delta_0}\sum_{i=1}^{I}\sum_{j=1}^{J}\theta_{ij}\,q_{ij} + \left(\sum_{i=1}^{I}\sum_{j=1}^{J}\theta_{ij}\,q_{ij}\right)^2$$

$$= \left(T^{\delta_0}\right)^2 - 2T^{\delta_0}\sum_{i=1}^{I}\sum_{j=1}^{J}\theta_{ij}\,q_{ij} + \sum_{i=1}^{I}\sum_{j=1}^{J}\sum_{i'=1}^{I}\sum_{j'=1}^{J}\theta_{ij}\,\theta_{i'j'}\,q_{ij}\,q_{i'j'}. \tag{8.30}$$

Write $\iota_{ii'} = 1$ if $i = i'$ and $\iota_{ii'} = 0$ otherwise. In (8.17),

$$-\,\varsigma_{\alpha/2}\sum_{i=1}^{I}\left\{\left(\sum_{j=1}^{J}\theta_{ij}\,q_{ij}^2\right) - \left(\sum_{j=1}^{J}\theta_{ij}\,q_{ij}\right)^2\right\}$$

$$= -\varsigma_{\alpha/2}\sum_{i=1}^{I}\sum_{j=1}^{J}\theta_{ij}\,q_{ij}^2 + \sum_{i=1}^{I}\sum_{j=1}^{J}\sum_{i'=1}^{I}\sum_{j'=1}^{J}\iota_{ii'}\,\theta_{ij}\,\theta_{i'j'}\,\varsigma_{\alpha/2}\,q_{ij}\,q_{i'j'}. \tag{8.31}$$

Combining (8.30) and (8.31), we have

$$f_{\alpha/2}(\boldsymbol{\theta}) = \left(T^{\delta_0}\right)^2 - \sum_{i=1}^{I}\sum_{j=1}^{J}\theta_{ij}\,a_{ij} + \sum_{i=1}^{I}\sum_{j=1}^{J}\sum_{i'=1}^{I}\sum_{j'=1}^{J}\theta_{ij}\,\theta_{i'j'}\,b_{iji'j'}$$

where

$$a_{ij} = 2T^{\delta_0}q_{ij} + \varsigma_{\alpha/2}\,q_{ij}^2 \quad \text{and} \quad b_{iji'j'} = q_{ij}\,q_{i'j'}\left(1 + \varsigma_{\alpha/2}\,\iota_{ii'}\right), \tag{8.32}$$

thereby expressing $f_{\alpha/2}(\boldsymbol{\theta})$ explicitly as a quadratic function of $\boldsymbol{\theta}$. Let $\mathbf{H}$ be the $IJ \times IJ$ matrix with $b_{iji'j'}$ in row ij and column $i'j'$. Then, because $f_{\alpha/2}(\boldsymbol{\theta})$ is quadratic, $\mathbf{H}$ is the matrix of second derivatives of $f_{\alpha/2}(\boldsymbol{\theta})$. To prove that $f_{\alpha/2}(\boldsymbol{\theta})$ is convex, we need to show that $\mathbf{H}$ is positive semidefinite [31, Corollary 4.30]; that is, we need to prove that $\mathbf{v}^T\mathbf{H}\mathbf{v} \geq 0$ for every IJ-dimensional vector $\mathbf{v}$. Now,

$$\mathbf{v}^T\mathbf{H}\mathbf{v} = \sum_{i=1}^{I}\sum_{j=1}^{J}\sum_{i'=1}^{I}\sum_{j'=1}^{J} v_{ij}\, v_{i'j'}\, q_{ij}\, q_{i'j'} \left(1 + \varsigma_{\alpha/2}\, \iota_{ii'}\right) \tag{8.33}$$

$$= \left(\sum_{i=1}^{I}\sum_{j=1}^{J} v_{ij}\, q_{ij}\right)^2 + \varsigma_{\alpha/2} \sum_{i=1}^{I}\left(\sum_{j'=1}^{J} v_{ij}\, q_{ij}\right)^2 \geq 0,$$

proving the proposition. □

Remark 8.1 It is easy to see that, in general, $f_{\alpha/2}(\boldsymbol{\theta})$ is not strictly convex. For $f_{\alpha/2}(\boldsymbol{\theta})$ to be strictly convex, its second derivative matrix, $\mathbf{H}$, would need to be positive definite [31, Corollary 4.30], with $\mathbf{v}^T\mathbf{H}\mathbf{v} > 0$ for every IJ-dimensional vector $\mathbf{v} \neq \mathbf{0}$. A simple counterexample occurs if two q_{ij} in the same block are tied. In particular, if $q_{\ell m} = q_{\ell m'}$, take $v_{\ell m} = 1$, $v_{\ell m'} = -1$ and $v_{ij} = 0$ for all other ij; then (8.33) equals 0 for $\mathbf{v} \neq \mathbf{0}$.

Remark 8.2 The second derivative matrix, $\mathbf{H}$, is $IJ \times IJ$; so, even in the small example in Sect. 1.4 with $I = 406$ and $J = 4$, the matrix $\mathbf{H}$ contains $I^2J^2 =$ 2,637,376 numbers. For computations using $\mathbf{H}$, it is useful to note from (8.33) that $\mathbf{v}^T\mathbf{H}\mathbf{v}$ can be computed for any $\mathbf{v}$ from $2IJ + 1$ numbers, namely, $\varsigma_{\alpha/2}$, v_{ij} and q_{ij} for $i = 1, \ldots, I$ and $j = 1, \ldots, J$.

8.10 *Appendix: A CLT for Biased Treatment Assignment

*Central Limit Theorem for Weighted Rank Statistics Under (8.11)

The central limit theorem for the null distribution of a weighted rank statistic needs minor adjustments if it is to work for a biased treatment assignment mechanism (8.11), and the needed adjustments are supplied in this appendix, which may be skipped. A minor but useful added benefit of these adjustments is that they also allow for within-block ties among responses.

We want a central limit theorem that applies under H_0 as the number of blocks increases, $I \to \infty$, with J fixed, for any infinite sequence of probabilities $(\theta_{i1}, \ldots, \theta_{iJ})$, $i = 1, 2, \ldots$ that satisfy (8.6) or equivalently that satisfy (8.8)–(8.10). Under the null hypothesis, the weighted rank statistic is $T_I = \sum_{i=1}^{I}\sum_{j=1}^{J} Z_{ij}\, \phi\left(q_{ij}^*\right) a_i$, where a_i, $i = 1, 2, \ldots$ is a fixed sequence of constants, the q_{ij}^* are the within-block ranks of the r_{Cij} in block i with average ranks for ties, and $\phi(\cdot)$ is a function that is not constant on the possible values of q_{ij}^*. The goal is to show that

$$D_I = \frac{T_I - \mathrm{E}(T_I \mid \mathcal{F}_I, \mathcal{Z}_I)}{\sqrt{\mathrm{var}(T_I \mid \mathcal{F}_I, \mathcal{Z}_I)}}$$

converges in distribution to the standard normal distribution, $\Phi(\cdot)$, where $\mathcal{F}_I$ and $\mathcal{Z}_I$ signify $\mathcal{F}$ and $\mathcal{Z}$ for the first I blocks. Under H_0, the rank scores $q_{ij} = \phi\left(q_{ij}^*\right) a_i$ are functions of r_{Cij} which are fixed by conditioning on $\mathcal{F}_I$. If $a_i = 1$ for all i and $\phi\left(q_{ij}^*\right) = q_{ij}^*$, then T_I is the blocked Wilcoxon rank sum statistic. If $a_i = i$ and $\phi\left(q_{ij}^*\right) = q_{ij}^*$, then T_I is Quade's statistic in Sect. 2.6. Stephenson's [93] rank scores pick an integer $m \geq 1$ and use ranks $a_i = 0$ for $i = 1, \ldots, m-1$ and $a_i = \binom{i-1}{m-1}$ for $i \geq m$. Other ranks a_i may be used instead [69, 79].

In Sect. 2.8, under condition (2.16), the special central limit theorem of Hajek, Sidak, and Sen [32, §6.1.2] demonstrated that, in the absence of ties, the null distribution of a weighted rank statistic in a randomized block experiment is asymptotically normal as the number of blocks increases, $I \to \infty$. The goal is to extend this to the case where θ_{ij} need not equal $1/J$ but does satisfy (8.6).

*Some Notation

Write $V_i = \sum_{j=1}^{J} (Z_{ij} - \theta_{ij})\, \phi\left(q_{ij}^*\right)$, so $\mathrm{E}(V_i \mid \mathcal{F}_I, \mathcal{Z}_I) = 0$ and

$$\mathrm{var}(V_i \mid \mathcal{F}_I, \mathcal{Z}_I) = \left\{\sum_{j=1}^{J} \theta_{ij}\, \phi\left(q_{ij}^*\right)^2\right\} - \left\{\sum_{j=1}^{J} \theta_{ij}\, \phi\left(q_{ij}^*\right)\right\}^2 = \nu_{\theta i}^2, \text{ say.}$$

Then $T_I - \mathrm{E}(T_I \mid \mathcal{F}_I, \mathcal{Z}_I) = \sum_{i=1}^{I} a_i V_i$ has expectation zero, and $\mathrm{var}(T_I \mid \mathcal{F}_I, \mathcal{Z}_I) = \mathrm{var}\left(\sum_{i=1}^{I} a_i V_i \,\middle|\, \mathcal{F}_I, \mathcal{Z}_I\right) = \sum_{i=1}^{I} a_i^2 \nu_{\theta i}^2$.

Then

$$D_I = \frac{\sum_{i=1}^{I} a_i V_i}{\sqrt{\sum_{i=1}^{I} a_i^2 \nu_{\theta i}^2}}. \tag{8.34}$$

So, the task is to show that $\Pr(D_I \leq d \mid \mathcal{F}_I, \mathcal{Z}_I) \to \Phi(d)$ as $I \to \infty$, where $\Phi(\cdot)$ is the standard normal cumulative distribution. In a randomized block experiment (2.4) that is free of within-block ties, $\nu_{\theta i}^2$ does not change with i, as is also true in the proof in [32, §6.1.2]. In contrast, either (8.11) or within-block ties mean that $\nu_{\theta i}^2$ can change with i, and it is this possibility that needs to be addressed.

*The Variance $\nu_{\theta i}^2$ of V_i Is Uniformly Bounded

Let us say that block i is informative if $\nu_{\theta i}^2 > 0$ and uninformative if $\nu_{\theta i}^2 = 0$. For instance, if block i is completely tied, $r_{Ci1} = \cdots = r_{CiJ}$, then $q_{i1}^* = \cdots = q_{iJ}^*$ and $\nu_{\theta i}^2 = 0$; so, block i is uninformative. Subject to (8.8)–(8.10), the θ_{ij} are bounded away from 0 and 1, so block i is uninformative if and only if $\phi\left(q_{i1}^*\right) = \cdots = \phi\left(q_{iJ}^*\right)$.[21] If T_I is to be asymptotically normal, then we will need an increasing number of informative blocks with $a_i \neq 0$ as $I \to \infty$.

Lemma 8.1 *There are two numbers, $0 < \upsilon \leq \upsilon' < \infty$, such that*

$$\nu_{\theta i}^2 > 0 \text{ implies } \upsilon \leq \nu_{\theta i}^2 \leq \upsilon' \text{ for } i = 1, 2, \ldots. \tag{8.35}$$

Proof Write $\mathbf{q}_i^* = \left(q_{i1}^*, \ldots, q_{iJ}^*\right)$ for Wilcoxon's ranks in block i. There are finitely many possible values of $\mathbf{q}_i^*$, reflecting both the ordering of responses r_{Cij} and their various patterns of ties. Let Q be the finite set containing the possible values of $\mathbf{q}_i^*$. For instance, for $J = 3$, Q contains the six permutations of (1, 2, 3), plus the three permutations of (1.5, 1.5, 3), plus the three permutations of (1, 2.5, 2.5), plus (2, 2, 2). It is important that Q is a fixed and finite set as $I \to \infty$; that is, there is variability but not novelty as new $\mathbf{q}_i^*$ become available, in the sense that every new $\mathbf{q}_i^*$ is in the same old set Q. For any fixed $\mathbf{q}_i^*$, the quantity $\nu_{\theta i}^2$ is a nonnegative, continuous function of $\theta_{i1}, \ldots, \theta_{iJ}$. The possible values of $\theta_{i1}, \ldots, \theta_{iJ}$ are confined to a compact set (8.8)–(8.10); so, for each fixed $\mathbf{q}_i^* \in Q$, there is a minimum value $\upsilon_{\mathbf{q}_i^*}$ of $\nu_{\theta i}^2$, where $\upsilon_{\mathbf{q}_i^*} \geq 0$, and also a maximum value $\upsilon'_{\mathbf{q}_i^*}$ of $\nu_{\theta i}^2$, for all $\theta_{i1}, \ldots, \theta_{iJ}$ that satisfy (8.8)–(8.10). To complete the proof, define

$$\upsilon' = \max_{\mathbf{q}_i^* \in Q} \upsilon'_{\mathbf{q}_i^*} \text{ and } \upsilon = \min_{\left\{\mathbf{q}_i^* \in Q:\, \upsilon_{\mathbf{q}_i^*} > 0\right\}} \upsilon_{\mathbf{q}_i^*}.$$

[21] Some care is required here. First, if $a_i = 0$, then a weighted rank statistic may disregard an informative block; for instance, this typically happens for the first few blocks using Stephenson's [93] ranks. Certain rank scores [8, 53, 55] have $a_i = 0$ for a third or more of all blocks, yet can have remarkably good properties when used in sensitivity analyses [73]. The central limit theorem needs a growing number of informative blocks, $\nu_{\theta i}^2 > 0$, that also have $a_i \neq 0$. Second, Wilcoxon's ranks, q_{ij}^*, may be informative in a block, while $\phi\left(q_{ij}^*\right)$ is uniformative. An example follows. Define $\phi\left(q_{ij}^*\right) = 1$ if $q_{ij}^* = J$ and $\phi\left(q_{ij}^*\right) = 0$ otherwise; then T_I receives contribution a_i from block i only if the treated individual in block i has the unique maximum response in block i; otherwise, block i contributes zero. For this $\phi(\cdot)$, it can happen that $\phi\left(q_{i1}^*\right) = \cdots = \phi\left(q_{iJ}^*\right)$ due to a tie for the maximum, even if not all of the q_{ij}^* are equal.

*The Central Limit Theorem Under Biased Treatment Assignment

Recall that block i is uninformative if and only if it is completely tied, $\phi\left(q_{i1}^{*}\right)=\cdots=\phi\left(q_{iJ}^{*}\right)$, or equivalently if and only if $\nu_{\theta i}^{2}=0$. Write $g_i=1$ if block i is informative, and $g_i=0$ if block i is uninformative. Now, $\text{var}\left(T_I \mid \mathcal{F}_I, \mathcal{Z}_I\right)=\sum_{i=1}^{I} a_i^2\,\nu_{\theta i}^2$ receives zero from each block which is uninformative with $g_i=0$, and it also receives zero if T_I ignores this block with $a_i=0$. Write

$$L_I^2=\frac{\sum_{i=1}^{I} g_i\,a_i^2}{\max_{1\le i\le I} g_i\,a_i^2}.$$

Stated informally, if $L_I^2\to\infty$ as $I\to\infty$, then the statistic, T_I, does not ignore a growing number of informative blocks, and no one block dominates all the others.

Proposition 8.6 *Under H_0 and the distribution (8.11), if $L_I^2\to\infty$ as $I\to\infty$, then* $\Pr\left(D_I\ge d \mid \mathcal{F}_I, \mathcal{Z}_I\right)\to 1-\Phi(d)$ *for each d.*

Proof Write s_I^2 for $\text{var}\left(T_I \mid \mathcal{F}_I, \mathcal{Z}_I\right)=\sum_{i=1}^{I} a_i^2\,\nu_{\theta i}^2$. Trivially, $g_i=g_i^2$ because g_i is 0 or 1. Also, trivially $a_i^2\,\nu_{\theta i}^2=g_i\,a_i^2\,\nu_{\theta i}^2$, because $g_i=1$ if and only if $\nu_{\theta i}^2\neq 0$. These trivial substitutions will be made several times. Using the definition of g_i, Lemma 8.1 implies $\nu_{\theta i}^2\ge g_i\,\upsilon$. It follows that

$$\frac{s_I^2}{\max_{1\le i\le I} g_i\,a_i^2}\ge\frac{\upsilon\sum_{i=1}^{I} g_i\,a_i^2}{\max_{1\le i\le I} g_i\,a_i^2}=\upsilon\,L_I^2\to\infty \text{ as } I\to\infty. \tag{8.36}$$

Recall the finite set $\mathcal{Q}$ defined in the proof of Lemma 8.1. The quantity $\phi\left(q_{ij}^{*}\right)$ can take on only finitely many values: every $\phi\left(q_{ij}^{*}\right)$ equals $\phi\left(p_j\right)$ for some $\left(p_1,\ldots,p_J\right)\in\mathcal{Q}$ and some $1\le j\le J$. Also, $Z_{ij}-\theta_{ij}$ equals either $1-\theta_{ij}$ or $0-\theta_{ij}$; in particular, $\left|Z_{ij}-\theta_{ij}\right|\le 1$ from (8.10). Consequently, given $\left(\mathcal{F}_I, \mathcal{Z}_I\right)$ each random variable $V_i=\sum_{j=1}^{J}\left(Z_{ij}-\theta_{ij}\right)\phi\left(q_{ij}^{*}\right)$ has finite support, say $\Pr\left(V_i=w_{ik} \mid \mathcal{F}_I, \mathcal{Z}_I\right)=\pi_{ik}$ for values $w_{i1},\ldots,w_{iK_i}$. It follows that the V_i are uniformly bounded with

$$\max_{1\le i\le\infty,\,1\le k\le K_i}\left|w_{ik}\right|\le\max_{\mathbf{p}\in\mathcal{Q}}\max_{1\le j\le J}\left|\phi\left(p_j\right)\right|=w_{\max},\text{ say.} \tag{8.37}$$

In particular, if block i is uninformative—i.e., if $\nu_{\theta i}^2=0$—then $V_i=0$; so, in this case $K_i=1$ and $w_{i1}=0$. For $\varepsilon>0$, for block i in T_I, define

$$h_{Ii\varepsilon}=\sum_{k:\,|a_i w_{ik}|>\varepsilon s_I} a_i^2\,w_{ik}^2\,\pi_{ik}=\sum_{k:\,|g_i\,a_i\,w_{ik}|>\varepsilon s_I} g_i\,a_i^2\,w_{ik}^2\,\pi_{ik}, \tag{8.38}$$

where the second equality uses $w_{ik}^2=0$ if $g_i=0$. Then the Lindeberg form [9, §9.1, Theorem 1] of the central limit theorem says $\Pr\left(D_I\ge d \mid \mathcal{F}_I, \mathcal{Z}_I\right)\to 1-\Phi(d)$

as $I \to \infty$ for each d if $\left(\sum_{i=1}^{I} h_{Ii\varepsilon}\right)/s_I^2 \to 0$ for every $\varepsilon > 0$. In (8.38), simple rearrangements yield

$$\{k : |g_i\, a_i\, w_{ik}| > \varepsilon s_I\} = \left\{k : g_i\, w_{ik}^2 > \frac{\varepsilon^2\, s_I^2}{a_i^2}\right\}$$

$$\subseteq \left\{k : g_i\, w_{ik}^2 > \frac{\varepsilon^2\, s_I^2}{\max_{1\le \ell \le I} b_\ell\, a_\ell^2}\right\} \subseteq \left\{k : w_{ik}^2 > \varepsilon^2\, \upsilon\, L_I^2\right\},$$

where the final step uses (8.36). Combining this with (8.38) yields

$$h_{Ii\varepsilon} \le \sum_{k\,:\, w_{ik}^2 > \varepsilon^2\, \upsilon\, L_I^2} g_i\, a_i^2\, w_{ik}^2\, \pi_{ik}. \tag{8.39}$$

Recall that $L_I^2 \to \infty$, $\varepsilon > 0$, and $\upsilon > 0$; so, for sufficiently large I

$$\varepsilon^2\, \upsilon\, L_I^2 > w_{\max}^2 \ge w_{ik}^2 \text{ for all } w_{ik},$$

and consequently the right side of (8.39) is zero. Therefore, $\left(\sum_{i=1}^{I} h_{Ii\varepsilon}\right)/s_I^2 \to 0$ for every $\varepsilon > 0$, as required to complete the proof. □

Problems

8.1 Perform a Sensitivity Analysis in an Observational Study

In R, use the `aHDL` data in the `iTOS` package and the function `wgtRank` in the `weightedRank` package to reproduce a few of the bounds on P-values in Table 8.1.

8.2 Amplification

In R, use the `amplify` function in the `iTOS` package to check that $\Gamma = 1.25$ amplifies to $(\Lambda, \Psi) = (2, 2)$ and that $\Gamma = 2$ amplifies to $(\Lambda, \Psi) = (3, 5)$ and also to $(5, 3)$. To gracefully interpret $\Gamma = 1.5$, find a pair of integer values that amplify $\Gamma = 1.5$ into (Λ, Ψ). Do the same for $\Gamma = 5/3$. Do the same for $\Gamma = 4$. Make a plot of the amplification of $\Gamma = 5/3$ that is analogous to Fig. 8.2.

8.3 Sensitivity Analysis for Noether's Statistic in Matched Pairs

(This problem uses the notation and results of Problem 2.2.)

(i) In the case of matched pairs, $J = 2$, write Noether's statistic from Problem 2.2 in the form $T = \sum_{i=1}^{I}\sum_{j=1}^{2} Z_{ij}\, q_{ij}$. (Hint: Consider $i \in \mathcal{N}$ and $i \notin \mathcal{N}$ separately. What is q_{ij} for $i \notin \mathcal{N}$? Is $q_{i1} = q_{i2}$ for any $i \in \mathcal{N}$?)

(ii) Use (8.20) to show that the upper bound on the upper-tailed one-sided P-value from Noether's statistic is obtained from the binomial distribution with sample size $|\mathcal{N}|$ and probability of success $\Gamma/(1+\Gamma)$.

(iii) For large I, the value of f in Noether's statistic strongly affects its ability to distinguish a treatment effect without bias and a bias without a treatment effect. This will be discussed in Chap. 9, but for now, let us get a feeling for this in the example of light daily alcohol and HDL cholesterol from Sect. 1.4. From the aHDL data in the iTOS package, calculate $I = 406$ treated-minus-control matched-pair differences, Y_i, comparing the daily drinkers (D) and never-drinkers (N) as follows:

```
y<-aHDL$hdl[aHDL$grpL=="D"]- aHDL$hdl[aHDL$grpL=="N"].
```

Apply Noether's test to the 406 pair differences, Y_i, with f equal to 0, 1/3, and 2/3, for $\Gamma = 1$, 2.5, and 4. What are the upper bounds on one-sided, upper-tail P-values testing no effect against the alternative hypothesis that light alcohol consumption increases HDL cholesterol? For which values of f is rejection of H_0 insensitive to a bias of $\Gamma = 4$? How many pairs, $|\mathcal{N}|$, have their signs counted for $f = 0, 1/3, 2/3$? What proportion of those pairs have positive signs for $f = 0, 1/3, 2/3$? How do those sample proportions compare with $\Gamma/(1+\Gamma)$ for $\Gamma = 1, 2.5, 4$? Would it be fair to say that when $|Y_i|$ is large, Y_i is very likely to be positive?

(iv) Using the Y_i in part (ii) from aHDL, calculate the mean of Y_i divided by the standard deviation of Y_i. You should get a ratio of about 0.537. Replace the actual data, Y_i, by $I = 406$ observations from a normal distribution with mean 0.5 and standard deviation 1.

```
set.seed(1)
y2<-rnorm(406)+.5
```

Repeat the calculations from part (iii) using these simulated normal values. Try this again, but with $I = 2000$ pairs:

```
set.seed(1)
y2<-rnorm(2000)+.5
```

8.4 Sensitivity Analysis for Noether's Statistic Without Positivity

(This problem refers to Problems 2.2 and 8.3 and footnote 10 in this chapter.)

In matched pairs, $J = 2$, suppose that (a) $q_{ij} = 0$ or $q_{ij} = 1$, as is true for Noether's test in Problem 8.3 and for McNemar's test for binary responses R_{ij}, and (b) the null hypothesis $H_0 : \delta = \delta_0$ is true. Define $\mathcal{N} \subset \{1, \ldots, I\}$ to be the set of pairs i with $q_{i1} \neq q_{i2}$, and define $n = |\mathcal{N}|$ to be the number of such pairs. Let the test statistic be $T^{\delta_0} = \sum_{i \in \mathcal{N}} \sum_{j=1}^{2} Z_{ij}\, q_{ij}$, so only pairs $i \in \mathcal{N}$ are counted in the test statistic.

(i) In parallel with Problem 8.3(ii), show that the maximum tail probability in (8.19) for $\boldsymbol{\theta} \in B_\Gamma$ is given by the binomial distribution with sample size n and probability of success $\Gamma/(1+\Gamma)$.

(ii) For $i \in \mathcal{N}$, let $0 \leq \theta_i^{\ddagger} \leq 1$ be probabilities whose average is $\Gamma/(1+\Gamma) = (1/n) \sum_{i \in \mathcal{N}} \theta_i^{\ddagger}$. In parallel with (8.20), define $\theta_{i1}^{\ddagger} = \theta_i^{\ddagger}$ and $\theta_{i2}^{\ddagger} = 1 - \theta_i^{\ddagger}$ if $q_{i1} > q_{i2}$, or $\theta_{i1}^{\ddagger} = 1 - \theta_i^{\ddagger}$ and $\theta_{i2}^{\ddagger} = \theta_i^{\ddagger}$ if $q_{i1} < q_{i2}$. Such a $\theta_{ij}^{\ddagger}$ may violate positivity with $\theta_{ij}^{\ddagger} = 0$ or $\theta_{ij}^{\ddagger} = 1$, and even if it does not it may fall outside B_Γ. Show that there is a reasonable sense in which the binomial upper tail bound in part (i) above is conservative; i.e., the binomial distribution yields a larger upper tail probability than do these $\theta_{ij}^{\ddagger}$, even when they violate positivity. (This demonstration can be done in two ways, so pick one of them. In the first way, the two distributions, the binomial

and the distribution using $\theta^{\ddagger}_{ij}$, are each approximated by normal distributions with the same expectation and different variances. The second way works with the exact distributions; so, in that sense, it is more satisfying. For the second way, you will want to consult articles by Hoeffding [38] or Gleser [28]; then, armed with their results, the proof is easy.)
(iii) Optional: Compare your conclusions with those of Wang and Krieger [96].

8.5 Sensitivity Analysis for Other Statistics Without Positivity
Problem 8.4 concluded that the sensitivity analysis for matched pairs with $\boldsymbol{\theta} \in B_\Gamma$ actually provides a bound for some $\boldsymbol{\theta} \notin B_\Gamma$, namely, those with $\theta^{\ddagger}_i = \max(\theta_{i1}, \theta_{i2})$ such that $\Gamma/(1+\Gamma) \geq (1/n)\sum_{i\in\mathcal{N}} \theta^{\ddagger}_i$; however, this conclusion used properties of the binomial distribution and was restricted to statistics with $q_{ij} = 0$ or $q_{ij} = 1$. Does this conclusion hold more generally? Brown [8] and Markowski and Hettmansperger [53] proposed two-step test statistics for matched pairs, $J = 2$, in place of Noether's one-step statistic. In these statistics, $\min(q_{i1}, q_{i2}) = 0$ for $i = 1, \ldots, I$, and $\max(q_{i1}, q_{i2})$ is 0, 1 or 2. Let $\mathcal{N}_1 \subset \{1, \ldots, I\}$ be the pairs i with $1 = \max(q_{i1}, q_{i2})$, and let $\mathcal{N}_2 \subset \{1, \ldots, I\}$ be the pairs i with $2 = \max(q_{i1}, q_{i2})$. Suppose the null hypothesis $H_0 : \boldsymbol{\delta} = \boldsymbol{\delta}_0$ is true.
(i) Show that the sensitivity bound (8.19) for the statistic $T^{\boldsymbol{\delta}_0} = \sum_{i=1}^{I}\sum_{j=1}^{2} Z_{ij}\, q_{ij}$ is given by the distribution of a binomial random variable with sample size $|\mathcal{N}_1|$ plus two times an independent binomial random variable with sample size $|\mathcal{N}_2|$, both with probability of success $\Gamma/(1+\Gamma)$. (Hint: Use (8.20).)
(ii) Show that the bound in part (i) is also a bound for $\boldsymbol{\theta} \notin B_\Gamma$ providing $\Gamma/(1+\Gamma) \geq (1/|\mathcal{N}_1|)\sum_{i\in\mathcal{N}_1} \max(\theta_{i1}, \theta_{i2})$ and $\Gamma/(1+\Gamma) \geq (1/|\mathcal{N}_2|)\sum_{i\in\mathcal{N}_2} \max(\theta_{i1}, \theta_{i2})$. (The two options for proving this are basically the same as in Problem 8.4(ii), except you need also the result discussed in footnote 8 in this chapter.)
(iii) Show that the result you proved in part (ii) does not hold if the two conditions,

$$\Gamma/(1+\Gamma) \geq \frac{1}{|\mathcal{N}_1|}\sum_{i\in\mathcal{N}_1} \max(\theta_{i1}, \theta_{i2})$$

and

$$\Gamma/(1+\Gamma) \geq \frac{1}{|\mathcal{N}_2|}\sum_{i\in\mathcal{N}_2} \max(\theta_{i1}, \theta_{i2}),$$

are replaced by the single condition

$$\Gamma/(1+\Gamma) \geq \frac{1}{|\mathcal{N}_1 \cup \mathcal{N}_2|}\sum_{i\in\mathcal{N}_1\cup\mathcal{N}_2} \max(\theta_{i1}, \theta_{i2}).$$

(Hint: It suffices to consider the maximum expectation of $T^{\boldsymbol{\delta}_0}$.) [23, 30].

References

1. Ahmed, A.H.N., Leon, R., Proschan, F.: Generalized association, with applications in multivariate statistics. Ann. Stat. **9**, 168–176 (1981)
2. Bahadur, R.R.: Stochastic comparison of tests. Ann. Math. Stat. **31**(2), 276–295 (1960)
3. Bahadur, R.R.: Rates of convergence of estimates and test statistics. Ann. Math. Stat. **38**(2), 303–324 (1967)
4. Baiocchi, M., Small, D.S., Lorch, S., Rosenbaum, P.R.: Building a stronger instrument in an observational study of perinatal care for premature infants. J. Am. Stat. Assoc. **105**(492), 1285–1296 (2010)
5. Birch, M.W.: The detection of partial association, i: the 2×2 case. J. Roy. Stat. Soc. B **26**(2), 313–324 (1964)
6. Bonvini, M., Kennedy, E.H.: Sensitivity analysis via the proportion of unmeasured confounding. J. Am. Stat. Assoc. **117**, 1540–1550 (2022)
7. Bross, I.D.J.: Spurious effects from an extraneous variable. J. Chronic Diseases **19**(6), 637–647 (1966)
8. Brown, B.M.: Symmetric quantile averages and related estimators. Biometrika **68**(1), 235–242 (1981)
9. Chow, Y.S., Teicher, H.: Probability Theory: Independence, Interchangeability, Martingales, 2nd edn. Springer, New York (1988)
10. Conlon, J.C., Leon, R.V., Proschan, F., Sethuraman, J.: G-ordered functions in statistics. Tech. rep., Florida State University (1977)
11. Cornfield, J., Haenszel, W., Hammond, E.C., Lilienfeld, A.M., Shimkin, M.B., Wynder, E.L.: Smoking and lung cancer: Recent evidence and a discussion of some questions. J. Natl. Cancer Inst. **22**(1), 173–203 (1959)
12. Cornfield, J., Haenszel, W., Hammond, E.C., Lilienfeld, A.M., Shimkin, M.B., Wynder, E.L.: Smoking and lung cancer: recent evidence and a discussion of some questions (reprint from 1959 with new Discussion by D. R. Cox, J. P. Vandenbroucke, M. Zwahlen and J. B. Greenhouse). Int. J. Epidemiol. **38**(5), 1175–91 (2009)
13. Crump, R.K., Hotz, V.J., Imbens, G.W., Mitnik, O.A.: Dealing with limited overlap in estimation of average treatment effects. Biometrika **96**(1), 187–199 (2009)
14. Ding, P., VanderWeele, T.J.: Generalized Cornfield conditions for the risk difference. Biometrika **101**(4), 971–977 (2014)
15. Dorn, J., Guo, K.: Sharp sensitivity analysis for inverse propensity weighting via quantile balancing. J. Am. Stat. Assoc. **118**(544), 2645–2657 (2023)
16. Eaton, M.L.: A review of selected topics in multivariate probability inequalities. Ann. Stat. **10**, 11–43 (1982)
17. Ertefaie, A., Small, D.S., Rosenbaum, P.R.: Quantitative evaluation of the trade-off of strengthened instruments and sample size in observational studies. J. Am. Stat. Assoc. **113**(523), 1122–1134 (2018)
18. Fogarty, C.: Sensitivity analysis. In: Zubizarreta, J.R., Stuart, E.A., Small, D.S., Rosenbaum, P.R. (eds.) Handbook of Matching and Weighting Adjustments for Causal Inference, pp. 553–582. Chapman and Hall/CRC, Boca Raton (2023)
19. Fogarty, C.B.: Studentized sensitivity analysis for the sample average treatment effect in paired observational studies. J. Am. Stat. Assoc. **115**(531), 1518–1530 (2020)
20. Fogarty, C.B., Lee, K., Kelz, R.R., Keele, L.J.: Biased encouragements and heterogeneous effects in an instrumental variable study of emergency general surgical outcomes. J. Am. Stat. Assoc. **116**(536), 1625–1636 (2021)
21. Fogarty, C.B., Mikkelsen, M.E., Gaieski, D.F., Small, D.S.: Discrete optimization for interpretable study populations and randomization inference in an observational study of severe sepsis mortality. J. Am. Stat. Assoc. **111**(514), 447–458 (2016)
22. Fogarty, C.B., Small, D.S.: Sensitivity analysis for multiple comparisons in matched observational studies through quadratically constrained linear programming. J. Am. Stat. Assoc. **111**(516), 1820–1830 (2016)

23. Fogelin, R.J.: Pyrrhonian Reflections on Knowledge and Justification. Oxford University Press, New York (1994)
24. Gastwirth, J.L.: Methods for assessing the sensitivity of statistical comparisons used in Title VII cases to omitted variables. Jurimetrics J. **33**, 19 (1992)
25. Gastwirth, J.L., Krieger, A.M., Rosenbaum, P.R.: Dual and simultaneous sensitivity analysis for matched pairs. Biometrika **85**(4), 907–920 (1998)
26. Gastwirth, J.L., Krieger, A.M., Rosenbaum, P.R.: Asymptotic separability in sensitivity analysis. J. Roy. Stat. Soc. B **62**(3), 545–555 (2000)
27. Gastwirth, J.L., Krieger, A.M., Rosenbaum, P.R.: Cornfield's inequality. In: Encyclopedia of Biostatistics, vol. 2. Wiley Online Library (2005)
28. Gleser, L.J.: On the distribution of the number of successes in independent trials. Ann. Probab. **3**, 182–188 (1975)
29. Greenhouse, S.W.: Jerome Cornfield's contributions to epidemiology. Biometrics (Supplement Volume) **38**, S33–S45 (1982)
30. Grice, H.P.: Aspects of Reason. Oxford University Press, New York (2001)
31. Güler, O.: Foundations of Optimization. Springer, Berlin (2010)
32. Hajek, J., Sidak, Z., Sen, P.K.: Theory of Rank Tests. Academic Press, New York (1999)
33. Hammond, E.C.: Smoking in relation to mortality and morbidity. Findings in first thirty-four months of follow-up in a prospective study started in 1959. J. Natl. Cancer Inst. **32**(5), 1161–1188 (1964)
34. Hansen, B.B., Rosenbaum, P.R., Small, D.S.: Clustered treatment assignments and sensitivity to unmeasured biases in observational studies. J. Am. Stat. Assoc. **109**(505), 133–144 (2014)
35. Heng, S., Small, D.S., Rosenbaum, P.R.: Finding the strength in a weak instrument in a study of cognitive outcomes produced by Catholic high schools. J. Roy. Stat. Soc. Ser. A **183**(3), 935–958 (2020)
36. Hernán, M.A., Brumback, B., Robins, J.M.: Marginal structural models to estimate the joint causal effect of nonrandomized treatments. J. Am. Stat. Assoc. **96**(454), 440–448 (2001)
37. Hernan, M.A., Robins, J.M.: Letter (Hernan & Robins) and Reply (Lin, Psaty and Kronmal): Assessing the sensitivity of regression results to unmeasured confounders in observational studies. Biometrics **55**, 1316–1317 (1999)
38. Hoeffding, W.: On the distribution of the number of successes in independent trials. Ann. Math. Stat. **27**, 713–721 (1956)
39. Hollander, M., Proschan, F., Sethuraman, J.: Functions decreasing in transposition and their applications in ranking problems. Ann. Stat. **5**, 722–733 (1977)
40. Hsu, J., Small, D., Rosenbaum, P.R.: Effect modification and design sensitivity in observational studies. J. Am. Stat. Assoc. **108**(501), 135–148 (2013)
41. Hsu, J., Zubizarreta, J.R., Small, D., Rosenbaum, P.R.: Strong control of the familywise error rate in observational studies that discover effect modification by exploratory methods. Biometrika **102**(4), 767–782 (2015)
42. Huang, M.Y.: Sensitivity analysis for the generalization of experimental results. J. Roy. Stat. Soc. Ser. A (2024). https://doi.org/10.1093/jrsssa/qnae012
43. Imbens, G.W., Rosenbaum, P.R.: Robust, accurate confidence intervals with a weak instrument: quarter of birth and education. J. Roy. Stat. Soc. Ser. A **168**(1), 109–126 (2005)
44. Jin, Y., Ren, Z., Candès, E.J.: Sensitivity analysis of individual treatment effects: A robust conformal inference approach. Proc. Natl. Acad. Sci. **120**(6), e2214889120 (2023)
45. Joiner, B.L.: The median significance level and other small sample measures of test efficacy. J. Am. Stat. Assoc. **64**, 971–985 (1969)
46. Kamae, T., Krengel, U., O'Brien, G.L.: Stochastic inequalities on partially ordered spaces. Ann. Probab. **5**(6), 899–912 (1977)
47. Lee, K., Small, D.S., Hsu, J.Y., Silber, J.H., Rosenbaum, P.R.: Discovering effect modification in an observational study of surgical mortality at hospitals with superior nursing. J. Roy. Stat. Soc. Ser. A: Stat. Soc. **181**(2), 535–546 (2018)
48. Lee, K., Small, D.S., Rosenbaum, P.R.: A powerful approach to the study of moderate effect modification in observational studies. Biometrics **74**(4), 1161–1170 (2018)

49. Li, F., Mattei, A., Mealli, F.: Evaluating the causal effect of university grants on student dropout: Evidence from a regression discontinuity design using principal stratification. Ann. Appl. Stat. **9**, 1906–1931 (2015)
50. Lin, D.Y., Psaty, B.M., Kronmal, R.A.: Assessing the sensitivity of regression results to unmeasured confounders in observational studies. Biometrics **54**, 948–963 (1998)
51. MacMahon, B., Yen, S., Trichopoulos, D., Warren, K., Nardi, G.: Coffee and cancer of the pancreas. N. Engl. J. Med. **304**(11), 630–633 (1981)
52. Maritz, J.S.: A note on exact robust confidence intervals for location. Biometrika **66**(1), 163–170 (1979)
53. Markowski, E.P., Hettmansperger, T.P.: Inference based on simple rank step score statistics for the location model. J. Am. Stat. Assoc. **77**(380), 901–907 (1982)
54. McCandless, L.C., Gustafson, P., Levy, A.: Bayesian sensitivity analysis for unmeasured confounding in observational studies. Stat. Med. **26**(11), 2331–2347 (2007)
55. Noether, G.E.: Some simple distribution-free confidence intervals for the center of a symmetric distribution. J. Am. Stat. Assoc. **68**(343), 716–719 (1973)
56. Robins, J.M., Rotnitzky, A., Scharfstein, D.O.: Sensitivity analysis for selection bias and unmeasured confounding in missing data and causal inference models. In: Halloran, M.E., Berry, D. (eds.) Statistical Models in Epidemiology, the Environment, and Clinical Trials, pp. 1–94. Springer, New York (2000)
57. Rosenbaum, P.R.: Sensitivity analysis for certain permutation inferences in matched observational studies. Biometrika **74**(1), 13–26 (1987)
58. Rosenbaum, P.R.: Sensitivity analysis for matched case-control studies. Biometrics **47**, 87–100 (1991)
59. Rosenbaum, P.R.: Some poset statistics. Ann. Stat. **19**(2), 1091–1097 (1991)
60. Rosenbaum, P.R.: Hodges-Lehmann point estimates of treatment effect in observational studies. J. Am. Stat. Assoc. **88**(424), 1250–1253 (1993)
61. Rosenbaum, P.R.: Quantiles in nonrandom samples and observational studies. J. Am. Stat. Assoc. **90**(432), 1424–1431 (1995)
62. Rosenbaum, P.R.: Reduced sensitivity to hidden bias at upper quantiles in observational studies with dilated treatment effects. Biometrics **55**(2), 560–564 (1999)
63. Rosenbaum, P.R.: Effects attributable to treatment: Inference in experiments and observational studies with a discrete pivot. Biometrika **88**(1), 219–231 (2001)
64. Rosenbaum, P.R.: Attributing effects to treatment in matched observational studies. J. Am. Stat. Assoc. **97**(457), 183–192 (2002)
65. Rosenbaum, P.R.: Covariance adjustment in randomized experiments and observational studies. Stat. Sci. **17**(3), 286–327 (2002)
66. Rosenbaum, P.R.: Observational Studies, 2nd edn. Springer, New York (2002)
67. Rosenbaum, P.R.: Exact confidence intervals for nonconstant effects by inverting the signed rank test. Am. Stat. **57**(2), 132–138 (2003)
68. Rosenbaum, P.R.: Sensitivity analysis for M-estimates, tests, and confidence intervals in matched observational studies. Biometrics **63**(2), 456–464 (2007)
69. Rosenbaum, P.R.: A new U-statistic with superior design sensitivity in matched observational studies. Biometrics **67**(3), 1017–1027 (2011)
70. Rosenbaum, P.R.: An exact adaptive test with superior design sensitivity in an observational study of treatments for ovarian cancer. Ann. Appl. Stat. **6**, 83–105 (2012)
71. Rosenbaum, P.R.: Optimal matching of an optimally chosen subset in observational studies. J. Comput. Graph. Stat. **21**(1), 57–71 (2012)
72. Rosenbaum, P.R.: Weighted M-statistics with superior design sensitivity in matched observational studies with multiple controls. J. Am. Stat. Assoc. **109**(507), 1145–1158 (2014)
73. Rosenbaum, P.R.: Bahadur efficiency of sensitivity analyses in observational studies. J. Am. Stat. Assoc. **110**(509), 205–217 (2015)
74. Rosenbaum, P.R.: Sensitivity analysis for stratified comparisons in an observational study of the effect of smoking on homocysteine levels. Ann. Appl. Stat. **12**(4), 2312–2334 (2018)
75. Rosenbaum, P.R.: Design of Observational Studies, 2nd edn. Springer, New York (2020)

76. Rosenbaum, P.R.: A statistic with demonstrated insensitivity to unmeasured bias for 2× 2× S tables in observational studies. Stat. Med. **41**(19), 3758–3771 (2022)
77. Rosenbaum, P.R.: Can we reliably detect biases that matter in observational studies? Stat. Sci. **38**, 440–457 (2023)
78. Rosenbaum, P.R.: Sensitivity analyses informed by tests for bias in observational studies. Biometrics **79**, 475–487 (2023)
79. Rosenbaum, P.R.: Bahadur efficiency of observational block designs. J. Am. Stat. Assoc. **119**(547), 1871–1881 (2024)
80. Rosenbaum, P.R., Krieger, A.M.: Sensitivity of two-sample permutation inferences in observational studies. J. Am. Stat. Assoc. **85**(410), 493–498 (1990)
81. Rosenbaum, P.R., Rubin, D.B.: Assessing sensitivity to an unobserved binary covariate in an observational study with binary outcome. J. Roy. Stat. Soc. Ser. B (Methodological) **45**(2), 212–218 (1983)
82. Rosenbaum, P.R., Rubin, D.B.: The bias due to incomplete matching. Biometrics **41**, 103–116 (1985)
83. Rosenbaum, P.R., Silber, J.H.: Amplification of sensitivity analysis in matched observational studies. J. Am. Stat. Assoc. **104**(488), 1398–1405 (2009)
84. Rosenbaum, P.R., Silber, J.H.: Sensitivity analysis for equivalence and difference in an observational study of neonatal intensive care units. J. Am. Stat. Assoc. **104**(486), 501–511 (2009)
85. Rosenbaum, P.R., Small, D.S.: An adaptive Mantel–Haenszel test for sensitivity analysis in observational studies. Biometrics **73**(2), 422–430 (2017)
86. Scharfstein, D.O., Rotnitzky, A., Robins, J.M.: Adjusting for nonignorable drop-out using semiparametric nonresponse models. J. Am. Stat. Assoc. **94**(448), 1096–1120 (1999)
87. Schlesselman, J.J.: Assessing effects of confounding variables. Am. J. Epidemiol. **108**(1), 3–8 (1978)
88. Schwartz, S., Li, F., Reiter, J.P.: Sensitivity analysis for unmeasured confounding in principal stratification settings with binary variables. Stat. Med. **31**(10), 949–962 (2012)
89. Shaked, M., Shanthikumar, J.G.: Stochastic Orders. Springer, New York (2007)
90. Shepherd, B.E., Gilbert, P.B., Jemiai, Y., Rotnitzky, A.: Sensitivity analyses comparing outcomes only existing in a subset selected post-randomization, conditional on covariates, with application to HIV vaccine trials. Biometrics **62**(2), 332–342 (2006)
91. Small, D.S., Rosenbaum, P.R.: War and wages: The strength of instrumental variables and their sensitivity to unobserved biases. J. Am. Stat. Assoc. **103**(483), 924–933 (2008)
92. Smith, L.H., VanderWeele, T.J.: Simple sensitivity analysis for control selection bias. Epidemiology (Cambridge, Mass.) **31**(5), e44 (2020)
93. Stephenson, W.R.: A general class of one-sample nonparametric test statistics based on subsamples. J. Am. Stat. Assoc. **76**(376), 960–966 (1981)
94. VanderWeele, T.J., Ding, P.: Sensitivity analysis in observational research: introducing the E-value. Ann. Internal Med. **167**(4), 268–274 (2017)
95. Wacholder, S., Silverman, D.T., McLaughlin, J.K., Mandel, J.S.: Selection of controls in case-control studies: Ii. types of controls. Am. J. Epidemiol. **135**(9), 1029–1041 (1992)
96. Wang, L., Krieger, A.M.: Causal conclusions are most sensitive to unobserved binary covariates. Stat. Med. **25**(13), 2257–2271 (2006)
97. Warshaw, A.L., Castillo, C.F.d.: Pancreatic carcinoma. N. Engl. J. Med. **326**(7), 455–465 (1992)
98. Wolfe, D.A.: A characterization of population weighted-symmetry and related results. J. Am. Stat. Assoc. **69**(347), 819–822 (1974)
99. Yu, B., Gastwirth, J.L.: The use of the 'reverse cornfield inequality' to assess the sensitivity of a non-significant association to an omitted variable. Stat. Med. **22**(21), 3383–3401 (2003)
100. Yu, B., Gastwirth, J.L.: Sensitivity analysis for trend tests: application to the risk of radiation exposure. Biostatistics **6**(2), 201–209 (2005)
101. Zhao, Q.: On sensitivity value of pair-matched observational studies. J. Am. Stat. Assoc. **114**, 713–722 (2019)
102. Zhao, Q., Small, D.S., Bhattacharya, B.B.: Sensitivity analysis for inverse probability weighting estimators via the percentile bootstrap. J. Roy. Stat. Soc. Ser. B **81**(4), 735–761 (2019)

Chapter 9
Design Sensitivity and the Choice of Statistical Methods

Abstract Design sensitivity is a number, $\widetilde{\Gamma}$; it is the limiting sensitivity to unmeasured bias as the sample size increases. It contrasts two situations: (i) a favorable situation with a treatment effect and no unmeasured bias in treatment assignment and (ii) an unfavorable situation with no treatment effect and a bias in treatment assignment. Can these two situations be distinguished in a large observational study? Consider the upper bound on the P-value testing the null hypothesis of no treatment effect in the presence of a bias of at most Γ. That bound is tending to 0 as $I \to \infty$ if the sensitivity analysis is performed with $\Gamma < \widetilde{\Gamma}$, but it is tending to 1 with $\Gamma > \widetilde{\Gamma}$. In a given favorable situation, a wise choice of test statistic can increase $\widetilde{\Gamma}$. An unwise choice of test statistic may lead to a claim that an observational study is sensitive to small unmeasured biases when that claim is untrue.

9.1 What Is Design Sensitivity?

Protection From Bias in the Absence of a Treatment Effect

Chapter 2 discussed a randomized block experiment having I blocks, J individuals per block, with one treated individual and $J - 1$ controls in each block. In a randomized block experiment, each person j in block i has probability $1/J$ of being the one treated individual in block i, and treatments are assigned independently in distinct blocks. In slightly more formal notation, $\theta_{ij} = \Pr\left(Z_{ij} = 1 \mid \mathcal{F}, \mathcal{Z}\right) = 1/J = \overline{\theta}_{ij}$ for $i = 1, \ldots, I$, $j = 1, \ldots, J$. In Chap. 2, an α-level test of $H_0 : \boldsymbol{\delta} = \boldsymbol{\delta}_0$ was derived from randomized treatment assignment, without sampling or distributional assumptions; then, the test was extended to composite hypotheses, and inverted for estimates and confidence sets. The test of $H_0 : \boldsymbol{\delta} = \boldsymbol{\delta}_0$ was obtained by applying the test of the hypothesis of no effect, $H_0 : \boldsymbol{\delta} = \mathbf{0}$, to the adjusted responses, $R_{ij}^{\delta_0} = R_{ij} - Z_{ij}\,\delta_{0ij}$. For this reason, it suffices in this chapter to discuss $H_0 : \boldsymbol{\delta} = \mathbf{0}$.

© The Author(s), under exclusive license to Springer Nature Switzerland AG 2025
P. R. Rosenbaum, *An Introduction to the Theory of Observational Studies*,
Springer Texts in Statistics, https://doi.org/10.1007/978-3-031-90494-3_9

The central problem in observational studies is that there is no reason to believe that θ_{ij} equals $1/J$ in the absence of randomized treatment assignment. Recall from (8.7) that $\boldsymbol{\theta}$ is the $I \times J$ matrix of θ_{ij}, and $\overline{\boldsymbol{\theta}}$ is the $I \times J$ matrix of $\overline{\theta}_{ij} = 1/J$. The sensitivity analysis in Chap. 8 considered departures from randomized treatment assignment, $\boldsymbol{\theta} \neq \overline{\boldsymbol{\theta}}$, expressed in terms of sets B_Γ of $\boldsymbol{\theta}$'s for $\Gamma \geq 1$, as defined in Sect. 8.2 by either (8.6) or (8.8)–(8.10). If a randomization test at $\overline{\boldsymbol{\theta}}$ rejects $H_0 : \boldsymbol{\delta} = \mathbf{0}$ at level α, then the sensitivity analysis asks: What magnitude Γ of departure from randomized assignment, $\boldsymbol{\theta} \neq \overline{\boldsymbol{\theta}}$, would need to be present for $H_0 : \boldsymbol{\delta} = \mathbf{0}$ to be accepted at level α? The sensitivity analysis in Chap. 8 controls the probability of a certain kind of error. Rejection of the null hypothesis $H_0 : \boldsymbol{\delta} = \mathbf{0}$ at level α for all $\boldsymbol{\theta} \in B_\Gamma$ means: If H_0 is true, then there is at most a probability of α that H_0 will be rejected if the bias in treatment assignment is at most Γ. For example, in the alcohol and HDL cholesterol example in Table 8.1, there is no bias of magnitude $\Gamma \leq 6$ that leads to acceptance of H_0 at level $\alpha = 0.05$, providing the statistic U878 is used. A bias of $\Gamma = 6$ would have explained away the effect of smoking on lung cancer in Hammond's [18] study [41, Table 4.1], one of the sturdiest findings in epidemiology.

The Favorable Situation: A Treatment Effect in the Absence of Bias

Controlling the probability of rejecting H_0 when H_0 is true is, of course, important, but we need more than this. The probability of rejecting H_0 would be zero if we simply declined to reject H_0 no matter what data we observed, and that would not be satisfactory. Suppose that H_0 is false and there is no bias in treatment assignment, so $\boldsymbol{\theta} = \overline{\boldsymbol{\theta}}$; then, we are eager to reject H_0. After all, in this case, the observed responses, R_{ij}, and assigned treatments, Z_{ij}, are associated because the treatment does actually cause its ostensible effects. Call this the favorable situation—$H_0 : \boldsymbol{\delta} = \mathbf{0}$ is false and there is no unmeasured bias, $\boldsymbol{\theta} = \overline{\boldsymbol{\theta}}$. We are eager to reject H_0 in a favorable situation.[1]

In an observational study, if we were in a favorable situation, then we could not know it. If we were in a favorable situation, we would see that R_{ij} and Z_{ij} are associated, but that association might be due to either $\boldsymbol{\delta} \neq \mathbf{0}$ or $\boldsymbol{\theta} \neq \overline{\boldsymbol{\theta}}$ or both.

---

[1] If $\boldsymbol{\delta} \neq \mathbf{0}$ and $\boldsymbol{\theta} \neq \overline{\boldsymbol{\theta}}$, then we are ambivalent about rejecting H_0. If $\boldsymbol{\delta}$ is close to $\mathbf{0}$, but $\boldsymbol{\theta}$ is far from $\overline{\boldsymbol{\theta}}$, then we might be nearly certain to reject the false hypothesis $H_0 : \boldsymbol{\delta} = \mathbf{0}$, but only because of large biases in treatment assignment. In this case, a randomized experiment might have a negligible chance of rejecting $H_0 : \boldsymbol{\delta} = \mathbf{0}$. More bias in treatment assignment—a larger difference between $\boldsymbol{\theta}$ and $\overline{\boldsymbol{\theta}}$ –might increase the power to reject $H_0 : \boldsymbol{\delta} = \mathbf{0}$ when it is false, but we can be at most ambivalent about rejecting a false H_0 because of increased bias in treatment assignment. Favorable situations are used to evaluate the performance of competing statistical methods or research designs. For that purpose, we prefer situations in which we are not ambivalent about our goals. If there is bias and no treatment effect, then we do not want to reject $H_0 : \boldsymbol{\delta} = \mathbf{0}$, but if there is a treatment effect and no bias, then we do want to reject H_0, and in both situations we are not ambivalent. It is easy to compute the properties of test procedures when $\boldsymbol{\delta} \neq \mathbf{0}$ and $\boldsymbol{\theta} \neq \overline{\boldsymbol{\theta}}$, but we do not know what sense to make of those properties once we have computed them.

Given that we cannot recognize a favorable situation when we are in one, we want statistical procedures that will perform well given the data available. The best we could hope to say in a favorable situation is that rejection of H_0 is insensitive to small and moderately large biases, Γ. Achieving the best we can hope for in favorable situations is the goal of Chaps. 9–11. Table 8.1 suggests that the choice of test statistic may be important for this goal, and that is the topic of the current chapter.

To repeat, Chap. 8 was concerned with the stochastic behavior of a sensitivity analysis when $H_0 : \boldsymbol{\delta} = \mathbf{0}$ is true and $\boldsymbol{\theta} \in B_\Gamma$ for $\Gamma > 1$. In Chaps. 9–11, we are still interested in the stochastic behavior of the same procedures, but not under the premises used to derive those procedures; rather, we are interested in the behavior of those procedures in favorable situations with $\boldsymbol{\delta} \neq \mathbf{0}$ and $\boldsymbol{\theta} = \overline{\boldsymbol{\theta}}$. This is analogous to saying that Chap. 8 concerned the behavior of a test when the null hypothesis is true, and Chaps. 9–11 concern the behavior of the same test when the null hypothesis is false; however, this is only an analogy, because $\boldsymbol{\delta} = \mathbf{0}$ and $\boldsymbol{\theta} \in B_\Gamma$ in Chap. 8 is replaced by $\boldsymbol{\delta} \neq \mathbf{0}$ and $\boldsymbol{\theta} = \overline{\boldsymbol{\theta}}$ in Chaps. 9–11. Unlike hypothesis testing in randomized experiments—unlike the procedures in Chap. 2—the sensitivity analysis cannot simply say that there is overwhelming evidence against $H_0 : \boldsymbol{\delta} = \mathbf{0}$. The sensitivity analysis in Chap. 8 might say: there is overwhelming evidence against $H_0 : \boldsymbol{\delta} = \mathbf{0}$ unless $\boldsymbol{\theta} \notin B_\Gamma$ for some moderately large value of Γ. Will the sensitivity analysis say this when, unknown to us, the data actually come from a favorable situation with $\boldsymbol{\delta} \neq \mathbf{0}$ and $\boldsymbol{\theta} = \overline{\boldsymbol{\theta}}$?

The answer to this question will come in two forms. The first form is the design sensitivity. In a favorable situation, as the number of blocks increases, $I \longrightarrow \infty$, there is typically a value, $\widetilde{\Gamma}$, called the design sensitivity, such that the probability of rejecting $H_0 : \boldsymbol{\delta} = \mathbf{0}$ tends to 1 for all $\boldsymbol{\theta} \in B_\Gamma$ for all $\Gamma < \widetilde{\Gamma}$, whereas the probability of rejecting $H_0 : \boldsymbol{\delta} = \mathbf{0}$ tends to 0 for some $\boldsymbol{\theta} \in B_\Gamma$ for all $\Gamma > \widetilde{\Gamma}$. Expressing the same idea in different terms, as $I \longrightarrow \infty$, the P-value bounds in (8.19) and Table 8.1 tend to 0 for $\Gamma < \widetilde{\Gamma}$ and to 1 for $\Gamma > \widetilde{\Gamma}$. In Table 8.1, see, for instance, the P-value bound of 0.9994 for the stratified Wilcoxon statistic at $\Gamma = 6$. In brief, $\widetilde{\Gamma}$ is the limiting sensitivity to unmeasured biases as $I \longrightarrow \infty$. Two test statistics may have different design sensitivities in the same favorable situation, leading us to prefer certain test statistics over others. This first form of answer, design sensitivity, is discussed in Chaps. 9–10.

The second form is the Bahadur [2, 3] relative efficiency of two test statistics in the same favorable situation, and it is discussed in Chap. 11. Pick a Γ below the smaller of the two design sensitivities of the two test statistics. At this Γ, the P-value bounds in (8.19) for the two statistics are both tending to zero as $I \longrightarrow \infty$. We may ask: Which P-value is tending to zero more quickly as I increases? The answer to this question is Bahadur's measure of relative efficiency applied to P-value bounds from a sensitivity analyses. In Table 8.1, the P-value bound for Wilcoxon's statistic is small for $\Gamma = 3.5$, but the other statistics have smaller P-value bounds at $\Gamma = 3.5$. The Bahadur efficiency provides useful information when I is not extremely large. The Bahadur efficiency of a statistic tends to zero as Γ increases to the design sensitivity, $\widetilde{\Gamma}$, of this statistic.

Put in the simplest terms, it is easy to simulate data from a favorable situation with $\boldsymbol{\delta} \neq \mathbf{0}$ and $\boldsymbol{\theta} = \overline{\boldsymbol{\theta}}$ and then perform a sensitivity analysis from Chap. 8 on the simulated data. If we did that many times in many situations, we would begin to learn which statistical methods and research designs are best for distinguishing actual causal effects, $\boldsymbol{\delta} \neq \mathbf{0}$ with no bias $\boldsymbol{\theta} = \overline{\boldsymbol{\theta}}$, from biased treatment assignment with no causal effect, $\boldsymbol{\delta} = \mathbf{0}$ with $\boldsymbol{\theta} \neq \overline{\boldsymbol{\theta}}$. The goal in Chaps. 9–11 is to develop some large sample criteria that will present a simpler and clearer picture than we are likely to obtain by an enormous variety of simulations. A few simulations will check or illustrate asymptotic results.

An Illustration of Design Sensitivity in Matched Pairs

In matched pairs, $J = 2$, let $Y_i = (Z_{i1} - Z_{i2})(R_{i1} - R_{i2})$ be the treated-minus-control pair difference in outcomes in pair i, so $Y_i = r_{Ti1} - r_{Ci2}$ if $Z_{i1} = 1 = 1 - Z_{i2}$, and $Y_i = r_{Ti2} - r_{Ci1}$ if $Z_{i2} = 1 = 1 - Z_{i1}$. In Chap. 8, under the hypothesis of no effect, $H_0 : \boldsymbol{\delta} = \mathbf{0}$, the pair difference is $Y_i = (2Z_{i1} - 1)(r_{Ci1} - r_{Ci2}) = \pm |r_{Ci1} - r_{Ci2}|$, but the calculation of the design sensitivity assumes this null hypothesis is false. Instead, $\mathcal{F}$ is assumed to have been sampled from a favorable situation with a treatment effect, where given $\mathcal{F}$ and $\mathbf{Z} \in \mathcal{Z}$, treatment assignment is randomized within pairs, so $\theta_{ij} = \Pr\left(Z_{ij} = 1 \,\middle|\, \mathcal{F}, \mathcal{Z}\right) = 1/2 = \overline{\theta}_{ij}$. The question is: How will the sensitivity analysis in Chap. 8 behave in this favorable situation?

To consider the simplest case, suppose the Y_i are independently sampled from a normal distribution with expectation τ and variance 1, $Y_i \sim N(\tau, 1)$; so, the expectation of a pair difference divided by its standard deviation is τ.[2] Suppose that H_0 is tested using Wilcoxon's signed rank statistic, which is the same as Quade's statistic in matched pairs, $J = 2$. Based on a calculation discussed in Sect. 9.3, the design sensitivity in this case is $\widetilde{\Gamma} = 3.17$. So, in this case, if a sensitivity analysis is performed with $\Gamma < \widetilde{\Gamma} = 3.17$, then the upper bound (8.19) on the P-value tends to zero as $I \to \infty$, but if $\Gamma > \widetilde{\Gamma} = 3.17$, then the bound on the P-value tends to 1. In words, for sufficiently large I, the null hypothesis H_0 of no effect will be rejected in this favorable situation for $\Gamma < 3.17$ and not rejected for $\Gamma > 3.17$. To illustrate this property, let us take a sample of size $I = 10^6$ pair differences and perform the sensitivity analysis with $\Gamma = 3.1 < 3.17 = \widetilde{\Gamma}$ and with $\Gamma = 3.2 > 3.17 = \widetilde{\Gamma}$.[3] The upper bound on the P-value is 1.11×10^{-16} at $\Gamma = 3.1$ and is 0.9998 at $\Gamma = 3.2$.

---

[2] Equivalently, assume $r_{Ti1} - r_{Ci2} \sim N(\tau, 1)$ and $r_{Ti2} - r_{Ci1} \sim N(\tau, 1)$, and a coin is flipped to set $Y_i = r_{Ti1} - r_{Ci2}$ with probability $1/2$ or $Y_i = r_{Ti2} - r_{Ci1}$ with probability $1/2$. Here, $r_{Ti1} - r_{Ci2}$ and $r_{Ti2} - r_{Ci1}$ refer to the same two people in pair i, so $r_{Ti1} - r_{Ci2}$ and $r_{Ti2} - r_{Ci1}$ may be dependent; however, such a dependence does not affect the distribution of the observable quantity Y_i.

[3] For $I = 10^6$, it speeds computation to use the explicit optimizing $\boldsymbol{\theta}$ in (8.20), as implemented in the `senWilcox` and `senU` functions in the R package `DOS2` associated with [54]. You can reproduce these calculations as follows:

```
set.seed(1)
y<-rnorm(1000000)+.5
DOS2::senWilcox(y,gamma=3.1)
DOS2::senWilcox(y,gamma=3.2).
```

Viewed as a function of Γ, as $I \to \infty$, the P-value bound is converging to a step function, with a single step up from 0 to 1 at $\widetilde{\Gamma} = 3.17$. In small sample sizes, the sensitivity value $\Gamma^{\bullet}$ in Sect. 8.6 is a random variable: it makes a wobbly approach, mostly upwards, to $\widetilde{\Gamma}$ as I increases.

If Y_i is not normally distributed, then $\widetilde{\Gamma}$ changes somewhat. To compare distributions that have different variances, consider the case in which the expectation $\mathrm{E}(Y_i)$ of Y_i is τ times its standard deviation $\sqrt{\mathrm{var}(Y_i)}$, as above. Specifically, $Y_i = \tau\sqrt{\mathrm{var}(\varepsilon_i)} + \varepsilon_i$ where ε_i's are I independent observations from either the logistic distribution or a t-distribution with 4 degrees of freedom. For the standard normal, logistic, and t-distributions, $\sqrt{\mathrm{var}(\varepsilon_i)}$ is 1 for the normal, $\sqrt{\pi^2/3} \doteq 1.814$ for the logistic distribution, and $\sqrt{\upsilon/(\upsilon-2)}$ for a t-distribution with $\upsilon \geq 3$ degrees of freedom, or $\sqrt{4/(4-2)} \doteq 1.414$ for $\upsilon = 4$. These distributions have longer tails than the normal distribution. At $\tau = 1/2$, as above, $\widetilde{\Gamma} = 3.40$ for the logistic distribution and $\widetilde{\Gamma} = 3.91$ for the t-distribution with 4 degrees of freedom [52, Table 2].

In the cases above, the design sensitivity $\widetilde{\Gamma}$ is an increasing function of τ. As $\tau \to 0$, the design sensitivity $\widetilde{\Gamma} \to 1$; that is, effects of negligible size, $\tau \doteq 0$, are sensitive to biases of negligible size $\Gamma \doteq 1$.

In a given favorable situation, changing the test statistic can have a substantial effect on the design sensitivity. As above, let $\tau = 1/2 = \mathrm{E}(Y_i)/\sqrt{\mathrm{var}(Y_i)}$, and consider the four statistics in Table 8.1. In Table 8.1, with matched pairs, $J = 2$, the blocked Wilcoxon statistic is the sign-test statistic and Quade's statistic is Wilcoxon's signed rank statistic as discussed above. In the paired normal case, the four statistics in Table 8.1 have design sensitivities of $\widetilde{\Gamma} = 2.24$ for the sign-test, $\widetilde{\Gamma} = 3.17$ for Wilcoxon's signed rank statistic, $\widetilde{\Gamma} = 4.20$ for U868, and $\widetilde{\Gamma} = 5.08$ for U878. Using U878 with the same normal sample as above, the upper bound (8.19) on the P-value is 0 to machine precision at $\Gamma = 3.2$, is 0.000848 at $\Gamma = 5$, and is 0.907 at $\Gamma = 5.1$.[4] In that sense, Wilcoxon's signed rank statistic exaggerates sensitivity to unmeasured biases for normally distributed Y_i.

Both U868 and U878 give less emphasis to pairs with small $|Y_i|$ and limited but more emphasis to pairs with large $|Y_i|$. This strategy worked for the normal distribution with its short tails. Does the same strategy work with the longer tailed logistic distribution and the t-distribution with 4 degrees of freedom? With $\tau = 1/2 = \mathrm{E}(Y_i)/\sqrt{\mathrm{var}(Y_i)}$, as above, U868 and U878 have, respectively, design sensitivities $\widetilde{\Gamma} = 4.24$ and $\widetilde{\Gamma} = 4.68$ for the logistic distribution and $\widetilde{\Gamma} = 4.73$ and $\widetilde{\Gamma} = 4.89$ for the t-distribution with 4 degrees of freedom [52, Table 2]. So, U878 continues to have a larger—hence better—design sensitivity $\widetilde{\Gamma}$ than Wilcoxon's signed rank statistic with these two longer tailed distributions, but its margin of victory is smaller.

[4] Continuing the previous footnote with the same y, the computations are:
```
DOS2::senU(y,gamma=3.2,m=8,m1=7,m2=8)
DOS2::senU(y,gamma=5,m=8,m1=7,m2=8)
DOS2::senU(y,gamma=5.2,m=8,m1=7,m2=8)
```

*Effect Sizes in Distributions With Different Shapes

A long tradition [10] in psychology and some other social sciences defines an effect size as the expected effect divided by the standard deviation. This tradition is informal motivation for the above comparison that fixes $\tau = \mathrm{E}(Y_i)/\sqrt{\mathrm{var}(Y_i)}$ when comparing data from a normal distribution, a logistic distribution, and a t-distribution. Fixing this standardized measure, τ, is fairly reasonable for the mean, $\overline{R}_t - \overline{R}_c = I^{-1}\sum_{i=1}^{I} Y_i$, as an estimator or test statistic in Sect. 2.6, but of course, in randomized experiments, the mean is less efficient than the signed rank statistic for data from the logistic distribution and the t-distribution with 4 degrees of freedom.

In this book, effect sizes with different error distributions are "equated" by equating $\tau = \mathrm{E}(Y_i)/\sqrt{\mathrm{var}(Y_i)}$, that is, by equating the expected effect on a single treated-minus-control matched pair difference, Y_i, measured in units of the standard deviation of that pair difference. This measure, τ, is familiar. It is useful in situations that are not extreme. Moreover, the standardized measure, τ, avoids silly comparisons, such as the comparison of standard—or "pretty"—forms of the normal and logistic distributions, which have variances 1 and $\pi^2/3 = 3.29$, respectively. At least with τ, we compare normal and logistic distributions with the same variance.

Additionally, focusing on a single treated-minus-control matched-pair difference, Y_i, is helpful when comparing block designs with blocks of different sizes. A block design with I blocks of size J supplies $J - 1$ correlated treated-minus-control pair differences, $(Z_{ij} - Z_{ij'})(R_{ij} - R_{ij'})$ with $(Z_{ij} - Z_{ij'}) \neq 0$, each of which has the distribution of a single matched pair difference, Y_i. An investigator with blocks of size J could instead have blocks of size $J - 1$ by randomly discarding one control in each block, or blocks of size $J-2$ by random discarding two controls, . . . , or matched pairs by randomly discarding $J - 2$ controls, and in all of these cases the behavior of a single treated-minus-control pair difference, Y_i, would not change. True, for $J > 2$ the pair differences in a block are correlated because they share the same treated individual, and we will need to take account of that. But if the effect size in a block design is defined in terms of a single matched-pair difference, Y_i, then we can hold the effect size constant as we ask: (i) How valuable is it to increase J? (ii) For fixed IJ, how does an increase in block size, J, compare with an increase in the number of blocks, I? Is it better to have $I = 1500$ matched pairs with $IJ = 1500 \times 2 = 3000$ people, or $I = 1000$ blocks of size $J = 3$, also with $IJ = 1000 \times 3 = 3000$ people?

Nonetheless, comparing shifts in a normal and a t-distribution using $Y_i = \tau\sqrt{\mathrm{var}(\varepsilon_i)} + \varepsilon_i$ has some limitations that are discussed in this brief subsection. For the t-distribution with 1 or 2 degrees of freedom, $\mathrm{var}(Y_i)$ does not exist, so one cannot hold $\tau = \mathrm{E}(Y_i)/\sqrt{\mathrm{var}(Y_i)}$ constant. The t-distribution with 1 degree of freedom is the Cauchy distribution.

For the signed rank statistic (and many other robust statistics), it is easy to compute the design sensitivity, whether or not $\mathrm{var}(Y_i)$ exists [54, §15.3.2]. That is, if we use a robust test statistic, then design sensitivity is not a fragile concept, like an expectation or a variance. If the pair differences, Y_i, are independent observations from a continuous distribution, then for the signed rank statistic the design sensitivity is

$$\widetilde{\Gamma} = \frac{\Pr\left(Y_i + Y_j > 0\right)}{1 - \Pr\left(Y_i + Y_j > 0\right)} \text{ for } i \neq j. \tag{9.1}$$

In particular, for the standard normal and standard Cauchy cumulative distributions, $\Phi(\cdot)$ and $\Upsilon(\cdot)$, respectively, the design sensitivities are

$$\widetilde{\Gamma} = \frac{\Phi\left(\sqrt{2}\tau\right)}{1 - \Phi\left(\sqrt{2}\tau\right)} \text{ if } Y_i - \tau \sim \Phi(\cdot), \tag{9.2}$$

and

$$\widetilde{\Gamma} = \frac{\Upsilon(\tau)}{1 - \Upsilon(\tau)} \text{ if } Y_i - \tau \sim \Upsilon(\cdot), \text{ respectively.} \tag{9.3}$$

Of course, $\left(Y_i + Y_j\right) > 0$ if and only if $\left(Y_i + Y_j\right)/2 > 0$. In the normal case, $\left(Y_i + Y_j\right)/2 \sim N\left(\tau, \frac{1}{2}\right)$ yielding (9.2). The average of two independent Cauchy random variables is itself a Cauchy random variable [63], so $\left\{(Y_i - \tau) + \left(Y_j - \tau\right)\right\}/2 \sim \Upsilon(\cdot)$, yielding (9.3). For a shift of $\tau = 1/2$ in (9.2) for the normal distribution, $\widetilde{\Gamma} = 3.17$ as above, whereas in (9.3) for the Cauchy distribution the design sensitivity is $\widetilde{\Gamma} = 1.84$. Alas, it is not clear how to compare these values because the scale of the Cauchy distribution is not comparable to that of the normal distribution.

For $p > 1/2$, McNeill and Tukey [35] compare the scale and shape of a continuous distribution $F(\cdot)$ symmetric about zero to that of the standard normal distribution using

$$s_p = \frac{F^{-1}(p) - F^{-1}(1-p)}{\Phi^{-1}(p) - \Phi^{-1}(1-p)},$$

which is the ratio of their interquartile ranges for $p = 0.75$ and the ratio of the central 90% intervals for $p = 0.95$. Note that $s_p = 1$ for all $0 < p < 1$ if $F(\cdot)$ is the standard normal distribution, $\Phi(\cdot)$, and $s_p = \sigma$ for all $0 < p < 1$ if $F(\cdot)$ is $N(0, \sigma^2)$.

A sturdy substitute for $Y_i = \tau\sqrt{\text{var}(\varepsilon_i)} + \varepsilon_i$ when $\varepsilon_i \sim F(\cdot)$ is $Y_i = \tau s_p + \varepsilon_i$. This does work, of course, but s_p can vary dramatically with p, thereby limiting its utility in the current context. Consider the design sensitivity of Wilcoxon's signed rank statistic, which is $\widetilde{\Gamma} = 3.17$ for $Y_i = \tau + \varepsilon_i$ when $\tau = 1/2$ and $\varepsilon_i \sim N(0, 1)$. With $\tau = 1/2$ and $F(\cdot) = \Upsilon(\cdot)$ in the Cauchy case, $s_{0.75} = 1.483$ for $p = 0.75$ yielding $\tau s_p = 0.741$ and a design sensitivity of $\widetilde{\Gamma} = 2.37$, while $s_{0.95} = 3.838$ for $p = 0.95$, yielding $\tau s_p = 1.919$ and a design sensitivity of $\widetilde{\Gamma} = 5.54$. It is easy to compute design sensitivities for Cauchy distributions, and these are correct statements about Cauchy distributions. These correct statements about Cauchy distributions do not stand in a simple relation to correct statements about the normal distribution.

Fortunately, our main interest in this chapter is the comparison of different statistics in the same favorable situation, not in the comparison of different favorable situations. In the previous subsection, compared to other statistics in Table 8.1, it was important that U878 had higher—hence better—design sensitivity than competing statistics for the normal distribution, the logistic distribution, and the t-distribution with four degrees of freedom. The differences among these three distributions were interesting but less central when picking a test statistic with large $\widetilde{\Gamma}$ for all three distributions.

9.2 Some Simple Calculations of Design Sensitivity

The Simplest Nontrivial Case: The Sign Test

As is commonly true in statistics, the calculation of a theoretical quantity, such as $\widetilde{\Gamma}$, is simple in some circumstances, still simple in other circumstances if you know a trick or two (e.g., (9.1)), more difficult but still feasible in other circumstances, and at times dependent on intense computation in challenging circumstances. It is useful to acquire some experience in each of these circumstances. In Sect. 9.2, we become acquainted with design sensitivity by considering very simple cases.

By far the simplest case is the sign test for matched pairs, $J = 2$. Admittedly, calculating $\widetilde{\Gamma}$ for the sign test for $Y_i \sim N(\tau, 1)$ merely adds one more reason to an already long list of very good reasons for avoiding the sign test.

With $J = 2$ for matched pairs, the one treated-minus-control pair difference in block i is $Y_i = \left(Z_{ij} - Z_{ij'}\right)\left(R_{ij} - R_{ij'}\right)$, and under $H_0 : \boldsymbol{\delta} = \mathbf{0}$ this becomes $Y_i = (Z_{i1} - Z_{i2})(r_{Ci1} - r_{Ci2})$, or $Y_i = (2Z_{i1} - 1)(r_{Ci1} - r_{Ci2}) = \pm |r_{Ci1} - r_{Ci2}|$ using $Z_{i1} + Z_{i2} = 1$. Write $\text{sgn}(a) = 1$ if $a > 0$ and $\text{sgn}(a) = 0$ if $a \leq 0$. Then, the sign test statistic is the number of positive pair differences, $T = \sum_{i=1}^{I} \text{sign}(Y_i)$. Because we will evaluate $\widetilde{\Gamma}$ for continuous favorable situations, I will ignore the possibility of ties, $Y_i = 0$, because this occurs with probability zero. In practice, a small adjustment allows for some $Y_i = 0$, but that adjustment is not needed when discussing continuous distributions. As always, the completely general hypothesis $H_0 : \boldsymbol{\delta} = \boldsymbol{\delta}_0$ could be tested by calculating $R_{ij}^{\delta_0} = R_{ij} - Z_{ij}\,\delta_{0ij}$, which equals r_{Cij} if $H_0 : \boldsymbol{\delta} = \boldsymbol{\delta}_0$ is true, and then applying the sign test to $R_{ij}^{\delta_0}$.

We need to determine two distributions for T: (i) the conditional distribution of T given $(\mathcal{F}, \mathcal{Z})$ in Chap. 8 under H_0 with no treatment effect and with a bias in treatment assignment of at most Γ and (ii) the distribution of T in a favorable situation with a treatment effect and no bias in treatment assignment, $\Pr(\mathbf{Z} = \mathbf{z} \mid \mathcal{F}, \mathcal{Z}) = |\mathcal{Z}|^{-1} = J^{-I} = 2^{-I}$. We are hoping to use T to distinguish these situations for small or moderate Γ, so we need to know the distributions we are trying to distinguish. The next paragraph addresses (i), and the paragraph after that addresses (ii).

Writing $q_{i1} = \text{sgn}(r_{Ci1} - r_{Ci2})$ and $q_{i2} = \text{sgn}(r_{Ci2} - r_{Ci1})$, so $q_{i1} = 1 - q_{i2}$, the sign test $H_0 : \boldsymbol{\delta} = \mathbf{0}$ becomes $T = \sum_{i=1}^{I} \text{sgn}(Y_i) = \sum_{i=1}^{I} \sum_{j=1}^{2} Z_{ij}\, q_{ij}$. In Proposition 8.1, q_{ij} is fixed by conditioning on $(\mathcal{F}, \mathcal{Z})$. Using (8.20) and (8.21) to evaluate (8.19), we see that under H_0 with $\boldsymbol{\theta} \in B_\Gamma$ the distribution of T is bounded by two binomial distributions:

$$\sum_{k=a}^{I} \binom{I}{k} \left(\frac{1}{1+\Gamma}\right)^{k} \left(\frac{\Gamma}{1+\Gamma}\right)^{I-k} \leq \Pr(T \geq a \mid \mathcal{F}, \mathcal{Z}) \leq \sum_{k=a}^{I} \binom{I}{k} \left(\frac{\Gamma}{1+\Gamma}\right)^{k} \left(\frac{1}{1+\Gamma}\right)^{I-k}, \tag{9.4}$$

with the consequence that T/I is likely to be inside or near the closed interval:

$$\left[\frac{1}{1+\Gamma}, \frac{\Gamma}{1+\Gamma}\right] \tag{9.5}$$

in the sense that

$$\Pr\left(\frac{T}{I} \notin \left[\frac{1}{1+\Gamma} - \varepsilon, \frac{\Gamma}{1+\Gamma} + \varepsilon\right]\right) \rightarrow 0 \quad \text{for } \varepsilon > 0 \text{ as } I \rightarrow \infty. \tag{9.6}$$

In a favorable situation in which $\tau > 0$ and the $Y_i - \tau$ are independently drawn from the standard normal cumulative distribution, $\Phi(\cdot)$, the sign statistic $T = \sum_{i=1}^{I} \text{sgn}(Y_i)$ has a binomial distribution with probability of success $\Pr(Y_i > 0) = \Pr(Y_i - \tau > -\tau) = 1 - \Phi(-\tau) = \Phi(\tau) > 1/2$; moreover, T/I converges in probability to $\Phi(\tau)$ as $I \rightarrow \infty$.

For sufficiently large I, we can eventually reject H_0 for all $\boldsymbol{\theta} \in B_\Gamma$ providing $\Phi(\tau)$ is not in the interval (9.5), that is, providing $\Phi(\tau) > \Gamma/(1+\Gamma)$. Solving the equation $\Phi(\tau) = \Gamma/(1+\Gamma)$, we conclude that the design sensitivity is $\widetilde{\Gamma} = \Phi(\tau)/\{1 - \Phi(\tau)\}$. For $\tau = 1/2$, the design sensitivity is $\widetilde{\Gamma} = 2.24$, much lower (i.e., worse) than the design sensitivity for Wilcoxon's signed rank statistic, $\widetilde{\Gamma} = 3.17$.

In parallel, in a favorable situation in which $\tau > 0$ and the $Y_i - \tau$ are independently sampled from a continuous cumulative distribution $F(\cdot)$ that is symmetric about zero, the sign statistic $T = \sum_{i=1}^{I} \text{sgn}(Y_i)$ is binomial with probability of success $F(\tau)$. The design sensitivity is $\widetilde{\Gamma} = F(\tau)/\{1 - F(\tau)\}$. An interesting case is the Cauchy distribution, $\Upsilon(\cdot)$, or equivalently the t-distribution with 1 degree of freedom, where $\widetilde{\Gamma} = \Upsilon(\tau)/\{1 - \Upsilon(\tau)\} = 1.84$ for $\tau = 1/2$. If you read the starred subsection of Sect. 9.1, then you remember the Cauchy formula $\widetilde{\Gamma} = \Upsilon(\tau)/\{1 - \Upsilon(\tau)\}$ as (9.3), where it was the design sensitivity for Wilcoxon's signed rank test, rather than for the sign test. Wilcoxon's signed rank test and the sign test are equally effective if $Y_i - \tau$ are sampled from $\Upsilon(\cdot)$; more precisely, they have the same design sensitivity.[5]

In Sect. 9.1, design sensitivities were compared for several distributions with the same value of $\tau = \text{E}(Y_i)/\sqrt{\text{var}(Y_i)}$ by taking $Y_i = \tau\sqrt{\text{var}(\varepsilon_i)} + \varepsilon_i$ when $\varepsilon_i \sim F(\cdot)$, where $F(\cdot)$ is continuous and symmetric about zero. This cannot be done for the Cauchy distribution, because the distribution has neither an expectation nor a variance, but it can be done for various other distributions. The design sensitivity

[5] This occurs because the Wilcoxon signed rank statistic differs only slightly from a U-statistic that determines the proportion of positive Walsh averages [32, Appendix Example 6], that is, positive $(Y_i + Y_j)/2$ for $i < j$. The average of two Cauchy random variables has the same distribution as a single Cauchy random variable, so $\Pr\{(Y_i + Y_j)/2 > 0\} = \Pr(Y_i > 0)$.

of the sign test is then $\widetilde{\Gamma} = F\left(\tau\sqrt{\mathrm{var}(\varepsilon)}\right) / \left\{1 - F\left(\tau\sqrt{\mathrm{var}(\varepsilon)}\right)\right\}$. For the logistic distribution with $\sqrt{\mathrm{var}(\varepsilon)} = \sqrt{\pi^2/3}$ and $\tau = 1/2$, the design sensitivity of the sign test is $\widetilde{\Gamma} = 2.48$, again much worse than for Wilcoxon's signed rank statistic with $\widetilde{\Gamma} = 3.40$.

In short, viewed from the perspective of design sensitivity, the sign test is not a wise choice in the situations considered.

A Small Change to the Sign Test Increases $\widetilde{\Gamma}$

When the sample size is large, a small adjustment to the sign test produces a statistic with substantially higher (i.e., better) design sensitivity. The statistic is due to Noether [37] and was developed further by Markowski and Hettmansperger [34]. Noether's statistic appeared in Problems 2.2 and 8.3. Design sensitivity will be calculated in testing $H_0 : \boldsymbol{\delta} = \mathbf{0}$ when the Y_i's are independent observations from a continuous, strictly increasing cumulative distribution, $G(\cdot)$; however, see Problem 2.2 for ties, other null hypotheses, and additional detail. Rank the $|Y_i|$ from 1 to I. Pick a number $0 \leq f < 1$, and let $\mathcal{N} \subset \{1, 2, \ldots, I\}$ be the indices i of the pairs with ranks of fI or more. Write $|\mathcal{N}|$ for the number of elements of $\mathcal{N}$, so $|\mathcal{N}|$ is approximately $I/3$ for $f = 2/3$.[6] Under H_0, the absolute pair difference is $|Y_i| = |r_{Ci1} - r_{Ci2}|$, and this is fixed by conditioning on $(\mathcal{F}, \mathcal{Z})$; so, $\mathcal{N}$ is also fixed under H_0. For $i \in \mathcal{N}$, define q_{ij} as in the sign test, $q_{i1} = \mathrm{sgn}(r_{Ci1} - r_{Ci2})$ and $q_{i2} = \mathrm{sgn}(r_{Ci2} - r_{Ci1})$, with $\mathrm{sgn}(a) = 1$ if $a > 0$ and $\mathrm{sgn}(a) = 0$ if $a \leq 0$. For $i \notin \mathcal{N}$, define $q_{ij} = 0$ for $j = 1, 2$. Noether's statistic is

$$T = \sum_{i=1}^{I} \sum_{j=1}^{2} Z_{ij}\, q_{ij} = \sum_{i \in \mathcal{N}} \sum_{j=1}^{2} Z_{ij}\, q_{ij};$$

so, it is the sum of $|\mathcal{N}|$ binary variables in both the sensitivity analysis and the favorable situation.

The sensitivity analysis here is similar to the sensitivity analysis for the sign test, but with a reduced sample size, $|\mathcal{N}|$. As in the sign test, (8.20) and (8.21) are used to evaluate (8.19). In parallel with the sign test, under H_0 with $\boldsymbol{\theta} \in B_\Gamma$, the sensitivity bounds for Noether's statistic are binomial but with sample size $|\mathcal{N}|$,

$$\sum_{k=a}^{|\mathcal{N}|} \binom{|\mathcal{N}|}{k} \left(\frac{1}{1+\Gamma}\right)^{k} \left(\frac{\Gamma}{1+\Gamma}\right)^{|\mathcal{N}|-k} \leq \Pr(T \geq a \mid \mathcal{F}, \mathcal{Z})$$

$$\leq \sum_{k=a}^{|\mathcal{N}|} \binom{|\mathcal{N}|}{k} \left(\frac{\Gamma}{1+\Gamma}\right)^{k} \left(\frac{1}{1+\Gamma}\right)^{|\mathcal{N}|-k}, \tag{9.7}$$

[6] Noether suggested $f = 1/3$ with a view to efficiency in randomized experiments. Larger values of f, such as $f = 2/3$, are better for design sensitivity for many but not all distributions $G(\cdot)$.

so as $I \to \infty$, $T/|\mathcal{N}|$ tends to be inside or near the interval (9.5), and T/I tends to be near or between $(1-f)/(1+\Gamma)$ and $\Gamma(1-f)/(1+\Gamma)$.

Now, consider the behavior of T in the favorable situation, with $Y_i \sim G(\cdot)$ and $\theta_{ij} = 1/2$. That is, we need to know something about the limiting behavior as $I \to \infty$ of T/I when Y_i's are independent observations from $G(\cdot)$ and there is no bias in treatment assignment, $\boldsymbol{\theta} = \overline{\boldsymbol{\theta}}$. For $y \geq 0$, define $L(y) = G(y) - G(-y) = \Pr(|Y| \leq y)$, and define ξ as the solution to $L(\xi) = f$, or equivalently $\xi = L^{-1}(f)$. In words, $L(\cdot)$ is the continuous distribution of $|Y|$ and ξ is its fth quantile. Let $\vartheta = 1 - G(\xi)$; then, trivially, $\vartheta = \Pr(Y \geq \xi) = \Pr(Y \geq \xi \text{ and } |Y| \geq \xi)$.

Here is an equivalent way to compute Noether's statistic. Let $\lceil a \rceil$ denote the smallest integer greater than or equal to a. Sort the $|Y_i|$ into increasing order, and write $\widehat{\xi}$ for the $\lceil fI \rceil$th-order statistic of the $|Y_i|$; so $\widehat{\xi}$ is a consistent estimate of ξ. Noether's statistic is the number of positive Y_i among those Y_i that have $|Y_i| \geq \widehat{\xi}$. Consequently, as $I \to \infty$ in the favorable situation, the statistic T/I converges to ϑ.

If we reject H_0 for large values of Noether's statistic, T, then for large enough I we will reject H_0 for all $\boldsymbol{\theta} \in B_\Gamma$ if $\vartheta > \Gamma(1-f)/(1+\Gamma)$. Solving for Γ in the equation $\vartheta = \Gamma(1-f)/(1+\Gamma)$ yields the design sensitivity [48, Proposition 1]:

$$\widetilde{\Gamma} = \frac{\vartheta}{(1-f) - \vartheta}, \tag{9.8}$$

which agrees with the sign test for $f = 0$.

If Y_i is normally distributed with expectation 1/2 and variance 1, then $\widetilde{\Gamma} = 3.17$ for Wilcoxon's signed rank test, $\widetilde{\Gamma} = 2.24$ for the sign test with $f = 0$, and $\widetilde{\Gamma} = 4.97$ for Noether's test with $f = 2/3$. Noether's test with $f = 2/3$ is much better than both the sign test and Wilcoxon's signed rank test in terms of design sensitivity. If Y_i is normally distributed with expectation 1/3 and variance 1, then the design sensitivities are all smaller, but they order the three statistics in the same way: $\widetilde{\Gamma} = 2.14$ for Wilcoxon's signed rank test, $\widetilde{\Gamma} = 1.71$ for the sign test with $f = 0$, and $\widetilde{\Gamma} = 2.80$ for Noether's test with $f = 2/3$. In these normal favorable situations, Noether's statistic with $f = 2/3$ has ignored 2/3 of the Y_i with small $|Y_i|$, but nonetheless has larger design sensitivity. This is less surprising than it might sound, because $\widetilde{\Gamma}$ refers to a limit as $I \to \infty$.

How does Noether's statistic perform in the alcohol and HDL cholesterol data in Sect. 1.4, where $I = 406$ rather than ∞? To extract pairs, $J = 2$, from this block design with $J = 4$, compare $I = 406$ daily drinkers (D) to $I = 406$ never drinkers (N) in terms of HDL cholesterol. In a one-sided test of no effect, the sign test has an upper bound on the P-value of 0.054 at $\Gamma = 2.1$, Wilcoxon's test has a bound P-value of 0.045 at $\Gamma = 2.75$, and Noether's statistic with $f = 2/3$ has a bound P-value of 0.045 at $\Gamma = 3.1$. So, the pattern of design sensitivities for normal data occurs also in the data in Sect. 1.4. Indeed, Noether's statistic with $f = 0.9$ has a bound P-value of 0.046 at $\Gamma = 4.4$. How does this happen? Among the $I - \lceil fI \rceil = 406 - \lceil 0.9 \times 406 \rceil = 40 = |\mathcal{N}|$ pair differences Y_i with the largest $|Y_i|$, 37 have $Y_i > 0$ and 3 have $Y_i < 0$, where $37/40 = 0.925$, and a binomial with probability $\Gamma/(1+\Gamma) = 4.4/(1+4.4) = 0.815$ is not likely to produce such a one-sided division of signs.

Table 9.1 Design sensitivities of Noether's statistic for t-distributions with 3, 4, or 5 degrees of freedom and the normal distribution. In all cases, the expectation of a matched pair difference, Y_i, is half the standard deviation of Y_i. In each row, the highest design sensitivity is in **bold**

	f				
Distribution	0	1/3	2/3	0.90	0.99
t_3	3.44	5.21	**5.77**	4.34	2.25
t_4	2.86	4.15	**5.10**	4.60	2.81
t_5	2.66	3.80	4.94	**4.98**	3.45
Normal	2.24	3.12	4.97	9.34	**23.10**

Table 9.1 shows the design sensitivity $\widetilde{\Gamma}$ of five versions of Noether's statistic in four favorable situations. The sign test, $f = 0$, has low design sensitivity in all four favorable situations, and $f = 2/3$ is much better than the sign test in all four situations. The normal distribution favors larger values of f, even $f = 0.99$, but we should be skeptical about this. For the longer-tailed t-distributions, $\widetilde{\Gamma}$ is smaller at $f = 0.99$ than at $f = 2/3$. More importantly, in the cholesterol data in Sect. 1.4 where $I = 406$, taking $f = 0.99$ means considering only 4 of 406 pairs, and little can be concluded based on 4 pairs even if the Y_i are normal. The efficiency calculations in Chap. 11 will consider $\widetilde{\Gamma}$ and I jointly.

In terms of design sensitivity, Noether's statistic with $f = 2/3$ is a big improvement over both the sign test and Wilcoxon's signed rank test. It is essentially a weighted rank statistic, $T = t(\mathbf{Z}, \mathbf{R}) = \sum_{i=1}^{I} \sum_{j=1}^{J} Z_{ij}\, q_{ij}$ with $q_{ij} = \phi\left(q_{ij}^{*}\right) \varphi\{b_i/(I+1)\}$, for $J = 2$ in which the φ-function is a step function with a single step up from 0 to 1 at f. Notably, for $J = 2$, the $\varphi(\cdot)$ functions in Fig. 8.1 for U868 and U878 are smooth functions that also give little weight to Y_i with small $|Y_i|$.

The Blocked Wilcoxon Rank Sum Statistic

The sign test is essentially the same as the blocked Wilcoxon rank sum statistic in matched pairs, or equivalently in blocks of size $J = 2$. What happens when $J > 2$?

Consider the favorable situation in which

$$\theta = \overline{\theta} \quad \text{and} \quad R_{ij} = \beta_i + Z_{ij}\,\tau + \varepsilon_{ij}, \text{, with } \varepsilon_{ij} \sim F(\cdot), \tag{9.9}$$

$i = 1, \ldots, I$, $j = 1, \ldots, J$, where the ε_{ij} are independent and $F(\cdot)$ is a continuous distribution.[7] Under (9.9), if $Z_{ij} = 1$ and $Z_{ij'} = 0$, then $Y_{ijj'} = R_{ij} - R_{ij'} = \tau + \varepsilon_{ij} - \varepsilon_{ij'}$ is a treated-minus-control matched-pair difference, and it is symmetrically distributed about τ. There are $J - 1$ such differences in block i, each with the same marginal distribution, but they are dependent because they compare the same

[7] In thinking about (9.9), recall the discussion in Chap. 2 of our inability to distinguish (2.25) and (2.26) using observable data.

Table 9.2 Design sensitivities, $\widetilde{\Gamma}$, for the blocked Wilcoxon rank sum statistic, for normal errors with effect τ in units of the standard deviation of a single treated-minus-control matched pair difference

J	2	3	4	5	6
$\tau = 1/2$	2.24	2.86	3.48	3.61	3.75
$\tau = 1/3$	1.71	2.06	2.29	2.34	2.45

treated individual, ij, to $J-1$ independent controls ij' with $j' \neq j$. Let $\varsigma = \Pr\left(Y_{ijj'} > 0 \middle| Z_{ij} + Z_{ij'} = 1\right)$, where $Y_{ijj'}$ is a treated-minus-control pair difference from (9.9).

The rank of the one treated response in block i is one plus the number of controls with lower responses; it has expectation $1 + (J-1)\varsigma$, which becomes $(J+1)/2$ when $\tau = 0$ and $\varsigma = 1/2$. The expectation of the blocked Wilcoxon rank sum statistic, T, in this favorable situation is $I\{1 + (J-1)\varsigma\}$.

In Chap. 8, under $H_0 : \boldsymbol{\delta} = \mathbf{0}$ with $\boldsymbol{\theta} \in B_\Gamma$, the maximum expectation of T given $(\mathcal{F}, \mathcal{Z})$ is $I\overline{\mu}_\Gamma$ where μ_Γ is given by $\overline{\mu}_i$ in (8.26) of Definition 8.1. Here, $\overline{\mu}_i$ is the same for all blocks i, because the ranks, $1, 2, \ldots, J$ are the same for all i. The design sensitivity $\widetilde{\Gamma}$ is the solution Γ to the equation[8] [43, §4]:

$$\{1 + (J-1)\varsigma\} = \overline{\mu}_\Gamma. \tag{9.10}$$

The dependence among the $J-1$ treated-minus-control pair differences, $Y_{ijj'}$, in block i does not affect (9.10), because both sides are simply expectations.

For comparison with the paired case, $J = 2$, consider situations in which each treated-minus-control pair difference is $Y_{ijj'} = \tau\sqrt{\mathrm{var}\left(\epsilon_{ijj'}\right)} + \epsilon_{ijj'}$ where $\epsilon_{ijj'} = \varepsilon_{ij} - \varepsilon_{ij'}$, so that $\tau = \mathrm{E}\left(Y_{ijj'}\right)/\sqrt{\mathrm{var}\left(Y_{ijj'}\right)}$ and τ is the effect in units of the standard deviation of a single matched pair difference. Formulated in this way, (9.10) yields the previously calculated design sensitivity for the sign test when $J = 2$.

For normal errors, Table 9.2 shows design sensitivities for blocks of size $J = 2, 3, \ldots, 6$. Notably, $\widetilde{\Gamma}$ increases with the block size, J. Even in a randomized experiment, the Pitman relative efficiency of Wilcoxon's blocked rank sum statistic improves with increasing block size [36]; so, the full implications of Table 9.2 are not immediately obvious [50]. The pattern in Table 9.2 will be discussed again in Chap. 10.

[8] This equation is derived from (8.26) where $\overline{\sigma}_i = \overline{\sigma}_\Gamma$ and $\overline{\mu}_i = \mu_\Gamma$ are both constant, the same for all i. In the favorable situation, T/I converges in probability to $\{1 + (J-1)\varsigma\}$. In expression (8.26) with $a = T$, $\sum \overline{\mu}_i = I\mu_\Gamma$, and $\sqrt{\sum \overline{\sigma}_i^2} = \overline{\sigma}_\Gamma\sqrt{I}$, the P-value in (8.26) tends to 0 if $\{1 + (J-1)\varsigma\} > \mu_\Gamma$ or to 1 if $\{1 + (J-1)\varsigma\} < \mu_\Gamma$.

9.3 Design Sensitivities for Some Practical Methods

Attaining High Design Sensitivity Within Families of Test Statistics

In Sect. 9.2, the concept of design sensitivity was introduced using simple existing methods requiring only simple calculations to determine $\widetilde{\Gamma}$; however, aside from Noether's statistic with moderately large f, such as $f = 2/3$, the methods in Sect. 9.2 did not achieve high design sensitivity. In the current section, methods are built to have high design sensitivity. The methods discussed here use rank tests, but similar design sensitivities can be achieved with analogous tests derived from Peter Huber's m-estimates [50, 51].

Noether's statistic is the exception in Sect. 9.2 in part because it is not a single statistic, but rather a family of statistics as f varies. Where Noether [37] achieved good Pitman efficiency in a randomized experiment at $f = 1/3$, impressive design sensitivity was found in Sect. 9.2 at $f = 2/3$, albeit with worse Pitman efficiency in a randomized experiment. This conclusion suggests a general strategy: consider a broad family of statistics that is anchored by a few familiar statistics, and compare the design sensitivity (and, in Chap. 11, the efficiency) of members of that family. In Noether's family, the familiar statistic was the sign test, but the sign test exhibits poor efficiency even in randomized experiments. For matched pairs, $J = 2$, the problem with Noether's family is not with its best members, some of which are quite good, but rather its uncompetitive anchor, namely, the sign test.

Another interesting family for matched pairs is discussed in the problems at the end of the chapter. Unlike Noether's statistic, this family takes not one but two steps, from 0 to 1 and then from 1 to 2. For instance, Bruce Brown [9] suggested steps at $f_1 = 1/3$ and $f_2 = 2/3$, and his procedure is competitive with Wilcoxon's signed rank test in randomized experiments, but has higher design sensitivity in observational studies [48, Prop. 1 and Table 2]. Edward Markowski and Thomas Hettmansperger [34] consider a range of values of (f_1, f_2), some of which yield high design sensitivity. One can also take more than two steps, or steps of unequal sizes, not 1 and 2 [16, 17]. With two steps, the null randomization distribution and sensitivity bounds are provided by a weighted sum of two independent binomial random variables (see Problem 8.5); so, computation of the design sensitivity resembles the computation in Sect. 9.2 for Noether's statistic [48, Proposition 1].

In contrast, the family of test statistics considered here is anchored by both the sign test and the Wilcoxon signed rank test for matched pairs, $J = 2$, and for blocks with $J > 2$ it is anchored by both the blocked Wilcoxon rank sum test and Quade's test [47, 57]. The four tests in Table 8.1 and Fig. 8.1 are members of this family. The family also includes the statistics proposed by Robert Stephenson [67]. Stephenson's tests are close to the optimal randomization test when only a subset of treated individuals respond to treatment [11, 44, 54, Ch. 17]. The family of test statistics considered here has several advantages: (i) two of its familiar anchors, Wilcoxon's signed rank test and Quade's test, exhibit competitive performance in randomized experiments; (ii) it includes analogous tests for $J = 2$ and for $J > 2$;

(iii) it permits adaptive inference, as described in Sect. 9.5; and (iv) as discussed in Chap. 11, its large sample efficiency in sensitivity analyses is known [52, 57].

A Family of Weighted Rank Statistics

The statistics in the current section are weighted rank statistics from Sect. 2.6 that are essentially the same as $T = t(\mathbf{Z}, \mathbf{R}) = \sum_{i=1}^{I} \sum_{j=1}^{J} Z_{ij} q_{ij}$ with $q_{ij} = \phi\left(q_{ij}^*\right) \varphi\{b_i/(I+1)\}$, where $\phi(\cdot)$ and $\varphi(\cdot)$ are two functions, and b_i is the rank of within-block range w_i in (2.11).[9]

The between-block weight function $\varphi(\cdot)$ has domain $[0, 1]$ and has a shape determined by three integers, $1 \le \underline{m} \le \overline{m} \le m$. In Fig. 8.1, U868 denotes $(m, \underline{m}, \overline{m}) = (8, 6, 8)$ and U878 denotes $(m, \underline{m}, \overline{m}) = (8, 7, 8)$. In Fig. 8.1, $\varphi(p) = 1$ for the sign test for $J = 2$ or for the blocked Wilcoxon rank sum test for $J \ge 2$; it will turn out to be $(m, \underline{m}, \overline{m}) = (1, 1, 1)$. Also, $\varphi(p) = p$ for Wilcoxon's signed rank test for $J = 2$ or for Quade's test for $J \ge 2$; it will turn out to be $(m, \underline{m}, \overline{m}) = (2, 2, 2)$.

The function $\varphi(\cdot)$ is

$$\varphi(p) = \sum_{\ell=\underline{m}}^{\overline{m}} \binom{m}{\ell} p^{\ell-1} (1-p)^{m-\ell}. \tag{9.11}$$

Clearly, $\varphi(p)$ is constant for $(m, \underline{m}, \overline{m}) = (1, 1, 1)$ and $\varphi(p)$ is proportional to p for $(m, \underline{m}, \overline{m}) = (2, 2, 2)$.

The family (9.11) is useful because it contains several familiar anchors plus many functions $\varphi(\cdot)$ with varied properties. In all cases, $\varphi(\cdot)$ is a polynomial of order $m-1$ and is nonnegative and bounded on its domain $[0, 1]$. The function $\varphi(\cdot)$ is monotone increasing in Fig. 8.1, but for $(m, \underline{m}, \overline{m}) = (8, 6, 7)$ the weight function $\varphi(\cdot)$ is redescending—it is near zero on $\left[0, \frac{1}{5}\right]$, increases gradually until about $\frac{4}{5}$, and then declines gradually back to zero [47, Figure 2]. For pairs, $J = 2$, weights $(m, \underline{m}, \overline{m}) = (8, 6, 7)$ have higher design sensitivity, $\widetilde{\Gamma}$, than the increasing φ-functions (8, 6, 8) and (8, 7, 8) for long-tailed errors, such as the t-distribution with 2 degrees of freedom [47, Table 3]. The φ-function (8, 5, 8) has the same high Pitman efficiency for normal errors as Wilcoxon's signed rank statistic, but (8, 5, 8) has higher design sensitivity [47, Tables 1 and 3]. Stephenson's [67] test differs negligibly from $(m, \underline{m}, \overline{m}) = (m, m, m)$, and for $m \ge 3$ the φ-function is proportional

[9] For discussion of test statistics that are "essentially the same," see Problem 2.7. In Sect. 9.3, for blocks of size $J > 2$, the within-block rank scores are $\phi\left(q_{ij}^*\right) = q_{ij}^*$, or $1, \ldots, J$, but for matched pairs, $J = 2$, they are $\phi\left(q_{ij}^*\right) = q_{ij}^* - 1$ or 0, 1. This change for $J = 2$ is tradition, nothing more—sign and signed rank tests for pairs traditionally use 0 or 1, but statistics with block sizes $J > 2$ traditionally rank $1, \ldots, J$—however, adhering to tradition does not affect the properties of the test statistic.

to p^{m-1}, so it is increasing and convex on its domain $[0, 1]$, unlike $(8, 6, 8)$ and $(8, 7, 8)$, which resemble a lazy S.

Because $\varphi(\cdot)$ in (9.11) is a polynomial in p with compact domain $[0, 1]$, $\varphi(\cdot)$ achieves its minimum, say $\underline{\kappa}$, and its maximum, say $\overline{\kappa}$; so, $\varphi(\cdot)$ maps $[0, 1]$ onto $\left[\underline{\kappa}, \overline{\kappa}\right]$. For $m = 1$, there is equality: $1 = \underline{\kappa} = \overline{\kappa}$; otherwise, $\underline{\kappa} = 0$ and $\overline{\kappa} > 0$. The case $m = 1$ is needed but exceptional; so, from now on, I will write κ for the maximum, $\overline{\kappa}$, and I will not again mention $\underline{\kappa}$, as it is zero in all cases except $m = 1$. For ease of visual comparisons in graphs, $\varphi(\cdot)/\kappa$ is plotted, not $\varphi(\cdot)$. For instance, $\varphi(\cdot)/\kappa$ is plotted in Fig. 8.1.

*Origin of the Function $\varphi(\cdot)$ in (9.11)

This entirely optional and slightly technical subsection addresses a curiosity that you may or may not have: Where does the strange function (9.11) come from? Is it just a way of generating lines and S-shaped curves like those in Fig. 8.1? Or does (9.11) have a deeper meaning? Is there any reason to prefer (9.11) to other S-shaped curves? Can (9.11) generate curves very different from those in Fig. 8.1? If so, what do they look like and are they useful? Here are two types of answers, one for a person who wants to skip this section, the other for a person who is inclined to read it.

For the person who would like to skip this section, let me say that any φ-function that looked much the same as the functions in Fig. 8.1 would have much the same properties. You can take Fig. 8.1 as the primary description of U868 and U878, skip this section, and encounter no difficulties later on in this book.

For the person who is inclined to read this section, let me say that the φ-function in (9.11) has a number of useful properties that I will not use in this book. Moreover, the form (9.11) is connected to a long sequence of useful technical results in statistics dating back to 1948, results that are still useful today, results that I believe have been underused in causal inference. In 1948, Wassily Hoeffding [22] showed (i) that the subject of "nonparametric inference" had been misnamed, because there are "nonparametric parameters" that exist for (essentially) every probability distribution, (ii) that there is a "best" unbiased estimator of each of his nonparametric parameters, and (iii) the estimator is, under very mild conditions, asymptotically normal.

The lines and S-shapes in Fig. 8.1 are only some of the shapes that (9.11) can produce; see Fig. 9.1. The φ-function $(m, \underline{m}, \overline{m}) = (8, 8, 8)$ is one of Stephenson's [67] statistics, and it is particularly effective if the treatment has no effect on most treated people but strongly affects an unknown subpopulation [11, 44]; in this situation, U888 has a high design sensitivity [54, Ch. 17]. The redescending curve U877 has a large design sensitivity $\widetilde{\Gamma}$ when the errors are from a t-distribution with 2, 3, or 4 degrees of freedom [47, Table 3]. Adding together two φ-functions with the same m produces a compromise between their shapes, as in U878+U877: it redescends slightly, but does not return to zero.

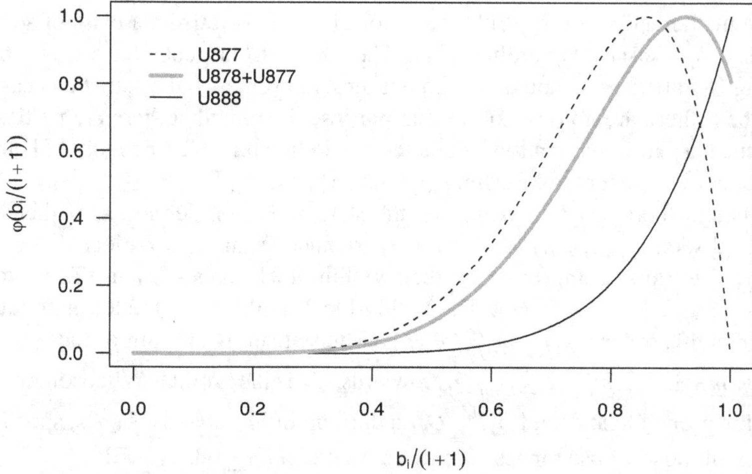

Fig. 9.1 Other shapes, besides lines and S-shapes, that can be produced by the φ-function in (9.11), $(m, \underline{m}, \overline{m})$. To aid visual comparisons, each curve has been scaled to have a maximum of 1

I said that I thought Hoeffding's [22] ideas—namely, his U-statistics—and their later development by other authors, are underused in causal inference. By this, I mean two things. First, the current literature on causal inference tries to use expected causal effects as "nonparametric parameters," but this is pointlessly limiting and not quite correct. It is not quite correct because, in general, expectations are not "nonparametric parameters," but instead are quite fragile as parameters [4]. Expected causal effects cannot describe certain kinds of important causal effects that can exist in principle and do exist in practice. A focus on expected causal effects is pointlessly limiting in leading us away from other nonparametric causal parameters that are useful. For example, a tiny expected treatment effect can be insensitive to large biases Γ if the effect is zero for most people, but is large for a small unknown subset of people [54, Ch. 17]. Think of two boxplots, treated and control, describing a large sample, with similar quartiles or boxes, similar means, but the treated boxplot has an unambiguously longer upper tail. As another example, certain standard U-statistics are interpretable as causal parameters in the presence of interference between units ([42, §6] and [45]). More generally, a causal effect may be defined in terms of the effect on its kernel [40, §4]. Second, U-statistics often have asymptotically normal distributions under nonlocal alternatives—that is, when the treatment effect is not trivially small—and only nonlocal alternatives can be insensitive to nontrivial biases $\Gamma > 1$.

The mathematical form (9.11) has its origin in a U-statistic, a class of statistics proposed by Wassily Hoeffding [22]. The form (9.11) generalizes a number of existing U-statistics. Although ties do not present problems, the statistic is easier to describe if there are no ties; so, for that purpose, assume that there are no ties. For an elementary introduction to U-statistics, see Lehmann [32, Appendix §5], and for more about U-statistics see Serfling [62, Ch. 5] or Lee [28].

Although there are $I > m$ blocks, the statistic is first defined as if there were only m blocks, $i = 1, \ldots, m$; then, it is extended from m to I blocks. Sort these m blocks into increasing order by their within-block ranges, w_i in (2.11), so that after sorting, $w_1 < \cdots < w_m$. The within-block rank of the treated individual in block ℓ in this order is $Q_\ell = \sum_{j=1}^{J} Z_{\ell j} q_{\ell j}^*$. The statistic is the sum of these Q_ℓ's for $\ell \in \{\underline{m}, \underline{m}+1, \ldots, \overline{m}\}$, or $\sum_{\ell=\underline{m}}^{\overline{m}} Q_\ell$. In words, Q_ℓ is the familiar Wilcoxon rank sum statistic for one block ℓ, and $\sum_{\ell=\underline{m}}^{\overline{m}} Q_\ell$ is the sum of $\overline{m} - \underline{m} + 1$ of Q_ℓ's, specifically the sum of those whose ranges w_i have ranks $\ell \in \{\underline{m}, \underline{m} + 1, \ldots, \overline{m}\}$.

For example, with m blocks, U878 or $(m, \underline{m}, \overline{m}) = (8, 7, 8)$ is $Q_7 + Q_8$, that is, the sum of the two within-block ranks for the $2 = 8 - 7 + 1$ blocks with the largest ranges w_i. Similarly, U868 is $Q_6 + Q_7 + Q_8$. The blocked Wilcoxon rank sum statistic, $(m, \underline{m}, \overline{m}) = (1, 1, 1)$, looks at $m = 1$ block and equals Q_1. For $J = 2$ and $m = 2$, the U-statistic associated with Wilcoxon's signed rank statistic [32, Example A21] is $(m, \underline{m}, \overline{m}) = (2, 2, 2)$ or Q_2, and for $J > 2$ it yields a U-statistic closely approximating Quade's [38] ranks. Stephenson's [67] statistic, $(m, \underline{m}, \overline{m}) = (m, m, m)$ is Q_m.

The statistic defined for m blocks is called the kernel of the U-statistic. With $I > m$ blocks, there are $\binom{I}{m}$ ways to pick m blocks, or $\binom{406}{8}$ ways to pick $m = 8$ blocks of the $I = 406$ blocks in the example in Sect. 1.4. The U-statistic is the average of the kernel computed from all $\binom{I}{m}$ sets of m blocks.

To compute the U-statistic with I blocks, rank the I block ranges, w_i, from 1 to I, and let a_i be the rank of w_i. In how many of the $\binom{I}{m}$ sets of m blocks is w_i the ℓth largest range? We can pick $\ell - 1$ ranges smaller than w_i in $\binom{a_i-1}{\ell-1}$ ways, and we can pick $m - \ell$ ranges larger than w_i in $\binom{I-a_i}{m-\ell}$ ways; so, there are

$$\binom{a_i - 1}{\ell - 1} \times \binom{I - a_i}{m - \ell}$$

sets of m blocks in which w_i is the ℓth largest. It follows that the U-statistic sums over ℓ and averages over i:

$$U = \binom{I}{m}^{-1} \sum_{i=1}^{I} Q_i \sum_{\ell=\underline{m}}^{\overline{m}} \binom{a_i - 1}{\ell - 1} \times \binom{I - a_i}{m - \ell}.$$

If we multiply by I, then the between-block rank for block i in U is

$$\varphi^{\dagger}(a_i) = I \times \binom{I}{m}^{-1} \sum_{\ell=\underline{m}}^{\overline{m}} \binom{a_i - 1}{\ell - 1} \times \binom{I - a_i}{m - \ell},$$

so $U = I^{-1}\sum_{i=1}^{I} Q_i\,\varphi^{\dagger}(a_i)$. What is the relationship between $\varphi^{\dagger}(a_i)$ and $\varphi(p)$ in (9.11)? As $I \to \infty$ the ratio $\varphi(p_i)/\varphi^{\dagger}(a_i)$ for $p_i = a_i/I$ tends to one [47, Lemma 1]. So, for practical purposes, the U-statistic, $U = I^{-1}\sum_{i=1}^{I} Q_i\,\varphi^{\dagger}(a_i)$, and the weighted rank statistic $T = \sum_{i=1}^{I} Q_i\,\varphi(p_i)$ are almost the same. Note that $T = \sum_{i=1}^{I} Q_i\,\varphi(p_i)$ does not involve large combinatorial coefficients, so T can be computed for large I.

Calculating Design Sensitivity for the Statistic $(m, \underline{m}, \overline{m})$

As is typical, computing the design sensitivity of a one-sided test starts by computing the limits of two expectations of the test statistic. The test rejects H_0 when T is large. The first limit μ^* is computed under a favorable model with an effect and no bias, $\boldsymbol{\theta} = \overline{\boldsymbol{\theta}}$, such as the model (9.9). The second limit is the limiting maximum expectation $\mu_{\Gamma}^{\triangledown}$ of T computed under a sensitivity model with biased treatment assignment $\boldsymbol{\theta} \in B_{\Gamma}$ but with no treatment effect. Because $B_{\Gamma} \subset B_{\Gamma'}$ for $\Gamma < \Gamma'$, $\mu_{\Gamma}^{\triangledown}$ becomes larger as Γ increases. The design sensitivity $\widetilde{\Gamma}$ solves the equation $\mu^* = \mu_{\Gamma}^{\triangledown}$ for Γ. Equation (9.10) was a simple example.

The statistic must be scaled so it has a limit as $I \to \infty$, but for a weighted rank statistic $T = \sum_{i=1}^{I} \varphi\{b_i/(I+1)\}\sum_{j=1}^{J} Z_{ij}\,\phi\left(q_{ij}^*\right)$ this simply means replacing T by T/I. For a continuous distribution of errors, as in (9.9), there are no ties, and this slightly simplifies the work at several stages. In particular, every block i has q_{ij}^*'s that are some rearrangement of $1, 2, \ldots, J$, and the b_i are always some rearrangement of $1, 2, \ldots, I$.

Proposition 9.1 *Assume that the R_{ij} are untied. If $H_0 : \boldsymbol{\delta} = \mathbf{0}$ is true and $\boldsymbol{\theta} \in B_{\Gamma}$, then $T/I = \frac{1}{I}\sum_{i=1}^{I} \varphi\{b_i/(I+1)\}\sum_{j=1}^{J} Z_{ij}\,\phi\left(q_{ij}^*\right)$ has maximum expectation:*

$$\max_{\boldsymbol{\theta}\in B_{\Gamma}} \mathrm{E}\left(T/I \mid \mathcal{F}, \mathcal{Z}\right) = \frac{\overline{\mu}_{\Gamma}}{I}\sum_{i=1}^{I} \varphi\{i/(I+1)\} \tag{9.12}$$

where $\overline{\mu}_{\Gamma}$ is the maximum expectation of $\sum_{j=1}^{J} Z_{ij}\,\phi(j)$ over $(\theta_{i1}, \ldots, \theta_{iJ})$ that satisfy $1 = \sum_{j=1}^{J} \theta_{ij}$ and $\Gamma^{-1} \le \theta_{ij}/\theta_{ij'} \le \Gamma$ for each $j \ne j'$.

Proof As $H_0 : \boldsymbol{\delta} = \mathbf{0}$ is true, the range w_i in (2.11) is a function of $\mathbf{R} = \mathbf{r}_C$, which is fixed by conditioning on $(\mathcal{F}, \mathcal{Z})$ in (9.12), so b_i and $\varphi\{b_i/(I+1)\}$ are also fixed. Because $\varphi\{b_i/(I+1)\}$ is fixed, the contribution to T from block i satisfies

$$\mathrm{E}\left(\varphi\{b_i/(I+1)\}\sum_{j=1}^{J} Z_{ij}\,\phi\left(q_{ij}^*\right)\,\middle|\, \mathcal{F}, \mathcal{Z}\right)$$

$$= \varphi\{b_i/(I+1)\}\,\mathrm{E}\left(\sum_{j=1}^{J} Z_{ij}\,\phi\left(q_{ij}^*\right)\,\middle|\, \mathcal{F}, \mathcal{Z}\right),$$

so to maximize (9.12), it suffices to maximize $\mathrm{E}\left(\sum_{j=1}^{J} Z_{ij}\,\phi\left(q_{ij}^{*}\right)\middle|\,\mathcal{F},\,\mathcal{Z}\right)$ one block at a time subject to $1=\sum_{j=1}^{J}\theta_{ij}$ and $\Gamma^{-1}\leq\theta_{ij}/\theta_{ij'}\leq\Gamma$ for each $j\neq j'$. □

Now, $\varphi:[0,\,1]\rightarrow[0,\,\kappa]$ is the polynomial (9.11), and consequently in (9.12),

$$\mu_{\Gamma}^{\nabla}=\lim_{I\rightarrow\infty}\frac{\overline{\mu}_{\Gamma}}{I}\sum_{i=1}^{I}\varphi\left\{i/(I+1)\right\}=\overline{\mu}_{\Gamma}\int_{0}^{1}\varphi\left(p\right)\,dp. \tag{9.13}$$

Although μ_{Γ}^{∇} must be computed for many Γ to solve $\mu^{*}=\mu_{\Gamma}^{\nabla}$ for Γ, the integral in (9.13) is computed only once.

In some instances, there is a formula for the expectation, μ^{*}, in the favorable situation, as discussed in the starred subsection of Sect. 9.1. In all cases, μ^{*} can be determined with any desired precision by Monte Carlo integration, that is, by simulating one large sample of size I from the favorable situation and computing T/I. For example, one might compute T/I from one sample of size I from the model (9.9).

Numerical Values of the Design Sensitivity

Table 9.3 reports design sensitivities [57, Table 1] for the four statistics or φ-functions that were used in Table 8.1 and depicted in Fig. 8.1. In Table 9.3, there are $J-1$ controls in each block, for $J=2,\,3,\,4,\,5$; so, $J=2$ refers to matched pairs and may be compared with Noether's statistic in Table 9.1. The errors in the favorable situation (9.9) are either normally distributed or t-distributed with 5 degrees of freedom. In all cases, a treated-minus-control pair difference in any block i has $\mathrm{E}\left(Y_{ijj'}\right)/\sqrt{\mathrm{var}\left(Y_{ijj'}\right)}=1/2$; so, for $J=2,\,3,\,4,\,5$, the first row of Table 9.2 equals the first four entries in the first row of Table 9.3.

Table 9.3 Design sensitivities for four weighted rank statistics in blocks of size $J=2,\,3,\,4,\,5$. In all cases, a treated-minus-control matched pair difference has expectation equal to half its standard deviation

	Normal errors				t_5 errors			
$\varphi(\cdot)$	J=2	J=3	J=4	J=5	J=2	J=3	J=4	J=5
Wilcoxon	2.2	2.9	3.5	3.6	2.5	3.2	4.0	4.3
Quade	3.2	3.8	4.4	4.8	3.4	4.0	4.7	5.2
U868	4.2	4.6	5.2	5.8	4.4	4.5	5.1	5.7
U878	5.1	5.1	5.7	6.4	4.8	4.7	5.2	5.8

Notably, for both the normal and t_5 distributions, the largest design sensitivity is for U878 and $J=5$ with $J-1=5-1=4$ controls. The statistic U878 still has the largest design sensitivity for pairs, $J=2$, but is only slightly better than Noether's statistic with $f=2/3$ in Table 9.1. The calculated pattern in Table 9.3

anticipates the pattern in data in Table 8.1; however, the true situation in Table 8.1 is a matter of speculation. In parallel with Table 9.2, if $\mathrm{E}\left(Y_{ijj'}\right)/\sqrt{\mathrm{var}\left(Y_{ijj'}\right)} = 1/3$ rather than $1/2$, then $\widetilde{\Gamma}$ is smaller but the qualitative pattern is fairly similar [57, Table 2]. Design sensitivities for other φ-functions are available for matched pairs [47, 52].[10]

In brief, both J and $\varphi(\cdot)$ strongly affect the limiting sensitivity $\widetilde{\Gamma}$ to unmeasured bias in a given sampling situation, and the investigator has complete control of $\varphi(\cdot)$ and may be able to increase J during research design.

Limitations of Design Sensitivity

Design sensitivity is a useful concept with some limitations. Several limitations follow.

- Design sensitivity $\widetilde{\Gamma}$ is a limit as the sample size increases, $I \to \infty$. For sufficiently large I, it will correctly order statistics in terms of sensitivity to unmeasured bias. For small I, however, conclusions are likely to be sensitive to a Γ well below $\widetilde{\Gamma}$ due to sampling uncertainty. That is, for finite I the sample sensitivity value $\Gamma^{\bullet}$ in Sect. 8.6 is typically below $\widetilde{\Gamma}$. The relative efficiency of two statistics at $\Gamma < \widetilde{\Gamma}$ need not prefer the statistic with the larger design sensitivity if I is small. For the normal distribution with $J = 4$ in Table 9.3, U868 has design sensitivity 5.2, below the design sensitivity of 5.7 for U878, but if the sensitivity analysis is performed with $\Gamma = 2$, then the Bahadur relative efficiency of U878 to U868 is 0.93, as discussed in Chap. 11. In the normal situation just considered, U868 is likely to outperform U878 at $\Gamma = 2$, but U878 will definitely outperform U868 at $\Gamma = 5.5$.[11] It is useful to know $\widetilde{\Gamma}$, but it is also useful to know Bahadur relative efficiency at $\Gamma < \widetilde{\Gamma}$, as developed in Chap. 11.
- Design sensitivity is concerned with distinguishing a nontrivial treatment effect, say τ, from a nontrivial bias, Γ. In contrast, Pitman efficiency lets $\tau \to 0$ as $I \to \infty$; however, every trivially small treatment effect, $\tau \doteq 0$, is sensitive to trivially small biases, $\Gamma \doteq 1$. If the only problem in observational studies was an inability to distinguish infinitesimal treatment effects from infinitesimal biases in treatment assignment, then there would be no problems of practical importance. In actual fact, it is often difficult to distinguish nontrivial effects from nontrivial biases. These considerations have two consequences. First, most of the results and intuition we have built up from calculating Pitman efficiency in randomized experiments is of little help in observational studies. Second, in observational studies, the numerical magnitude of the effect—whether measured

[10] Design sensitivities are also available for various block sizes, J, for the permutation distribution [33] of Huber's M-statistics [50, 51].

[11] Partly for this reason, U868 is the default in the `wgtRank` function in the `weightedRank` package in R.

by τ or something else—matters for the relative performance of two tests even as $I \rightarrow \infty$.

- We should be cautious about extrapolating patterns seen in numerical tables of design sensitivities. For instance, for each $\varphi(\cdot)$ and both error distributions in Table 9.3, the design sensitivity increases with the block size J.[12] However, this is not true in general. If $\mathrm{E}\left(Y_{ijj'}\right) / \sqrt{\mathrm{var}\left(Y_{ijj'}\right)} = 1/3$ rather than $1/2$, then the design sensitivity with $J - 1 = 5 - 1 = 4$ controls is slightly below or equal to the design sensitivity with $J - 1 = 4 - 1 = 3$ controls [57, Tables 1 and 2].
- Some design sensitivities in Table 9.3 are vastly better than others. The most popular statistic in Table 9.3, Wilcoxon's widely used blocked rank sum statistic, has consistently low $\widetilde{\Gamma}$. However, there is, as yet, no optimality theory for design sensitivity, and the values in Table 9.3 are not optimal even for the situations considered. In practice, we do not know either the effect size or the error distribution; so, from a practical point of view, the relative optimality achieved by adaptive inference in Sect. 9.5 is likely to be of more importance than optimality for a single known sampling distribution. You can see this in Table 9.1 where an unreasonable choice of $f = 0.99$ yields an amazing design sensitivity for normal errors; however, $f = 0.99$ is quite poor for errors from the t-distribution with 3, 4 or 5 degrees of freedom, where the reasonable choice of $f = 2/3$ is much better. Also, $f = 0.99$ discards 99% of the matched pairs; so, a goal of optimizing $\widetilde{\Gamma}$ for normal errors is not a reasonable goal.

9.4 What Aspects of a Statistic Lead to High Design Sensitivity?

Why does U878 have higher design sensitivity than the other $\varphi(\cdot)$ in Fig. 8.1? Why does Noether's statistic with $f = 2/3$ have high design sensitivity in Table 9.1 even for long tailed distributions? Why in Table 9.1 does Noether's statistic have $\widetilde{\Gamma} = 4.97$ with $f = 2/3$ and $\widetilde{\Gamma} = 23.10$ with $f = 0.99$ for the normal distribution, but $\widetilde{\Gamma} = 5.77$ with $f = 2/3$ and $\widetilde{\Gamma} = 2.24$ with $f = 0.99$ for the t-distribution with 3 degrees of freedom? Can we make some sense of these patterns?

Consider the case of $J = 2$, that is, treated-minus-control matched pair differences, Y_i. In Fig. 9.2, the Y_i have a normal distribution with expectation $1/2$ and variance 1, that is, $Y_i \sim N\left(\frac{1}{2}, 1\right)$.

The behavior of a signed rank statistic depends upon a function introduced by Albers, Bickel, and van Zwet [1], namely,

$$\mathrm{abz}(y) = \Pr(Y > 0 \mid |Y| = y) \text{ for } y \geq 0. \tag{9.14}$$

Consider this probability twice, once with a bias and no treatment effect—$\boldsymbol{\delta} = \mathbf{0}$ and $\boldsymbol{\theta} \in B_{\Gamma}$—and a second time with a treatment effect and no bias, $\boldsymbol{\theta} = \overline{\boldsymbol{\theta}}$.

---

[12] Actually, even in Table 9.3, there is one exception: for t_5 errors, using U878, the design sensitivity declines from 4.8 to 4.7 moving from $J = 2$ to $J = 3$ and then rises for larger J.

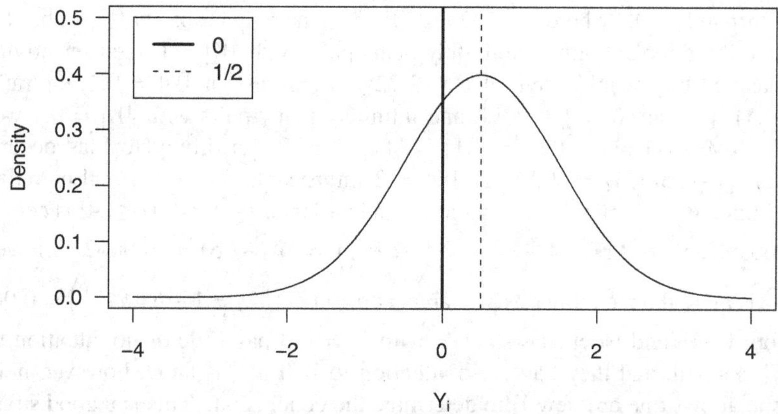

Fig. 9.2 For matched pairs, $J = 2$, a normal distribution of treated-minus-control matched pair differences, Y_i, with expectation 1/2 and variance 1 is shown. The dashed vertical line is at $E(Y_i) = 1/2$

If $\boldsymbol{\delta} = \mathbf{0}$, then $r_{Tij} = r_{Cij}$; so, a treated-minus-control pair difference, Y_i, compares two r_{Cij}, but perhaps the larger r_{Cij} is more likely to be selected for treatment. Under $H_0 : \boldsymbol{\delta} = \mathbf{0}$ and $\boldsymbol{\theta} \in B_\Gamma$ in the sensitivity model in Chap. 8, the treated-minus-control pair difference is $Y_i = (Z_{i1} - Z_{i2})(r_{Ci1} - r_{Ci2})$ can be asymmetrically distributed about zero only because of selection bias, that is, only because $\boldsymbol{\theta} \neq \overline{\boldsymbol{\theta}}$, and more specifically only because $\theta_{i1} \neq \theta_{i2}$. Under $H_0 : \boldsymbol{\delta} = \mathbf{0}$ and $\boldsymbol{\theta} \in B_\Gamma$, the pair difference $Y_i = (Z_{i1} - Z_{i2})(r_{Ci1} - r_{Ci2})$ is positive with probability at most $\Gamma/(1+\Gamma)$, because

$$\frac{1}{1+\Gamma} \leq \theta_{ij} = \Pr\left(Z_{ij} = 1 \,\middle|\, \mathcal{F}, \mathcal{Z}\right) \leq \frac{\Gamma}{1+\Gamma}.$$

Moreover, if $\boldsymbol{\delta} = \mathbf{0}$, then $|Y_i| = |(Z_{i1} - Z_{i2})(r_{Ci1} - r_{Ci2})| = |r_{Ci1} - r_{Ci2}|$ is fixed by conditioning on $\mathcal{F}$. If $\boldsymbol{\delta} = \mathbf{0}$ and $\Gamma = 2$, then

$$\frac{1}{\Gamma} \leq \frac{\Pr(Y > 0 \mid |Y| = y)}{\Pr(Y < 0 \mid |Y| = y)} \leq \Gamma. \tag{9.15}$$

Suppose instead that $\boldsymbol{\theta} = \overline{\boldsymbol{\theta}}$ and $Y_i \sim N(\tau, 1)$, as in Fig. 9.2 where $\tau = 1/2$. Then

$$\frac{\Pr(Y > 0 \mid |Y| = y)}{\Pr(Y < 0 \mid |Y| = y)} = \frac{\text{abz}(y)}{1 - \text{abz}(y)} = \frac{\text{n}(y-\tau)}{\text{n}(-y-\tau)}, \tag{9.16}$$

where $\text{n}(\cdot)$ is the standard normal density function.

Fix $|Y_i| = y > 0$. If the ratio in (9.16) is larger than Γ at this y, then positive Y_i occur at this $|Y_i| = y$ too frequently to be explained by a bias of Γ in (9.15). Conversely, if (9.16) is at most Γ, then the frequency of positive Y_i at this $|Y_i| = y$ could be explained by a bias of Γ.

Return to Fig. 9.2 where $\tau = 1/2$. At $|Y_i| = 1$, the ratio is $\text{abz}(1)/\{1 - \text{abz}(1)\} = 2.72$, so if we looked only at infinitely many pairs with $|Y_i| = 1$, then sensitivity to unmeasured bias would occur at $\Gamma = 2.72$. In contrast, at $|Y_i| = 0.1$, the ratio is $\text{abz}(0.1)/\{1 - \text{abz}(0.1)\} = 1.11$, and infinitely many pairs with $|Y_i| = 0.1$ would be sensitive to a bias of $\Gamma = 1.11$. At $|Y_i| = 2$, sensitivity to bias occurs at $\text{abz}(2)/\{1 - \text{abz}(2)\} = 7.39$. Is $|Y_i| = 2$ improbable for the normal cumulative distribution $\Phi(y - \tau)$ with expectation τ and variance 1? Well, $Y_i \le -2$ is certainly improbable, with $\Pr(Y_i \le -2) = \Phi\left(-2 - \frac{1}{2}\right) = \Phi(-2.5) = 0.0062$. However, $Y_i \ge 2$ is more than ten times as probable with $\Pr(Y_i \ge 2) = 1 - \Phi\left(2 - \frac{1}{2}\right) = 0.0668$.

Both U878 and Noether's statistic with $f = 2/3$ pay little or no attention to Y_i if $|Y_i|$ is small, and they pay close attention to Y_i if $|Y_i|$ is large; however, neither statistic allows one or a few Y_i to determine the conclusion. This is a good strategy for increasing $\widetilde{\Gamma}$ when $\text{abz}(y)$ increases as y increases. Consider a positive additive effect, $\tau > 0$. In this case, $\text{abz}(y) \to 1$ as $y \to \infty$ for the normal distribution, and $\text{abz}(y)$ is monotone increasing to an asymptote less than 1 for the logistic and double exponential distributions; however, $\text{abz}(y)$ is redescending—it rises, then falls—for the Cauchy distribution [46, Figure 2]. For $J = 3$, a similar pattern occurs for the expected within-block rank, $\text{E}\left(\sum_{j=1}^{J} Z_{ij}\, q_{ij}^{*} \middle| w_i\right)$, of the treated individual [57, Figure 2] when plotted against the within-block range w_i in (2.11). In Table 9.1, recall that $\widetilde{\Gamma}$ was not monotone increasing in f for Noether's statistic when the distribution of errors had long tails. As noted earlier, for matched pairs, the redescending φ-function U867 has high design sensitivity for long tailed distributions. In general, to achieve high design sensitivity, $\varphi(\cdot)$ should be large where $\text{abz}(y)$ in (9.14) is large and for long-tailed distributions that may be in their shoulders rather than their extreme tails.

We have seen this pattern before in the alcohol and HDL cholesterol example. Recall that, from the discussion in Sect. 9.2 of Noether's test applied to this example, 37 of the 40 largest $|Y_i|$ had $Y_i > 0$, where $I = 406$ and $40/406 \doteq 10\%$. As $37/40 = 0.925$, among the 40 largest $|Y_i|$, positive Y_i occurred $.925/(1 - .925) = 12.33$ times more often than negative Y_i. How does that compare to Fig. 9.2? Because $0.9 = \Phi(1.839 - 1/2) - \Phi(-1.839 - 1/2)$, the upper 10% point of the $|Y_i|$ for the distribution in Fig. 9.2 is 1.839. So, $\text{abz}(1.839)/\{1 - \text{abz}(1.839)\} = 6.29$, rather than 12.33. In both cases, insensitivity to larger Γ is found at upper quantiles of $|Y_i|$.

9.5 Adaptive Inference

Testing One Hypothesis Twice

As is evident from Table 9.1, given a choice of two test statistics, the statistic with the larger design sensitivity $\widetilde{\Gamma}$ will vary with the favorable situation. Is it possible to always have the larger design sensitivity of two or more specified statistics? Perhaps surprisingly, the answer is yes [23,48,49,57].

When testing $H_0 : \delta = \delta_0$ with $\theta \in B_\Gamma$ at a specific $\Gamma \geq 1$, compute two upper bounds on the P-value, $P_{1\Gamma}$ and $P_{2\Gamma}$, from two test statistics, $T_1^{\delta_0}$ and $T_2^{\delta_0}$, having design sensitivities $\widetilde{\Gamma}_1$ and $\widetilde{\Gamma}_2$ in a particular favorable situation. If $H_0 : \delta = \delta_0$ and $\theta \in B_\Gamma$ are true, then $P_{1\Gamma}$ and $P_{2\Gamma}$ are each valid bounds on the P-value; so, for every $\alpha \in [0, 1]$,

$$\Pr(P_{1\Gamma} \leq \alpha \mid \mathcal{F}, \mathcal{Z}) \leq \alpha \quad \text{and} \quad \Pr(P_{2\Gamma} \leq \alpha \mid \mathcal{F}, \mathcal{Z}) \leq \alpha. \tag{9.17}$$

Our goal is to have a test statistic with design sensitivity $\max\left(\widetilde{\Gamma}_1, \widetilde{\Gamma}_2\right)$, even though we do not know whether $\widetilde{\Gamma}_1 > \widetilde{\Gamma}_2$ or $\widetilde{\Gamma}_1 \leq \widetilde{\Gamma}_2$ in the particular favorable situation in which we find ourselves.

Define $P^*_{\min\Gamma} = \min(P_{1\Gamma}, P_{2\Gamma})$. By the definition of design sensitivity, as $I \to \infty$, if $\Gamma < \widetilde{\Gamma}_1$, then $P_{1\Gamma} \to 0$, and if $\Gamma < \widetilde{\Gamma}_2$, then $P_{2\Gamma} \to 0$; so if $\Gamma < \max\left(\widetilde{\Gamma}_1, \widetilde{\Gamma}_2\right)$, then $P^*_{\min\Gamma} \to 0$. Now, $P^*_{\min\Gamma}$ is not a P-value, as (9.17) does not rule out the possibility that $\Pr\left(P^*_{\min\Gamma} \leq \alpha\right) > \alpha$; however, $P^*_{\min\Gamma}$ is a statistic, so we can obtain a valid P-value from a bound on the null distribution of $P^*_{\min\Gamma}$.

The simplest, but not the best, approach is to apply the Bonferroni inequality. A simple but conservative approach applies the Bonferroni inequality to (9.17):

$$\begin{aligned} \Pr\left(2P^*_{\min\Gamma} \leq \alpha \,\middle|\, \mathcal{F}, \mathcal{Z}\right) &= \Pr\left(P^*_{\min\Gamma} \leq \alpha/2 \,\middle|\, \mathcal{F}, \mathcal{Z}\right) \\ &= \Pr(P_{1\Gamma} \leq \alpha/2 \text{ or } P_{2\Gamma} \leq \alpha/2 \mid \mathcal{F}, \mathcal{Z}) \leq \alpha; \end{aligned} \tag{9.18}$$

so, $2P^*_{\min\Gamma}$ is a valid P-value bound when testing $H_0 : \delta = \delta_0$ with $\theta \in B_\Gamma$. If $\Gamma < \max\left(\widetilde{\Gamma}_1, \widetilde{\Gamma}_2\right)$, then $2P^*_{\min\Gamma} \to 0$; so, the valid P-value bound $2P^*_{\min\Gamma}$ has design sensitivity $\max\left(\widetilde{\Gamma}_1, \widetilde{\Gamma}_2\right)$. The only problem is that the bound, $2P^*_{\min\Gamma}$, could be made smaller.

This Bonferroni method is quite conservative, unlike many applications of the Bonferroni inequality to nearly independent statistics. Because $T_1^{\delta_0}$ and $T_2^{\delta_0}$ are two statistics testing the same null hypothesis using the same data, $T_1^{\delta_0}$ and $T_2^{\delta_0}$ can be highly correlated, and it is in this situation that the Bonferroni inequality is quite conservative.

A better approach uses a bivariate distribution or limiting distribution of $\left(T_1^{\delta_0}, T_2^{\delta_0}\right)$ when $H_0 : \delta = \delta_0$ with $\theta \in B_\Gamma$ to determine the bound on the probability distribution $\Pr\left(P^*_{\min\Gamma} \leq p \,\middle|\, \mathcal{F}, \mathcal{Z}\right)$. For certain weighted rank statistics, including those in Table 8.1, for large I, the required bound is obtained from a bivariate normal distribution [57, §5], as explained later in Sect. 9.5.

First, let us consider an example.

Adaptive Inference for Alcohol and HDL Cholesterol

For the daily alcohol and HDL cholesterol example in Sect. 1.4 and Table 8.1, the adaptive tests of $H_0 : \delta = \delta_0$ with $\boldsymbol{\theta} \in B_\Gamma$ are shown in Table 9.4. The first two rows of Table 9.4 report the bounds on P-values using $U868$ and U878 separately. In this example, results obtained from U878 are insensitive to a larger bias, $\Gamma = 6$ with P-value 0.0456 for U878 rather than 0.1340 for U868. The third row of Table 9.4 is $P^*_{\min\Gamma}$, which happens to be the P-value for U878; however, $P^*_{\min\Gamma}$ is not a P-value. It would be dishonest to do several tests and report the smallest of several P-values as if it were a true P-value. If the Bonferroni inequality is used to correct for testing one hypothesis twice, then the combined test is insensitive to a bias of $\Gamma = 5.5$ with $2P^*_{\min\Gamma} = 0.0348$. If instead the joint distribution of U868 and U878 is used, then the adaptive P-value is 0.0359 at $\Gamma = 5.75$. Not shown in Table 9.4, the adaptive P-value is 0.050 at $\Gamma^\bullet = 5.938$. So, the adaptive procedure is only slightly behind the procedure, U878, that reported greatest insensitivity to unmeasured bias. A result of Robert Berk and Douglas Jones [7] says that the adaptive procedure is very close to the better procedure in large samples. The Berk-Jones theorem is discussed in Sect. 11.4.

Table 9.4 Adaptive inference using both U868 and U878 for the alcohol and HDL cholesterol example. The values shown are upper bounds on P-values from U868 and U878, their minimum, the Bonferroni adjusted minimum—i.e., twice the minimum—and the adaptive P-value that uses the joint distribution of the two statistics

	Γ						
	1	3	4	5	5.5	5.75	6
U868	0.0000	0.0000	0.0003	0.0154	0.0537	0.0880	0.1340
U878	0.0000	0.0000	0.0001	0.0050	0.0174	0.0291	0.0456
Minimum	0.0000	0.0000	0.0001	0.0050	0.0174	0.0291	0.0456
Bonferroni	0.0000	0.0000	0.0003	0.0101	0.0348	0.0581	0.0913
Adaptive	0.0000	0.0000	0.0002	0.0065	0.0218	0.0359	0.0555

The correlation between U868 and U878 is very high in Table 9.4, about 0.97. If we are trying to achieve the better performance of two tests, perhaps we should pick two tests that are not so similar. The statistic U888 is Stephenson's [67] test based on subsamples of size 8. The blocked version of Stephenson's test goes even further than U878 in focusing on blocks with large ranges, and its $\varphi(\cdot)$ function is convex, so it is still accelerating upwards when we reach the block whose range w_i has rank $b_i = I$. Consequently, U888 is not the best choice for distributions with long tails, such as the t-distribution with 2 or 3 degrees of freedom [47, Table 3]. In Sect. 1.4, however, U888 performs well. Used alone, its P-value bound is 0.0410 at $\Gamma = 6.3$. Using both U868 and U888 adaptively, the P-value bound is 0.0500 at $\Gamma^\bullet = 6.15$. The correlation between U868 and U888 is 0.84. In practice, before doing the analysis, either U868 or U888 might outperform the other. In a large sample, the adaptive test is expected to perform only slightly worse than the stronger performer.

*Adaptive Inference for Matched Pairs, $J = 2$

In this and the next subsection, the limiting distribution of $P^*_{\min\Gamma}$ is obtained. It is a little easier to do this for matched pairs, $J = 2$, which are discussed in this subsection, than for blocks of size $J > 2$, which are discussed in the next subsection.

Recall that $P^*_{\min\Gamma}$ in Table 9.4 is not a P-value; however, it is a statistic. The limiting distribution of $P^*_{\min\Gamma}$ lets us derive an actual P-value from $P^*_{\min\Gamma}$ as the probability that $P^*_{\min\Gamma}$ is as small or smaller than its observed value. These P-values appeared in the bottom row of Table 9.4, and they were smaller than the conservative P-values, $\min\left(2P^*_{\min\Gamma}, 1\right)$, that are provided by the Bonferroni inequality. As is often true, issues are simplest for matched pairs [49] where a weighted rank statistic is simply a general signed rank statistic and the sensitivity bound is found at the $\boldsymbol{\theta} \in B_\Gamma$ given by (8.20). As always, we can reduce testing $H_0 : \boldsymbol{\delta} = \boldsymbol{\delta}_0$ to testing $H_0 : \boldsymbol{\delta} = \mathbf{0}$ by replacing $\mathbf{R}$ by $\mathbf{R}^{\boldsymbol{\delta}_0}$; so, throughout both this subsection and the next subsection, assume $H_0 : \boldsymbol{\delta} = \mathbf{0}$ is true.

For $J = 2$, consider testing $H_0 : \boldsymbol{\delta} = \mathbf{0}$ using two signed rank statistics, T_k, $k = 1, 2$, where rejection occurs for large values of T_k. For pairs, $J = 2$, Wilcoxon's within-block ranks, q^*_{ij}, are 1 or 2, but it is simpler to work with $q^{**}_{ij} = q^*_{ij} - 1$ which are 0 or 1. More precisely, if $|R_{i1} - R_{i2}| \neq 0$, set $q^{**}_{ij} = 1$ if $R_{ij} = \max(R_{i1}, R_{i2})$, and in all other cases set $q^{**}_{ij} = 0$. A signed rank statistic has the form $T_k = \sum_{i=1}^{I} \varphi_k \{b_i/(I + 1)\} \sum_{j=1}^{2} Z_{ij}\, q^{**}_{ij}$, where b_i is the rank of $|R_{i1} - R_{i2}|$, with average ranks for ties, and $\varphi_k : [0, 1] \to [0, \kappa]$, as in Fig. 8.1.[13] An important consideration here is that T_1 and T_2 apply different weights, $\varphi_1 \{b_i/(I + 1)\}$ or $\varphi_2 \{b_i/(I + 1)\}$, to the same binary variables $\sum_{j=1}^{2} Z_{ij}\, q^{**}_{ij}$. For $J = 2$, this will be important because (T_1, T_2) are then jointly stochastically largest at one $\boldsymbol{\theta} \in B_\Gamma$, namely, the $\boldsymbol{\theta}$ given by (8.20).

Because $H_0 : \boldsymbol{\delta} = \mathbf{0}$ is true, $R_{ij} = r_{Cij}$ is fixed by conditioning on $\mathcal{F}$; so, everything that depends only on $R_{ij} = r_{Cij}$ is fixed, including b_i, $\max(R_{i1}, R_{i2}) = \max(r_{Ci1}, r_{Ci2})$, q^{**}_{ij}, and the scores $\varphi_k \{b_i/(I + 1)\} = \varphi_{ik}$, say. That is, under H_0, the statistic $T_k = \sum_{i=1}^{I} \varphi_{ik} \sum_{j=1}^{2} Z_{ij}\, q^{**}_{ij}$ is the sum of fixed scores φ_{ik} for which the random variable $\sum_{j=1}^{2} Z_{ij}\, q^{**}_{ij}$ equals 1.

Under H_0 and $\boldsymbol{\theta} \in B_\Gamma$, the stochastically largest distribution of each $\sum_{j=1}^{2} Z_{ij}\, q^{**}_{ij}$ occurs at the $\boldsymbol{\theta} \in B_\Gamma$ given by (8.20); so, the stochastically largest distribution of (T_1, T_2) also occurs at (8.20). Now, (T_1, T_2) converges in distribution to a bivariate normal distribution if $\lambda_1 T_1 + \lambda_2 T_2$ converges to a univariate normal distribution for every $(\lambda_1, \lambda_2) \neq (0, 0)$ by the Cramer-Wold device [39, 2c.5(iv)]. Of course, $\lambda_1 T_1 + \lambda_2 T_2$ is itself a signed rank statistic with score function $\lambda_1 \varphi_1(\cdot) + \lambda_2 \varphi_2(\cdot)$; that is,

$$\lambda_1 T_1 + \lambda_2 T_2 = \sum_{i=1}^{I} (\lambda_1 \varphi_{i1} + \lambda_2 \varphi_{i2}) \sum_{j=1}^{2} Z_{ij}\, q^{**}_{ij}.$$

[13] This implicitly handles within-block ties as follows: if $|R_{i1} - R_{i2}| = 0$, then $q^{**}_{i1} = q^{**}_{i2} = 0$ and $0 = \sum_{j=1}^{2} Z_{ij}\, q^{**}_{ij}$; otherwise, if $|R_{i1} - R_{i2}| \neq 0$, then $\sum_{j=1}^{2} Z_{ij}\, q^{**}_{ij}$ is 1 or 0 depending upon the value of the treatment assignment $Z_{i1} = 1 - Z_{i2}$ in pair i.

Consequently, Proposition 8.6 applies to each $a_i = \lambda_1\varphi_{i1} + \lambda_2\varphi_{i2}$ at every $\boldsymbol{\theta} \in B_\Gamma$, and in particular at the $\boldsymbol{\theta}$ given by (8.20). Under H_0 at the $\boldsymbol{\theta}$ in (8.20), as $I \to \infty$, for reasonable $\varphi_1(\cdot)$ and $\varphi_2(\cdot)$,

$$\left\{\frac{T_1 - \mathrm{E}(T_1 \mid \mathcal{F}, \mathcal{Z})}{\sqrt{\mathrm{var}(T_1 \mid \mathcal{F}, \mathcal{Z})}}, \frac{T_2 - \mathrm{E}(T_2 \mid \mathcal{F}, \mathcal{Z})}{\sqrt{\mathrm{var}(T_2 \mid \mathcal{F}, \mathcal{Z})}}\right\} \xrightarrow{D} N\left(\begin{bmatrix} 0 & 0 \end{bmatrix}, \begin{bmatrix} 1 & \varsigma \\ \varsigma & 1 \end{bmatrix}\right), \tag{9.19}$$

where $\mathrm{E}(T_k \mid \mathcal{F}, \mathcal{Z})$ and $\mathrm{var}(T_k \mid \mathcal{F}, \mathcal{Z})$ are given by Proposition 8.2, and

$$\mathrm{cov}(T_1, T_2 \mid \mathcal{F}, \mathcal{Z}) = \left(\sum_{i=1}^{I} \varphi_{i1}\,\varphi_{i2} \sum_{j=1}^{2} \theta_{ij}\, q_{ij}^{**}\right) - \mathrm{E}(T_1 \mid \mathcal{F}, \mathcal{Z})\,\mathrm{E}(T_2 \mid \mathcal{F}, \mathcal{Z}),$$

$$\varsigma = \frac{\mathrm{cov}(T_1, T_2 \mid \mathcal{F}, \mathcal{Z})}{\sqrt{\mathrm{var}(T_1 \mid \mathcal{F}, \mathcal{Z})}\sqrt{\mathrm{var}(T_2 \mid \mathcal{F}, \mathcal{Z})}}.$$

At the $\boldsymbol{\theta}$ in (8.20), write

$$D = \max\left\{\frac{T_1 - \mathrm{E}(T_1 \mid \mathcal{F}, \mathcal{Z})}{\sqrt{\mathrm{var}(T_1 \mid \mathcal{F}, \mathcal{Z})}}, \frac{T_2 - \mathrm{E}(T_2 \mid \mathcal{F}, \mathcal{Z})}{\sqrt{\mathrm{var}(T_2 \mid \mathcal{F}, \mathcal{Z})}}\right\}.$$

As $P^*_{\min\Gamma}$ was computed from the two normal approximations to the distributions of T_1 and T_2—that is, from the two marginal distributions of (8.20)—it follows that $P^*_{\min\Gamma} = 1 - \Phi(D)$, where $\Phi(\cdot)$ is the standard normal cumulative distribution. Fix a number d, and consider the lower left quadrant of the plane whose upper right corner is at the point (d, d). Denote by $\mathfrak{R}_\varsigma(d)$ the probability that the bivariate normal distribution (9.19) attaches to that quadrant, that is, the probability of the event that both coordinates in (9.19) are less than d.[14] For large I, $\Pr(D \ge d \mid \mathcal{F}, \mathcal{Z})$ is approximated by $1 - \mathfrak{R}_\varsigma(d)$. Consequently, the limiting distribution of $P^*_{\min\Gamma}$ under H_0 at $\boldsymbol{\theta}$ in (8.20) is

$$\begin{aligned} \Pr\left(P^*_{\min\Gamma} \le p \mid \mathcal{F}, \mathcal{Z}\right) &= \Pr\left\{D \ge \Phi^{-1}(1-p) \mid \mathcal{F}, \mathcal{Z}\right\} \\ &\to 1 - \mathfrak{R}_\varsigma\left\{\Phi^{-1}(1-p)\right\}. \end{aligned}$$

*Adaptive Inference for Blocks, $J > 2$

With blocks of size $J > 2$, there is no longer a single $\boldsymbol{\theta} \in B_\Gamma$ given by (8.20) that provides a stochastically largest distribution for (T_1, T_2). Instead, asymptotic separability in Definition 8.1 is used to place a bound on the P-value [52, §5].

---

14 In R, this is easy to calculate using the `mvtnorm` package. The `wgtRanktt` function in the `weightedRank` package does all of the required calculations.

Now, T_1 and T_2 are each weighted rank statistics, but with different weights attached to the ranks b_i of the within-block range w_i in (2.11); that is, for $k = 1$, 2, $T_k = \sum_{i=1}^{I} \sum_{j=1}^{J} Z_{ij}\, q_{ijk}$ with $q_{ijk} = \phi\left(q_{ij}^*\right) \varphi_k \{b_i/(I+1)\}$, or equivalently $T_k = \sum_{i=1}^{I} \varphi_k \{b_i/(I+1)\} \sum_{j=1}^{J} Z_{ij}\, \phi\left(q_{ij}^*\right)$. Importantly, $\sum_{j=1}^{J} Z_{ij}\, \phi\left(q_{ij}^*\right)$ is the same for T_1 and T_2; only $\varphi_k \{b_i/(I+1)\}$ changes with k. This is the situation in Tables 8.1 and 9.4, where $\phi\left(q_{ij}^*\right) = q_{ij}^*$. Because T_1 and T_2 differ only in $\varphi_1 \{b_i/(I+1)\}$ and $\varphi_2 \{b_i/(I+1)\}$, which are fixed under $H_0 : \boldsymbol{\delta} = \mathbf{0}$ by conditioning upon $\mathcal{F}$, the separable approximation in Definition 8.1 calculates different $\overline{\mu}_{ik}$ and $\overline{\sigma}_{ik}^2$ for T_k, $k = 1, 2$, using their different $\varphi_k \{b_i/(I+1)\}$, but it calculates them at the same $\boldsymbol{\theta} \in \mathfrak{B}_\Gamma$ with $(\theta_{i1}, \ldots, \theta_{iJ})$ having the form (8.22).[15] Write $\boldsymbol{\theta}_s$ for the $\boldsymbol{\theta} \in \mathfrak{B}_\Gamma$ that provides the separable bound for both T_1 and T_2. Replacing $\boldsymbol{\theta}$ in (8.20) by $\boldsymbol{\theta}_s$, the remainder of the argument from the previous subsection is unchanged.

For example, consider the computation of the adaptive P-value 0.0555 for $\Gamma = 6$ in Table 9.4. There, $P_{\min\Gamma}^* = 0.04562505$ from U878. We want $\Pr\left(P_{\min\Gamma}^* \leq 0.04562505 \,\middle|\, \mathcal{F}, \mathcal{Z}\right)$ under H_0 at $\Gamma = 6$ computed at $\boldsymbol{\theta}_s$. The correlation is found to be $\varsigma = 0.9663405$. Then $\Phi^{-1}(1 - 0.04562505) = 1.688840$. Of course, 1.688840 is simply the standardized deviate associated with U878. The bivariate normal (9.19) attaches probability $\Re_\varsigma\left\{\Phi^{-1}(1-p)\right\} = \Re_\varsigma\{1.688840\} = 0.9445061$ to the lower left quadrant of the plane, $[-\infty, 1.688840] \times [-\infty, 1.688840]$, and $1 - \Re_\varsigma\left\{\Phi^{-1}(1-p)\right\} = 1 - 0.9445061 = 0.05549386$ is the adaptive P-value in Table 9.4.[16]

*Further Aspects of Adaptive Inference to Increase $\widetilde{\Gamma}$

So far, the discussion has focused on adaptive inference with $K = 2$ tests, T_1 and T_2, that attach different weights to the ranks b_i of the within-block ranges w_i in (2.11). A similar approach works with $K \geq 2$ tests, and it has been used with $K = 12$ tests [49, Table 3]. All of the K tests must use the same within-block ranks, $\sum_{j=1}^{J} Z_{ij}\, \phi\left(q_{ij}^*\right)$, but the scoring of the blocks need not focus on the within-

[15] More precisely, let $\overline{\mu}_i$ and $\overline{\sigma}_i^2$ be the expectation and variance of $\sum_{j=1}^{J} Z_{ij}\, \phi\left(q_{ij}^*\right)$ determined by the separable approximation in Definition 8.1. Then $\overline{\mu}_{ik} = \sum_{i=1}^{I} \overline{\mu}_i\, \varphi_k \{b_i/(I+1)\}$ and $\overline{\sigma}_{ik}^2 = \sum_{i=1}^{I} \overline{\sigma}_i^2\, \varphi_k^2 \{b_i/(I+1)\}$ for $k = 1, 2$. Also, the covariance of $\left(T_1^{\delta_0}, T_2^{\delta_0}\right)$ is $\sum_{i=1}^{I} \overline{\sigma}_i^2\, \varphi_1 \{b_i/(I+1)\}\, \varphi_2 \{b_i/(I+1)\}$. If there are no ties within blocks, then the q_{ij}^* are a permutation of $1, 2, \ldots, J$ for each i, with the consequence that $\overline{\mu}_i$ and $\overline{\sigma}_i^2$ do not vary with the block i, so the correlation ς between $T_1^{\delta_0}$ and $T_2^{\delta_0}$ does not depend upon $\overline{\mu}_i$ and $\overline{\sigma}_i^2$, so it also does not depend upon Γ.

[16] In the `mvtnorm` package in R, compute:

```
sig <-matrix(c(1,0.9663405,0.9663405,1),2,2)
1-pmvnorm(upper=c(1.688840,1.688840),sigma=sig)
```

The `wgtRanktt` function in the `weightedRank` package does all of the required calculations for the adaptive P-value.

block range w_i. The within-block rank, $\sum_{j=1}^{J} Z_{ij}\,\phi\left(q_{ij}^{*}\right)$, is unchanged by strictly increasing transformations of R_{ij}, but the within-block ranges w_i are affected; so, T_1 might analyze R_{ij} while T_2 might analyze $\log\left(R_{ij}\right)$. Sometimes, the treatment in block i has a dose v_i. Statistic T_1 might ignore the doses, while statistic T_2 might include the dose in the pair or block weights [12]. Most simply, some other measure of within-block dispersion measure might replace the within-block range w_i; for instance, the gap—the difference between $\max_{1\le j\le J} R_{ij}$ and the average of the remaining R_{ij} in block i—has higher design sensitivity in some settings [56]. One example with $K = 12$ tests used various test statistics, with or without doses, with or without a log-transformation, and yet the adaptive test was almost as insensitive to bias as knowing a priori the best choice of test [49, Table 3].

For simple test statistics, an adaptive test may have a tractable exact distribution [48, 61]. Adaptive inference is not confined to rank tests and is applicable to the permutation distribution of weighted M-statistics [51]. The efficiency of adaptive inference for $\Gamma < \min\left(\widetilde{\Gamma}_1, \widetilde{\Gamma}_2\right)$ is discussed in Chap. 11.

9.6 *Further Reading

Power of a sensitivity analysis for finite I: Design sensitivity $\widetilde{\Gamma}$ refers to the limit as $I \to \infty$ of the power to reject H_0 with $\boldsymbol{\theta} \in B_\Gamma$ in a particular favorable situation: the power tends to one if $\Gamma < \widetilde{\Gamma}$ or to zero if $\Gamma > \widetilde{\Gamma}$. For certain test statistics and finite I, it is possible to compute the actual power of a sensitivity analysis in a favorable situation [43, 54, 68]. This may be useful when planning an observational study and considering alternative sample sizes.

Conditioning to increase design sensitivity: For blocks of size $J \geq 3$, a conditioning tactic can further increase design sensitivity [58]. Instead of examining all I blocks, the inference focuses on a subset of the I blocks, and it is a conditional inference given the information used to determine the subset. For brevity, call a block "decisive" if the treated individual has either the highest or lowest response in the block. Attention focuses on decisive blocks. Suppose that the treatment has an effect that increases the responses of treated individuals. Then, in a favorable situation, a treated individual may have the highest response in a block, but it is improbable that the treated individual will have a lower response than $J-1$ controls; so, a larger bias Γ is required to explain this observable pattern of responses.

Effect modification and design sensitivity: Effect modification refers to a treatment effect that varies in size as a function of measured covariates. Effect modification can be an important fact on its own terms, but it can also affect sensitivity to unmeasured biases. Often, a larger treatment effect yields a larger design sensitivity. When there is effect modification, the design sensitivity $\widetilde{\Gamma}$ may be larger in a subpopulation defined by measured covariates, and various strategies have been proposed to make use of this fact; see Jesse Hsu et al. [24, 25] and Kwonsang Lee et al. [29–31]. Generally, there is a multiple testing problem of some kind when examining several or many subpopulations; however, that problem becomes smaller as $I \longrightarrow \infty$ without affecting the design sensitivity, because $\widetilde{\Gamma}$ is a limit as $I \longrightarrow \infty$. The practical problem is to achieve the design sensitivity found in a subpopulation with a larger treatment effect, yet not pay an exorbitant price when correcting for multiple testing to find that population. One can pay no price at the risk of not finding the best subpopulation [25], or a high price with the certainty of finding the best subpopulation [24], or a moderate price by restricting attention to subpopulations that are not complex, for instance, that divide one population into two subpopulations in a variety of ways [31]. For an application in which effect modification occurred in a consequential way, see Silber et al. [65, Table 5].

Instruments and design sensitivity: Weak instruments or instrumental variables are invariably sensitive to small biases that even slightly invalidate the instrument, so strong instruments are preferred [66]. Strategies have been proposed for strengthening an instrument or increasing its design sensitivity [5, 6, 13, 14, 21, 26, 27, 69].

Large but rare treatment effects: Some treatments have dramatic effects on a small and unpredictable portion of the population and no effect on everyone else, so the average treatment effect is small but the effect on responders is large. The locally most powerful rank test against this alternative hypothesis [11, 44] resembles the statistic of Stephenson [67], which in turn resembles a statistic of the form $(m, \underline{m}, \overline{m}) = (m, m, m)$ in (9.11). In a favorable situation defined by this alternative hypothesis, the statistic $(m, \underline{m}, \overline{m}) = (m, m, m)$ can have a large design sensitivity, $\widetilde{\Gamma}$, even when the average treatment effect is small [54, Ch. 17]. In particular, $(m, \underline{m}, \overline{m}) = (8, 8, 8)$ is depicted in Fig. 9.1. See also the work of Siyu Heng and colleagues [20, 21]. For an application in which this issue played an important role, see the study by José Zubizarreta and colleagues [73].

Sample splitting for planning an analysis: It is sometimes possible to trade a small part of the data for a better analytic plan that is insensitive to larger unmeasured biases. As the biases do not diminish as $I \longrightarrow \infty$ but the standard error does diminish, this may be a worthwhile trade when I is large. Suppose that the I blocks are randomly divided into a planning sample of size, say, $I/10$, and an analysis sample of size, say, $9I/10$. The analysis sample is set aside for the moment. Analysis of the planning sample leads to a plan for a primary analysis of the analysis sample. The planning sample is then discarded, and the primary analysis is conducted using the analysis sample. As $I \longrightarrow \infty$, the loss of $I/10$ blocks is without consequence so far as $\widetilde{\Gamma}$ is concerned. However, a better plan for analysis may have a larger $\widetilde{\Gamma}$. This strategy is discussed and illustrated by Ruth Heller et al. [19] and Kai Zhang et al. [70].

Sensitivity analysis with many outcomes, but only a few affected outcomes: The Bonferroni inequality may be applied to the upper bounds on P-values for several or many outcomes, but it is somewhat conservative, for certain technical reasons [60, §4.5]. Colin Fogarty and Dylan Small [15] directly remove this conservative element. When there are many outcomes, an alternative approach due to Qingyuan Zhao and colleagues [72] develops an idea of Marina Bogomolov and Ruth Heller [8]. The approach is called "cross-screening," and it is most suitable when you suspect that only a few of the many outcomes are substantially affected by the treatment—that is, when you are looking for a small number of large needles in a very big haystack. Essentially, cross-screening controls the family-wise error rate in the presence of a bias of at most $\Gamma > 1$ using a tactic that greatly reduces the number of outcomes, exploiting the fact that many unaffected outcomes are likely to have large P-value bounds even for a Γ only modestly larger than 1, say for $\Gamma = 1.25$.

Adaptive inference: In Sect. 9.5, an adaptive inference used the data to select from two or a few test statistics. There [64] have been several attempts to make an adaptive choice among a large number of test statistics [23, 53, 55]. A treatment effect is said to be aberrant if the treatment causes an individual to exhibit a response outside the normal range of responses, and it is sometimes important to separate the hypothesis of no aberrant effects from the more familiar and encompassing hypothesis $H_0 : \boldsymbol{\delta} = \mathbf{0}$ of no effect [59]. Siyu Heng and colleagues study adaptive inference in the context of aberrant treatment effects [20].

Design sensitivity and instruments: The choice of statistic also affects studies with instruments (or instrumental variables). Siyu Heng and colleagues [21] compare statistics of the form (9.11) and "two-stage least squares" or the Wald estimator in matched pairs, $J = 2$, finding substantial differences in design sensitivity. Also important is the strength of the instrument and the degree of success achieved by efforts to strengthen an instrument [5, 13].

Problems

9.1 Checking Design Sensitivity for $J = 2$ Using Simulation

(i) In R, do the simulations in this chapter's Footnotes 3 and 4 to check the stated design sensitivities.
(ii) In part (i), you were essentially determining Qingyuan Zhao's [71] sensitivity value $\Gamma^{\bullet}$ from Sect. 8.6 for one very large I, namely, $I = 10^6$. At $I = 10^6$, there is very little sampling variability in $\Gamma^{\bullet}$. Continuing part (i), for Wilcoxon's signed rank statistic and for U878, simulate several sensitivity values $\Gamma^{\bullet}$ for $I = 100$ and $I = 1000$.

9.2 Checking Design Sensitivity for Noether's Statistic
For $J = 2$, using $I = 10^7$ and the same seed as in Problem 9.1(i), check by simulation that the design sensitivity of Noether's paired test with $f = 2/3$ is $\widetilde{\Gamma} = 4.966$ for normal Y_i with $\tau = 1/2$. (Hint: Use `binom.test` in the `stats` package in R.)

9.3 Calculating Design Sensitivity for Noether's Statistic
(i) For $J = 2$, $\tau = 1/2$, and a t-distribution with 3 degrees of freedom, demonstrate that the design sensitivity of Noether's statistic is $\widetilde{\Gamma} = 5.774$ with $f = 2/3$.
(ii) For $J = 2$, $\tau = 1/2$, and a t-distribution with 3 degrees of freedom, calculate the design sensitivity $\widetilde{\Gamma}$ of Noether's statistic is with $f = 1/2$.
(ii) For $J = 2$, $\tau = 1/2$, plot $\widetilde{\Gamma}$ versus f for the normal distribution and the t-distributions with 10, 5, and 3 degrees of freedom.

9.4 The abz(y) **Function and** $\widetilde{\Gamma}$ **for** $J = 2$
(i) Plot the abz(y) function in (9.14) for several favorable situations, such as $Y_i \sim N(1/2, 1)$, a logistic Y_i scaled to have expectation 1/2 and variance 1, and a t-distribution with 5 degrees of freedom, also scaled to have expectation 1/2 and variance 1. (Solution: [46, Figure 2].)
(ii) Find some (doubtless not entirely satisfactory) way to add the Cauchy distribution to your plot in part (i). (For a not entirely satisfactory solution, see [46, Figure 2].)
(iii) Compare the shapes in your plots of the abz-function to the shapes in Figs. 8.1 and 9.1. Guess which φ-functions would have large design sensitivities $\widetilde{\Gamma}$ when paired with the distributions you have considered.
(iv) Use the `senU` function in the `DOS2` package in R to simulate a few examples to check your guesses in part (iii).
(v) (Optional/a bit harder) Enough already with simulations! Find a formula for $\widetilde{\Gamma}$ in the paired cases, $J = 2$, that we have been considering, and determine numerical values of $\widetilde{\Gamma}$. (Two very different solutions [46, (8)] and [47, Prop. 1]. For numerical values [47, Table 3])

References

1. Albers, W., Bickel, P.J., van Zwet, W.R.: Asymptotic expansions for the power of distribution free tests in the one-sample problem. Ann. Stat. **4**, 108–156 (1976)
2. Bahadur, R.R.: Stochastic comparison of tests. Ann. Math. Stat. **31**(2), 276–295 (1960)
3. Bahadur, R.R.: Rates of convergence of estimates and test statistics. Ann. Math. Stat. **38**(2), 303–324 (1967)
4. Bahadur, R.R., Savage, L.J.: The nonexistence of certain statistical procedures in nonparametric problems. Ann. Math. Stat. **27**(4), 1115–1122 (1956)
5. Baiocchi, M., Small, D.S., Lorch, S., Rosenbaum, P.R.: Building a stronger instrument in an observational study of perinatal care for premature infants. J. Am. Stat. Assoc. **105**(492), 1285–1296 (2010)
6. Baiocchi, M., Small, D.S., Yang, L., Polsky, D., Groeneveld, P.W.: Near/far matching: a study design approach to instrumental variables. Health Services Outcomes Res. Methodol. **12**, 237–253 (2012)

7. Berk, R.H., Jones, D.H.: Relatively optimal combinations of test statistics. Scand. J. Stat. **5**, 158–162 (1978)
8. Bogomolov, M., Heller, R.: Discovering findings that replicate from a primary study of high dimension to a follow-up study. J. Am. Stat. Assoc. **108**(504), 1480–1492 (2013)
9. Brown, B.M.: Symmetric quantile averages and related estimators. Biometrika **68**(1), 235–242 (1981)
10. Cohen, J.: The statistical power of abnormal-social psychological research: a review. J. Abnormal Soc. Psychol. **65**(3), 145 (1962)
11. Conover, W.J., Salsburg, D.S.: Locally most powerful tests for detecting treatment effects when only a subset of patients can be expected to "respond" to treatment. Biometrics **44**, 189–196 (1988)
12. van Eeden, C.: An analogue, for signed rank statistics, of Jureckova's asymptotic linearity theorem for rank statistics. Ann. Math. Stat. **43**(3), 791–802 (1972)
13. Ertefaie, A., Small, D.S., Rosenbaum, P.R.: Quantitative evaluation of the trade-off of strengthened instruments and sample size in observational studies. J. Am. Stat. Assoc. **113**(523), 1122–1134 (2018)
14. Fogarty, C.B., Lee, K., Kelz, R.R., Keele, L.J.: Biased encouragements and heterogeneous effects in an instrumental variable study of emergency general surgical outcomes. J. Am. Stat. Assoc. **116**(536), 1625–1636 (2021)
15. Fogarty, C.B., Small, D.S.: Sensitivity analysis for multiple comparisons in matched observational studies through quadratically constrained linear programming. J. Am. Stat. Assoc. **111**(516), 1820–1830 (2016)
16. Gastwirth, J.L.: On robust procedures. J. Am. Stat. Assoc. **61**(316), 929–948 (1966)
17. Groeneveld, R.A.: Asymptotically optimal group rank tests for location. J. Am. Stat. Assoc. **67**(340), 847–849 (1972)
18. Hammond, E.C.: Smoking in relation to mortality and morbidity. Findings in first thirty-four months of follow-up in a prospective study started in 1959. J. Natl. Cancer Inst. **32**(5), 1161–1188 (1964)
19. Heller, R., Rosenbaum, P.R., Small, D.S.: Split samples and design sensitivity in observational studies. J. Am. Stat. Assoc. **104**(487), 1090–1101 (2009)
20. Heng, S., Kang, H., Small, D.S., Fogarty, C.B.: Increasing power for observational studies of aberrant response: an adaptive approach. J. Roy. Stat. Soc. B **83**(3), 482–504 (2021)
21. Heng, S., Small, D.S., Rosenbaum, P.R.: Finding the strength in a weak instrument in a study of cognitive outcomes produced by Catholic high schools. J. Roy. Stat. Soc. Ser. A **183**(3), 935–958 (2020)
22. Hoeffding, W.: A class of statistics with asymptotically normal distribution. Ann. Math. Stat. **19**(3), 293–325 (1948)
23. Howard, S.R., Pimentel, S.D.: The uniform general signed rank test and its design sensitivity. Biometrika **108**(2), 381–396 (2021)
24. Hsu, J., Small, D., Rosenbaum, P.R.: Effect modification and design sensitivity in observational studies. J. Am. Stat. Assoc. **108**(501), 135–148 (2013)
25. Hsu, J., Zubizarreta, J.R., Small, D., Rosenbaum, P.R.: Strong control of the familywise error rate in observational studies that discover effect modification by exploratory methods. Biometrika **102**(4), 767–782 (2015)
26. Keele, L., Harris, S., Pimentel, S.D., Grieve, R.: Stronger instruments and refined covariate balance in an observational study of the effectiveness of prompt admission to intensive care units. J. Roy. Stat. Soc. Ser. A **183**(4), 1501–1521 (2020)
27. Keele, L., Morgan, J.W.: How strong is strong enough? strengthening instruments through matching and weak instrument tests. Ann. Appl. Stat. **10**, 1086–1106 (2016)
28. Lee, A.J.: U-Statistics: Theory and Practice. Chapman and Hall/CRC, Boca Raton (1990)
29. Lee, K., Small, D.S., Dominici, F.: Discovering heterogeneous exposure effects using randomization inference in air pollution studies. J. Am. Stat. Assoc. **116**(534), 569–580 (2021)
30. Lee, K., Small, D.S., Hsu, J.Y., Silber, J.H., Rosenbaum, P.R.: Discovering effect modification in an observational study of surgical mortality at hospitals with superior nursing. J. Roy. Stat. Soc. Ser. A: Stat. Soc. **181**(2), 535–546 (2018)

31. Lee, K., Small, D.S., Rosenbaum, P.R.: A powerful approach to the study of moderate effect modification in observational studies. Biometrics **74**(4), 1161–1170 (2018)
32. Lehmann, E.L.: Nonparametrics. Holden-Day, San Francisco (1975)
33. Maritz, J.S.: A note on exact robust confidence intervals for location. Biometrika **66**(1), 163–170 (1979)
34. Markowski, E.P., Hettmansperger, T.P.: Inference based on simple rank step score statistics for the location model. J. Am. Stat. Assoc. **77**(380), 901–907 (1982)
35. McNeill, J.J., Tukey, J.W.: Higher-order diagnosis of two-way tables, illustrated on two sets of demographic empirical distributions. Biometrics **31**, 487–510 (1975)
36. Noether, G.E.: Efficiency of the Wilcoxon two-sample statistic for randomized blocks. J. Am. Stat. Assoc. **58**(304), 894–898 (1963)
37. Noether, G.E.: Some simple distribution-free confidence intervals for the center of a symmetric distribution. J. Am. Stat. Assoc. **68**(343), 716–719 (1973)
38. Quade, D.: Using weighted rankings in the analysis of complete blocks with additive block effects. J. Am. Stat. Assoc. **74**(367), 680–683 (1979)
39. Rao, C.R.: Linear Statistical Inference and Its Applications. Wiley, New York (1973)
40. Rosenbaum, P.R.: Effects attributable to treatment: Inference in experiments and observational studies with a discrete pivot. Biometrika **88**(1), 219–231 (2001)
41. Rosenbaum, P.R.: Observational Studies, 2nd edn. Springer, New York (2002)
42. Rosenbaum, P.R.: Exact confidence intervals for nonconstant effects by inverting the signed rank test. Am. Stat. **57**(2), 132–138 (2003)
43. Rosenbaum, P.R.: Design sensitivity in observational studies. Biometrika **91**(1), 153–164 (2004)
44. Rosenbaum, P.R.: Confidence intervals for uncommon but dramatic responses to treatment. Biometrics **63**(4), 1164–1171 (2007)
45. Rosenbaum, P.R.: Interference between units in randomized experiments. J. Am. Stat. Assoc. **102**(477), 191–200 (2007)
46. Rosenbaum, P.R.: Design sensitivity and efficiency in observational studies. J. Am. Stat. Assoc. **105**(490), 692–702 (2010)
47. Rosenbaum, P.R.: A new U-statistic with superior design sensitivity in matched observational studies. Biometrics **67**(3), 1017–1027 (2011)
48. Rosenbaum, P.R.: An exact adaptive test with superior design sensitivity in an observational study of treatments for ovarian cancer. Ann. Appl. Stat. **6**, 83–105 (2012)
49. Rosenbaum, P.R.: Testing one hypothesis twice in observational studies. Biometrika **99**(4), 763–774 (2012)
50. Rosenbaum, P.R.: Impact of multiple matched controls on design sensitivity in observational studies. Biometrics **69**(1), 118–127 (2013)
51. Rosenbaum, P.R.: Weighted M-statistics with superior design sensitivity in matched observational studies with multiple controls. J. Am. Stat. Assoc. **109**(507), 1145–1158 (2014)
52. Rosenbaum, P.R.: Bahadur efficiency of sensitivity analyses in observational studies. J. Am. Stat. Assoc. **110**(509), 205–217 (2015)
53. Rosenbaum, P.R.: A conditional test with demonstrated insensitivity to unmeasured bias in matched observational studies. Biometrika **107**(4), 827–840 (2020)
54. Rosenbaum, P.R.: Design of Observational Studies, 2nd edn. Springer, New York (2020)
55. Rosenbaum, P.R.: A statistic with demonstrated insensitivity to unmeasured bias for $2\times 2\times S$ tables in observational studies. Stat. Med. **41**(19), 3758–3771 (2022)
56. Rosenbaum, P.R.: A second evidence factor for a second control group. Biometrics **79**, 3968–3980 (2023)
57. Rosenbaum, P.R.: Bahadur efficiency of observational block designs. J. Am. Stat. Assoc. **119**(547), 1871–1881 (2024)
58. Rosenbaum, P.R.: A conditioning tactic that increases design sensitivity in observational block designs. J. Roy. Stat. Soc. B (2025). https://doi.org/10.1093/jrsssb/qkaf007
59. Rosenbaum, P.R., Silber, J.H.: Aberrant effects of treatment. J. Am. Stat. Assoc. **103**(481), 240–247 (2008)

60. Rosenbaum, P.R., Silber, J.H.: Sensitivity analysis for equivalence and difference in an observational study of neonatal intensive care units. J. Am. Stat. Assoc. **104**(486), 501–511 (2009)
61. Rosenbaum, P.R., Small, D.S.: An adaptive Mantel–Haenszel test for sensitivity analysis in observational studies. Biometrics **73**(2), 422–430 (2017)
62. Serfling, R.J.: Approximation Theorems of Mathematical Statistics. John Wiley & Sons, New York (2009)
63. Severini, T.A.: Elements of Distribution Theory. Cambridge University Press, New York (2005)
64. Shauly-Aharonov, M.: An exact test with high power and robustness to unmeasured confounding effects. Stat. Med. **39**(8), 1041–1053 (2020)
65. Silber, J.H., Rosenbaum, P.R., McHugh, M.D., Ludwig, J.M., Smith, H.L., Niknam, B.A., Even-Shoshan, O., Fleisher, L.A., Kelz, R.R., Aiken, L.H.: Comparison of the value of nursing work environments in hospitals across different levels of patient risk. JAMA Surgery **151**(6), 527–536 (2016)
66. Small, D.S., Rosenbaum, P.R.: War and wages: The strength of instrumental variables and their sensitivity to unobserved biases. J. Am. Stat. Assoc. **103**(483), 924–933 (2008)
67. Stephenson, W.R.: A general class of one-sample nonparametric test statistics based on subsamples. J. Am. Stat. Assoc. **76**(376), 960–966 (1981)
68. Ye, T., Small, D.S., Rosenbaum, P.R.: Dimensions, power and factors in an observational study of behavioral problems after physical abuse of children. Ann. Appl. Stat. **16**(4), 2732–2754 (2022)
69. Yu, R., Kelz, R., Lorch, S., Keele, L.J.: The risk of maternal complications after cesarean delivery: Near-far matching for instrumental variables study designs with large observational datasets. Ann. Appl. Stat. **17**(2), 1701–1721 (2023)
70. Zhang, K., Small, D.S., Lorch, S., Srinivas, S., Rosenbaum, P.R.: Using split samples and evidence factors in an observational study of neonatal outcomes. J. Am. Stat. Assoc. **106**(494), 511–524 (2011)
71. Zhao, Q.: On sensitivity value of pair-matched observational studies. J. Am. Stat. Assoc. **114**, 713–722 (2019)
72. Zhao, Q., Small, D.S., Rosenbaum, P.R.: Cross-screening in observational studies that test many hypotheses. J. Am. Stat. Assoc. **113**(523), 1070–1084 (2018)
73. Zubizarreta, J.R., Cerda, M., Rosenbaum, P.R.: Effect of the 2010 Chilean earthquake on post-traumatic stress: Reducing sensitivity to unmeasured bias through study design. Epidemiology **24**(1), 79 (2013)

Chapter 10
Study Design and Design Sensitivity

Abstract As the name suggests, design sensitivity was originally intended as a guide to the design of observational studies. This chapter considers three aspects of the design that affect the design sensitivity: (i) the block size, (ii) the exclusion of individuals who received small doses of treatment, and (iii) reducing the heterogeneity of treated-minus-control matched pair differences. Although references are given to theoretical results, the focus is on redesigning the study of alcohol and HDL cholesterol, noting the sensitivity to bias of alternative designs. Theoretical results differ by replacing actual data by a probability model with known properties and calculating the design sensitivity under various models.

10.1 Poor Designs Are Sensitive to Small Unmeasured Biases

Although a sensitivity analysis talks about unmeasured biases, it is computed from the observable data, so its stochastic behavior is governed by the distributions of observable quantities. Change the observable distributions by changing the study design and you change the sensitivity to unmeasured biases. Because design sensitivity $\widetilde{\Gamma}$ refers to the limit as the sample size increases, $I \to \infty$, a study design with an inferior $\widetilde{\Gamma}$ will be limited in what it can say no matter how large the sample becomes. Without guidance from statistical theory, mistakes in designing observational studies result in claims that the effects of a treatment are sensitive to small unmeasured biases, when a better study design would have reported insensitivity to larger unmeasured biases.

Recall from Chap. 9 that design sensitivity compares two situations, in effect: (i) a null or unfavorable situation in there is no treatment effect but there is a bias, $\boldsymbol{\theta} \in B_\Gamma$, in treatment assignment of magnitude at most Γ, and (ii) an alternative favorable situation in which there is a treatment effect and no bias in treatment assignment, $\boldsymbol{\theta} = \overline{\boldsymbol{\theta}} \in B_1$. In the unfavorable situation, we hope to avoid a claim that there is a

© The Author(s), under exclusive license to Springer Nature Switzerland AG 2025

P. R. Rosenbaum, *An Introduction to the Theory of Observational Studies*, Springer Texts in Statistics, https://doi.org/10.1007/978-3-031-90494-3_10

treatment effect, because there is none. In the favorable situation, we hope to find evidence of a treatment effect that is insensitive to small and moderate biases in treatment assignment, as measured by Γ. Of course, if we knew whether we were in the unfavorable or favorable situation, we would simply say that, but we cannot know this in an observational study. Better study designs and better methods of analysis correctly distinguish favorable from unfavorable situations for larger values of Γ.

Part III of my book [37, Part III], *Design of Observational Studies*, discusses ways to increase design sensitivity through decisions made during study design. That material is theoretical and not difficult, but it is about one hundred pages in length; so, I do not want to repeat it here. Rather than do that, Sect. 10.2 and Sect. 10.3 will do something not done in *Design of Observational Studies*; namely, they will take the study of light alcohol and HDL cholesterol in Sect. 1.4 and redesign it in two mistaken ways, thereby illustrating that mistaken designs end up reporting sensitivity to smaller unmeasured biases. Sections 10.2 and 10.3 describe the associated theory informally, with references to formal results. Sections 10.4 and 10.5 sketch two other topics in study design that affect sensitivity to unmeasured biases.

10.2 Block Size and Design Sensitivity

Block Size Affects Design Sensitivity

Table 9.3 has already considered one of the simplest decisions in study design that affects sensitivity to unmeasured bias, namely, the number of controls in a block with one treated individual and $J-1$ controls. With one exception in Table 9.3, for a fixed test statistic and favorable sampling situation, the design sensitivity $\widetilde{\Gamma}$ increases as J increases from $J = 2$ for pairs to $J = 5$ for 4 controls matched to each treated individual.[1] The exception is for U878 with errors from the t-distribution, where $\widetilde{\Gamma} = 4.8$ for $J = 2$ and $\widetilde{\Gamma} = 4.7$ for $J = 3$.

Before continuing, let us recall what this means in a tangible sense. Consider a favorable situation with normal errors and a treatment effect that equals half the standard deviation of a treated-minus-control pair difference, as in Table 9.3. Using U868 in Table 9.3, the design sensitivity is $\widetilde{\Gamma} = 4.2$ for matched pairs, $J = 2$, and is $\widetilde{\Gamma} = 5.8$ for blocks of size $J = 5$. Consider what happens if we perform a sensitivity analysis with $\Gamma = 5$, where $4.2 < 5 < 5.8$. If we simulate this favorable situation in Table 9.3, say with $I = 10000$ blocks of size $J = 5$, and we perform a sensitivity

[1] The situation is different in the less common case in which J is much larger than five. To benefit from increasing the block size much beyond $J = 5$, one needs to consider a larger class of test statistics. Suppose that the data come from a favorable situation with a midsized positive treatment effect. If $J = 3$ and block i has a large rank b_i for its within-block range (2.11), then it is fairly likely that the treated individual's response R_{ij} has rank $q^*_{ij} = 3$ in this block [39, Fig. 2]. In the same situation but with $J = 10$, it is less probable that the one treated individual has a higher response than all $J - 1 = 9$ controls; so, the within-block range is less successful at picking out blocks that clearly exhibit the treatment effect. Tardif [47] finds a similar pattern for the efficiency of weighted rank statistics in randomized block experiments.

using U868 at $\Gamma = 5$, then the upper bound on the one-sided P-value is 0.0084. If instead we use only the first control of the $J - 1$ controls, reducing J from 5 to 2, then the upper bound on the one-sided P-value is 1.0000. Obviously, there is less data with $J = 2$ than with $J = 5$, as there are $I \times (J - 1) = 10000 \times 1 = 10000$ controls with $J = 2$, but there are $I \times (J - 1) = 10000 \times 4 = 40000$ controls with blocks of size $J = 5$. However, if we simulate $I = 40000$ pairs with $J = 2$ in this favorable situation, then there is more data, namely, 40000 controls and 40000 treated individuals, rather than 10000 treated individuals. In this simulation the upper bound on the one-sided P-value is also 1.0000. In brief, it is the block structure, $J = 5$ rather than $J = 2$, not the sample size I, that increases $\widetilde{\Gamma}$.[2]

This pattern of design sensitivities is fairly intuitive. Having several controls matched to each treated individual provides more information useful in distinguishing treatment effects from biased treatment assignment. After all, in each block i, the treatment should affect the one treated individual and none of the controls.[3] Consider an unfavorable situation in which responses R_{ij} exhibit no treatment effect but there is biased treatment assignment, $\boldsymbol{\theta} \in B_\Gamma$, for $\Gamma > 1$. To be more specific, suppose that the R_{ij} in block i are independently sampled from the continuous distribution $F_i(\cdot)$ that may change with i.[4] A severe bias $\boldsymbol{\theta} \in B_\Gamma$ works to push one of the larger order statistics, $R_{i(1)} < R_{i(2)} < \cdots < R_{i(J)}$, from block i into the treated group with $Z_{ij} = 1$, where $1 = \sum_{j=1}^{J} Z_{ij}$ for each i. Contrast this with a favorable situation with $\boldsymbol{\theta} = \overline{\boldsymbol{\theta}} \in B_1$ in which $J - 1$ control responses are sampled from $F_i(r)$ and one treated response is sampled from $F_i(r - \tau)$ with $\tau > 0$.[5] In a pair, $J = 2$, a severe bias pushes $R_{i(2)}$ towards the treated group, as in (8.20); so, in a pair, both the unfavorable situation and the favorable situation leave behind a visible pattern in which the higher response, $R_{i(2)}$, is more likely to be the response of the treated individual than of the control. The situation is different when $J > 2$. In the unfavorable situation, the $R_{i(j)}$ are J order statistics from the same distribution, $F_i(\cdot)$, but in the favorable situation the $R_{i(j)}$ were derived from $J - 1$ observations from $F_i(r)$ and one observation from $F_i(r - \tau)$. For small $J > 2$, we intuitively expect the one treated individual to stand a bit apart from the $J - 1$ controls, and we expect this to be reflected, perhaps usefully, in the J order statistics, $R_{i(1)} < R_{i(2)} < \cdots < R_{i(J)}$.[6] Although this pattern will be

---

[2] The R code for this calculation follows:

```
set.seed(1)
y<-matrix(rnorm(50000),10000,5)
y[,1]<-y[,1]+(.5)*sqrt(2)
library(weightedRank)
wgtRank(y,gamma=5)
wgtRank(y[,1:2],gamma=5)
y<-matrix(rnorm(80000),40000,2)
y[,1]<-y[,1]+(.5)*sqrt(2)
wgtRank(y,gamma=5)
```

[3] At least, this is true in the absence of interference between units [17, 29, 46, 48].

[4] This is the null hypothesis $H_0^{\dagger}$ in Definition 3.1 in Sect. 3.2.

[5] This is $H_\tau^{\dagger}$ in Sect. 3.2.

[6] This is true in several formal senses. Of course, we expect the largest order statistic, $R_{i(J)}$ in block i to be larger if one observation is from $F_i(r - \tau)$ with $\tau > 0$ than if all J observations are from

seen clearly in a single block i only if τ is very large, a statistic can be designed to recognize this pattern in many blocks for smaller τ and distinguish this pattern from larger biases in treatment assignment [31, 32, 39].

We have seen this happen in theory in Table 9.3 and in the simulated example discussed above. Can we see it in the actual study in Sect. 1.4?

Comparing Two Designs for Alcohol and HDL Cholesterol

This section compares two versions of the study of alcohol and HDL cholesterol in Sect. 1.4. One version has $I = 406$ pairs or blocks of size $J = 2$ formed by picking at random one control from each block in the original study. The other version has $I' = 271$ blocks of size $J = 4$, formed by sampling 271 of the original 406 blocks of size 4. It seems fair to compare fewer blocks of size $J = 4$ to more pairs of size $J = 2$, but why is $I' = 271$ blocks of size $J = 4$ the correct number for a fair comparison?

For the sole purpose of equating I and I', consider a standard linear model for an $I \times J$ block design, where $R_{ij} = \beta_j + \tau Z_{ij} + \epsilon_{ij}$ with independent and identically distributed errors ϵ_{ij} having constant variance $\text{var}\left(\epsilon_{ij}\right) = \sigma^2$. In the absence of bias in treatment assignment, $\boldsymbol{\theta} = \overline{\boldsymbol{\theta}} \in B_1$, the treated-minus-control difference in mean responses,

$$\frac{1}{I}\sum_{i=1}^{I}\sum_{j=1}^{J} Z_{ij}\, R_{ij} - \frac{1}{I\,(J-1)}\sum_{i=1}^{I}\sum_{j=1}^{J}\left(1 - Z_{ij}\right) R_{ij},$$

has expectation τ and variance $\sigma^2\,\{1 + 1/(J-1)\}\,/I$. As $(1 + 1/3)\,/271 = 0.00492$ for $J = 4$ and $(1 + 1/1)\,/406 = 0.00493$ for $J = 2$, the treated-minus-control difference in means has the same standard error with $I = 406$ and $J = 2$ as it does with $I' = 271$ and $J' = 4$. In this specific and limited sense, the standard error alone views $(I = 406, J = 2)$ and $(I' = 271, J' = 4)$ as virtually equivalent. Are they equivalent in a sensitivity analysis?

For $(I = 406, J = 2)$ and $(I' = 271, J' = 4)$, Table 10.1 reproduces the calculations in Table 8.1 where there were 406 blocks of size 4. As in Table 8.1, Table 10.1 gives the upper bound (8.13) on the one-sided P-value testing the null hypothesis of no effect.

What would we expect to see in Table 10.1 if the design sensitivities in Table 9.3 are a useful guide? For $(I' = 271, J' = 4)$ on the right side of Table 10.1, we would expect the P-value bounds to be somewhat larger than those in Table 8.1 where there were 406 blocks, but otherwise we would expect a similar pattern. In contrast, for

---

$F_i\,(r)$. More subtly, $R_{i(J)}$ is stochastically larger in this favorable situation than if all J observations in block i are sampled from the same mixture distribution $\{(J-1)\,F_i\,(r) + F_i\,(r-\tau)\}\,/J$, so the mere knowledge that there is exactly one treated individual in the block changes the distribution of $R_{i(1)} < R_{i(2)} < \cdots < R_{i(J)}$; see David and Nagaraja [5, Theorem 5.2.1] and Sen [43]. Indeed, the configuration of $R_{i(1)} < R_{i(2)} < \cdots < R_{i(J)}$ provides information about the identity of the treated individual in the favorable situation, but not in the unfavorable situation [39, Fig. 2].

Table 10.1 Bounds on P-values for the hypothesis of no effect in the study of HDL cholesterol and light daily alcohol consumption. In each column, the most insensitive P-value ≤ 0.05 is in **bold**

	406 1-to-1 pairs				271 1-to-3 blocks			
Γ	Wilcoxon	Quade	U868	U878	Wilcoxon	Quade	U868	U878
1	0.000	0.000	0.000	0.000	0.000	0.000	0.000	0.000
2	**0.006**	**0.000**	0.000	0.000	0.000	0.000	0.000	0.000
3.5	0.994	0.233	**0.013**	0.003	**0.044**	0.001	0.000	0.000
4	1.000	0.584	0.064	0.015	0.224	0.008	0.001	0.001
4.5	1.000	0.851	0.182	**0.046**	0.532	**0.045**	0.007	0.004
5	1.000	0.963	0.359	0.106	0.799	0.143	**0.024**	0.014
5.5	1.000	0.993	0.552	0.198	0.937	0.310	0.063	**0.034**
6	1.000	0.999	0.720	0.311	0.985	0.511	0.131	0.069

($I = 406$, $J = 2$) on the left side of Table 10.1, we would expect to see sensitivity to smaller biases. By and large, Table 10.1 is consistent with these expectations, albeit with modest sampling fluctuations. For instance, at $\Gamma = 6$, U878 has a P-value bound of 0.0456 in Table 8.1 and a bound of 0.069 in Table 10.1. Indeed, with $J = 4$, increasing the number of blocks from 271 to 406 typically decreases the P-value bounds only slightly. In contrast, the change due to reducing J from 4 in Table 8.1 to 2 in Table 10.1 results in a dramatic change in sensitivity to unmeasured bias. Where U878 had a P-value bound of 0.0456 at $\Gamma = 6$ in Table 8.1, it has in Table 10.1 a bound of 0.046 at $\Gamma = 4.5$ for $J = 2$, but a bound of 0.004 at $\Gamma = 4.5$ for $J = 4$. Qualitatively similar patterns are seen as I and J change for the other three statistics, including Quade's statistic, which becomes Wilcoxon's signed rank statistic for $J = 2$.

In brief: in theory, in a simulated example, and in the actual data, an increase in the block size from $J = 2$ to $J = 4$ increased the value Γ at which the study becomes sensitive to unmeasured biases.

10.3 Do Intermediate Doses of Treatment Strengthen Design?

Dose-Response and Evidence Concerning Causal Effects

Epidemiologists have expressed a range of views about the relevance or otherwise of a dose-response relationship in an observational study of causal effects [13,41,49]. This debate is always interesting, but it is typically informal, without proof of a definite result under specific conditions.

In particular, this debate does not typically ask whether intermediate doses with intermediate effects have consequences for the degree of sensitivity to unmeasured biases. Section 10.3 focuses on this specific question.

Design Sensitivity Can Be Diluted by Low Doses of Treatment

In Sect. 1.4, the comparison of HDL cholesterol levels and light daily alcohol consumption involved $I = 406$ treated individuals in group D who drank at least five days a week (more precisely, on at least $5 \times 52 = 260$ days in the past year) and drank between 1 and 3 drinks on those days. Members of this group consumed a mean of 588 drinks in the past year, but one person in the group reported drinking $3 \times 365 = 1095$ drinks in the past year. Would it be useful to expand the treated group to include people who drank much less than 588 drinks in the past year?

Theoretical calculations suggest that, if intermediate doses produce intermediate effects, then the answer to this question is no. In these calculations, the design sensitivity $\widetilde{\Gamma}$ is largest if the study is confined to higher-dose treated individuals for whom the treatment effect is larger. The theoretical calculation comes in several forms. One form concerns matched pairs, $J = 2$, using Constance van Eeden [6]'s dose-weighted version of Wilcoxon's signed rank statistic [37, Proposition 18.1]; it says $\widetilde{\Gamma}$ is made larger by giving zero weight to low-dose pairs. A second form for $J \geq 2$ concerns a dose-weighted version of the blocked Wilcoxon rank sum statistic [27, §4, Table 3]; it also says that $\widetilde{\Gamma}$ is made larger by having a high-dose in every block. In large samples, these and similar calculations suggest that if an intermediate dose has an effect that is substantial but is also substantially smaller than a full dose, then the best weight to attach to individuals with intermediate doses is zero, providing the goal is to report insensitivity to small and moderate biases. This is not surprising: the size of the treatment effect has a strong influence on the design sensitivity, and the effect size is, by assumption, smaller with an intermediate dose. Obviously, a supporting analysis might satisfy our curiosity about the effects of intermediate doses, but it is reasonable to expect that this supporting analysis will be sensitive to smaller unmeasured biases than the primary analysis.

The first sensitivity analysis by Cornfield and colleagues [4] did not distinguish between the sensitivity of an inference and the design sensitivity—in effect, it did not distinguish Γ and $\widetilde{\Gamma}$—but it did discuss an aspect of the issue above about intermediate doses, saying:

> Cigarette smokers have a nine-fold greater risk of developing lung cancer than nonsmokers, while over-two-pack-a-day smokers have at least a 60-fold greater risk. Any characteristic proposed as a measure of the postulated cause common to both smoking status and lung-cancer risk must therefore be at least nine-fold more prevalent among cigarette smokers than among nonsmokers and at least 60-fold more prevalent among two-pack-a-day smokers.

Here, Cornfield et al. are saying that they found insensitivity to larger biases at higher doses.

When we do distinguish the sensitivity of an inference, Γ, from the design sensitivity, $\widetilde{\Gamma}$, the question takes on a slightly different form. Thinking that more data can never be a disadvantage, we might hope for a test statistic that can combine data from high and intermediate doses in such a way that intermediate doses do not reduce the design sensitivity.[7] Attaching intermediate weight to individuals with intermediate doses can increase power in a randomized experiment where $\theta = \overline{\theta} \in B_1$, but that is a different situation, because insensitivity to biased treatment assignment is not a concern in a randomized experiment.

The calculations in Sect. 10.3 use a dose-weighted rank statistic of the form $T = t(\mathbf{Z}, \mathbf{R}) = \sum_{i=1}^{I} \sum_{j=1}^{J} Z_{ij}\, q_{ij}$ with $q_{ij} = d_i\, \phi\left(q_{ij}^{*}\right) \varphi\left\{b_i/(I+1)\right\}$, where (i) $d_i \geq 0$ is a score for the dose of treatment given in block i, (ii) q_{ij}^{*} is the rank of R_{ij} in block i, ranking from 1 to J, (iii) b_i is the rank of the within-block range in block i, and (iv) $\phi(\cdot)$ and $\varphi(\cdot)$ are score functions. Taking $d_i = 1$ for all i yields the usual weighted rank statistic [39] in Sect. 2.6 and Chaps. 8 and 9. In the case of matched pairs, $J = 2$, this is the dose-weighted signed-rank statistic of Constance van Eeden [6]. When $\phi\left(q_{ij}^{*}\right) = q_{ij}^{*}$ and $\varphi\left\{b_i/(I+1)\right\} = 1$ for all i, this is the dose-weighted blocked Wilcoxon rank sum statistic [27].

A Larger Study of HDL Cholesterol Including Smaller Doses of Alcohol

Consider adding 197 additional treated individuals who drank one drink on 2 to 3 days each week or more precisely on between $104 = 2 \times 52$ and $156 = 3 \times 52$ days in the past year. These 197 individuals drank a mean of 128 drinks in the past year, much less than the mean of 588 drinks for the 406 individuals in group D in Sect. 1.4, but much more than the mean of 0 drinks for the 406 individuals in group N.

Each of these 197 additional treated individuals is matched to an unmatched member of either group N or group R in Table 1.1, again matching for sex, age, and education. Recall that control group R for "rarely" may have had a few alcoholic drinks during the past year.

Figure 10.1 shows age and education for the original 406 high-dose D-versus-N pairs and the 197 newly added low-dose matched pairs. It is no surprise that these 197 occasional drinkers and their matched controls differed in sex, age, and education from the 406 daily drinkers and their matched controls. In particular, on average the 197 occasional drinkers and their matched controls were about 4 years younger than the daily drinkers, had a little more education, and were 53% female rather than 34%

[7] Using adaptive inference, as in Sect. 9.5 and [30, 40], it is possible to do this, but one must adaptively choose between two or more statistics, one of which uses only the high-dose pairs or blocks. If the effect increases with the dose, then, as $I \to \infty$, the adaptive inference will eventually prefer the statistic that uses only the high-dose pairs or blocks; so, adaptive inference is not expected to increase design sensitivity in that specific situation. Adaptive inference does provide certain protections, however. In particular, if the effect does not materially increase with an increase in dose, or the effect is not monotone increasing in the dose, then an adaptive inference that includes statistics that pay little or no attention to doses may provide protection against these possibilities [30]. Another approach involves highly adaptive inference that can adapt to a dose-response relationship that is not monotone [36, 38]. Yet another approach uses two evidence factors in the sense of Chap. 13, one that uses doses and another that ignores them [18].

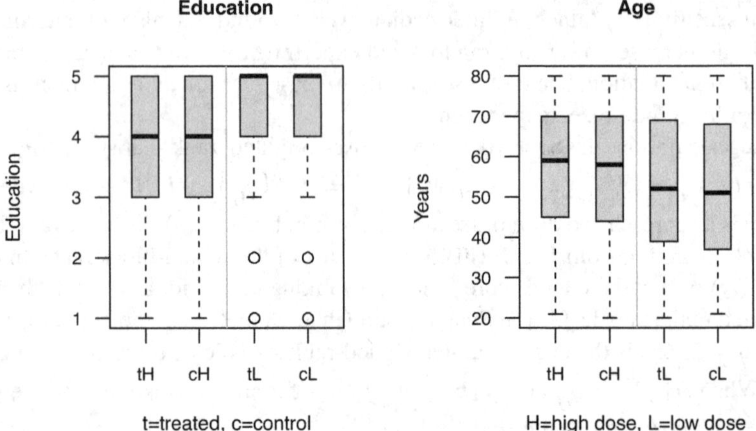

Fig. 10.1 Addition of 197 low-dose matched pairs to the $I = 406$ high-dose D-versus-N pairs in the study of light daily alcohol and HDL cholesterol. The low-dose pairs are slightly younger and have somewhat more education than the high-dose pairs. Also, the high-dose pairs are 34% female, but the low-dose pairs are 53% female

female. However, within each of the $406 + 197 = 603$ matched pairs, the treated and control individuals were similar in terms of these three covariates.

Figure 10.2 shows alcohol consumption and HDL cholesterol levels for the original 406 high-dose D-versus-N pairs and the newly added 197 low-dose matched pairs. Using the conventional one-sample Hodges-Lehmann estimate [14], the typical treated-minus-control pair difference in HDL cholesterol is almost twice as large in the 406 high-dose pairs as in the 197 low-dose pairs, even though the usual randomization-based P-value from Wilcoxon's signed rank test is below 0.0001 in both sets of matched pairs. Would increasing the sample size from 406 pairs to $603 = 406 + 197$ strengthen the inference if a suitable weight, d_i, were chosen for the low-dose pairs? Obviously, taking $d_i = 0$ for low-dose pairs entails excluding the 197 low-dose pairs, more or less as we have done all along, while taking $d_i = 1$ for all pairs simply adds them to the analysis without taking account of the lower dose in these pairs.[8]

Table 10.2 compares the sensitivity to bias with 197 additional pairs at intermediate doses, for various ways of weighting the intermediate doses. For the 406 pairs at full dose, $d_i = 1$ throughout Table 10.2. For the 197 pairs with intermediate doses,

[8] Why "more or less?" The ranks of the within-block ranges are slightly affected by the presence of the additional 197 intermediate pairs, even if $d_i = 0$ for these pairs.

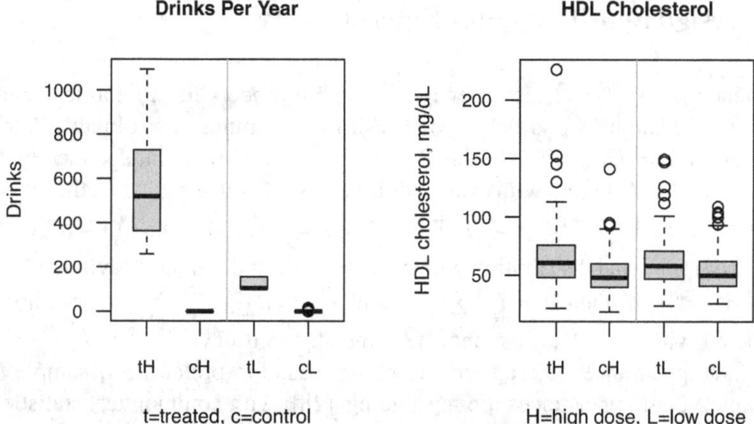

Fig. 10.2 Addition of 197 low-dose matched pairs to the $I = 406$ high-dose D-versus-N pairs in the study of light daily alcohol and HDL cholesterol. On average, treated individuals in high-dose pairs had 588 alcoholic drinks in the past year, while in low-dose pairs that had 128 drinks. The Hodges-Lehmann [14] estimate of the typical treated-minus-control pair difference in HDL cholesterol levels was 12.5 for high-dose pairs and 6.5 for low-dose pairs

Table 10.2 Upper bounds on the one-sided P-value testing the hypothesis H_0 of no treatment effect for various ways, d_i, of weighting the 197 pairs (of $603 = 406 + 197$ pairs) with intermediate doses of treatment, using either the Wilcoxon signed rank statistic or U868. Only U868 ignoring the 197 intermediate pairs, $d_i = 0$, rejects H_0 at the 0.05 level for $\Gamma = 4$. Bounds ≤ 0.05 are in **bold**

d_i	$\Gamma = 2.8$		$\Gamma = 3$		$\Gamma = 4$	
	Quade	U868	Quade	U868	Quade	U868
0.00	**0.0176**	**0.0001**	0.0537	**0.0006**	0.6702	**0.0428**
0.10	**0.0248**	**0.0002**	0.0746	**0.0009**	0.7635	0.0629
0.25	**0.0411**	**0.0004**	0.1184	**0.0016**	0.8690	0.1075
0.50	0.0892	**0.0011**	0.2271	**0.0045**	0.9591	0.2253
0.75	0.1681	**0.0032**	0.3676	**0.0122**	0.9882	0.3836
0.90	0.2281	**0.0059**	0.4551	**0.0209**	0.9943	0.4827
1.00	0.2714	**0.0087**	0.5109	**0.0291**	0.9964	0.5454

values 0.00, 0.1, 0.25, 0.50, 0.75, 0.90, and 1.00 are considered for d_i. Two statistics are considered, Wilcoxon's signed rank statistic and the statistic U868.[9]

Table 10.2 displays the upper bound on the one-sided P-value testing the null hypothesis of no effect, for three values of Γ. At $\Gamma = 4$, only U868 with $d_i = 0$ leads to rejection at the 0.05 level; that is, the least sensitive result is obtained by discarding the intermediate-dose pairs, as anticipated by theory. As one moves down any column in Table 10.2, the results become more sensitive to bias as more weight is given to the pairs with intermediate doses.

[9] Wilcoxon's signed rank statistic is Quade's statistic for pairs, $J = 2$. The statistic U868 is the default setting in the `wgtRank` function of the `weightedRank` package in R.

10.4 Design Sensitivity and Heterogeneity

In matched pairs, $J = 2$, consider two favorable models for a treatment effect in the absence of unmeasured biases, one with treated-minus-control pair differences in outcomes, $Y_i = (R_{i1} - R_{i2})(Z_{i1} - Z_{i2})$, $i = 1, \ldots, I$, that are independently drawn from a normal distribution with expectation τ and standard deviation σ, the other with pair differences $Y_i' = \left(R_{i1}' - R_{i2}'\right)(Z_{i1} - Z_{i2})$, $i = 1, \ldots, I'$, that are independently drawn from a normal distribution with expectation τ and standard deviation $\sigma' > \sigma$. If $I/I' = (\sigma/\sigma')^2$, then $\overline{Y} = I^{-1}\sum_{i=1}^{I} Y_i$ and $\overline{Y}' = (I')^{-1}\sum_{i=1}^{I'} Y_i'$ are both normally distributed with expectation τ and the same standard deviation $\sigma/\sqrt{I} = \sigma'/\sqrt{I'}$; so, to first appearances, there seems to be no reason to prefer the Y_i sample to the Y_i' sample. First appearances are misleading [28]: with common test statistics, the design sensitivity $\widetilde{\Gamma}$ for the Y_i sample is larger than the design sensitivity for the Y_i' sample; so, in that sense, Y_i is preferable to Y_i', even though $I < I'$. For example, using Wilcoxon's signed rank statistic, the design sensitivity [37, §16.2.4] for Y_i is

$$\widetilde{\Gamma} = \frac{\Phi\left(\sqrt{2}\frac{\tau}{\sigma}\right)}{1 - \Phi\left(\sqrt{2}\frac{\tau}{\sigma}\right)},$$

with an analogous formula for Y_i'. Notably, I does not enter into this formula for $\widetilde{\Gamma}$, but σ does; so, a smaller σ increases $\widetilde{\Gamma}$ even if purchased at the expense of a smaller sample. Table 10.3 shows how $\widetilde{\Gamma}$ varies with σ. Passing from σ to 0.9σ produces a meaningful increase in $\widetilde{\Gamma}$, while passing from σ to 0.5σ produces an enormous increase in $\widetilde{\Gamma}$, and these gains in $\widetilde{\Gamma}$ can occur despite a loss in sample size I needed to acquire more homogeneous pairs. Studies of twins or sibling pairs are familiar examples of trading a reduced sample size I for a decrease in heterogeneity σ, and there are many other ways to do this [37, §16.4].

Table 10.3 and similar tabulations for other distributions suggest the following strategy. Use some combination of techniques such as propensity scores, fine balance [25, 51], two-criteria matching [53], or cardinality matching [23] to balance covariates that must be balanced for an equitable comparison, but pair using a small subset of covariates highly predictive of the outcome to reduce heterogeneity of the

Table 10.3 In matched pairs, $J = 2$, design sensitivities, $\widetilde{\Gamma}$, for Wilcoxon's signed rank test applied to treated-minus-control matched-pair differences, $J = 2$, that are normal with expectation τ and standard deviation σ

σ	τ	
	1/2	1/3
1.00	3.17	2.14
0.90	3.63	2.33
0.75	4.78	2.78
0.50	11.71	4.78

pair differences Y_i. Pairing in two different ways the same balanced sample does not alter covariate balance, but it can alter the standard deviation of pair differences Y_i, thereby altering sensitivity to unmeasured biases [56].

10.5 Design Sensitivity and Multivariate Outcomes

It is common to have several outcomes, rather than one. For instance, in Sect. 1.5 and Fig. 1.8, there were three outcomes: diastolic and systolic blood pressure, plus their standardized combination. If several outcomes are all affected by the treatment in the same direction and to a similar degree, then a weighted combination of these outcomes may be more insensitive to bias than any one outcome is on its own; that is, the design sensitivity may be higher for the combination than for each of the components [27]. There are intermediate cases in which one outcome is more strongly affected than another outcome, so the best combination of outcomes has unequal weights attached to these outcomes. Indeed, a negative weight may increase design sensitivity if it is attached to an unaffected outcome that is positively correlated with an affected outcome [10, Table 4].

In a case study, Ting Ye and colleagues [50] consider three possible psychological outcomes of the physical abuse of children, namely, aggression, withdrawal, and depression. Although all three outcomes are elevated among abused children, depression as an isolated symptom is not characteristic of abuse, not specific to abuse; rather, aggression and withdrawal accompanied by depression are characteristic of abuse. After attending to issues of multiple testing, Ye and colleagues [50] find that insensitivity to unmeasured bias is greatest for a linear combination of outcomes that gives positive weight to aggression and withdrawal, and negative weight to depression, despite elevated rates of depression among abused children. Ye et al. [50, §7.3] conclude:

> A familiar clinical notion is "differential diagnosis." Which symptoms do the most to identify the cause? While depression may be elevated among abused children, . . . depression may have widely varied causes so that a comparison . . . emphasizing aggression may be more characteristic of abuse, more specific to abuse . . . In a sense, differential diagnosis and insensitivity to bias are opposite sides of the same coin: the more precisely we characterize the effect, the more strongly the effect so characterized tracks the cause, the more insensitive to bias is the association between cause and effect.

If several or many linear combinations of outcomes are examined, then one must control in some way for multiple testing. One approach uses a split sample: a small planning sample formulates a single combined outcome and the planning sample is discarded; then, that combined outcome is examined in a complementary, large analysis sample [10, 55]. A second approach uses Scheffé [21, 42] projections and looks at every linear combination of a few outcomes [34, 50]. Use of Scheffé projections secures the largest design sensitivity that can be produced by a linear combination of outcomes, and it has high power in large samples with two or three outcomes [50]. A third approach extends Scheffé's method by equitably sharing the correction for multiple testing between one linear combination of outcomes chosen a priori and examination of all possible linear combinations of outcomes [35, Proposition 2.1].[10]

Instead of combining outcomes, one may consider several outcomes with a correction for simultaneous testing. Colin Fogarty and Dylan Small [8] show that, with appropriate analysis, two or several uncombined outcomes may be less sensitive to bias than the outcomes would be if viewed one at a time, essentially because a single bias $\boldsymbol{\theta} \in B_\Gamma$ must explain all of the outcomes.

10.6 *Further Reading

The topic of this chapter is the focus of Part III of my book, *Design of Observational Studies*, where considerably more information may be found [37].

Effect modification: Effect modification means the magnitude or stability of a treatment effect varies predictably as a function of observed covariates. A larger or more stable treatment effect typically has a larger design sensitivity. Suppose that the treatment effect is larger or more stable in a subpopulation defined by measured covariates; then, rejection of the hypothesis of no treatment effect may be insensitive to larger unmeasured biases in that subpopulation [15]. If matching or blocking controls for a covariate that modifies the effect, then pairs or blocks at different levels of that covariate may be examined separately. Several methods exist for locating effect modifiers that affect sensitivity to unmeasured biases, while controlling for multiple testing [16, 19, 20].[11] Special forms of matching facilitate use of these methods [16,20]; so, it is best to plan the study in anticipation of a search for effect-modifiers.

Dose-response and design sensitivity: Sir Austin Bradford Hill [13] suggested that a dose-response relationship is a consideration relevant to a judgment about causality. Although five of Hill's considerations had been listed in the 1964 US Surgeon General's Report [2, Ch. 3, p. 20] *Smoking and Health*, the consideration of dose-response was not on the Surgeon General's list, and this consideration has remained controversial [41]. Arguably, the relevant question is whether a dose-response relationship increases insensitivity to unmeasured biases [26], or more precisely whether it increases the design sensitivity. Somewhat in parallel to Noether's [24] statistic for matched pair differences without doses, a nonparametric correlation measure called the cross-cut statistic dramatically increases design sensitivity by discarding intermediate doses, focusing instead on high and low doses [33, Table 3].[12] For example, a cross-cut statistic can have a design sensitivity of $\widetilde{\Gamma} = 32.1$ when computed from

[10] The methods in this paragraph are implemented in the `sensitivitymult` package in R.

[11] The method of Kwonsang Lee and colleagues [20] is implemented in the R package `submax`.

[12] The cross-cut statistic is implemented as `crosscut` and `crosscutplot` in the R package `DOS2`.

a normal distribution with correlation 0.3. The cross-cut statistic can be used with multiple cuts in adaptive inference [40, §6].

Zhang, Small, and Heng [54] develop an alternative approach to sensitivity analysis with doses of treatment.

Other considerations that affect design sensitivity: Many aspects of study design alter the design sensitivity [37, Part III], including (i) the definition of a case in a case-control study [44] or a case-case study [3], (ii) clustering of treatment assignments, when whole schools or whole medical practices are assigned to treatment or control [9,52], and (iii) the strength and strengthening of instruments or instrumental variables [1,7,11,12,45,57]. For an application of instrument strengthening, see the article by Mark Neuman and colleagues [22, Fig. 2].

Problems

10.1 Simulating the Influence of Heterogeneity on Design Sensitivity
In parallel with Sect. 10.4, in R, simulate I observations from a normal distribution with expectation $1/2$ and standard deviation $1/2$ and also $4I$ observations from a normal distribution with expectation $1/2$ and standard deviation 1; so, in both cases the variance of the mean pair difference is $1/(4I)$. Do this for $I = 100$. View your simulated samples as I or $4I$ treated-minus-control matched pair differences Y_i in a favorable situation; so, the treatment effect is 1/2 and there is no bias in treatment assignment. Now, use the `senWilcox` function in the `DOS2` package to do a sensitivity analysis for these two samples from two favorable situations, using Wilcoxon's signed rank statistic at $\Gamma = 3.3$. Compare the two upper bounds on the P-value testing the hypothesis of no treatment effect. Repeat the analysis with several values of Γ.

10.2 Design Sensitivity Refers to the Limit as $I \to \infty$
Repeat Problem 10.1 but with $I = 1000$ rather than $I = 100$. Repeat Problem 10.1 but with $I = 10000$ rather than $I = 100$.

10.3 Reduced Heterogeneity Combined with a Test Statistic with a Larger Design Sensitivity
Use the simulated data from Problem 10.2 with $I = 1000$, but replace Wilcoxon's signed rank test by the U-statistic U878, by replacing `senWilcox` by `senU`, which is also in the `DOS2` package. Perform the sensitivity analysis with $\Gamma = 3.3$, 6, and 10. Discuss the combined effect of reduced heterogeneity and a test statistic with a larger design sensitivity.

References

1. Baiocchi, M., Small, D.S., Lorch, S., Rosenbaum, P.R.: Building a stronger instrument in an observational study of perinatal care for premature infants. J. Am. Stat. Assoc. **105**(492), 1285–1296 (2010)
2. Bayne-Jones, S., Burdette, W.J., Cochran, W.G., Farber, E., Fieser, L., Furth, J., Hickam, J.B., LeMaistre, C., Schuman, L.M., Seevers, M.H.: Smoking and Health: Report of the Advisory Committee to the US Surgeon General. Public Health Service, US Government Printing Service, Washington, DC (1964). Reprinted by: D. Van Nostrand Company, Princeton, NJ. Page references are to this edition.
3. Chen, K., Ye, T., Small, D.S.: Sensitivity analysis for attributable effects in case^2 studies. Preprint arXiv:2405.16046 (2024)
4. Cornfield, J., Haenszel, W., Hammond, E.C., Lilienfeld, A.M., Shimkin, M.B., Wynder, E.L.: Smoking and lung cancer: Recent evidence and a discussion of some questions. J. Natl. Cancer Inst. **22**(1), 173–203 (1959)
5. David, H.A., Nagaraja, H.N.: Order Statistics, 3rd edn. John Wiley & Sons, New York (2003)
6. van Eeden, C.: An analogue, for signed rank statistics, of Jureckova's asymptotic linearity theorem for rank statistics. Ann. Math. Stat. **43**(3), 791–802 (1972)
7. Ertefaie, A., Small, D.S., Rosenbaum, P.R.: Quantitative evaluation of the trade-off of strengthened instruments and sample size in observational studies. J. Am. Stat. Assoc. **113**(523), 1122–1134 (2018)
8. Fogarty, C.B., Small, D.S.: Sensitivity analysis for multiple comparisons in matched observational studies through quadratically constrained linear programming. J. Am. Stat. Assoc. **111**(516), 1820–1830 (2016)
9. Hansen, B.B., Rosenbaum, P.R., Small, D.S.: Clustered treatment assignments and sensitivity to unmeasured biases in observational studies. J. Am. Stat. Assoc. **109**(505), 133–144 (2014)
10. Heller, R., Rosenbaum, P.R., Small, D.S.: Split samples and design sensitivity in observational studies. J. Am. Stat. Assoc. **104**(487), 1090–1101 (2009)
11. Heng, S., Small, D.S., Rosenbaum, P.R.: Finding the strength in a weak instrument in a study of cognitive outcomes produced by Catholic high schools. J. Roy. Stat. Soc. Ser. A **183**(3), 935–958 (2020)
12. Heng, S., Zhang, B., Han, X., Lorch, S.A., Small, D.S.: Instrumental variables: To strengthen or not to strengthen? J. Roy. Stat. Soc. Ser. A **186**(4), 852–873 (2023)
13. Hill, A.B.: The environment and disease: Association or causation? Proceedings of the Royal Society of Medicine **58**, 295–300 (1965)
14. Hodges, J., Lehmann, E.: Estimates of location based on rank tests. Ann. Math. Stat. **34**(2), 598–611 (1963)
15. Hsu, J., Small, D., Rosenbaum, P.R.: Effect modification and design sensitivity in observational studies. J. Am. Stat. Assoc. **108**(501), 135–148 (2013)
16. Hsu, J., Zubizarreta, J.R., Small, D., Rosenbaum, P.R.: Strong control of the familywise error rate in observational studies that discover effect modification by exploratory methods. Biometrika **102**(4), 767–782 (2015)
17. Hudgens, M.G., Halloran, M.E.: Toward causal inference with interference. J. Am. Stat. Assoc. **103**(482), 832–842 (2008)
18. Karmakar, B., Small, D.S., Rosenbaum, P.R.: Using evidence factors to clarify exposure biomarkers. Am. J. Epidemiol. **189**(3), 243–249 (2020)
19. Lee, K., Small, D.S., Hsu, J.Y., Silber, J.H., Rosenbaum, P.R.: Discovering effect modification in an observational study of surgical mortality at hospitals with superior nursing. J. Roy. Stat. Soc. Ser. A: Stat. Soc. **181**(2), 535–546 (2018)
20. Lee, K., Small, D.S., Rosenbaum, P.R.: A powerful approach to the study of moderate effect modification in observational studies. Biometrics **74**(4), 1161–1170 (2018)
21. Miller, R.G.: Simultaneous Statistical Inference. Springer, New York (1981)
22. Neuman, M.D., Rosenbaum, P.R., Ludwig, J.M., Zubizarreta, J.R., Silber, J.H.: Anesthesia technique, mortality, and length of stay after hip fracture surgery. J. Am. Med. Assoc. **311**(24), 2508–2517 (2014)

23. Niknam, B.A., Zubizarreta, J.R.: Using cardinality matching to design balanced and representative samples for observational studies. J. Am. Med. Assoc. **327**(2), 173–174 (2022)
24. Noether, G.E.: Some simple distribution-free confidence intervals for the center of a symmetric distribution. J. Am. Stat. Assoc. **68**(343), 716–719 (1973)
25. Pimentel, S.D., Kelz, R.R., Silber, J.H., Rosenbaum, P.R.: Large, sparse optimal matching with refined covariate balance in an observational study of the health outcomes produced by new surgeons. J. Am. Stat. Assoc. **110**(510), 515–527 (2015)
26. Rosenbaum, P.R.: Does a dose–response relationship reduce sensitivity to hidden bias? Biostatistics **4**(1), 1–10 (2003)
27. Rosenbaum, P.R.: Design sensitivity in observational studies. Biometrika **91**(1), 153–164 (2004)
28. Rosenbaum, P.R.: Heterogeneity and causality: Unit heterogeneity and design sensitivity in observational studies. Am. Stat. **59**(2), 147–152 (2005)
29. Rosenbaum, P.R.: Interference between units in randomized experiments. J. Am. Stat. Assoc. **102**(477), 191–200 (2007)
30. Rosenbaum, P.R.: Testing one hypothesis twice in observational studies. Biometrika **99**(4), 763–774 (2012)
31. Rosenbaum, P.R.: Impact of multiple matched controls on design sensitivity in observational studies. Biometrics **69**(1), 118–127 (2013)
32. Rosenbaum, P.R.: Weighted M-statistics with superior design sensitivity in matched observational studies with multiple controls. J. Am. Stat. Assoc. **109**(507), 1145–1158 (2014)
33. Rosenbaum, P.R.: The cross-cut statistic and its sensitivity to bias in observational studies with ordered doses of treatment. Biometrics **72**(1), 175–183 (2016)
34. Rosenbaum, P.R.: Using Scheffé projections for multiple outcomes in an observational study of smoking and periodontal disease. Ann. Appl. Stat. **10**, 1447–1471 (2016)
35. Rosenbaum, P.R.: Combining planned and discovered comparisons in observational studies. Biostatistics **21**(3), 384–399 (2020)
36. Rosenbaum, P.R.: A conditional test with demonstrated insensitivity to unmeasured bias in matched observational studies. Biometrika **107**(4), 827–840 (2020)
37. Rosenbaum, P.R.: Design of Observational Studies, 2nd edn. Springer, New York (2020)
38. Rosenbaum, P.R.: A statistic with demonstrated insensitivity to unmeasured bias for 2× 2× S tables in observational studies. Stat. Med. **41**(19), 3758–3771 (2022)
39. Rosenbaum, P.R.: Bahadur efficiency of observational block designs. J. Am. Stat. Assoc. **119**(547), 1871–1881 (2024)
40. Rosenbaum, P.R., Small, D.S.: An adaptive Mantel–Haenszel test for sensitivity analysis in observational studies. Biometrics **73**(2), 422–430 (2017)
41. Rothman, K.J., Greenland, S.: Causation and causal inference in epidemiology. Am. J. Public Health **95**(S1), S144–S150 (2005)
42. Scheffé, H.: A method for judging all contrasts in the analysis of variance. Biometrika **40**(1-2), 87–110 (1953)
43. Sen, P.K.: A note on order statistics for heterogeneous distributions. Ann. Math. Stat. **41**(6), 2137–2139 (1970)
44. Small, D.S., Cheng, J., Halloran, M.E., Rosenbaum, P.R.: Case definition and design sensitivity. J. Am. Stat. Assoc. **108**(504), 1457–1468 (2013)
45. Small, D.S., Rosenbaum, P.R.: War and wages: The strength of instrumental variables and their sensitivity to unobserved biases. J. Am. Stat. Assoc. **103**(483), 924–933 (2008)
46. Sobel, M.E.: What do randomized studies of housing mobility demonstrate? Causal inference in the face of interference. J. Am. Stat. Assoc. **101**(476), 1398–1407 (2006)
47. Tardif, S.: Efficiency and optimality results for tests based on weighted rankings. J. Am. Stat. Assoc. **82**(398), 637–644 (1987)
48. Tchetgen-Tchetgen, E.J., VanderWeele, T.J.: On causal inference in the presence of interference. Stat. Methods Med. Res. **21**(1), 55–75 (2012)
49. Weiss, N.S.: Inferring causal relationships: elaboration of the criterion of "dose-response". Am. J. Epidemiol. **113**(5), 487–490 (1981)

50. Ye, T., Small, D.S., Rosenbaum, P.R.: Dimensions, power and factors in an observational study of behavioral problems after physical abuse of children. Ann. Appl. Stat. **16**(4), 2732–2754 (2022)
51. Yu, R.: How well can fine balance work for covariate balancing? Biometrics **79**, 2346–2356 (2023)
52. Zhang, B., Heng, S., MacKay, E.J., Ye, T.: Bridging preference-based instrumental variable studies and cluster-randomized encouragement experiments: study design, noncompliance, and average cluster effect ratio. Biometrics **78**(4), 1639–1650 (2022)
53. Zhang, B., Small, D.S., Lasater, K.B., McHugh, M., Silber, J.H., Rosenbaum, P.R.: Matching one sample according to two criteria in observational studies. J. Am. Stat. Assoc. **118**, 1140–1151 (2022)
54. Zhang, J., Small, D.S., Heng, S.: Sensitivity analysis for matched observational studies with continuous exposures and binary outcomes. Biometrika **111**(4), 1349–1368 (2024)
55. Zhang, K., Small, D.S., Lorch, S., Srinivas, S., Rosenbaum, P.R.: Using split samples and evidence factors in an observational study of neonatal outcomes. J. Am. Stat. Assoc. **106**(494), 511–524 (2011)
56. Zubizarreta, J.R., Paredes, R.D., Rosenbaum, P.R.: Matching for balance, pairing for heterogeneity in an observational study of the effectiveness of for-profit and not-for-profit high schools in Chile. Ann. Appl. Stat. **8**(1), 204–231 (2014)
57. Zubizarreta, J.R., Small, D.S., Goyal, N.K., Lorch, S., Rosenbaum, P.R.: Stronger instruments via integer programming in an observational study of late preterm birth outcomes. Ann. Appl. Stat. **7**, 25–50 (2013)

Chapter 11
Efficiency of Sensitivity Analyses

Abstract Design sensitivity, $\widetilde{\Gamma}$, governs the performance of a sensitivity analysis in the limit as the sample size increases, $I \longrightarrow \infty$. In samples of moderate size, a sensitivity analysis may terminate at a Γ well below $\widetilde{\Gamma}$ due to sampling variability. The Bahadur efficiency of a sensitivity analysis compares the performance of two statistics at a Γ below the minimum of their two design sensitivities. The Bahadur slope of a test statistic drops to zero as Γ increases to $\widetilde{\Gamma}$. The best statistic in a randomization test—a test at $\Gamma = 1$—is often different from the best statistic for larger Γ, and the Bahadur relative efficiency provides insight into performance at intermediate values of Γ.

11.1 Design Sensitivity and Efficiency

Design Sensitivity Governs in Large Samples, But What About Smaller Samples?

In Chaps. 9 and 10, we saw that the upper bound on a P-value in a sensitivity analysis tends to zero as the sample size increases, $I \longrightarrow \infty$, if the sensitivity analysis is performed at Γ below the design sensitivity, $\widetilde{\Gamma}$, and it tends to one if $\Gamma > \widetilde{\Gamma}$. We also saw that $\widetilde{\Gamma}$ was strongly affected by the choice of study design and analytical methods; poor choices make $\widetilde{\Gamma}$ smaller. An investigator whose observational study is sensitive to small unmeasured biases may think this is an attribute of the treatment under study, not realizing that it is instead a consequence of mistakes in study design and analysis.

© The Author(s), under exclusive license to Springer Nature Switzerland AG 2025

P. R. Rosenbaum, *An Introduction to the Theory of Observational Studies*, Springer Texts in Statistics, https://doi.org/10.1007/978-3-031-90494-3_11

An important limitation of design sensitivity was noted at the end of Sect. 9.3. A bias is of constant size (or more precisely of "order 1") if it does not diminish as the sample size increases, $I \to \infty$.[1] The biases in observational studies are of constant size. Observational studies simultaneously face both biases of constant size and standard errors of order $1/\sqrt{I}$, so for large enough I, the bias is more important than the standard error; however, this is not entirely realistic for any finite I.

For large enough I, the design sensitivity $\widetilde{\Gamma}$ is a good guide in observational studies and the standard error is a poor guide. In truth, however, for finite I, we should pay attention to both the bias and the standard error, paying more and more attention to bias as $I \to \infty$, because the standard error is less and less of a problem as $I \to \infty$. To do this, we need to make small adjustments to the intuition we have built up when solving problems that are free of biases of constant size. The Bahadur efficiency of a sensitivity analysis is a useful tool here: it views design sensitivity through a telephoto lens, so that the bias and the standard error are simultaneously visible. As will be seen, the Bahadur efficiency drops to zero as $\Gamma \to \widetilde{\Gamma}$, so the telephoto lens provided by Bahadur efficiency and the wide-angle lens provided by design sensitivity depict the same landscape at different magnifications.

In simpler but less useful terms, if an estimator $\widehat{\tau}$ of a parameter τ has expectation $\mathrm{E}(\widehat{\tau}) = \overline{\tau}$ and variance ς^2/I, then $\widehat{\tau}$ has mean squared error (MSE):

$$\mathrm{E}\left\{(\widehat{\tau} - \tau)^2\right\} = \frac{\varsigma^2}{I} + (\overline{\tau} - \tau)^2 \,; \tag{11.1}$$

see Problem 11.1. If $\overline{\tau} \neq \tau$ and $\varsigma^2 > 0$, then for large enough I the squared bias $(\overline{\tau} - \tau)^2$ overwhelms the variance ς^2/I in (11.1). Although the contrast between a term of constant size, such as $\overline{\tau} - \tau$, and a standard error of order $1/\sqrt{I}$, such as $\varsigma/\sqrt{I}$, is clearly evident in (11.1), there are reasons to avoid using (11.1) as a guide to thinking about bias in observational studies, and these issues are summarized in the next optional subsection.

*Is the Mean Squared Error Helpful in Observational Studies?

Why is the mean squared error (11.1) inadequate as a guide to unmeasured biases in observational studies? There are several reasons.

First, treatment assignment plays no obvious role in (11.1), yet causal inference is challenging in observational studies because treatments were not randomly assigned.

[1] In various technical problems in statistics, there are biases that diminish with increasing sample sizes: a consistent estimator need not be an unbiased estimator. The consequences of a bias that diminishes as $I \to \infty$ vary depending upon how quickly the bias diminishes as I increases. Often, a bias that is of order $1/I$ is inconsequential, because the standard error is of order $1/\sqrt{I}$ and so it tends to be much larger than the bias for large I. All of this is a bit of a distraction in an observational study, where there is nothing to make biases smaller as the sample becomes larger. To avoid this distraction, I speak of a constant bias or a bias of constant size, rather than the more traditional bias of order 1.

Perhaps (11.1) has not quite discarded the baby with the bath water, but the baby's location is certainly obscure in (11.1).

Second, τ is not known. If unmeasured biases in treatment assignment are possible in an observational study—and unmeasured biases are *always* possible, if not likely, in an observational study—then τ is not identified and there is no consistent estimate of τ. In light of this, focusing on (11.1) might lead us to passively regret the fact that association does not imply causation in observational studies, because the bias is $\overline{\tau} - \tau$ and we have no consistent estimate of τ. Instead, we should take active and potentially constructive steps to distinguish meaningful treatment effects τ from nontrivial departures from randomized treatment assignment, Γ. This active strategy can work, has worked [8], and can be guided by statistical theory to work better.

11.2 Review of Relative Efficiency and Asymptotic Relative Efficiency

Relative Efficiency

Suppose that the null hypothesis, H_0, asserts that the I observations were independently sampled from a distribution $F(\cdot)$ and the alternative hypothesis, H_1, asserts that the distribution was $G(\cdot)$, not $F(\cdot)$. There are two test statistics, say T_I computed from I observations, and $T'_{I'}$ computed from I' observations. How can we make an equitable quantitative comparison of T_I and $T'_{I'}$? For this, we need both a concept of an equitable comparison and some quantitative unit of measure of relative performance.

For an equitable comparison, it seems natural to ask T_I and $T'_{I'}$ to do the same thing, accomplish the same task, and run the same race. In testing hypotheses, the same task consists of (i) having the same size, α, so that both tests reject H_0 when H_0 is true with probability α and (ii) having the same power, ϖ, so that both tests reject H_0 when H_1 is true with probability ϖ.

A test or test statistic, T_I, of H_0 against H_1 is said to be consistent if, for each $\alpha > 0$, the power ϖ tends to 1 as $I \to \infty$; otherwise, the test is inconsistent. If T_I is consistent but $T'_{I'}$ is inconsistent, that does seem to settle the matter: use T_I.[2] Having settled that situation, let us continue under the assumption that T_I and $T'_{I'}$ are both consistent.

With α, ϖ, $F(\cdot)$, and $G(\cdot)$ specified, it is possible in principle to determine the smallest sample size I such that T_I has size α and power $\geq \varpi$ in a test of $F(\cdot)$

[2] There are issues even with this seemingly mild statement. In a sensitivity analysis done at Γ, if T_I has design sensitivity $\widetilde{\Gamma}$ and T_I' has design sensitivity $\widetilde{\Gamma}'$, where $\widetilde{\Gamma} > \Gamma > \widetilde{\Gamma}'$, then this argument says to use T_I. That is correct only in sufficiently large samples, because we typically perform a sequence of sensitivity analyses for an increasing sequence of Γ's, stopping with the first Γ that leads to acceptance [26]. For this sequence, the relative performance of T_I and T_I' at smaller values of Γ matters too. It may be that T_I' has more power than T_I at $\Gamma^{\dagger} < \widetilde{\Gamma}'$ even though T_I' is inconsistent at $\Gamma > \widetilde{\Gamma}'$.

against $G(\cdot)$, and similarly the smallest sample size I' such that $T'_{I'}$ has size α and power $\geq \varpi$ in a test of $F(\cdot)$ against $G(\cdot)$. If $I < I'$, then T_I has won its race with $T'_{I'}$: it has accomplished the same task with fewer observations. If $I/I' = 1/2$, then T_I required half as much data to do the same task as $T'_{I'}$; so, T_I is twice as efficient as $T'_{I'}$ with $I'/I = 2$.

For example, in his nonparametric textbook, Erich Lehmann [17, §4.3] compared the efficiency of Wilcoxon's signed rank test, T_I, and the t-test, $T'_{I'}$, when $F(\cdot) = \Phi(\cdot)$ is a standard normal cumulative distribution with expectation 0 and variance one, and $G(\cdot)$ is a normal distribution with expectation τ and variance one; so, $G(y) = \Phi(y - \tau)$. The t-test has certain optimal properties in this case, so we expect to need a larger sample size I for the Wilcoxon test than for the t-test, $I/I' > 1$ and an efficiency of the Wilcoxon test relative to the t-test that is less than one, $I'/I < 1$. Lehmann [17, Table 4.4] then specifies a wide variety of sizes, α; powers, ϖ; and effects, τ, and for each combination (α, ϖ, τ) he calculates (I, I') obtaining the following relative efficiencies I'/I: 0.968, 0.967, 0.966, 0.965, 0.965, 0.964, 0.960, 0.959 0.957, 0.956, and 0.955. Lehmann makes two observations. First, although (α, ϖ, τ) vary widely, the relative efficiency I'/I is quite stable, hinting that, perhaps, I'/I is tending to some sort of limit that is not acutely dependent on all the details in (α, ϖ, τ). Second, with the deck stacked in favor of the t-test, the t-test does win but not by much. Once the concept of a limit is clarified in a certain way,[3] it turns out that the Wilcoxon test is more efficient than the t-test when the deck is not stacked in favor of the t-test, with I'/I near 1.1 when $F(\cdot)$ is a logistic distribution, or near 1.5 when $F(\cdot)$ is a double-exponential distribution [25, Table 5.4.7]. If $F(\cdot)$ is the $\epsilon \geq 0$ contaminated normal distribution comprised of a standard normal observation with probability $1 - \epsilon$ or a normal observation with standard deviation 3 with probability ϵ—that is, if $F(y) = (1 - \epsilon)\,\Phi(y) + \epsilon\,\Phi(y/3)$ and $G(y) = F(y - \tau)$—then the relative efficiency I'/I is close to 1 for $\epsilon = 0.01$, close to 1.1 for $\epsilon = 0.03$, close to 1.2 for $\epsilon = 0.05$, and close to 1.5 for $\epsilon = 0.15$ [14, Table 2.3]. Stated informally, if $I'/I = 1.5$, then the Wilcoxon test can accomplish with $I = 100$ observations what the t-test needs $I' = 150$ observations to accomplish.

Asymptotic Relative Efficiency

As Lehmann [17, Table 4.4] observed when comparing the Wilcoxon test and the t-test, for a wide variety of values of (α, ϖ, τ), the finite sample relative efficiency, I'/I, is almost constant. If I'/I approached a limit in large samples and if that limit did not depend upon (α, ϖ, τ), then that would be very convenient: we could compare T_I and $T'_{I'}$ once and for all using the limit, without much attention to all the details in (α, ϖ, τ). Alas, the situation is not quite that convenient.

The two sample sizes, I and I', typically increase if the effect size decreases, $\tau \to 0$, or if the size of the test decreases, $\alpha \to 0$, or if the power increases, $\varpi \to 1$,

[3] Clarified in the sense of Pitman efficiency, as discussed soon

or if both $\alpha \longrightarrow 0$ and $\varpi \longrightarrow 1$. If the ratio I'/I tends to a limit, then that limit is the asymptotic relative efficiency or ARE [33, Ch. 10], where Pitman [21] efficiency lets $\tau \longrightarrow 0$, Bahadur [1,2] efficiency lets $\alpha \longrightarrow 0$, Hodges-Lehmann [15] efficiency lets $\varpi \longrightarrow 1$, and Chernoff [7] efficiency lets $\alpha \longrightarrow 0$ and $\varpi \longrightarrow 1$. For reviews of asymptotic relative efficiency, see Groeneboom and Oosterhoff [11,12], Nikitin [20] and Serfling [33, Ch. 10]. The material in Sect. 11.2 is standard and is adapted from these reviews.

By far, the most widely used measure of asymptotic relative efficiency is Pitman efficiency, in which I'/I may tend to a limit as $\tau \longrightarrow 0$. The limiting comparisons of I'/I quoted in the previous section were Pitman efficiencies.

Pitman efficiency is less useful in observational studies than in randomized experiments. Every small treatment effect is sensitive to small biases: letting $\tau \longrightarrow 0$ typically entails $\widetilde{\Gamma} \longrightarrow 1$. A study with an infinitesimal treatment effect is sensitive to an infinitesimal departure from randomized treatment assignment. Somewhat more precisely, in a favorable situation, with a treatment effect and no unmeasured bias in treatment assignment, $\boldsymbol{\theta} = \overline{\boldsymbol{\theta}}$, as the treatment effect becomes smaller, the study becomes sensitive to smaller biases, and the design sensitivity, $\widetilde{\Gamma}$, declines to 1.

In truth, we have no real interest in infinitesimal treatment effects; rather, we wish to distinguish meaningful treatment effects from nontrivial biases in treatment assignment. If every observational study ever conducted of an infinitesimal treatment effect had failed to provide firm evidence of a nonzero effect, then the total absolute error over this finite list of studies would be infinitesimally small. Our concern is, or should be, to recognize treatment effects of meaningful size and to design observational studies so that such effects cannot easily be attributed to small or moderate biases in treatment assignment.

Again, Bahadur efficiency determines the limit of I'/I as $\alpha \longrightarrow 0$ for fixed τ and ϖ; so, unlike Pitman efficiency, it does not direct attention to situations that are inevitably sensitive to small biases, $\widetilde{\Gamma} \doteq 1$.

Bahadur Asymptotic Relative Efficiency

Fix τ and ϖ, and let α_I be the size of the test of the test of H_0 against H_1 when the sample size is I. So, α_I is a number computed from properties of the statistic T_I under the distributions $F(\cdot)$ and $G(\cdot)$. Now, imagine an infinite sequence of independent observations drawn from $G(\cdot)$, where the first I observations are used to compute the P-value, say P_I, using T_I to test H_0 against H_1. At the risk of belaboring the point: α_I, $I = 1, 2, \ldots$ is a sequence of real numbers, whereas P_I, $I = 1, 2, \ldots$ is a sequence of random variables.

Perhaps surprisingly, as $I \to \infty$, under mild conditions, two quantities derived from α_I and P_I converge in appropriate senses to the same constant:

$$-\frac{2}{I}\log(\alpha_I) \to b \tag{11.2}$$

$$-\frac{2}{I}\log(P_I) \to b, \tag{11.3}$$

where the constant b is called the Bahadur [1, 2] slope. The convergence in (11.2) refers to an ordinary limit in the sense of calculus. The convergence in (11.3) may be either convergence in probability, in which case b is called the weak Bahadur slope, or convergence with probability one, in which case b is called the strong Bahadur slope. A strong Bahadur slope is a promise about the infinite sequence $P_1, P_2, \ldots$, saying the sequence exhibits the convergence (11.3) with probability one, whereas a weak Bahadur slope is a promise about what will be approximately true with high probability in one sample of size I, providing I is large enough.

In typical cases, b does not depend upon the power, ϖ for $0 < \varpi < 1$. This is part of what makes (11.2) and (11.3) surprising: (11.2) is a sequence of constants that depend upon ϖ, and (11.3) makes no explicit mention of ϖ; yet, the transformed constants and the transformed random variables converge to the same limit, b. For discussion of the relationship between (11.2) and (11.3), see Raghavachari [24, Theorem 2] and Groeneboom and Oosterhoff [12, p. 136].

Informally rearranging (11.2) and (11.3) yields

$$\alpha_I \approx \exp(-bI/2) \text{ and } P_I \approx \exp(-bI/2),$$

saying that α_I and P_I are declining to zero as $I \to \infty$ at an exponential rate determined by b. Informally rearranging (11.2) in a different way gives $I \approx -\frac{2}{b}\log(\alpha_I)$, which is half of what is needed for a calculation of relative efficiency. These informal rearrangements motivate a formal definition.

Suppose that a second test statistic, $T'_{I'}$, has Bahadur slope b' when testing H_0 against H_1. Then the Bahadur asymptotic relative efficiency of T_I versus $T'_{I'}$ is defined to be b/b'. The ratio may be understood in several ways: (i) a comparison of the rates at which the P-values decline to zero; (ii) a comparison of the rates at which the sizes, α_I, tend to zero; and (iii) the limiting ratio of the sample sizes, I'/I, needed to achieve the same power and size.

The calculation of a Bahadur slope involves what are called "large-deviation probabilities"; however, in their statistical applications, these might more naturally be called probabilities of fixed deviations in large samples. Consider independent observations, $W_1, W_2, \ldots$, from the same distribution with expectation zero and variance one. Suppose that we asked: What is the probability that the mean, $I^{-1}\sum_i^I W_i$, of the first I independent observations is greater than 1/2? As $I \to \infty$, that is question about a "large-deviation probability," and theorems about large deviations refer to the rate at which such probabilities decline to zero with increasing I. For the simplest large deviation theorem for binomial probabilities, see Feller [10, §7.6]. Taking account of a few details, these rates are Bahadur slopes. There are a number of such large deviation results for the mean of independent and identically distributed random variables, but they are not very helpful for the problems discussed in this book. More helpful are several results involving the moment generating function of T_I and its limiting behavior, specifically Sievers' [35] theorem and its extensions [18, 22, 23]. For a concise summary, see Groeneboom and Oosterhoff [11, Theorem 3.2].

Bahadur Relative Efficiency of a Sensitivity Analysis

A sensitivity analysis is actually a test of a composite null hypothesis, such as (i) $H_0 : \boldsymbol{\delta} = \mathbf{0}$ with $\boldsymbol{\theta} \in B_\Gamma$, or (ii) $H_0 : \boldsymbol{\delta} = \tau_0 \mathbf{1}$ with $\boldsymbol{\theta} \in B_\Gamma$ for fixed τ_0 or (iii) $H_0 : \boldsymbol{\delta} = \boldsymbol{\delta}_0$ with $\boldsymbol{\theta} \in B_\Gamma$ for fixed $\boldsymbol{\delta}_0$. It is a composite hypothesis whose component simple null hypotheses fix a particular $\boldsymbol{\theta} \in B_\Gamma$. As such, the main elements of Bahadur efficiency do not require substantial changes. Rejection of the null hypothesis occurs if each component is rejected, that is, if the upper bound on the P-value is sufficiently small. A Bahadur slope b refers to the rate at which the upper bound on the P-value declines to zero for a fixed $\Gamma < \widetilde{\Gamma}$.

The matched paired case, $J = 2$, is simplest. In this case, the upper bound on the P-value is determined at a single $\boldsymbol{\theta} \in B_\Gamma$, namely, (8.20). Under H_0, the I pairs are independent, and each pair contributes a random quantity that can take two possible values with probabilities determined by (8.20), so it is straightforward to determine the moment generating function; see Problem 11.3. One must verify that the moment generating function has certain limits as $I \to \infty$ and that these limits satisfy certain regularity conditions. Also needed is the limiting expectation of the test statistic in the favorable situation, with a treatment effect and no bias in treatment assignment, $\boldsymbol{\theta} = \overline{\boldsymbol{\theta}}$. Although there are a few details [29], the calculation of the Bahadur slope of a sensitivity analysis is essentially an application of Sievers' [35] theorem and its extensions [18, 22, 23].

The case of blocks larger than pairs, $J > 2$, adds an additional technical issue, namely, that there is no single $\boldsymbol{\theta} \in B_\Gamma$ that is fixed a priori that yields a stochastically largest distribution for a weighted rank statistic, T_I, such as Quade's statistic. In the end, this is not a big problem. However, it does take an additional step involving the separable approximation in Definition 8.1 to realize that this is not a big problem [30, Remark 4]. Essentially, the moment generating function is evaluated at the $\boldsymbol{\theta} \in B_\Gamma$ determined by the separable approximation and, after that, things proceed as in the paired case [31].

11.3 The Relative Efficiency of Competing Sensitivity Analyses

Comparing Competing Test Statistics

Table 11.1 compares the relative efficiency of the four statistics used in an example in Table 8.1. Instead of comparing the performance of statistics in an example, where the true situation is unknown, Table 11.1 compares performance under a model in which the true situation is known. This is one important use of models: to compare the performance of statistical procedures under a variety of known conditions—see "Tukey's Advice about Assumptions" in Sect. 2.8.

Table 11.1 compares four favorable situations, that is, four block models (9.9) with no bias in treatment assignment. In Table 11.1, a treatment effect shifts a treated-minus-control pair difference by $\tau = \frac{1}{2}$ or $\tau = \frac{1}{3}$ times the standard deviation of that pair difference, with errors that are either from the normal distribution or a t-distribution with 5 degrees of freedom. The block size in Table 11.1 is $J = 4$, but analogous tables for other block sizes and other favorable situations are available [31]. For each favorable situation, for each statistic, Table 11.1 gives the design sensitivity, $\widetilde{\Gamma}$, and a Bahadur relative efficiency for several values of Γ. The denominator for the Bahadur relative efficiency is the statistic U868, so the column for U868 is always 1.000.[4]

Table 11.1 Bahadur efficiency relative to U868 in sensitivity analyses performed with $\Gamma = 1, 1.5, 2, 3$ and 4 for blocks of size $J = 4$. The treatment effect is τ times the standard deviation of a matched pair difference. The Bahadur slope tends to 0 as $\Gamma \to \widetilde{\Gamma}$ and relative efficiency tends to 0 (or possibly to 0/0) . The best result in each favorable situation is in **bold**

		Normal errors				t_5 errors			
		Wilcoxon	Quade	U868	U878	Wilcoxon	Quade	U868	U878
					$\tau = 1/2$				
Γ	$\widetilde{\Gamma}$	3.5	4.4	5.2	**5.7**	4.0	4.7	5.1	**5.2**
1		1.08	**1.21**	1.00	0.85	**1.38**	1.35	1.00	0.77
1.5		0.83	**1.11**	1.00	0.89	1.19	**1.29**	1.00	0.78
2		0.58	**1.01**	1.00	0.93	1.00	**1.23**	1.00	0.79
3		0.15	0.76	1.00	**1.04**	0.56	**1.07**	1.00	0.81
4		0.00	0.23	1.00	**1.41**	0.00	0.65	**1.00**	0.89
					$\tau = 1/3$				
Γ	$\widetilde{\Gamma}$	2.3	2.8	3.2	**3.5**	2.6	3.0	**3.2**	**3.2**
1		1.06	**1.20**	1.00	0.86	**1.36**	1.34	1.00	0.77
1.5		0.64	**1.03**	1.00	0.92	1.05	**1.24**	1.00	0.79
2		0.16	0.77	1.00	**1.05**	0.58	**1.07**	1.00	0.81
3		0.00	0.00	1.00	**3.09**	0.00	0.00	1.00	**1.20**

[4] In calculating relative efficiencies, it is important that the statistic T' in the denominator have reasonably high design sensitivity, because the Bahadur slope approaches 0 as Γ increases to $\widetilde{\Gamma}$: a relative efficiency of $0/b'$ is interpretable if $b' > 0$, but a relative efficiency of $0/0$ tells us little. The statistic U868 is the default option in the `wgtRank` function in the `weightedRank` package in R.

Table 11.1 tells us much more than we learned from the design sensitivity alone. The statistic U878 has the largest design sensitivity, $\widetilde{\Gamma}$, in all situations, and that is good advice for Γ near $\widetilde{\Gamma}$, but U878 is never best in Table 11.1 for randomization tests, $\Gamma = 1$, or for a sensitivity analysis performed at $\Gamma = 1.5$. For $\tau = \frac{1}{3}$ with normal errors, U878 has design sensitivity $\widetilde{\Gamma} = 3.5$ and a relative efficiency of 3.09 compared to U868 in a sensitivity analysis performed at $\Gamma = 3$, whereas the blocked Wilcoxon statistic and Quade's statistic have relative efficiency of 0, because $\Gamma = 3 > \widetilde{\Gamma}$. A relative efficiency of 3.09 means that U868 needs $I/I' = 3.09$ times as many blocks to equal the performance of U878. Nonetheless, in this favorable situation, Quade's statistic is more efficient than the others for $\Gamma = 1$ and $\Gamma = 1.5$. Quade's statistic performs well for smaller Γ with errors from the t-distribution, falling behind only as Γ approaches its somewhat lower design sensitivity, $\widetilde{\Gamma}$.

Fix $\boldsymbol{\delta}_0$, possibly $\boldsymbol{\delta}_0 = \mathbf{0}$ or $\boldsymbol{\delta}_0 = \tau_0\mathbf{1}$. The common practice is to test the sequence of composite hypotheses, "$H_0 : \boldsymbol{\delta} = \boldsymbol{\delta}_0$ with $\boldsymbol{\theta} \in B_\Gamma$," for an increasing sequence of Γ's, starting with $\Gamma = 1$, stopping the testing at the first Γ at which the composite hypothesis is not rejected at level α. Because $B_\Gamma \subset B_{\Gamma'}$ for $\Gamma < \Gamma'$, hypothesis ($H_0 : \boldsymbol{\delta} = \boldsymbol{\delta}_0$ with $\boldsymbol{\theta} \in B_\Gamma$) is false whenever hypothesis ($H_0 : \boldsymbol{\delta} = \boldsymbol{\delta}_0$ with $\boldsymbol{\theta} \in B_{\Gamma'}$) is false. Consequently, this is a sound approach to multiple testing [26]: it falsely rejects at least one true hypothesis ($H_0 : \boldsymbol{\delta} = \boldsymbol{\delta}_0$ with $\boldsymbol{\theta} \in B_\Gamma$) with probability at most α.[5] When $\boldsymbol{\delta} = \boldsymbol{\delta}_0$, in very large samples, this process will likely terminate at a Γ slightly below $\widetilde{\Gamma}$; however, in smaller samples, it may terminate much sooner, at a Γ far below $\widetilde{\Gamma}$. In smaller samples, Table 11.1 suggests that testing might terminate at a larger Γ if we do not use the test statistic with the largest design sensitivity.

In very large samples, design sensitivity is the decisive consideration. What should be done in samples of moderate size? One approach, perhaps the most principled approach, uses adaptive inference [13, 16, 27, 28, 31, 32], as discussed in Sects. 9.5 and 11.4. Adaptive inference is principled in the specific sense that no guessing is involved, so a lucky guess does not arouse skepticism. A simple alternative to adaptive inference that is compatible with Table 11.1 is to begin testing at $\Gamma = 1$ using a test statistic with good performance at $\Gamma = 1$, perhaps Quade's statistic, and to use a different test statistic for $\Gamma > 1$, perhaps U868.

Comparing Competing Study Designs

Bahadur efficiency can be used to compare study designs rather than test statistics. Table 11.2 compares efficiency with blocks of various sizes [31]. In each case, the comparison in the denominator of the Bahadur efficiency is matched pairs, $J = 2$. The treatment effects τ and error distributions are as in Table 11.1. Efficiency is

[5] The proof of this is straightforward and immediate. Let $\Gamma^{\natural}$ be the smallest $\Gamma \geq 1$ such that ($H_0 : \boldsymbol{\delta} = \boldsymbol{\delta}_0$ with $\boldsymbol{\theta} \in B_\Gamma$) is true; possibly $\Gamma^{\natural} = \infty$ because some $\theta_{ij} = 0$. Because testing occurs in order of increasing Γ and stops at the first acceptance, rejection of at least one true hypothesis ($H_0 : \boldsymbol{\delta} = \boldsymbol{\delta}_0$ with $\boldsymbol{\theta} \in B_\Gamma$) occurs if and only if ($H_0 : \boldsymbol{\delta} = \boldsymbol{\delta}_0$ with $\boldsymbol{\theta} \in B_{\Gamma^{\natural}}$) is rejected, and this isolated rejection occurs with probability at most α.

Table 11.2 Bahadur efficiency of U868 with various block sizes $J = 2, 3, 4, 5$ compared to matched pairs, $J = 2$, in a sensitivity analysis performed with $\Gamma = 2$. The left half compares U868 to itself at $J = 2$. The right half compares U868 to Wilcoxon's signed rank statistic (SRS) at $J = 2$

	U868 versus U868 at $J = 2$				U868 versus SRS at $J = 2$			
	$\tau = 1/2$		$\tau = 1/3$		$\tau = 1/2$		$\tau = 1/3$	
J	Normal	t_5	Normal	t_5	Normal	t_5	Normal	t_5
2	1.00	1.00	1.00	1.00	1.58	1.26	8.08	3.05
3	1.37	1.23	2.14	1.66	2.16	1.55	17.26	5.07
4	1.83	1.63	3.07	2.29	2.89	2.04	24.81	6.98
5	1.76	1.56	2.88	2.13	2.77	1.96	23.26	6.49

evaluated for an analysis at $\Gamma = 2$. Unlike Table 10.1, the number of blocks I is not reduced when J is larger; rather, Table 11.2 compares I pairs to I blocks of size $J \geq 2$.

The left side of Table 11.2 compares U868 used in blocks of size $J = 2, 3, 4, 5$ to U868 used in pairs, $J = 2$. For each test statistic, blocks of size $J = 4$ are much more efficient than pairs. Efficiency is not monotone in the block size: $J = 5$ is slightly less efficient than $J = 4$.

The right side of Table 11.2 contemplates the combined effect of two mistakes, namely, use of pairs, $J = 2$, rather than larger blocks, $J > 2$, and use of Wilcoxon's signed rank statistic (SRS) rather than a statistic, U868, with a larger design sensitivity. An asymptotic relative efficiency of 24.81 for $J = 4$ means that each block of size $J = 4$ using U868 contributes about the same as nearly 25 pairs using Wilcoxon's signed rank test.

In brief, the decisions made in design and analysis strongly affect the degree to which an observational study is sensitive to unmeasured biases.

11.4 Adaptive Inference and Bahadur Efficiency

The Berk-Jones Theorem

Although Tables 11.1 and 11.2 and other similar tables [29, 31] provide some unambiguous guidance, they point to no one uniformly best method. Adaptive inference, as discussed in Sect. 9.5, lets the data speak to the issue [13,16,27,28,31, 32]; for instance, it lets the data choose the test statistic, say T_1 or T_2, when testing $H_0 : \boldsymbol{\delta} = \boldsymbol{\delta}_0$ with $\boldsymbol{\theta} \in B_\Gamma$.

As in Sect. 9.5, at a specified $\Gamma \geq 1$, the two upper bounds on P-values, $P_{1\Gamma}$ and $P_{2\Gamma}$, are computed from T_1 and T_2. Their minimum, $P^*_{\min\Gamma} = \min(P_{1\Gamma}, P_{2\Gamma})$, is not a valid P-value because in most cases $\Pr\left(P^*_{\min\Gamma} \leq \alpha \,\middle|\, \mathcal{F}, \mathcal{Z}\right) > \alpha$. However, $P^*_{\min\Gamma}$ is a statistic, and if its distribution can be determined when $H_0 : \boldsymbol{\delta} = \boldsymbol{\delta}_0$ with $\boldsymbol{\theta} \in B_\Gamma$, then a valid P-value, say $P_{\min\Gamma}$, may be derived from its null distribution, using either the exact joint distribution of (T_1, T_2) or an approximation to that distribution

[27, 28, 31].[6] As noted in Sect. 9.5, this adaptive method has design sensitivity $\max\left(\widetilde{\Gamma}_1, \widetilde{\Gamma}_2\right)$, where T_1 has design sensitivity $\widetilde{\Gamma}_1$ and T_2 has design sensitivity $\widetilde{\Gamma}_2$. So, in the limit, as $I \to \infty$, the investigator secures the better design sensitivity of T_1 and T_2 without knowing which statistic has design sensitivity $\max\left(\widetilde{\Gamma}_1, \widetilde{\Gamma}_2\right)$.

A theorem of Robert Berk and Douglas Jones [4] says more than this. At $\Gamma < \min\left(\widetilde{\Gamma}_1, \widetilde{\Gamma}_2\right)$, let $b_{\Gamma 1}$ and $b_{\Gamma 2}$ be the Bahadur slopes of T_1 and T_2. At such a Γ, Table 11.1 shows that the statistic with the larger design sensitivity may have the smaller Bahadur slope. More precisely, if $\widetilde{\Gamma}_1 = \max\left(\widetilde{\Gamma}_1, \widetilde{\Gamma}_2\right) > \min\left(\widetilde{\Gamma}_1, \widetilde{\Gamma}_2\right) = \widetilde{\Gamma}_2$, then T_1 is the better choice for a sensitivity analysis at Γ if $\widetilde{\Gamma}_1 > \Gamma > \widetilde{\Gamma}_2$, because at this Γ we have $b_{\Gamma 1} > b_{\Gamma 2} = 0$; however, T_2 may be nonetheless the better choice at a $\Gamma < \min\left(\widetilde{\Gamma}_1, \widetilde{\Gamma}_2\right)$ because at this Γ we may possibly have $0 < b_{\Gamma 1} < b_{\Gamma 2}$. This sort of reversal happens several times in Table 11.1, for example, for Quade's statistic and U878 with normal errors and $\tau = 1/2$.

The Berk-Jones [4] theorem says that the Bahadur slope of the adaptive procedure is $\max\left(b_{\Gamma 1}, b_{\Gamma 2}\right)$ at each Γ. Stated informally, the adaptive procedure makes the right choice between T_1 and T_2 even when reversals occur as Γ increases; that is, even if the plots of $b_{\Gamma 1}$ and $b_{\Gamma 2}$ against Γ cross [29, Fig. 2], the adaptive procedure has Bahadur slope $\max\left(b_{\Gamma 1}, b_{\Gamma 2}\right)$. This is a statement about asymptotic relative efficiency, $b_{\Gamma 1}/b_{\Gamma 2}$.

Simulations

Simulations corroborate the asymptotic theory, suggesting that the adaptive procedure lags only slightly behind knowing the better procedure a priori. If T_2 is the better test at a given Γ, with $b_{\Gamma 1}/b_{\Gamma 2} < 1$, then simulations suggest that the adaptive procedure produces P-values, $P_{\min \Gamma}$, slightly above $P_{2\Gamma}$ but very close to it [31, §5.3]. In particular, consider 10,000 simulated normal favorable situations, each with $I = 500$ blocks of size $J = 3$ and $\tau = 1/2$. A one-sided sensitivity analysis is performed testing the hypothesis of no effect with $\Gamma = 3$. The design sensitivities, $\widetilde{\Gamma}$, of the blocked Wilcoxon rank sum statistic, U868, and U878 are 2.9, 4.6, and 5.1, and the Bahadur efficiencies at $\Gamma = 3$ relative to U868 are 0.00, 1.00, and 1.21, respectively [31, Table 1]. Consequently, we expect negligible power from Wilcoxon's statistic and better performance from U878 than from U868. Is that expectation realized with $I = 500$ blocks replicated 10,000 times? Because simulated power is a binomial proportion, the standard error of a simulated power is at most $\sqrt{0.5 \times 0.5/10000} = 0.005$.

Using the blocked Wilcoxon statistic as T_1 and U868 as T_2 in adaptive inference, so $b_{\Gamma 1}/b_{\Gamma 2} = 0$ at $\Gamma = 3$, the power of T_1 was 0.1%, the power of T_2 was 92%,

---

[6] The function `wgtRanktt` in the `weightedRank` package in `R` implements adaptive inference for the tests in Table 11.1.

and the power of the adaptive procedure was 87% [31, §5.3]. Whenever the null hypothesis was rejected by the adaptive procedure, it was rejected based on T_2. The median difference in the P-values, $P_{\min \Gamma} - P_{2\Gamma}$, was 0.0018. It is better to use T_2 based on a priori considerations, such as asymptotic results in Table 11.1, but the adaptive procedure, $P_{\min \Gamma}$, is only slightly behind the better procedure, $P_{2\Gamma}$.

Using U868 as T_1 and U878 as T_2 in adaptive inference, so $b_{\Gamma 1}/b_{\Gamma 2} = 1/1.21$ at $\Gamma = 3$, the power of T_1 was 92% as above, the power of T_2 was 96%, and the power of the adaptive procedure was 95%. The median difference in the P-values, $P_{\min \Gamma} - P_{2\Gamma}$, was 0.00026.

These simulations are consistent with the asymptotic Berk-Jones [4] theorem in studies with $I = 500$ blocks.

*The Informal Intuition Behind Adaptive Inference

Why does the adaptive procedure work almost as well as knowing that T_2 is better than T_1 at a particular Γ? Some informal intuition follows. See Berk and Jones [4] for a proof of the Berk-Jones theorem.

Add a subscript I, so $P_{1\Gamma I}$ and $P_{2\Gamma I}$ are the P-value bounds based on a study with I blocks, and $\mathcal{F}_I$, $\mathcal{Z}_I$ also refer to this study with I blocks. Suppose that $b_{\Gamma 2}$ and $b_{\Gamma 1}$ are weak Bahadur slopes and $b_{\Gamma 2} > b_{\Gamma 1}$ at a particular Γ, so

$$-\frac{2}{I}\log\left(P_{1\Gamma I}\right) \xrightarrow{P} b_{\Gamma 1} \text{ and } -\frac{2}{I}\log\left(P_{2\Gamma I}\right) \xrightarrow{P} b_{\Gamma 2} \text{ as } I \to \infty, \tag{11.4}$$

where $\xrightarrow{P}$ denotes convergence in probability.

Knowing (11.4), an omniscient investigator would use T_2. Suppose that $\overline{\alpha} = \Pr\left(P_{2\Gamma I} \le \overline{\alpha} \mid \mathcal{F}_I, \mathcal{Z}_I\right)$ for all $0 < \overline{\alpha} < 1$. Fix an α, $0 < \alpha < 1$, that you might use in inference, perhaps $\alpha = 0.05$ or $\alpha = 0.001$. The omniscient investigator will reject the null hypothesis at this Γ if $P_{2\Gamma I} \le \alpha$, thereby obtaining a test of size $\alpha = \Pr\left(P_{2\Gamma I} \le \alpha \mid \mathcal{F}_I, \mathcal{Z}_I\right)$. Not knowing that $b_{\Gamma 2} > b_{\Gamma 1}$, we would like to use as a test statistic $P^*_{\min \Gamma I} = \min\left(P_{1\Gamma I}, P_{2\Gamma I}\right)$ in a test of size α, but to achieve size α we must reject when $P^*_{\min \Gamma I} \le \alpha^*_I$, where

$$\begin{aligned} \alpha &= \Pr\left(P^*_{\min \Gamma I} \le \alpha^*_I \,\middle|\, \mathcal{F}_I, \mathcal{Z}_I\right) \\ &= \Pr\left(P_{2\Gamma I} \le \alpha^*_I \,\middle|\, \mathcal{F}_I, \mathcal{Z}_I\right) + \Pr\left(P_{2\Gamma I} > \alpha^*_I \text{ and } P_{1\Gamma I} \le \alpha^*_I \,\middle|\, \mathcal{F}_I, \mathcal{Z}_I\right) \\ &\ge \Pr\left(P_{2\Gamma I} \le \alpha^*_I \,\middle|\, \mathcal{F}_I, \mathcal{Z}_I\right) = \alpha^*_I. \end{aligned}$$

Let $\mathcal{B}_I$ be the "bad" event $\left\{P_{2\Gamma I} > \alpha^*_I \text{ and } P_{1\Gamma I} \le \alpha^*_I\right\}$, so that

$$\alpha - \alpha^*_I = \Pr\left(P_{2\Gamma I} > \alpha^*_I \text{ and } P_{1\Gamma I} \le \alpha^*_I \,\middle|\, \mathcal{F}_I, \mathcal{Z}_I\right) = \Pr\left(\mathcal{B}_I \mid \mathcal{F}_I, \mathcal{Z}_I\right) \tag{11.5}$$

is the penalty that we must pay for our lack of omniscience, that is for using $P^*_{\min \Gamma I}$ as a test statistic rather than T_2. How large is the probability in (11.5)? How often is $P_{1\Gamma I} \leq \alpha_I^* < P_{2\Gamma I}$ by luck given that $b_{\Gamma 2} > b_{\Gamma 1}$? Let $\epsilon = (b_{\Gamma 2} - b_{\Gamma 1})/3 > 0$, and let $\mathcal{E}_I$ be the event that

$$-\frac{2}{I}\log(P_{1\Gamma I}) < b_{\Gamma 1} + \epsilon \text{ and } -\frac{2}{I}\log(P_{2\Gamma I}) > b_{\Gamma 2} - \epsilon.$$

Because of (11.4), it follows that $\Pr(\mathcal{E}_I \mid \mathcal{F}_I, \mathcal{Z}_I) \to 1$ as $I \to \infty$. Also, if $\mathcal{E}_I$ occurs, then $\mathcal{B}_I$ does not occur, so $\Pr(\mathcal{B}_I \mid \mathcal{F}_I, \mathcal{Z}_I) \to 0$ in (11.5). Consequently, $\alpha - \alpha_I^* \to 0$ as $I \to \infty$; so, the penalty for a lack of omniscience in (11.5) becomes negligible. As $\alpha > 0$ is fixed, it is also true that $(\alpha - \alpha_I^*)/\alpha \to 0$ as $I \to \infty$; so, the penalty becomes a negligible part of the size α of the omniscient investigator's test.

11.5 *Further Reading

Bahadur efficiency in general: Bahadur efficiency was introduced by Raj Bahadur [1–3]. van der Vaart [36, §14.4] provides a concise introduction. Sievers' [35] theorem and its extensions [18, 22, 23] were important in this chapter; they are discussed by Groeneboom and Oosterhoff [11, Theorem 3.2]. Bahadur efficiency is discussed by Groeneboom and Oosterhoff [11, 12], Nikitin [20] and Serfling [33, Ch. 10]. Large deviation theorems, including the Gärtner-Ellis theorem, are discussed by Bucklew [6] and Dembo and Zeitouni [9]. The Gärtner-Ellis theorem resembles Sievers' theorem.

Bahadur efficiency of sensitivity analyses: This chapter is largely based on two of my articles [29, 31].

Problems

11.1 Mean Squared Error.
Prove the familiar fact (11.1). (Hint: In (11.1), separate the bias and the variance using

$$\mathrm{E}\{(\widehat{\tau} - \tau)^2\} = \mathrm{E}[\{(\widehat{\tau} - \overline{\tau}) + (\overline{\tau} - \tau)\}^2],$$

remembering that $\widehat{\tau}$ has expectation $\overline{\tau}$.)

11.2 Efficiency of Noether's Statistic in Sensitivity Analyses
This problem continues Problem 8.3(ii) when testing $H_0 : \tau = 0$, where you demonstrated that the upper bound on the P-value from Noether's statistic in matched pairs is given by a certain binomial distribution with fixed sample size $|\mathcal{N}|$ and probability of success $\Gamma/(1+\Gamma)$. Recall that Problem 8.3 continued Problem 2.2, as you will need some details and notation from that earlier problem also. Assume in this problem that there are no ties, so that the I treated-minus-control pair differences, Y_i, $i = 1, \ldots, I$, are never zero, never tied, and their absolute values are never tied. Consequently,

Noether's statistic is the number of positive Y_i among the $|\mathcal{N}| = \lceil f\, I \rceil$ differences Y_i with the largest $|Y_i|$, where $\lceil f\, I \rceil$ is the smallest integer greater than or equal to $f\, I$. There are several intermediate quantities used in the computation of the Bahadur slope. Problem 11.2 asks you to determine a few of these quantities and to think about others. A complete calculation with numerical comparisons of efficiency with other statistics is available if you are interested [29]. Incidentally, Thomas Severini [34, §4.3] provides an introduction to moment generating functions. The **optional** part of this problem is more difficult and asks you to refer to other books for specifics about Bahadur efficiency calculations.

(i) The calculation of the Bahadur efficiency uses the moment generating function of the distribution that provides the upper bound on the P-value at a specific Γ. In this case, that is the moment generating function of a particular binomial distribution. Find the moment generating function of the number of successes in that binomial distribution.

(ii) In Problem 2.2, Noether's statistic becomes the sign statistic if $f = 0$; then, $|\mathcal{N}| = I$ and the signs of all I of the matched-pair differences, Y_i, are counted in Noether's statistic. Consider the following favorable situation: there is no bias in treatment assignment, $\boldsymbol{\theta} = \overline{\boldsymbol{\theta}}$, and the Y_i are independent normal random variables with expectation $\tau > 0$ and variance 1. What is the expectation of the sign statistic in this favorable situation? What is the distribution of the sign statistic in this favorable case? (Hint: What is the probability that a sign is positive? Are the signs independent?)

(iii) Optional. At this point, you have the inputs you need to determine the Bahadur slope for the sign statistic in this favorable situation when conducting a sensitivity analysis at Γ. At this point, you could calculate a Bahadur slope in the usual way. See van der Vaart [36, §14.4] and in particular his Example 14.24. Essentially, you need a slope when comparing two binomials with different probabilities of success, and, for this, Chernoff [7, Example 3] or Serfling [33, §10.3.2, Example B] fill in a few details. An alternative approach is to skip this optional problem and move immediately to a more general solution in Problem 11.3.

11.3 Moment Generating Function for General Signed Rank Statistics

(i) In Problem 11.2(i), you determined the moment generating function of a sum of $|\mathcal{N}| = \lceil f\, I \rceil$ independent trials that scored a 1 with probability $\Gamma/(1+\Gamma)$ and a 0 with probability $1/(1+\Gamma)$, consistent with the $\boldsymbol{\theta}$ given in (8.20). Suppose that the I binary trials were multiplied by nonnegative constants, $a_i \geq 0$, $i = 1, \ldots, I$ before calculating the sum of the I terms. What is the moment generating function of this new sum?

(ii) Show that your answer to Problem 11.3(i) provides an alternative way of obtaining the moment generating function of Noether's statistic at the $\boldsymbol{\theta}$ given in (8.20). (Hint: How should you define $a_i \geq 0$, $i = 1, \ldots, I$?)

(iii) Optional. You now have what you need to compute Bahadur slopes and Bahadur relative efficiencies for sensitivity analyses for general signed-rank statistics in matched pairs, $J = 2$. For example, you could compare various versions of Noether's statistic, varying f, Wilcoxon's signed rank statistic, U868, and U878, or other statistics [29]. In doing this, you would use Sievers' [35] theorem and its extensions

[18, 22, 23]. See Groeneboom and Oosterhoff [11, Theorem 3.2] for a statement of this theorem. Implicitly, Sievers' theorem places restrictions on the behavior of the constants, a_i, as $I \to \infty$. (Solution: [29, Prop. 2].)

11.4 Adaptive Inference Using Noether's Statistic
(i) Let T_1 be Noether's statistic with f_1 and let T_2 be Noether's statistic with f_2, where $f_1 < f_2$. Under the hypothesis of no effect in the presence of a bias of at most Γ, describe the joint distribution of T_1 and T_2 under the hypothesis of no effect at the θ given in (8.20). (Hint: T_1 counts all the pairs counted by T_2 plus some more. What is the distribution of $T_1 - T_2$ at the θ given in (8.20)?)
(ii) How would your answers to (i) change if you replaced T_1 by the statistic $T_3 = 2 \times T_2 + (T_1 - T_2)$? The statistic T_3 is discussed by Brown [5] and Markowski and Hettmansperger [19].
(iii) Consider adaptive inference in this case [27, 29]. Suppose that you knew the design sensitivity and Bahadur efficiency of T_1, T_2, and T_3 when used alone. How would they determine the design sensitivity and Bahadur efficiency of an adaptive choice of T_1 or T_2? What about an adaptive choice of T_3 or T_2? (A brief, easy, conceptual answer suffices.)

References

1. Bahadur, R.R.: Stochastic comparison of tests. Ann. Math. Stat. **31**(2), 276–295 (1960)
2. Bahadur, R.R.: Rates of convergence of estimates and test statistics. Ann. Math. Stat. **38**(2), 303–324 (1967)
3. Bahadur, R.R.: Some Limit Theorems in Statistics. SIAM, Philadelphia (1971)
4. Berk, R.H., Jones, D.H.: Relatively optimal combinations of test statistics. Scand. J. Stat. **5**, 158–162 (1978)
5. Brown, B.M.: Symmetric quantile averages and related estimators. Biometrika **68**(1), 235–242 (1981)
6. Bucklew, J.A.: Introduction to Rare Event Simulation. Springer, New York (2004)
7. Chernoff, H.: A measure of asymptotic efficiency for tests of a hypothesis based on the sum of observations. Ann. Math. Stat., 493–507 (1952)
8. Cornfield, J., Haenszel, W., Hammond, E.C., Lilienfeld, A.M., Shimkin, M.B., Wynder, E.L.: Smoking and lung cancer: Recent evidence and a discussion of some questions. J. Natl. Cancer Inst. **22**(1), 173–203 (1959)
9. Dembo, A., Zeitouni, O.: Large Deviations and Applications. Springer, New York (2010)
10. Feller, W.: An Introduction to Probability Theory and its Applications, vol. 1. Wiley, New York (1968)
11. Groeneboom, P., Oosterhoff, J.: Bahadur efficiency and probabilities of large deviations. Statistica Neerlandica **31**(1), 1–24 (1977)
12. Groeneboom, P., Oosterhoff, J.: Bahadur efficiency and small-sample efficiency. Int. Stat. Rev. **49**, 127–141 (1981)
13. Heng, S., Kang, H., Small, D.S., Fogarty, C.B.: Increasing power for observational studies of aberrant response: An adaptive approach. J. Roy. Stat. Soc. B **83**(3), 482–504 (2021)
14. Hettmansperger, T.P.: Statistical Inference Based on Ranks. Wiley, New York (1984)
15. Hodges Jr, J.L., Lehmann, E.L.: The efficiency of some nonparametric competitors of the t-test. Ann. Math. Stat., 324–335 (1956)

16. Howard, S.R., Pimentel, S.D.: The uniform general signed rank test and its design sensitivity. Biometrika **108**(2), 381–396 (2021)
17. Lehmann, E.L.: Nonparametrics. Holden-Day, San Francisco (1975)
18. Lynch, J.: A curious converse of Siever's theorem. Ann. Probab. **6**(1), 169–173 (1978)
19. Markowski, E.P., Hettmansperger, T.P.: Inference based on simple rank step score statistics for the location model. J. Am. Stat. Assoc. **77**(380), 901–907 (1982)
20. Nikitin, Y.: Asymptotic Efficiency of Nonparametric Tests. Cambridge University Press, New York (1995)
21. Noether, G.E.: On a theorem of Pitman. Ann. Math. Stat. **26**, 64–68 (1955)
22. Plachky, D.: On a theorem of G. L. Sievers. Ann. Math. Stat. **42**(4), 1442–1443 (1971)
23. Plachky, D., Steinebach, J.: A theorem about probabilities of large deviations with an application to queuing theory. Periodica Mathematica Hungarica **6**(4), 343–345 (1975)
24. Raghavachari, M.: On a theorem of Bahadur on the rate of convergence of test statistics. Ann. Math. Stat. **41**, 1695–1699 (1970)
25. Randles, R.H., Wolfe, D.A.: Introduction to the Theory of Nonparametric Statistics. Wiley, New York (1979)
26. Rosenbaum, P.R.: Testing hypotheses in order. Biometrika **95**(1), 248–252 (2008)
27. Rosenbaum, P.R.: An exact adaptive test with superior design sensitivity in an observational study of treatments for ovarian cancer. Ann. Appl. Stat. **6**, 83–105 (2012)
28. Rosenbaum, P.R.: Testing one hypothesis twice in observational studies. Biometrika **99**(4), 763–774 (2012)
29. Rosenbaum, P.R.: Bahadur efficiency of sensitivity analyses in observational studies. J. Am. Stat. Assoc. **110**(509), 205–217 (2015)
30. Rosenbaum, P.R.: Sensitivity analysis for stratified comparisons in an observational study of the effect of smoking on homocysteine levels. Ann. Appl. Stat. **12**(4), 2312–2334 (2018)
31. Rosenbaum, P.R.: Bahadur efficiency of observational block designs. J. Am. Stat. Assoc. **119**(547), 1871–1881 (2024)
32. Rosenbaum, P.R., Small, D.S.: An adaptive Mantel–Haenszel test for sensitivity analysis in observational studies. Biometrics **73**(2), 422–430 (2017)
33. Serfling, R.J.: Approximation Theorems of Mathematical Statistics. Wiley, New York (2009)
34. Severini, T.A.: Elements of Distribution Theory. Cambridge University Press, New York (2005)
35. Sievers, G.L.: On the probability of large deviations and exact slopes. Ann. Math. Stat. **40**, 1908–1921 (1969)
36. van der Vaart, A.W.: Asymptotic Statistics. Cambridge University Press, New York (2000)

Part IV
Quasi-Experimental Devices

Perception is not something that
happens to us. It is something we do.

Could there be an entirely inactive,
an *inert* perceiver?

The invariant structure of reality unfolds
in the active exploration of appearances.

Alva Noë
Action in Perception, pp. 1, 12, 85

What goes on in science is not that we try to have
theories that accommodate our experiences;
it's closer that we try to have experiences
that adjudicate among our theories.

Jerry A. Fodor
The Dogma That Didn't Bark

You must find the way from where you are
to where the issue is decided.

Ludwig Wittgenstein
Philosophical Remarks, p. 77

Chapter 12
Known Effects in Observational Studies

> Properly conducted inductive research corrects its own premises.
>
> Charles Sanders Peirce 1898
> The First Rule of Logic [35, p. 44]

Abstract Unmeasured bias in observational studies is often gauged by estimating effects that we think we know. Is a treatment associated with an outcome it should not affect? Is a treatment positively associated with an outcome for which a negative effect is anticipated? Information of this kind can inform a sensitivity analysis.

12.1 Outcomes Unaffected by Treatment

Methylmercury in the Study of Light Daily Drinking

In Sect. 1.4, in the study of HDL cholesterol and light daily consumption of alcohol, there is a secondary outcome—a quantity measured after treatment—that we thought alcohol should not affect, namely, blood levels of methylmercury, a neurotoxin. The World Health Organization [62] and the US Centers for Disease Control [58] both conclude that methylmercury in humans almost invariably reflects the consumption of fish or shellfish containing methylmercury. Pedersen et al. [34] looked for methylmercury in alcoholic beverages, but found little or no evidence of it; see also Dressler et al. [15]. About inorganic mercury (Hg) and methylmercury (MeHg), the US National Academy of Sciences [59, pp. 15–16] writes:

> Conversion of inorganic Hg to MeHg occurs primarily in microorganisms especially in aquatic systems. Once in its methylated form, Hg bioaccumulates up the food chain; the

© The Author(s), under exclusive license to Springer Nature Switzerland AG 2025
P. R. Rosenbaum, *An Introduction to the Theory of Observational Studies*,
Springer Texts in Statistics, https://doi.org/10.1007/978-3-031-90494-3_12

> microorganisms are consumed by fish, and the smaller fish are consumed by larger fish. Such bioaccumulation can result in very high concentrations of MeHg in some fish, which are one of the main sources of human and piscivorous wildlife exposure to MeHg.

So, there is reason to doubt that elevated methylmercury levels are caused by light daily drinking.

The US National Health and Nutrition Examination Survey (NHANES) measured methylmercury levels for a subsample of survey participants. The matching in Sect. 1.4 controlled also for membership in this subsample; that is, treated individuals with methylmercury levels were matched to controls with methylmercury levels, yielding 200 blocks with methylmercury levels and 206 blocks without them. For the 200 blocks with methylmercury levels, Figs. 1.4 and 1.5 depict methylmercury levels by alcohol group. Because numerical results in this chapter refer only to the 200 blocks with methylmercury levels, the results differ slightly from related results in other chapters that use all 406 = 200 + 206 blocks.

In Fig. 1.4, daily drinkers have higher methylmercury levels than each of the three control groups. Presumably, this indicates a diet containing more fish and shellfish than in the control groups. A diet containing more fish and shellfish must also differ in other respects. If fish and shellfish are added to an otherwise unchanged diet, then the new diet has added calories and protein and certain fats found in seafood. If servings of fish substitute for other foods, say for servings of red meat, then the new diet is only partially characterized by what is added.

The pattern for HDL cholesterol on the left in Fig. 1.5 seems to resemble the pattern on the right for methylmercury. Should we doubt that the pattern for HDL cholesterol is caused by alcohol given that we do doubt that the similar pattern for methylmercury is caused by alcohol?

Affected and Unaffected Outcomes

Suppose that the potential outcomes are bivariate vectors, $\mathbf{r}_{Tij} = \left(r_{Tij1}, r_{Tij2}\right)$, $\mathbf{r}_{Cij} = \left(r_{Cij1}, r_{Cij2}\right)$, $\mathbf{R}_{ij} = \left(R_{ij1}, R_{ij2}\right) = Z_{ij}\,\mathbf{r}_{Tij} + \left(1 - Z_{ij}\right)\,\mathbf{r}_{Cij}$, where the first coordinate is the HDL cholesterol level and the second coordinate is the methylmercury level. Most of the discussion in earlier chapters spoke of a scalar outcome, but the main results about propensity scores, the principal unobserved covariate, and sensitivity analyses carry over to the bivariate or multivariate outcomes with minor changes. For instance, the principal unobserved covariate is $\zeta = \Pr(Z = 1 \mid \mathbf{x}, \mathbf{r}_C, \mathbf{r}_T)$.

The new element is that we have reason to think that the treatment does not affect the second coordinate—that a daily drink of alcohol does not cause an increase in methylmercury—so that $r_{Tij2} = r_{Cij2}$. The new element is that we have reason to think that the boxplot on the right of Fig. 1.5 is produced by biased treatment assignment in the absence of a causal effect. In other words we have reason to believe that Fisher's hypothesis of no treatment is true for the second coordinate of the bivariate outcome. Can that information be used to gauge the magnitude of bias in treatment assignment that is present?

There are now two test statistics, $T_1^{\delta_0}$ testing $H_0 : \delta = \delta_0$ for the possibly affected first outcome, where $\delta_{ij} = r_{Tij1} - r_{Cij1}$, and T_2 testing what we know, namely, $r_{Tij2} = r_{Cij2}$ for the second outcome. For instance, $T_1^{\delta_0}$ and T_2 might be two weighted rank statistics, each with the properties discussed in Chap. 2, Sect. 4.4, and Chap. 8. Although there are two statistics, there is only one treatment assignment, Z_{ij}, for any individual and hence just one θ_{ij} that conditions on the vector of potential outcomes $\left(\mathbf{r}_{Tij}, \mathbf{r}_{Cij}\right)$ in $\mathcal{F}$.

The logic in Chap. 2 said: if Fisher's hypothesis H_0 of no treatment were true of an outcome in a randomized block experiment, then an α-level randomization test would reject this hypothesis with probability at most α. In other words, knowing that $\boldsymbol{\theta} = \overline{\boldsymbol{\theta}}$ in a randomized experiment permits a test of the hypothesis of no treatment effect, H_0. Chapter 2 tested the conjunction hypothesis, $\left(\boldsymbol{\theta} = \overline{\boldsymbol{\theta}} \text{ and } H_0\right)$, knowing that $\boldsymbol{\theta} = \overline{\boldsymbol{\theta}}$ because treatments were randomly assigned. Moreover, in Sect. 4.4, this same conclusion would be true if treatment assignment were ignorable given the observed covariates and if the blocking had controlled the propensity score, because these premises would imply that treatment assignment is ignorable given the blocks, i.e., that $\boldsymbol{\theta} = \overline{\boldsymbol{\theta}}$. We can turn this logic around, testing $\left(\boldsymbol{\theta} = \overline{\boldsymbol{\theta}} \text{ and } H_0\right)$, while knowing that H_0 is true for the unaffected outcome, $r_{Tij2} = r_{Cij2}$. If we know Fisher's hypothesis H_0 of no effect is true of an unaffected outcome in a blocked observational study and if an α-level blocked randomization test rejects the conjunction hypothesis, $\left(\boldsymbol{\theta} = \overline{\boldsymbol{\theta}} \text{ and } H_0\right)$, then we have evidence that treatment assignment is not ignorable given the blocks; that is, we have rejected $H_0' : \boldsymbol{\theta} = \overline{\boldsymbol{\theta}}$. Having an outcome that is unaffected by the treatment creates a test of the null hypothesis $H_0' : \boldsymbol{\theta} = \overline{\boldsymbol{\theta}}$ of ignorable treatment assignment [37].

In brief, the task is to coordinate two tests, a test of $H_0 : \delta = \delta_0$ using $T_1^{\delta_0}$ computed from the first outcome and a test of $H_0' : \boldsymbol{\theta} = \overline{\boldsymbol{\theta}}$ using T_2 computed from the second, unaffected outcome. In the example, the task is to make a coordinated appraisal of the two sides of Fig. 1.5. The left panel of Fig. 1.5 for HDL cholesterol may reflect either a treatment effect or biased treatment assignment or both, but the right panel for methylmercury provides focused information about possible bias in treatment assignment.

Properties of Tests for Bias Using Unaffected Outcomes

The following claims about the test based on T_2 are fairly intuitive, and it is not difficult to state them formally and prove them [38,39]. As has been true all along, the $I \times J$ block design was formed by matching for a function, $\mathbf{h}(\mathbf{x})$, of the observed covariates, $\mathbf{x}$, so that each block contains one treated individual and $J - 1$ controls.[1]

[1] The claims hold under more general conditions, as discussed in the cited references, but are described here in the special case of the $I \times J$ block design so that no additional notation is needed.

Suppose that treatment assignment would have been strongly ignorable given both the observed covariates $\mathbf{x}$ and a scalar unobserved covariate u, so that

$$0 < \Pr(Z = 1 \mid \mathbf{x}, u) = \Pr(Z = 1 \mid \mathbf{x}, \mathbf{r}_C, \mathbf{r}_T) = \zeta < 1.$$

In the $I \times J$ block design, treatment assignment is governed by (8.11), where θ_{ij} is what remains of ζ_{ij} having blocked for $\mathbf{h}(\mathbf{x}_{ij})$ and having conditioned on $\mathbf{Z} \in \mathcal{Z}$; so, $\theta_{ij} \neq 1/J$ for some ij when treatment assignment is ignorable given $(\mathbf{x}, u)$, but not ignorable given $\mathbf{h}(\mathbf{x})$ alone. Because the second outcome is unaffected, with $r_{Tij2} = r_{Cij2} = R_{ij2}$, it suffices to refer to r_{Cij2} in the claims below.

- The randomization test of no effect on an unaffected outcome r_{Cij2} is a valid test of the null hypothesis that $\theta_{ij} = 1/J$ for all ij, or equivalently, the null hypothesis that treatment assignment is ignorable given the blocks derived from matching for $\mathbf{h}(\mathbf{x})$. As always, a level α test of some hypothesis H_0 is valid if the probability is at most α that the test rejects H_0 when H_0 is true.
- For any test statistic in a large class of statistics, including the statistics in Table 8.1, a one-sided test is unbiased against alternatives in which, within blocks, θ_{ij} is positively associated with r_{Cij2} [38, Thm. 1 and Prop. 1]. As always, a test is unbiased against a set of alternative hypotheses if its power equals or exceeds its level α for all alternatives in this set. Stated informally, an unbiased test is pointed in the right direction.
- The power of these tests increases as the association between the unaffected outcome r_{Cij2} and θ_{ij} becomes stronger [38, Prop. 2].
- Within blocks, the visible association between the unaffected outcome r_{Cij2} and the treatment Z_{ij} is weaker, or harder to detect, than the corresponding invisible association between u_{ij} and Z_{ij} would have been had it been observed.[2] In other words, the visible manifestation of biased treatment assignment in r_{Cij2} is a weak echo of its origin in biased treatment assignment that depends on u_{ij}.

These claims are useful in indicating that tests for biased treatment assignment may be appraised with many of the same tools generally used to appraise the performance of statistical tests. The claims contain an implicit warning, however. The claims helpfully move us away from pure significance tests, that is, tests considered solely in terms of their properties when the null hypothesis is true. The claims helpfully move us to consider a test's ability to distinguish a null hypothesis from one or many specific alternative hypotheses. The implicit warning is that a test of ignorable treatment assignment may or may not have good performance against the alternatives that should be of greatest concern.

Consider these issues in the context of methylmercury as an outcome unaffected by consuming alcohol, $R_{ij2} = r_{Tij2} = r_{Cij2}$. Higher levels of methylmercury, R_{ij2}, in daily drinkers are presumably an excellent indicator of an imbalance in an unobserved covariate u_{ij} measuring the consumption of species of fish that contain high levels of methylmercury, such as swordfish and shark. Other species of fish, such as salmon

[2] More precisely, after adjustment for $\mathbf{x}$, the Kullback-Leibler [25] information in r_{Cij2} is at most equal to, and is typically much less than, theKullback-Leibler information in u_{ij} [39, §4.3].

and sardines, contain much less methylmercury. So, methylmercury is, at best, an oblique indicator of an unobserved covariate u_{ij} measuring the consumption of fish. Methylmercury is an even more oblique indicator of dietary differences relevant to HDL cholesterol, because a person may avoid fish by eating steak instead, or by eating lentils instead. The implicit warning is that we cannot expect adjustments for R_{ij2} to remove the bias from the most relevant u_{ij}. Adjusting for R_{ij2} in place of u_{ij} is analogous to shutting off the fire alarm in lieu of putting out the fire.

Magnitudes of Bias Needed to Explain Associations

The simplest comparison concerns the magnitudes of bias needed to separately explain the two panels of Fig. 1.5, for HDL cholesterol and methylmercury. This comparison is not completely satisfactory, because it ignores the relationship between the potentially affected outcome and the unaffected outcome, that is, the relationship between HDL cholesterol and methylmercury. Better methods are discussed in Sects. 12.2 and 12.3, and these methods say more by taking account of the relationship between the two coordinates of the bivariate outcome $\mathbf{R}_{ij}$.

Before examining the data, there was no reason to expect a particular direction of association between methylmercury and daily drinking, so a two-sided test seems appropriate. To simplify comparisons between outcomes and methods in Sects. 12.1–12.3, all tests in this chapter are two-sided and use Quade's statistic applied to the 200 blocks that record methylmercury levels. In other words, at a given $\boldsymbol{\theta} \in B_\Gamma$, hypotheses are rejected at level α if (8.16) occurs, rather than if (8.18) occurs.

It is convenient to make use of the 0.05-level sensitivity value, $\Gamma^{\bullet}$, as proposed by Qingyuan Zhao's [64]. Recall from Sect. 8.6 that $\Gamma^{\bullet}$ is the random value of Γ such that the null hypothesis H_0 has a P-value bound of 0.05. In this chapter, the value $\Gamma^{\bullet}$ refers to rejection of H_0 in a two-sided 0.05-level test using Quade's statistic for all $\boldsymbol{\theta} \in B_{\Gamma^{\bullet}}$ but not for some $\boldsymbol{\theta} \in B_\Gamma$ for every $\Gamma > \Gamma^{\bullet}$.

Keep in mind that comparisons in Fig. 1.5 involve the 200 blocks in which methylmercury was measured, not all of the $I = 406$ blocks in which only HDL cholesterol was measured. Therefore, analyses for HDL cholesterol differ slightly from analyses in other chapters that use all 406 blocks.[3]

Examining the left and right sides of Fig. 1.5 separately, the sensitivity value is $\Gamma^{\bullet} = 3.614$ for HDL-cholesterol and is $\Gamma^{\bullet} = 1.993$ for methylmercury. In words, the unaffected outcome, methylmercury, has rejected the hypothesis of ignorable treatment assignment, $H_0' : \boldsymbol{\theta} = \overline{\boldsymbol{\theta}}$, and indeed has rejected at level $\alpha = 0.05$ all $\boldsymbol{\theta} \in B_\Gamma$ for $\Gamma \leq 1.993$. Not only is ignorable treatment assignment implausible, but so

[3] As discussed in Chap. 9, as $I \to \infty$, the sensitivity value $\Gamma^{\bullet}$ converges in probability to a constant $\widetilde{\Gamma}$ called the design sensitivity [42]; however, $\Gamma^{\bullet}$ tends to approach $\widetilde{\Gamma}$ unsteadily from below, just as the lower endpoint of a consistent confidence interval tends to converge to the true parameter from below. If you take a random sample of 200 blocks from $I = 406$ blocks, then you expect $\Gamma^{\bullet}$ to be somewhat smaller with 200 blocks than with 406 blocks, even though the data are just a smaller sample from the same population.

are all small and moderately large deviations from ignorable treatment assignment, namely, all $\boldsymbol{\theta} \in B_\Gamma$ for $\Gamma \leq 1.993$. The methylmercury comparison provides strong evidence that the true treatment assignment probabilities $\boldsymbol{\theta}$ are not in $B_{1.993}$, but rather are in B_Γ for some $\Gamma > 1.993$.

Despite this, the conclusion about HDL cholesterol stands unaltered. The hypothesis of no effect of daily drinking on HDL cholesterol is rejected for all $\boldsymbol{\theta} \in B_{3.614}$ and is not rejected for some $\boldsymbol{\theta} \in B_\Gamma$ for every $\Gamma > 3.614$. As it stands, that statement requires no amendment, because $B_{1.993} \subset B_{3.614}$. To say more, attention must turn to the relationship between HDL cholesterol levels and methylmercury levels.

The pattern seen in this example is not inevitable. The reverse pattern is also possible. There are examples in which the smallest bias Γ that can explain the behavior of the unaffected outcome, $R_{ij2} = r_{Tij2} = r_{Cij2}$, is larger than needed to explain away the possible effects on the primary outcome [9].

12.2 Did the Test For Bias Increase Insensitivity to Bias?

Testing a Single Vector of Treatment Assignment Probabilities $\boldsymbol{\theta}$

With knowledge that $R_{ij2} = r_{Tij2} = r_{Cij2}$ is unaffected by treatment, it is possible to use R_{ij2} to test $H_0' : \boldsymbol{\theta} = \boldsymbol{\theta}_0$ for any specific $\boldsymbol{\theta}_0$, simply by using T_2 in (8.16) computed at $\boldsymbol{\theta}_0$. Indeed, every $\boldsymbol{\theta}_0 \in B_{1.993}$ was tested and rejected in this way in Sect. 12.1. Alas, as discussed in Sect. 12.1, the biased assignment probabilities $\boldsymbol{\theta} \in B_{1.993}$ are not especially interesting biased treatment assignments $\boldsymbol{\theta}$, because rejection of the hypothesis of no effect on HDL cholesterol, R_{ij1}, is insensitive to all biases $\boldsymbol{\theta} \in B_{3.614} \supset B_{1.993}$. What are the interesting and potentially troubling biased treatment assignment probabilities $\boldsymbol{\theta}$?

The interesting and troubling $\boldsymbol{\theta}$s are those in the set $\mathcal{J}$ of boundary points of $B_{3.614}$ such that (8.16) holds as an equality.[4] At those troubling boundary points in $\mathcal{J}$, the smallest increase in Γ would lead to acceptance of the null hypothesis of no effect of alcohol on HDL cholesterol. Are these $\boldsymbol{\theta}_0 \in \mathcal{J}$ plausible in light of the pattern of methylmercury levels? In the study in Sect. 1.4, methylmercury is of interest only indirectly as a tool for shedding light on the comparison of HDL cholesterol levels of light daily drinkers and controls.

Although the hypothesis of no effect of alcohol on HDL cholesterol is just barely rejected for a few troubling boundary points $\boldsymbol{\theta}_0 \in \mathcal{J} \subset B_\Gamma$ with $\Gamma = 3.614$, none of these boundary points is plausible as the true $\boldsymbol{\theta}$ in light of the pattern of methylmercury levels. As we will see in a moment, to be compatible with the pattern of methylmercury levels and also explain the higher HDL cholesterol levels among light daily drinkers, the treatment assignment probabilities $\boldsymbol{\theta}$ must lie in a B_Γ with

[4] This interesting and troubling set $\mathcal{J}$ of biases [46] was discussed in Sect. 8.6 in its final subsection. However, that subsection of Sect. 8.6 has an asterisk, and you do not need to read it to read Sect. 12.2.

$\Gamma > 3.614$ and not in $B_{3.614}$. Not only does the pattern of methylmercury levels in Fig. 1.5 not weaken the conclusion about the effects on HDL cholesterol, but instead it strengthens that conclusion. Although rejection of no effect on HDL cholesterol is indeed sensitive to some $\boldsymbol{\theta} \in B_{3.615} \supset B_{3.614}$, those $\boldsymbol{\theta}$s are themselves rejected when tested using methylmercury levels.

Conceptually, for each $\boldsymbol{\theta}_0 \in \mathcal{J}$, the standardized absolute deviate on the left side of (8.16) is computed from the unaffected outcome $R_{ij2} = r_{Tij2} = r_{Cij2}$—here, from the methylmercury levels. In (8.16) and similar expressions, substitute the score q'_{ij} computed from the unaffected R_{ij2} for the score q_{ij} computed from the possibly affected R_{ij1}. Then, (8.16) computed from R_{2ij} is used to test $H'_0 : \boldsymbol{\theta} = \boldsymbol{\theta}_0$ for each $\boldsymbol{\theta}_0 \in \mathcal{J}$. The question is whether the $\boldsymbol{\theta}_0 \in \mathcal{J}$ that barely reject the hypothesis of no effect on R_{ij1} are themselves rejected by the testing using the unaffected outcome, R_{2ij}.

In the example using Quade's statistic, for $\boldsymbol{\theta}_0 \in \mathcal{J}$, the minimum absolute deviate (8.16) testing $H'_0 : \boldsymbol{\theta} = \boldsymbol{\theta}_0$ is 5.30 yielding a maximum P-value of 1.17×10^{-7}. So, none of the $\boldsymbol{\theta} \in \mathcal{J}$ is actually plausible; it is virtually inconceivable that any of these $\boldsymbol{\theta}$'s could produce Fig. 1.5. There is a $\boldsymbol{\theta} \in B_\Gamma$ for every $\Gamma > 1.993$ that could produce the pattern for methylmercury on the right in Fig. 1.5, and there is another $\boldsymbol{\theta} \in B_\Gamma$ for $\Gamma = 3.614 + \varepsilon$ for every $\varepsilon > 0$ that could produce the pattern on left in Fig. 1.5, but for sufficiently small $\varepsilon > 0$ there is no $\boldsymbol{\theta} \in B_\Gamma$ for $\Gamma = 3.614 + \varepsilon$ that can simultaneously produce both sides of Fig. 1.5. If the difference in HDL cholesterol levels in Fig. 1.5 is not an effect of alcohol, then bias needs to be larger than $\Gamma = 3.614$.

In a situation like this, we say that there is no gap between the sensitivity analysis and the test for bias: at the point where the main comparison is becoming sensitive to bias, the test for bias is stepping in to reject the troubling boundary points $\boldsymbol{\theta}_0 \in \mathcal{J}$ that produce sensitivity to unmeasured bias [46]. When there is no gap, the test for bias is providing useful information.

The calculations are easiest to understand when $\mathcal{J}$ contains a single boundary point, $\mathcal{J} = \{\boldsymbol{\theta}_0\}$. This happens, for example, in matched pairs, $J = 2$, if the within-block ranks for the primary outcome are never tied, say $q_{i1} \neq q_{i2}$ for every i. In this case, the one boundary bias $\boldsymbol{\theta}_0$ is given by (8.20) with Γ set to the sensitivity value $\Gamma^\bullet = 3.614$. The two-sided deviate in (8.16) is computed at this $\boldsymbol{\theta}_0$.[5]

---

[5] The situation is only slightly more complicated when $J \geq 2$ or ties are present or both [46, Appendix]. This footnote makes reference to the starred subsection of Sect. 8.6 and in particular to its set $\mathcal{M}_\Gamma$, where $\mathcal{J} = \mathcal{M}_{\Gamma^\bullet}$; so, this footnote also qualifies for an asterisk or star. Unlike $J = 2$, with $J > 2$, there is no explicit formula for the $\boldsymbol{\theta} \in \mathcal{J} = \mathcal{M}_{\Gamma^\bullet}$ that achieve the sensitivity value, $\Gamma^\bullet$; so, the separable approximation in Definition 8.1 is used to determine the upper bound on the P-value for the primary outcome, here HDL cholesterol. All of the $\boldsymbol{\theta} \in \mathcal{J} = \mathcal{M}_{\Gamma^\bullet}$ give the same bound on the P-value for the primary outcome, but they may differ about the unaffected outcome, here methylmercury. Some q_{ij}'s for the primary outcome, here HDL cholesterol, may be tied; so, in the separable algorithm, when individuals j in block i are sorted into increasing order by their q_{ij}'s, the order statistics, $q_{i(1)} \leq \cdots \leq q_{i(J)}$, are well defined, but the identity of the person giving rise to $q_{i(j)}$ may be ambiguous. Write q'_{ij} for the score for the unaffected outcome for individual j in block i. Create not one but two orderings for the pairs $\left(q_{ij}, q'_{ij}\right)$ within block i. In order 1, sort

To produce Fig. 1.5 in the absence of an effect of alcohol on HDL cholesterol, the bias in treatment assignment needs to be larger than $\Gamma = 3.614$. How much larger? That question is answered in Sect. 12.3.

12.3 Sensitivity Analyses Informed by Tests for Bias

A Confidence Set Θ for θ

Which $\boldsymbol{\theta}_0$ are not rejected by a test for bias using an unaffected outcome, such as methylmercury levels? Define Θ to be the set of all $\boldsymbol{\theta}_0$ that are not rejected at level α' when testing $H_0' : \boldsymbol{\theta} = \boldsymbol{\theta}_0$ by (8.16) using an unaffected outcome $R_{ij2} = r_{Tij2} = r_{Cij2}$.[6] Then Θ is a set of $I \times J$ matrices $\boldsymbol{\theta}_0$ with

$$0 \leq \theta_{ij} \leq 1 \text{ for all } ij \text{ and } 1 = \sum_{j=1}^{J} \theta_{ij} \text{ for each } i. \tag{12.1}$$

From first principles, Θ is a $1 - \alpha'$ confidence set for $\boldsymbol{\theta}_0$; that is, when one true value $\boldsymbol{\theta}$ is tested, it is mistakenly rejected with probability at most α', so with probability at least $1 - \alpha'$ that does not happen and the random set Θ contains the true $\boldsymbol{\theta}$. As with the confidence set $\mathcal{D}$ for $\boldsymbol{\delta}$ in Sect. 2.10, the set Θ does not converge to a single $\boldsymbol{\theta}$, and indeed its dimension increases as $I \to \infty$. Nonetheless, Θ may provide useful information.

In parallel with (8.17) for the primary outcome R_{ij1}, there is a second function $f'_{\alpha/2}(\boldsymbol{\theta})$ for the unaffected outcome:

$$f'_{\alpha'/2}(\boldsymbol{\theta}) = \left(T_2 - \sum_{i=1}^{I}\sum_{j=1}^{J}\theta_{ij}\, q'_{ij}\right)^2 - \varsigma_{\alpha'/2}\sum_{i=1}^{I}\sum_{j=1}^{J}\left\{\theta_{ij}\left(q'_{ij}\right)^2 - \left(\sum_{j=1}^{J}\theta_{ij}\, q'_{ij}\right)^2\right\}. \tag{12.2}$$

---

by increasing q_{ij}, and if two or more q_{ij}'s are tied, sort within a tied group by increasing order of q'_{ij}. In order 2, sort by increasing q_{ij}, and if two or more q_{ij}'s are tied, sort within a tied group by decreasing order of q'_{ij}. In the separable algorithm, each order produces a $\boldsymbol{\theta}_0$ using (8.22). Among $\boldsymbol{\theta}_0 \in \mathcal{J} = \mathcal{M}_{\Gamma^\bullet}$, order 1 makes it most difficult to use the unaffected outcome to reject $H_0' : \boldsymbol{\theta} = \boldsymbol{\theta}_0$ in the upper tail of (8.16). Among $\boldsymbol{\theta}_0 \in \mathcal{J} = \mathcal{M}_{\Gamma^\bullet}$, order 2 makes it most difficult to use the unaffected outcome to reject $H_0' : \boldsymbol{\theta} = \boldsymbol{\theta}_0$ in the lower tail of (8.16). So, compute both of these one-sided P-values testing $H_0' : \boldsymbol{\theta} = \boldsymbol{\theta}_0$, double the smaller of the two one-sided P-values, and report the minimum of that value or 1 as the two-sided P-value for $H_0' : \boldsymbol{\theta} = \boldsymbol{\theta}_0$. It is not difficult to show that orders 1 and 2 provide the relevant bounds; see Propositions 1 and 2 and §5 of [49] or [41, §4.7.3].

[6] As always, when R_{ij2} replaces R_{ij1} in (8.16), and in similar expressions, the score q'_{ij} for R_{ij2} replaces the score q_{ij} for R_{ij1}. It is important that we have two test statistics of the form (8.16) involving the same Z_{ij} and the same θ_{ij} but different scores, q_{ij} or q'_{ij}.

In parallel with Proposition 8.3, a $\boldsymbol{\theta}$ satisfying (12.1) is included in the $1-\alpha'$ confidence set Θ if and only if $f'_{\alpha'/2}(\boldsymbol{\theta}) < 0$. In parallel with Proposition 8.4, $f'_{\alpha'/2}(\boldsymbol{\theta})$ is also a convex quadratic function of $\boldsymbol{\theta}$.

Strictly speaking, a $\boldsymbol{\theta}$ with $f'_{\alpha'/2}(\boldsymbol{\theta}) = 0$ is outside the confidence set, Θ, but barely so. Although there are some practical and important exceptions [4, 18], in most statistical work we do not distinguish a confidence interval, say [4.7, 5.3), from its closure, [4.7, 5.3], because it does not seem relevant to regard 5.29999 as plausible and 5.3 as implausible. When it is technically convenient, I will replace Θ by its closure $\overline{\Theta}$ without much discussion. The closure $\overline{\Theta}$ of Θ is the set of $\boldsymbol{\theta}$ satisfying (12.1) such that $f'_{\alpha'/2}(\boldsymbol{\theta}) \leq 0$.

Is There a Gap Between a Test for Bias and a Sensitivity Analysis?

Instead of worrying about all $\boldsymbol{\theta} \in B_\Gamma$, perhaps we should confine our worries to a possibly smaller set, $\boldsymbol{\theta} \in B_\Gamma \cap \Theta$. After all, values of $\boldsymbol{\theta} \in B_\Gamma$ that are not also in Θ have been rejected by the test for bias using the unaffected outcome. By definition of the sensitivity value, $\Gamma^\bullet$, the primary comparison is sensitive to some $\boldsymbol{\theta} \in B_\Gamma$ for all $\Gamma > \Gamma^\bullet$. The method in Sect. 12.2 asked whether the primary comparison involving HDL cholesterol is insensitive to all $\boldsymbol{\theta} \in B_\Gamma \cap \Theta$ for $\Gamma = \Gamma^\bullet + \varepsilon = 3.614 + \varepsilon$ for all sufficiently small $\varepsilon > 0$.

Equivalently, Sect. 12.2 asked whether the troubling boundary biases in $\mathcal{J}$ are all excluded from the confidence set Θ, in the sense that $\emptyset = \mathcal{J} \cap \Theta$. The notion of "no gap" was introduced in Sect. 12.2; it said, informally, that there is no gap between the sensitivity analysis and the test for bias if none of the most immediately troubling biases $\boldsymbol{\theta} \in \mathcal{J}$ is plausible. That informal definition may be replaced by a definition: if $\emptyset = \mathcal{J} \cap \Theta$, then there is "no gap" [46, Definition 3.1]. If $\emptyset \neq \mathcal{J} \cap \Theta$, then we gain nothing by restricting our worries to $\boldsymbol{\theta} \in B_\Gamma \cap \Theta \subseteq B_\Gamma$.

Informed Sensitivity Analyses

As noted in the previous subsection, if there is no gap, then the test for bias strengthens the sensitivity analysis by ruling out some $\boldsymbol{\theta}$s of magnitude greater than $\Gamma^\bullet$. To what precise extent is the sensitivity analysis strengthened? What is the largest Γ such that the primary comparison is insensitive to all $\boldsymbol{\theta} \in B_\Gamma \cap \overline{\Theta}$? If there is no gap, then we know this Γ is larger than $\Gamma^\bullet$. How much larger?

The answer requires some computation, but otherwise is not difficult. Recall that $f_{\alpha/2}(\boldsymbol{\theta})$ is defined in (8.17) and $f'_{\alpha'/2}(\boldsymbol{\theta})$ is defined in (12.2). Rejection of $H_0 : \boldsymbol{\delta} = \boldsymbol{\delta}_0$ in a two-sided α-level test is insensitive to all biased treatment assignments $\boldsymbol{\theta} \in B_\Gamma \cap \overline{\Theta}$

Table 12.1 Optimized uninformed and informed θ_{ij}'s for block $i = 5$ computed at $\Gamma = 3.614$ and Quade's ranks for HDL cholesterol and methylmercury. Note that $0.5464167/0.1511944 = 0.3916342/0.1083658 = 3.614$

Block i	Person j	Treatment Z_{ij}	HDL cholesterol	Methylmercury	Uninformed θ_{ij}	Informed θ_{ij}
5	1	1	2.71	2.18	0.1511944	0.3916342
5	2	0	0.90	0.54	0.1511944	0.1083658
5	3	0	1.80	1.64	0.1511944	0.1083658
5	4	0	3.61	1.09	0.5464167	0.3916342

if $f_{\alpha/2}(\boldsymbol{\theta}) \geq 0$ for all $\boldsymbol{\theta} \in B_\Gamma$ with $f'_{\alpha'/2}(\boldsymbol{\theta}) \leq 0$. In other words, solve the optimization problem

$$F^*_{\Gamma,\alpha/2} = \min_{\boldsymbol{\theta} \in B_\Gamma \cap \overline{\Theta}} f_{\alpha/2}(\boldsymbol{\theta}), \tag{12.3}$$

and reject H_0 in the presence of a bias of Γ if $F^*_{\Gamma,\alpha/2} \geq 0$. The optimization problem (12.3) minimizes a convex quadratic function, $f_{\alpha/2}(\boldsymbol{\theta})$, subject to linear equality and inequality constraints (8.8)–(8.10) and one convex quadratic constraint, namely, $f'_{\alpha'/2}(\boldsymbol{\theta}) \leq 0$.[7]

The hypothesis, $H_0 : \boldsymbol{\delta} = \mathbf{0}$, of no effect of light daily alcohol on HDL cholesterol levels in Sect. 1.4 is rejected at level $\alpha = 0.05$ for all $\boldsymbol{\theta} \in B_\Gamma$ with $\Gamma = \Gamma^\bullet = 3.614$. Confining the sensitivity analysis to the (closure of the) 95% confidence set, $\boldsymbol{\theta} \in \overline{\Theta}$, the hypothesis $H_0 : \boldsymbol{\delta} = \mathbf{0}$ is rejected for all $\boldsymbol{\theta} \in B_\Gamma \cap \overline{\Theta}$ for $\Gamma = 3.82$. So, the test for bias using methylmercury, R_{ij2}, found strong evidence of unmeasured confounding—i.e., strong evidence that $\boldsymbol{\theta} \neq \overline{\boldsymbol{\theta}}$—and yet taking account of that evidence only strengthened the evidence in support of an effect of light alcohol consumption on HDL cholesterol. Without the information provided by methylmercury, the HDL cholesterol comparison becomes sensitive at $\Gamma = 3.614$; however, with that information, it becomes sensitive at $\Gamma = 3.82$. In a matched pair, using the formula $\Gamma = (\Lambda\Delta + 1)/(\Gamma + \Delta)$ from Sect. 8.7, $\Gamma = 3.614$ is equivalent to $(\Lambda, \Delta) = (6, 8.7)$, while $\Gamma = 3.82$ is equivalent to $(\Lambda, \Delta) = (6, 10.1)$.[8]

In understanding the role of the test for bias in informing the sensitivity analysis, it is helpful to examine the 800-dimensional vectors $\boldsymbol{\theta}$ that minimize $f_{\alpha/2}(\boldsymbol{\theta})$ subject to (8.8)–(8.10) with and without the constraint $f'_{\alpha'/2}(\boldsymbol{\theta}) \leq 0$. The uninformed sensitivity analysis ignores methylmercury and is not constrained to satisfy $f'_{\alpha'/2}(\boldsymbol{\theta}) \leq 0$, while the informed sensitivity analysis insists that $f'_{\alpha'/2}(\boldsymbol{\theta}) \leq 0$ to simultaneously produce both sides of Fig. 1.5. For $\Gamma = 3.614$, Table 12.1 shows the uninformed and informed θ_{ij} for block $i = 5$, the first block in which they differ. Uninformed

[7] The R package `informedSen` solves this optimization problem using `gurobi` [48]. It is quick with 200 blocks of size $J = 4$ in the HDL cholesterol example, where $\boldsymbol{\theta}$ has dimension $200 \times 4 = 800$.

[8] This example used $\alpha = \alpha' = 0.05$ in two-sided tests. There are other options. For instance, taking $\alpha + \alpha' = 0.05$ ensures that the chance that either Θ fails to cover $\boldsymbol{\theta}$ or H_0 is falsely rejected is at most 0.05. This perspective views $\boldsymbol{\theta}$ as a nuisance parameter when testing H_0 and applies the method of Berger and Boos [5]. The requirement that $\alpha + \alpha' = 0.05$ has both advantages and disadvantages [48, §5.2].

Table 12.2 Correlation between HDL cholesterol, methylmercury, and the optimizing θ_{ij} with (informed by) or without (uninformed by) the quadratic constraint $f'_{\alpha'/2}(\boldsymbol{\theta}) \leq 0$. The values for HDL cholesterol and methylmercury are Quade's ranks centered to have mean zero in each block i

	HDL	Methylmercury	Informed θ_{ij}	Uninformed θ_{ij}
HDL	1.000			
Methylmercury	0.132	1.000		
Informed θ_{ij}	0.687	0.397	1.000	
Uninformed θ_{ij}	0.676	0.071	0.745	1.000

by methylmercury, at the optimum, the uninformed θ_{ij} has given the largest possible probability to person $j = 4$ in block $i = 5$, because this person has the largest rank for HDL cholesterol. The informed θ_{ij} has shared the largest probability between persons $j = 1$ and $j = 4$, because person $j = 1$ has the largest rank for methylmercury and a large rank for HDL cholesterol. The informed θ_{ij} is doing the best it can within $B_{3.614}$ to produce both sides of Fig. 1.5, while the uninformed θ_{ij} is only trying to produce the left panel of Fig. 1.5. In trying to produce both sides of Fig. 1.5, the informed θ_{ij} is struggling within $\boldsymbol{\theta} \in B_{3.614}$; it needs a larger Γ—it needs $\boldsymbol{\theta} \in B_{3.82}$—to produce both sides of Fig. 1.5.

Table 12.2 shows correlations involving the informed $\boldsymbol{\theta}$ and the uninformed $\boldsymbol{\theta}$. HDL cholesterol and methylmercury are represented in Table 12.2 by Quade's ranks centered to have mean zero in each block. Because $1 = \sum_{j=1}^{J} \theta_{ij}$ for each i, the mean of θ_{ij} is $1/J$ in every block. So, the correlations in Table 12.2 are analogous to partial correlations that have removed the between-block variation. In Table 12.2, the centered ranks for HDL cholesterol and methylmercury are correlated, but not strongly correlated; the correlation is 0.132. The uninformed θ_{ij} are only slightly correlated with methylmercury ranks (0.071), but the constraint $f'_{\alpha'/2}(\boldsymbol{\theta}) \leq 0$ forces that correlation up to 0.397. The informed and uninformed θ_{ij} have correlation 0.745, so the constraint $f'_{\alpha'/2}(\boldsymbol{\theta}) \leq 0$ has materially distracted θ_{ij} from the task of producing the left panel of Fig. 1.5.

In one sense, the finding of increased insensitivity to bias can seem to be almost inevitable, because $B_\Gamma \cap \overline{\Theta} \subseteq B_\Gamma$: a minimum of $f_{\alpha/2}(\boldsymbol{\theta})$ over $B_\Gamma \cap \overline{\Theta}$ cannot be smaller than a minimum of $f_{\alpha/2}(\boldsymbol{\theta})$ over B_Γ. However, increased insensitivity is not inevitable, because in many cases the two minima are equal. Again, the issue turns on whether there is a gap between the sensitivity analysis and the test for bias, that is, whether the confidence set excludes from consideration the troublesome boundary points of B_Γ, or formally whether $\emptyset = \mathcal{J} \cap B_\Gamma$.

The Covering Design Sensitivity

In parallel with the design sensitivity, $\widetilde{\Gamma}$, in Chap. 10, there is another quantity, $\widehat{\Gamma}$, called the covering design sensitivity. In a favorable situation with a treatment effect and no unmeasured bias in treatment assignment, $\boldsymbol{\theta} = \overline{\boldsymbol{\theta}}$, the design sensitivity $\widetilde{\Gamma}$

is the limiting sensitivity to unmeasured bias as $I \rightarrow \infty$. In parallel, but aided by an unaffected outcome $R_{ij2} = r_{Tij2} = r_{Cij2}$ to build a confidence set Θ for $\boldsymbol{\theta}$, the covering design sensitivity is the limit as $I \rightarrow \infty$ of the smallest Γ that can explain the pattern of both outcomes, R_{ij1} and R_{ij2}, in terms of biased treatment assignment, $\boldsymbol{\theta} \neq \overline{\boldsymbol{\theta}}$.

Calculations of the covering design sensitivity are available in several simple situations [46, §5]. Consider one simple situation. As has been the case throughout this chapter, the bivariate $\mathbf{R}_{ij}$ has a possibly affected primary outcome as its first coordinate, R_{i1}, and an unaffected outcome as its second coordinate, R_{i2}.[9] This situation has matched pairs, $J = 2$, and the treated-minus-control pair differences, $\mathbf{Y}_i = (\mathbf{R}_{i1} - \mathbf{R}_{i2})(Z_{i1} - Z_{i2})$, are bivariate normal with variances one, correlation ρ, and mean vector $\left(\frac{1}{2}, 0\right)$, so Y_{i1} has a treatment effect that is half its standard deviation in size, and Y_{i2} is unaffected with expectation zero.

The rank statistic, MH, for pair differences, Y_i, was proposed by Markowski and Hettmansperger [28] and was discussed in Problem 8.5 and Sect. 9.3. In the notation of Sect. 9.3, the version of the MH statistic used here has $f_1 = 0.4$ and $f_2 = 0.8$ and was suggested as best for normal data [28]. So, unlike Noether's statistic, this statistic assigns rank 0 to the 40% of pairs with the smallest $|Y_i|$, rank 2 to the 20% of pairs with the largest $|Y_i|$, and rank 1 to the remaining 40% of pairs.

The design sensitivity, $\widetilde{\Gamma}$, and covering design sensitivity, $\widehat{\Gamma}$, are both computed in the same favorable situation with a treatment effect and no unmeasured bias in treatment assignment. Unlike the design sensitivity, $\widetilde{\Gamma}$, the covering design sensitivity, $\widehat{\Gamma}$ takes account of the additional information provided by the unaffected outcome. In this situation, if $\rho = 0$, then $\widetilde{\Gamma} = \widehat{\Gamma} = 3.90$. Because the design sensitivity $\widetilde{\Gamma}$ is based on an analysis that ignores R_{ij2}, it is unchanged when ρ changes. At $\rho = 0.25$, the covering design sensitivity is $\widehat{\Gamma} = 4.34$, while at $\rho = 0.5$ it is $\widehat{\Gamma} = 5.01$.

The design sensitivity, $\widetilde{\Gamma}$, and covering design sensitivity, $\widehat{\Gamma}$, have been compared in additional simple situations with various statistics [46, Table 3]. In particular, it seems best to use different statistics for the test for bias and for the test for effect. If the test for bias uses different rank scores in [46, Table 3], then $\widehat{\Gamma} = 4.50$ at $\rho = 0.25$ and $\widehat{\Gamma} = 5.54$ at $\rho = 0.5$. This pattern is also evident in simulations [46, Table 2].

In large samples, the unaffected outcome can substantially increase the magnitude of bias in treatment assignment, Γ, that would need to be present to explain away the observed associations as something other than a treatment effect.

---

[9] The situations discussed here are labeled "MH, methods 1 and 2, N, $\tau = 1/2$" in [46, Table 3].

12.4 *Further Reading

Quasi-experimental devices: Unlike a sensitivity analysis, a quasi-experimental device introduces some new element of data intended to shed light on unmeasured biases in observational studies. Known effects are one such device, but there are many others. Quasi-experimental devices were first studied systematically by Donald T. Campbell [10, 11] and his colleagues [12, 52]. There are several reviews of quasi-experimental devices [1, 3, 23, 31, 36, 43, 51, 55], as well as detailed reviews of specific devices [7, 13, 14, 21, 56]. Books about causal inference in observational studies often devote a chapter or more to quasi-experimental devices [2, 22, 44, 47].

One concept with many names: In the literature of several fields, known effects are also called "control constructs," "control outcomes," "negative control outcomes," and "placebo outcomes," and that literature provides a wide variety of interesting examples and methods [16, 20, 26, 27, 29, 30, 32, 37, 38, 40, 41, 46, 48, 53, 57, 65]. Karmakar and colleagues [24] use known effects to construct two evidence factors in case-control studies, where the known effect yields two types of cases.

Hill's consideration of "specificity": Sir Austin Bradford Hill [19] suggested that a treatment associated with few effects was more plausibly the cause of those effects than a treatment associated with many effects. Kenneth Rothman and Sander Greenland [50] are critical of the idea that counting associations is a reliable guide to causality. In a short, interesting article, Noel Weiss [60] views known effects of various kinds as rehabilitating Sir Austin Bradford Hill's concept of the "specificity of an effect," while removing its problematic aspects. Specificity has played an important role in some observational studies [54].

Effects of known direction: A known effect need not be an effect known to be a zero effect. Sometimes the direction of an effect is known, even though the magnitude of the effect is not known ([41, §6.5] and [45, §5.2.4]). Often, "no effect" is a boundary case of an effect known to be nonnegative, as in Sect. 2.9. There are a number of interesting examples from economics [6, 8] and public health [63].

Choice of test statistics: For simplicity, this chapter used Quade's statistic in two-sided tests, both in tests for a treatment effect and in tests for unmeasured bias using an unaffected outcome. This is a simple choice, but not the best choice. The logic in Chaps. 9 and 11 suggested certain test statistics for use in sensitivity analyses of tests for a treatment effect, but that logic says nothing about testing for bias using an unaffected outcome. As noted in the discussion of the covering design sensitivity in Sect. 12.3, different test statistics should be used in the test for effect based on (r_{Tij1}, r_{Cij1}) and the test for bias based on the unaffected outcome (r_{Tij2}, r_{Cij2}) [46, Tables 2 and 3].

Problems

12.1 Sensitivity Value, $\Gamma^{\bullet}$

Focus on the 200 blocks with data on methylmercury levels in the HDL cholesterol example. Check that the sensitivity value in the HDL cholesterol example is $\Gamma^{\bullet} = 3.614$ in a 0.05-level two-sided test using Quade's statistic.

12.2 Problem 12.1, Continued

Using the same data as in Problem 12.1, determine the sensitivity value $\Gamma^{\bullet}$ if Quade's ranks are replaced by (i) Wilcoxon's within-block ranks and (ii) the U-statistic (8,6,8) ranks, which is the default in the `wgtRank` function.

12.3 Problems 12.1 and 12.2, Continued

Problems 12.1 and 12.2 used the 200 blocks that had data on methylmercury; however, these problems did not use the data on methylmercury. To gain insight into the behavior of the sensitivity value $\Gamma^{\bullet}$ as I increases, repeat Problems 12.1 and 12.2 using all $I = 406$ blocks in `aHDL`.

12.4 Use the `informedSen` Package in R

Install `gurobi` and `informedSen`. Perform a sensitivity analysis informed by a test for bias by following the steps in the example in the documentation for `informedSen`. That example uses an M-statistic rather than a rank statistic.

12.5 Two Unaffected Outcomes

Suppose that you had a 3-dimensional outcome, $\mathbf{R}_{ij}$, in which R_{ij2} and R_{ij3} are both unaffected outcomes. Propose a method to conduct a sensitivity analysis for R_{ij1} informed by both R_{ij2} and R_{ij3}. (For an easy solution, see [48, §5.2].)

References

1. Angrist, J.D., Krueger, A.B.: Empirical strategies in labor economics. In: O. Ashenfelter, D. Card (eds.) Handbook of Labor Economics, vol. 3, pp. 1277–1366. Elsevier, New York (1999)
2. Angrist, J.D., Pischke, J.S.: Mostly Harmless Econometrics: An Empiricist's Companion. Princeton University Press, Princeton, NJ (2009)
3. Athey, S., Imbens, G.W.: The state of applied econometrics: Causality and policy evaluation. J. Econ. Perspect. **31**(2), 3–32 (2017)
4. Bauer, P., Kieser, M.: A unifying approach for confidence intervals and testing of equivalence and difference. Biometrika **83**(4), 934–937 (1996)
5. Berger, R.L., Boos, D.D.: P values maximized over a confidence set for the nuisance parameter. J. Am. Stat. Assoc. **89**(427), 1012–1016 (1994)
6. Bernanke, B.S.: The macroeconomics of the Great Depression: A comparative approach. In: Essays on the Great Depression, pp. 5–37. Princeton University Press, Princeton, NJ (2009). Reprinted from the Journal of Money, Credit and Banking, 1995
7. Bertrand, M., Duflo, E., Mullainathan, S.: How much should we trust differences-in-differences estimates? Quart. J. Econ. **119**(1), 249–275 (2004)

8. Bound, J.: The health and earnings of rejected disability insurance applicants. Am. Econ. Rev. **81**, 482–503 (1989)
9. Brumberg, K., Ellis, D.E., Small, D.S., Hennessy, S., Rosenbaum, P.R.: Using natural strata when examining unmeasured biases in an observational study of neurological side effects of antibiotics. J. Roy. Stat. Soc. C (Appl. Stat.) **72**(2), 314–329 (2023)
10. Campbell, D.T.: Factors relevant to the validity of experiments in social settings. Psychol. Bull. **54**(4), 297–312 (1957)
11. Campbell, D.T.: Methodology and Epistemology for Social Science: Selected Papers. University of Chicago Press, Chicago (1988)
12. Campbell, D.T., Stanley, J.C.: Experimental and Quasi-experimental Designs for Research. Rand McNally, Chicago (1966)
13. Cattaneo, M.D., Idrobo, N., Titiunik, R.: A Practical Introduction to Regression Discontinuity Designs. Cambridge University Press, New York (2019)
14. Cattaneo, M.D., Titiunik, R.: Regression discontinuity designs. Annu. Rev. Econ. **14**(1), 821–851 (2022)
15. Dressler, V.L., Santos, C.M.M., Antes, F.G., Bentlin, F.R.S., Pozebon, D., Flores, E.M.M.: Total mercury, inorganic mercury and methyl mercury determination in red wine. Food Analyt. Methods **5**, 505–511 (2012)
16. Eggers, A.C., Tuñón, G., Dafoe, A.: Placebo tests for causal inference. Am. J. Polit. Sci. **68**, 1106–1121 (2024)
17. Fodor, J.A.: The dogma that didn't bark (A fragment of a naturalized epistemology). Mind **100**(2), 201–220 (1991)
18. Goeman, J.J., Solari, A., Stijnen, T.: Three-sided hypothesis testing: simultaneous testing of superiority, equivalence and inferiority. Statist. Med. **29**(20), 2117–2125 (2010)
19. Hill, A.B.: The environment and disease: Association or causation? Proc. Roy. Soc. Med. **58**, 295–300 (1965)
20. Hu, J.K., Tchetgen Tchetgen, E.J., Dominici, F.: Using negative controls to adjust for unmeasured confounding bias in time series studies. Nature Rev. Methods Primers **3**, 66 (2023)
21. Imbens, G., Lemieux, T.: The regression discontinuity design: Theory and applications. J. Economet. **142**, 611–614 (2008)
22. Imbens, G.W., Rubin, D.B.: Causal Inference in Statistics, Social, and Biomedical Sciences. Cambridge University Press, New York (2015)
23. Imbens, G.W., Wooldridge, J.M.: Recent developments in the econometrics of program evaluation. J. Econ. Literat. **47**(1), 5–86 (2009)
24. Karmakar, B., Doubeni, C.A., Small, D.S.: Evidence factors in a case-control study with application to the effect of flexible sigmoidoscopy screening on colorectal cancer. Ann. Appl. Stat. **14**(2), 829–849 (2020)
25. Kullback, S., Leibler, R.A.: Information and sufficiency. Ann. Math. Stat. **22**(1), 79–86 (1951)
26. Kundu, S., Ding, P., Li, X., Wang, J.: Sensitivity analysis for the test-negative design. Preprint arXiv:2406.06980 (2024)
27. Lipsitch, M., Tchetgen, E.T., Cohen, T.: Negative controls: A tool for detecting confounding and bias in observational studies. Epidemiology **21**(3), 383 (2010)
28. Markowski, E.P., Hettmansperger, T.P.: Inference based on simple rank step score statistics for the location model. J. Am. Stat. Assoc. **77**(380), 901–907 (1982)
29. Mattei, A., Li, F., Mealli, F.: Exploiting multiple outcomes in bayesian principal stratification analysis with application to the evaluation of a job training program. Ann. Appl. Stat. **7**, 2336–2360 (2013)
30. Mealli, F., Pacini, B.: Using secondary outcomes to sharpen inference in randomized experiments with noncompliance. J. Am. Stat. Assoc. **108**(503), 1120–1131 (2013)
31. Meyer, B.D.: Natural and quasi-experiments in economics. J. Bus. Econ. Stat. **13**(2), 151–161 (1995)
32. Miao, W., Geng, Z., Tchetgen Tchetgen, E.J.: Identifying causal effects with proxy variables of an unmeasured confounder. Biometrika **105**(4), 987–993 (2018)
33. Noë, A.: Action in Perception. MIT Press, Cambridge, MA (2004)

34. Pedersen, G.A., Mortensen, G.K., Larsen, E.H.: Beverages as a source of toxic trace element intake. Food Addit. Contamin. **11**(3), 351–363 (1994)
35. Peirce, C.S.: The First Rule of Logic. In: The Essential Peirce, Volume 2: Selected Philosophical Writings (1893-1913). Indiana University Press, Bloomington, IN (1992)
36. Reichardt, C.S.: Quasi-experimentation: A Guide to Design and Analysis. Guilford Publications, New York (2019)
37. Rosenbaum, P.R.: From association to causation in observational studies: The role of tests of strongly ignorable treatment assignment. J. Am. Stat. Assoc. **79**(385), 41–48 (1984)
38. Rosenbaum, P.R.: On permutation tests for hidden biases in observational studies. Ann. Stat. **17**(2), 643–653 (1989)
39. Rosenbaum, P.R.: The role of known effects in observational studies. Biometrics **45**, 557–569 (1989)
40. Rosenbaum, P.R.: Detecting bias with confidence in observational studies. Biometrika **79**(2), 367–374 (1992)
41. Rosenbaum, P.R.: Observational Studies, 2nd edn. Springer, New York (2002)
42. Rosenbaum, P.R.: Design sensitivity in observational studies. Biometrika **91**(1), 153–164 (2004)
43. Rosenbaum, P.R.: How to see more in observational studies: Some new quasi-experimental devices. Annu. Rev. Stat. Appl. **2**, 21–48 (2015)
44. Rosenbaum, P.R.: Observation and Experiment: An Introduction to Causal Inference. Harvard University Press, Cambridge, MA (2017)
45. Rosenbaum, P.R.: Design of Observational Studies, 2nd edn. Springer, New York (2020)
46. Rosenbaum, P.R.: Can we reliably detect biases that matter in observational studies? Stat. Sci. **38**, 440–457 (2023)
47. Rosenbaum, P.R.: Causal Inference. MIT Press, Cambridge, MA (2023)
48. Rosenbaum, P.R.: Sensitivity analyses informed by tests for bias in observational studies. Biometrics **79**, 475–487 (2023)
49. Rosenbaum, P.R., Krieger, A.M.: Sensitivity of two-sample permutation inferences in observational studies. J. Am. Stat. Assoc. **85**(410), 493–498 (1990)
50. Rothman, K.J., Greenland, S.: Causation and causal inference in epidemiology. Am. J. Public Health **95**(S1), S144–S150 (2005)
51. Salzberg, A.J.: Removable selection bias in quasi-experiments. Am. Stat. **53**(2), 103–107 (1999)
52. Shadish, W., Cook, T.D., Campbell, D.T.: Experimental and Quasi-experimental Designs for Generalized Causal Inference. Houghton Mifflin Boston, MA (2002)
53. Shi, X., Miao, W., Tchetgen Tchetgen, E.: A selective review of negative control methods in epidemiology. Current Epidemiol. Rep. **7**, 190–202 (2020)
54. Silber, J.H., Rosenbaum, P.R., Reiter, J.G., Jain, S., Hill, A.S., Hashemi, S., Brown, S., Olfson, M., Ing, C.: Exposure to operative anesthesia in childhood and subsequent neurobehavioral diagnoses: A natural experiment using appendectomy. Anesthesiology **141**(3), 489–499 (2024)
55. Stuart, E.A., Rubin, D.B.: Best practices in quasi-experimental designs. In: Best Practices in Quantitative Methods. Sage (2008)
56. Stuart, E.A., Rubin, D.B.: Matching with multiple control groups with adjustment for group differences. J. Educ. Behav. Stat. **33**(3), 279–306 (2008)
57. Tchetgen Tchetgen, E.: The control outcome calibration approach for causal inference with unobserved confounding. Am. J. Epidemiol. **179**(5), 633–640 (2014)
58. US Centers for Disease Control: Mercury (2009). https://www.cdc.gov/biomonitoring/pdf/Mercury-FactSheet.pdf (Accessed 3 July 2023).
59. US National Research Council: Toxicological Effects of Methylmercury. National Academies Press, Washington, DC (2000)
60. Weiss, N.S.: Can the "specificity" of an association be rehabilitated as a basis for supporting a causal hypothesis? Epidemiology **13**(1), 6–8 (2002)
61. Wittgenstein, L.: Philosophical Remarks. University of Chicago Press, Chicago (1980)
62. World Health Organization: Mercury and Health (2017). Https://www.who.int/news-room/fact-sheets/detail/mercury-and-health (Accessed 3 July 2023)

63. Wright, M.A., Wintemute, G.J., Rivara, F.P.: Effectiveness of denial of handgun purchase to persons believed to be at high risk for firearm violence. Am. J. Public Health **89**(1), 88–90 (1999)
64. Zhao, Q.: On sensitivity value of pair-matched observational studies. J. Am. Stat. Assoc. **114**, 713–722 (2019)
65. Zhou, Y., Tang, D., Kong, D., Wang, L.: Promises of parallel outcomes. Biometrika **111**(2), 537–550 (2024)

Chapter 13
Evidence Factors for Two Control Groups

We may add force to these experiments
by others of a different kind.

David Hume, 1748
An Enquiry Concerning Human Understanding [22, p. 38]

Abstract This chapter introduces a general technique, evidence factors, in its simplest application, namely, the evaluation of the new information provided by a second control group. The rationale underlying the use of multiple control groups is briefly reviewed. A study has two evidence factors if it permits two essentially independent tests of hypotheses about treatment effects, where the unmeasured biases that affect one test do not affect the other, even though both tests may be biased. Because the two tests are essentially independent, they may be combined using meta-analytic tools as if they came from unrelated studies of unrelated data, even though they actually reanalyze the same data from two orthogonal perspectives. A good test for the second evidence factor is found with the aid of design sensitivity and Bahadur efficiency.

13.1 Multiple Control Groups

What Do We Learn From a Second Control Group?

The two alcohol examples in Sects. 1.4 and 1.5 both had multiple control groups. What is the role of a second control group?

© The Author(s), under exclusive license to Springer Nature Switzerland AG 2025

P. R. Rosenbaum, *An Introduction to the Theory of Observational Studies*,
Springer Texts in Statistics, https://doi.org/10.1007/978-3-031-90494-3_13

We could always have two control groups rather than one by using random numbers to split one control group at random into two groups, but surely nothing is learned by doing that. Whatever is wrong with the first random control group is equally wrong with the second one. If two control groups are to serve any purpose, they must differ in some consequential way. But in what way? Presumably, multiple control groups are intended to speak to the issue of unmeasured bias in treatment assignment, but how do they do that? What can you learn, and what can you not learn, from multiple control groups?

More to the point, once you have multiple control groups, what *have* you learned from them? If we wanted to measure, in quantitative terms, the completely *new* information actually provided by the addition of a second control group—the new information about unmeasured biases—how would we go about it? Do certain patterns in data lead to an increase in insensitivity to unmeasured bias? Do certain patterns entirely eliminate certain counterclaims that refer to certain specific unmeasured biases?

Control by Systematic Variation

Attributing the idea to Morton Bitterman [5], Donald Campbell [7, 8] suggested selecting multiple control groups according to the principle of "control by systematic variation." If an important covariate is unmeasured, perhaps it is possible to find two control groups that are expected to differ substantially with respect to this covariate. If outcomes are similar in two such control groups, but are very different in the treated group, then that tends to undermine the counterclaim asserting that imbalances in this covariate account for the ostensible effect of the treatment [44, 45].

In Sect. 1.4, the three control groups currently drank little alcohol, but their past relationships to alcohol were very different. Members of group N had fewer than 12 drinks in their life, while members of group B had a period in their life when they engaged in binge drinking on most days. This certainly shows a different past relationship with alcohol, but it suggests different attitudes about behaviors and substances that may affect health. Table 13.1 summarizes some differences among the four groups that were mentioned in Sect. 1.4. The *P*-values in Table 13.1 are from William Cochran's [9] Q-statistic for binary variables and Milton Friedman's [16] statistic for continuous variables.

Table 13.1 Comparison of the four groups in the study of alcohol and HDL cholesterol

Variable		Alcohol group				
D=daily, N=never, R=rarely, B=past binge		D	N	R	B	P-value
Ever tried marijuana or hashish?	%	73	9	25	75	0.0000000
Ever tried cocaine, heroin, meth?	%	29	4	4	37	0.0000000
Methylmercury in blood (μg/L)	M	1.12	0.54	0.56	0.56	0.0000008
Been to dentist in past year?	%	67	58	57	48	0.0000006

Notably in Table 13.1, the four groups are very different. Former binge drinkers—group B—resemble the treated group of daily drinkers, D, in answers to "Ever tried marijuana or hashish?" and to a lesser degree in answers to "Ever tried cocaine, heroin, meth?" However, groups D and B are far apart in answers to "Been to dentist in past year?" Groups never, N, and rarely, R, differ most from each other in their answers to "Ever tried marijuana or hashish?", but they differ in many ways from groups D and B. So, the four groups are very different in ways that are ill-defined. And yet, it seems unlikely that trying marijuana once or visiting the dentist have much to do with HDL cholesterol levels, except perhaps as indirect markers for lifestyle differences that are not directly indicated in Table 13.1.

Most worrisome in Table 13.1 is the difference in methylmercury. That difference likely reflects the consumption of fish containing methylmercury, which may in turn reflect a diet that differs in other respects as well, as discussed in Sect. 1.4.[1] This difference is worrisome because, whatever it signifies, group D has high levels of methylmercury, while control groups N, R, and B are lower and similar, so whatever is signified by methylmercury has not been systematically varied in the three control groups. Nonetheless, the analyses in Chap. 12 shed some light on the matter, and that light did nothing to undermine, and indeed went some ways to buttressing, the evidence that alcohol increases HDL cholesterol.

Despite the differences in Table 13.1, Fig. 1.3 indicates that HDL cholesterol tracks current alcohol consumption, not the differences among the control groups N, R, and B. Because the three control groups systematically vary certain lifestyle differences, yet the control groups have similar HDL cholesterol levels despite these variations, it becomes more difficult to attribute the higher HDL cholesterol levels among light daily drinkers to these lifestyle differences. Reasoning of this kind can be formalized [44–46, Ch. 8] or developed informally [53, pp. 145–154].

13.2 Boxplots of Two Evidence Factors

Binge Drinking and Blood Pressure

Before considering statistical properties of the two evidence factors for two control groups, it is helpful to draw some pictures. For this purpose, turn from the study in Sect. 1.4 to the second alcohol example in Sect. 1.5, where the treatment is current binge drinking and the outcome is increased blood pressure.

In the study of current binge drinking and blood pressure in Sect. 1.5, a treated group B of frequent binge drinkers was compared to two control groups. Recall the definitions of these two control groups. Group N—for never—did not binge at all in the past year and drank alcohol on at most one day a week in the last year, and there was no time in their lives when they binged almost every day. Control group

[1] It is not possible to change a diet in just one respect [12]. If fish is substituted for red meat, then the composition of fats in the diet is changed. If fish is added to an otherwise unchanged diet, then calories and protein are increased, and the percent of calories from carbohydrates is decreased.

P engaged in binge drinking in the past, but quit. In group P, individuals did have a period in their lives when they engaged in binge drinking almost every day, but they did not engage in binge drinking at any time in the past year and drank alcohol on at most one day a week during the past year. The blood pressure in these three groups is depicted in Fig. 1.9, and it is notably higher in group B than in groups N and P; moreover, groups N and P look similar.

Presumably, a study with one control group would compare groups B and N. In the way investigators commonly design studies, group P is an addition if it is included at all. Basic comparisons compare a treated group to untreated controls, not to people who quit the treatment long ago. Tables 9.2, 10.1, and 11.2 suggest it is better to have triples than pairs, but this is a different issue—we could have taken two controls from group N and none from P—and this different issue will be considered separately in Sect. 13.6.

Is the treated group B more similar to group N or group P? Groups B and P did both have a period of frequent binge drinking, so in that sense they are similar to each other and different from N. On the other hand, groups B and N did what they did and kept doing it, but perhaps with a great heave of the will, individuals in group P ended an addictive behavior. Maybe the people in group P are quite remarkable, unlike most of us, unlike the people in groups B and N who do in the future what they have done in the past.

If group P is an addition, if a study with one control group would have used group N as the control, then it is natural to want to see that study, before the addition of P, namely, the comparison of matched pairs of B and N. If we accept that, then ask: What is the entirely new information provided by P?

Plots of Two Evidence Factors

As will be seen in later sections, the entirely new information compares group P to the pooled group composed of both B and N. That information does not overlap with the information in the comparison of groups B and N.[2] For the combined blood pressure measure comparison in Sect. 1.5, this new information is depicted in

[2] A reader familiar with the use of orthogonal contrasts in balanced one-way analysis of variance with Gaussian errors [60, §12.9] may note an analogy with the two contrasts $B-N$ and $(B+N)-P$. This analogy is useful as motivation, but limited. The independence of orthogonal contrasts is dependent upon Gaussian errors and balanced designs, neither of which play an important role in evidence factors. Closer to evidence factors in this respect is the discussion by John Marden [37]. The linear model does not separate treatment effects and bias from nonrandom treatment assignment, but that is the goal with evidence factors. Many evidence factors have nothing to do with contrasts among groups, but rather with the factorization of a design symmetry into a subsymmetry and its cosets [55, Ch. 11]. For B-N-P, the symmetry is the symmetric group acting on three letters. This group of $3! = 6$ permutations has a subgroup of 2 permutations that transpose B and N and a cyclic subgroup of 3 permutations that rotate B-N-P, where both subgroups contain the identity, and $2 \times 3 = 6$. These two subgroups form the evidence factors that are discussed in this chapter. In other contexts, evidence factors come from a permutation group, a subgroup, and the cosets of that subgroup [55, Ch. 12].

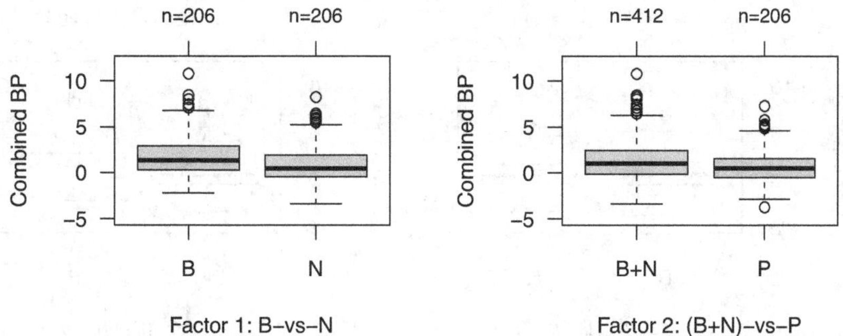

Fig. 13.1 Two evidence factors in the study of binge drinking. The outcome on the vertical axis is the combined blood pressure measure or "combined BP"

the right panel of Fig. 13.1, while the left panel is the conventional comparison of groups B and N.

Notably in Fig. 13.1, B is higher than N on the left, and the combination of B and N is higher than P on the right. This is, of course, what we would expect to see if binge drinking increased blood pressure and there was no bias in treatment assignment: on the left in Fig. 13.1, B would be higher than N because of the treatment effect, and on the right, the merged group, B∪N, would be higher than P because half the people in B∪N are binge drinkers. In each block i, we expect one member of B∪N to be affected by the treatment and the other member to be unaffected. Groups B and N are not distinguished on the right in Fig. 13.1 because that information has already been used on the left in Fig. 13.1, and we are currently asking: What new information, not used before, has been added by the second control group, P?

What do we expect to see in Fig. 13.1 if there were no effect caused by binge drinking, but there is selection bias in the division of individuals into three groups? The answer depends upon the nature of the selection bias.

Recall the distinction between a causal effect and a selection bias. In Chap. 2, Fisher's hypothesis of no effect meant $R_{ij} = r_{Tij} = r_{Cij}$ for all i and j, so that given $\mathcal{F}$, $\mathcal{Z}$ the three order statistics, $R_{i(1)} \leq R_{i(2)} \leq R_{i(3)}$, in block i are fixed, are functions of $\mathcal{F}$, not varying with the group to which an individual is assigned. In a randomized experiment in the absence of an effect, R_{ij} and $R_{i(1)} \leq R_{i(2)} \leq R_{i(3)}$ do not predict group membership. In Sect. 3.2, the hypothesis of no effect meant that R_{ij} was independently sampled from a continuous distribution $F_i(\cdot)$ for all i and j, which implied that the only valid level-α test of this null hypothesis in a randomized experiment is Fisher's randomization test. Under either null hypothesis, in an observational study, there is selection bias in the assignment to groups if the conditional probability of being in group B, N, or P depends upon $\mathcal{F}$ or equivalently upon the order statistics $R_{i(1)} \leq R_{i(2)} \leq R_{i(3)}$.

So, suppose that there is no treatment effect in either of these senses, but there is a selection bias. Suppose that the selection bias is due to an unobserved covariate u_{ij} that is associated with higher blood pressure, that is, higher R_{ij}. What do we expect to see in this case in a figure analogous to Fig. 13.1? If B, N, and P had the same

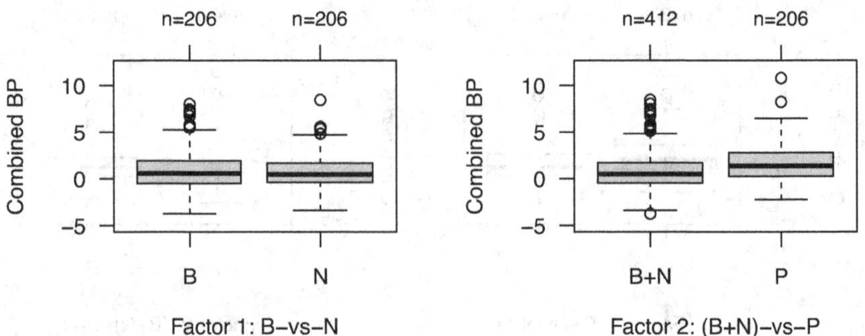

Fig. 13.2 Simulated example built from the actual data in Fig. 13.1 by biased allocation of the within-block order statistics, with a 0.6 chance that the largest order statistic is in group P, followed by random allocation to groups B and N of the order statistics not picked for group P. This is $(\Gamma, \Upsilon) = (1, 3)$

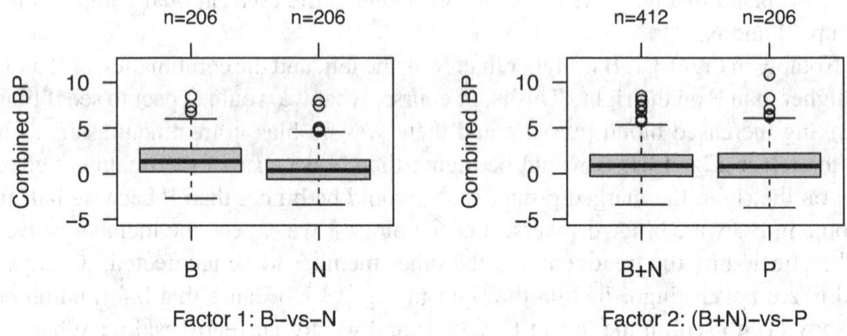

Fig. 13.3 Simulated example built from the actual data in Fig. 13.1 by biased allocation of the within-block order statistics, with a random order statistic given to group P, followed by allocation of the larger remaining order statistics to B with probability 0.75. This is $(\Gamma, \Upsilon) = (3, 1)$

distribution of u_{ij}, then we expect to see parallel boxplots in both factors, on the left and right of Fig. 13.1. If B and N had the same distribution of u_{ij} but P was different, then we expect parallel boxplots in factor 1, but different boxplots in factor 2. Figure 13.2 is a simulated example in which the $I = 206$ within-block order statistics in Fig. 13.1 were allocated to artificial groups B, N, and P with a selection bias affecting only group P. This selection bias is clearly evident in Fig. 13.2; moreover, Fig. 13.2 is not compatible with a treatment effect in the absence of bias because of factor 1.

Conversely, if P had the same distribution of u_{ij} as the union of groups B and N, but a selection bias acted on the union of groups B and N to place higher u_{ij}'s into group B, then we expect different boxplots in factor 1 and parallel boxplots in factor 2. Figure 13.3 is a simulated example in which the $I = 206$ within-block order statistics in Fig. 13.1 were allocated to artificial groups B, N, and P picking a random individual for P and, from the remaining two individuals, picking the larger order statistic for B with probability 0.75. Again, selection bias is clearly evident in Fig.

13.3; moreover, Fig. 13.3 is not compatible with a treatment effect in the absence of bias because of factor 2.

Selection bias in both factors is possible, so Fig. 13.1 renders implausible certain simple forms of selection bias, but it does not eliminate selection bias as a possible explanation of the ostensible effect of the treatment. Selection bias in both factors is examined using a sensitivity analysis in Sect. 13.4.

13.3 Factors of Randomization Tests

Independent Analyses of the Same Randomized Experiment

Evidence factors provide insight into unmeasured biases in observational studies. Consequently, evidence factors are of little or no use in randomized experiments, where unmeasured biases in treatment assignment are avoided by randomly allocating treatments. Nonetheless, the behavior of evidence factors in randomized experiments provides a starting point for understanding their uses in observational studies.

In the following conceptual discussion, simplify slightly by assuming that there are no ties among responses in the same block i, that is, $R_{ij} \neq R_{ij'}$ for $j \neq j'$. Define a "null randomized experiment" as follows: (i) there is no treatment effect, so $R_{ij} = r_{Cij}$ does not change when ij is assigned to one group rather than another; (ii) each individual ij has probability $1/3$ of being assigned to the second control group; (iii) conditionally given that ij is not assigned to the second control group, this individual has probability $1/2$ of being assigned to the treated group; and (iv) random assignments in distinct blocks, $i \neq i'$, are independent. There are $3! = 6$ possible treatment assignments in block i, and each has probability $(1/3)(1/2) = 1/6$. Let A_i be the rank—1, 2, or 3—of $R_{ij} = r_{Cij}$ for the individual assigned to the second control group, and let B_i be the rank—1 or 2—of $R_{ij} = r_{Cij}$ for the individual assigned to the treated group among the two individuals not assigned to the second control group. Here, A_i and B_i are called partial ranks.

In a null randomized experiment, it is easy to see that A_i and B_i are independent. After all, whatever value A_i takes, B_i has probability 1/2 of being 1 and 1/2 of being 2. This is a special case of an old result of Alfred Renyi that is nicely described with various applications by Khursheed Alam [1].[3]

In a null randomized experiment, $\sum_{i=1}^{I} A_i$ is the blocked Wilcoxon rank sum statistic in Sect. 2.6 comparing the second control group to the combination of the first two groups—as in the right or second factor in Fig. 13.1—and $\sum_{i=1}^{I} B_i$ is the blocked Wilcoxon rank sum statistic (or effectively the sign statistic) comparing the treated group and the first control group—as in the left or first factor in Fig. 13.1. Moreover, the two test statistics, $\sum_{i=1}^{I} A_i$ and $\sum_{i=1}^{I} B_i$, are independent in a null

[3] This is also true if $J > 3$ and $J - 1$ rather than 2 partial ranks are computed [1], and it is true much more generally [37,55].

randomized experiment: the value of $\sum_{i=1}^{I} A_i$ does nothing to predict the value of $\sum_{i=1}^{I} B_i$. This is slightly surprising, as $2I$ of the $3I$ individuals in the experiment are used in both $\sum_{i=1}^{I} A_i$ and $\sum_{i=1}^{I} B_i$. It is almost as if one experiment of size $3I$ has become two unrelated experiments of sizes $3I$ and $2I$, for a total effective sample size of $5I$, despite using many of the same people twice. Indeed, in testing H_0, we could compute the two P-values, one from $\sum_{i=1}^{I} A_i$ and the other from $\sum_{i=1}^{I} B_i$, and combine them using meta-analytic techniques as if they came from independent experiments. This is true, also, if A_i and B_i are replaced by $\rho(A_i)$ and $\phi(B_i)$ for functions $\rho(\cdot)$ and $\phi(\cdot)$. For instance, for $J = 3$, it will be useful in Sect. 13.5 to consider the function $\rho(\cdot)$ of within-block ranks, 1, 2, 3, defined by $\rho(1) = 1$, $\rho(2) = 2$, $\rho(3) = 5$.

The conclusions of the previous paragraph would be more useful if the blocked Wilcoxon rank sum statistic were itself more useful. However, similar results apply to other statistics, including weighted rank statistics, which are cousins of Wilcoxon's signed rank statistic, rather than of his rank sum statistic. In Sect. 2.6, a weighted rank statistic attached weight $\varphi\{b_i/(I+1)\}$ to block i, where b_i was the rank of the within-block range (2.11). In a null randomized experiment, $\sum_{i=1}^{I} \rho(A_i)\ \varrho\{b_i/(I+1)\}$ and $\sum_{i=1}^{I} \phi(B_i)\ \varphi\{b_i/(I+1)\}$ are independent weighted rank statistics.[4] There are many variations on this theme that yield either exact or approximate independence for a wide variety of test statistics [51,55].

Some Notation for Two Control Groups in Blocks of Size $J = 3$

With blocks of size $J = 3$, let $S_{ij} = 1$ for the one individual assigned to the second control group and $S_{ij} = 0$ for other individuals, so $1 = \sum_{i=1}^{J} S_{ij}$ for each i. Then $A_i = \sum_{i=1}^{J} S_{ij}\, q_{ij}^*$ where the q_{ij}^*'s are the usual ranks of R_{ij} within block i. Let $Z_{ij} = 1$ for the one individual assigned to the treated group, $Z_{ij} = 0$ for other individuals, so $Z_{ij}\, S_{ij} = 0$ and $1 = \sum_{i=1}^{J} Z_{ij}$. In brief, treatments are assigned so that

$$1 = \sum_{i=1}^{J} S_{ij} \text{ and } 1 = \sum_{i=1}^{J} Z_{ij} = \sum_{i=1}^{J} Z_{ij}\left(1 - S_{ij}\right) \text{ for } i = 1, \ldots, I. \tag{13.1}$$

Let $\mathcal{E}$ denote the event (13.1) that occurs by design. Write $\mathbf{S}$ for the $I \times 3$ matrix of S_{ij} and $\mathbf{Z}$ for the $I \times 3$ matrix of Z_{ij}. In a null randomized experiment, the group assignments, $\left(S_{ij}, Z_{ij}\right)$, in distinct blocks are independent, and within block i assignments are governed by $\Pr\left(S_{ij} = 1 \,\middle|\, \mathcal{F}, \mathcal{E}\right) = 1/3$ for all ij, and $\Pr\left(Z_{ij} = 1 \,\middle|\, \mathbf{S} = \mathbf{s}, \mathcal{F}, \mathcal{E}\right) = 1/2$ providing $s_{ij} = 0$.

---

[4] In a null randomized experiment, $\max_{1\le j\le 3} R_{ij} - \min_{1\le j\le 3} R_{ij}$ equals $\max_{1\le j\le 3} r_{Cij} - \min_{1\le j\le 3} r_{Cij}$; so, it is fixed by conditioning on $\mathcal{F}$, and $\varrho\{b_i/(I+1)\}$ and $\varphi\{b_i/(I+1)\}$ are also fixed, not varying with the random assignments of individuals to groups. The independence of $\sum_{i=1}^{I} \rho(A_i)\ \varrho\{b_i/(I+1)\}$ and $\sum_{i=1}^{I} \phi(B_i)\ \varphi\{b_i/(I+1)\}$ then follows from the independence of A_i and B_i.

The randomization distribution for the first factor, the **Z**-factor, is always conditional on the selection of individuals for the second control group, **S** = **s**. It is best to view the second factor as tested given $\mathcal{F}$, $\mathcal{E}$ and the first factor as tested conditionally given **S** = **s**, $\mathcal{F}$, $\mathcal{E}$. Viewed in this way, the first factor may condition on everything that has been fixed by the event **S** = **s**, and this enlarges the class of tests that may be used for the first factor. Consider the simplest example. We might wish to use Wilcoxon's signed rank test for the first factor, but this uses the range or absolute difference of the two R_{ij}'s for the two individuals with $S_{ij} = 0$, rather than the range of the three R_{ij}'s in block i. So, given **S** = **s**, define $q'_{ij} = 0$ if $s_{ij} = 1$, and for the two individuals with $s_{ij} = 0$ define q'_{ij} to be the partial rank, 1 or 2, of their R_{ij}. Given **S** = **s**, define b'_i to be the rank of the range of R_{ij}'s for the two individuals with $s_{ij} = 0$. The small but important issue here is that b_i is fixed by conditioning on $\mathcal{F}$, $\mathcal{E}$, but b'_i is not; however, b'_i is fixed by conditioning on **S** = **s**, $\mathcal{F}$, $\mathcal{E}$. So, conditionally given **S** = **s**, the quantities $B_i = \sum Z_{ij}\, q'_{ij}$ and b'_i are well defined, and the statistic for the first factor can use $\sum_{i=1}^{I} \phi(B_i)\, \varphi\{b'_i/(I+1)\}$ rather than $\sum_{i=1}^{I} \phi(B_i)\, \varphi\{b_i/(I+1)\}$. Under H_0, if the ranges are untied, then $\sum_{i=1}^{I} \rho(A_i)\, \varrho\{b_i/(I+1)\}$ and $\sum_{i=1}^{I} \phi(B_i)\, \varphi\{b'_i/(I+1)\}$ are independent given $(\mathcal{F}, \mathcal{E})$ in a null randomized experiment, despite substituting b'_i for b_i.[5]

Randomization Analysis of the Binge Drinking Example

Returning to the binge drinking comparison in Sect. 1.5, consider testing the hypothesis H_0 of no treatment effect on the combined blood pressure measurement using the two factors depicted in Fig. 13.1. The current section analyzes the data as if individuals were randomly assigned to groups binge B, never N, and past binge drinking P. In Sect. 13.4, each factor has a sensitivity analysis.

Using the statistic U868 in both factors yields a P-value of 0.00000627 from the first factor on the left in Fig. 13.1 and a P-value of 0.000340 for the second factor on the right in Fig. 13.1. These P-values would be independent in a null randomized trial, so each would constitute fairly strong evidence against H_0.

Figures 13.2 and 13.3 create a situation in which one factor departs from randomized treatment assignment but the other does not. Because both P-values are so small, 0.00000627 and 0.000340, the situations depicted in Figs. 13.2 and 13.3 could not plausibly explain the higher blood pressures among frequent binge drinkers; rather, both control groups must be biased—both factors must be biased—to produce Fig. 13.1 if H_0 is true. Stated informally, to produce Fig. 13.1 in the absence of a treatment effect, there has to be something seriously wrong with both control groups.

[5] Ties make the argument a bit more detailed, but they present no problems. Indeed, in the general discussion of evidence factors, ties play no role, essentially because the important aspects of evidence factors are not closely connected to rank statistics [55]. For example, the permutation distribution of rank statistics may be replaced by the permutation distribution of M-statistics [51].

Zahkin and colleagues [69] combine independent P-values by taking the product of those P-values that are less than or equal to some threshold, ι. They determined the distribution of the truncated product for independent uniform random variables. By definition, the statistic is 1 if there are no P-values that are less than or equal to ι. For $\iota = 1$, the method becomes Fisher's method of combining P-values using their product. Here, a threshold of $\iota = 0.2$ is used; see Problem 13.5.[6] In sensitivity analyses, upper bounds on P-values are often close to one, and consequently, the truncated product method tends to have more power in sensitivity analyses [21].

Using the truncated product of P-values to combine the P-values from the two factors yields a combined P-value of 4.12×10^{-8}, much smaller than either 0.00000627 or 0.000340 for the two factors separately. This will become more important in Sect. 13.4 where a sensitivity analysis is performed for each factor, and these are combined.

Stated more precisely, the analysis above used $\sum_{i=1}^{I} \rho(A_i)\ \varrho\{b_i/(I+1)\}$ for factor two to compare group P to the combined group B∪N in matched triples with b_i as the rank of the block range (2.11), and then, given **S**, it used $\sum_{i=1}^{I} \phi(B_i)\ \varphi\{b_i^{'}/(I+1)\}$ in matched pairs to compare group B and group N with $b_i^{'}$ as the rank of the within-pair range. Use of U868 means that $\varphi(\cdot)$ and $\varrho(\cdot)$ are both the U868 curve in Fig. 8.1.

Combining Independent P-values

What does it mean for one random vector, say $\mathbf{V}$, to be larger than another random vector, $\mathbf{V}^*$? Stochastic ordering of random variables was defined in the usual way in Sect. 8.5, but how can this definition be extended to random vectors? A function $g : \mathbb{R}^K \to \mathbb{R}$ of a K-dimensional real vector $\mathbf{v}$ is said to be monotone increasing if $g(\mathbf{v}) \geq g(\mathbf{v}^*)$ whenever $v_1 \geq v_1^*, \ldots, v_K \geq v_K^*$. By definition [32, 38, 59], $\mathbf{V}$ is stochastically larger than $\mathbf{V}^*$ if $\mathrm{E}\{g(\mathbf{V})\} \geq \mathrm{E}\{g(\mathbf{V}^*)\}$ for all monotone increasing functions $g(\cdot)$ for which the expectations exist.

A valid P-value testing a null hypothesis H_0 has the property that, for every α, the P-value is below α with probability at most α when H_0 is true; that is, the P-value is stochastically larger than a random variable that is uniformly distributed on the interval $[0, 1]$.

A variety of methods exist for combining K independent valid P-values—say, $\mathbf{P}^* = (P_1^*, \ldots, P_K^*)$—that each test the same null hypothesis H_0.[7] The combination produces one valid P-value testing H_0 from $\mathbf{P}^*$. Typically these methods define

[6] This is the default in the `truncatedP` function of the `sensitivitymv` package in R.

[7] This "same" null hypothesis H_0 may be the conjunction of K distinct hypotheses, $H_1, \ldots, H_K$; that is, H_0 may assert that $H_1, \ldots, H_K$ are all true. Using $\wedge$ to denote logical "and,"then H_0 may assert that $H_1 \wedge H_2 \wedge \cdots \wedge H_K$ is true. That is, if P_k is the P-value testing H_k, we view each P_k as a P-value testing the "same" hypothesis $H_0 = H_1 \wedge H_2 \wedge \cdots \wedge H_K$. If $P_k \leq \alpha$ with probability at most α when H_k is true, then $P_k \leq \alpha$ with probability at most α when H_0 is true, because H_k is true whenever H_0 is true. An interesting and useful variation is a partial conjunction hypothesis

a new statistic, $g : [0,1]^K \rightarrow \mathbb{R}$, that is a monotone increasing function, and ask whether $g(\mathbf{P}^*)$ is surprisingly small; that is, a new P-value is computed from the statistic $g(\mathbf{P}^*)$, where H_0 is rejected if $g(\mathbf{P}^*)$ is small. It seems natural to insist that the combining function, $g(\cdot)$, be monotone increasing: if the P_k^*'s become larger, then there is less evidence against H_0.

For example, Fisher [15] combined independent P-values using their product, $g(\mathbf{P}^*) = \prod_{k=1}^{K} P_k^*$. Zahkin and colleagues [69] specified a fixed threshold, $0 < \iota \leq 1$, and defined the truncated product of P-values, $g(\mathbf{P}^*)$, to be 1 if $P_k^* > \iota$ for all k and otherwise defined $g(\mathbf{P}^*)$ to be the product of all the P_k that were $\leq \iota$. Dudbridge and Koeleman [13] combine independent P-values by using their rank truncated product, $g(\mathbf{P}^*)$, defined to be the product of the L-smallest of the P-values, for some fixed $L \leq K$. The truncated product becomes Fisher's method if $\iota = 1$ and the rank truncated product becomes Fisher's method if $L = K$. The Bahadur efficiency of various combining functions $g(\cdot)$ has been compared [4].

Let $\mathbf{U} = (U_1, \ldots, U_K)$ be a K-dimensional vector of independent random variables uniformly distributed on $[0,1]$. Suppose that $g : [0,1]^K \rightarrow \mathbb{R}$ is a specified monotone increasing function. Then $\Pr\{g(\mathbf{U}) \leq c\} = 1 - \Pr\{g(\mathbf{U}) > c\}$ is well defined; moreover, for certain $g(\cdot)$ the distribution $\Pr\{g(\mathbf{U}) \leq c\}$ has a recognizable form; see Problems 13.3–13.4. The distribution $\Pr\{g(\mathbf{U}) \leq c\}$ is used to obtain a single combined P-value from a vector of K independent valid P-values, $\mathbf{P}^* = \left(P_1^*, \ldots, P_K^*\right)$, by the following reasoning. For an event E, write $\chi(E) = 1$ if E occurs and $\chi(E) = 0$ if E does not occur. Because $g(\cdot)$ is monotone increasing, $\chi\{g(\cdot) > c\}$ is also monotone increasing. Also, $\Pr\{g(\mathbf{U}) > c\} = \mathrm{E}[\chi\{g(\mathbf{U}) > c\}]$. Consequently, if $\mathbf{P} = (P_1, \ldots, P_K)$ is stochastically larger than $\mathbf{U}$, then

$$\begin{aligned} \Pr\{g(\mathbf{U}) > c\} &= \mathrm{E}[\chi\{g(\mathbf{U}) > c\}] \\ &\geq \mathrm{E}[\chi\{g(\mathbf{P}) > c\}] = \Pr\{g(\mathbf{P}) > c\}; \end{aligned} \tag{13.2}$$

so, $\Pr\{g(\mathbf{P}) \leq c\} \leq \Pr\{g(\mathbf{U}) \leq c\}$. Suppose that we determine c such that $\alpha = \Pr\{g(\mathbf{U}) \leq c\}$, and we reject H_0 when $g(\mathbf{P}) \leq c$; then the probability of rejecting H_0 when H_0 is true is at most α.

Dependent P-Values That Are Larger Than Uniform on $[0,1] \times [0,1]$

Importantly, (13.2) is true whenever $\mathbf{P}$ is stochastically larger than $\mathbf{U}$, whether or not the coordinates of $\mathbf{P}$ are independent. Unlike independent uniform random variables in $\mathbf{U}$ and the independent valid P-values in $\mathbf{P}^*$, the coordinates of $\mathbf{P}$ need not be independent for (13.2) to be true; rather, $\mathbf{P}$ must simply be stochastically larger than $\mathbf{U}$. In brief, if $\mathbf{P}$ is stochastically larger than $\mathbf{U}$, then the P-values in $\mathbf{P}$ may be combined using $g(\mathbf{P})$ as if they were independent despite their dependence.

of Yoav Benjamini and Ruth Heller [3] that asserts that at least L of the K hypotheses H_k are true. Bikram Karmakar and Dylan Small [27] examine the partial conjunction of evidence factors.

This issue is important because strict independence of evidence factors is limited to certain simple uses of particular rank statistics, whereas evidence factors in which $\mathbf{P}$ is dependent but stochastically larger than $\mathbf{U}$ are much more common and are not limited to rank statistics [51,55].

Valid P-values that are dependent yet stochastically larger than $\mathbf{U}$ commonly occur with evidence factors, because the same data are being analyzed several times. One P-value, say P_2, may depend upon $\mathbf{S}$ alone, as in factor 2 on the right in Fig. 13.1, while another P-value, say P_1, may depend on $(\mathbf{S}, \mathbf{Z})$ but use the conditional distribution of $\mathbf{Z}$ given $\mathbf{S}$ to obtain a valid conditional P-value, as in factor 1 on the left in Fig. 13.1. The P-values may be dependent because they both use the information in $\mathbf{S}$, yet P_1 remains a valid P-value for each possible realization $\mathbf{s}$ of $\mathbf{S}$. Recall the discussion earlier in this section of using Wilcoxon's signed rank statistic for factor 1 in Fig. 13.1, where the b_i' depend on $(\mathbf{S}, \mathbf{Z})$ but are fixed by conditioning on $\mathbf{S}$.

Consider the simplest case, $\mathbf{P} = (P_1, P_2)$. Suppose that P_2 is a valid P-value that is a function of $\mathbf{S}$, so that $\Pr(P_2 \le \alpha) \le \alpha$ for all $0 \le \alpha \le 1$ if H_0 is true. Suppose that for each value $\mathbf{s}$ of $\mathbf{S}$, P_1 is a valid P-value that is a function of $(\mathbf{S}, \mathbf{Z})$ and is computed from the conditional distribution of $\mathbf{Z}$ given $\mathbf{S}$, so that $\Pr(P_1 \le \alpha \mid \mathbf{S} = \mathbf{s}) \le \alpha$ for each $\mathbf{s}$ and for all $0 \le \alpha \le 1$ if H_0 is true. Then of course P_1 is a valid P-value: if H_0 is true, then

$$\Pr(P_1 \le \alpha) = \mathrm{E}\{\Pr(P_1 \le \alpha \mid \mathbf{S})\} \le \alpha, \tag{13.3}$$

because $\Pr(P_1 \le \alpha \mid \mathbf{S} = \mathbf{s}) \le \alpha$ for each $\mathbf{s}$; however, (P_1, P_2) may be dependent because both coordinates may depend on $\mathbf{S}$. Nonetheless, despite dependence, it may be shown that $\mathbf{P} = (P_1, P_2)$ is stochastically larger than $\mathbf{U} = (U_1, U_2)$, that is, stochastically larger than the uniform distribution on the unit square [55, Proposition 7.3.2].[8] As a consequence, the two P-values $\mathbf{P} = (P_1, P_2)$ may be combined using $g(\mathbf{P})$ as if they were independent despite their dependence.

[8] This is also true of $\mathbf{P} = (P_1, \ldots, P_K)$ for $K > 2$, providing P_k is computed from $V_1, \ldots, V_k$, and $\Pr(P_k \le \alpha \mid V_1, \ldots, V_{k-1}) \le \alpha$ for $k = 1, \ldots, K$ [55, Proposition 7.3.2]. There is even a sense in which it is true of a subset of the P-values, even if P-values not in this subset are invalid. Suppose that $\Pr(P_k \le \alpha \mid V_1, \ldots, V_{k-1}) \le \alpha$ for $k \in \mathcal{K} \subseteq \{1, \ldots, K\}$, but possibly $\Pr(P_\ell \le \alpha \mid V_1, \ldots, V_{\ell-1}) > \alpha$ for some $\ell \notin \mathcal{K}$. Then P_k for $k \in \mathcal{K}$ are jointly stochastically larger than U_k for $k \in \mathcal{K}$, even though P_k is computed from $V_1, \ldots, V_k$, and it is possible that $\Pr(P_\ell \le \alpha \mid V_1, \ldots, V_{\ell-1}) > \alpha$ for some $1 \le \ell < k$, $\ell \notin \mathcal{K}$ [55, Proposition 7.3.3]. Stated informally in words, the joint validity of several factors does not presuppose the validity of other factors. The proof uses either a result of Arthur Cohen and Harold Sackrowitz [10] or a similar result given in the text by Moshe Shaked and George Shanthikumar [59, Theorem 6.B.3].

13.4 Sensitivity Analysis with Evidence Factors

Biased Allocation in Either or Both Factors

In Sect. 13.3, in a null randomized experiment, group assignments, (S_{ij}, Z_{ij}), in distinct blocks are independent, and in each block i assignments are random in the sense that $\Pr\left(S_{ij}=1 \,\middle|\, \mathcal{F}, \mathcal{E}\right)=1/3$ for all ij, and $\Pr\left(Z_{ij}=1 \,\middle|\, \mathbf{S}=\mathbf{s}, \mathcal{F}, \mathcal{E}\right)=1/2$ providing $s_{ij}=0$. In an observational study, group assignments may be biased, with $\Pr\left(S_{ij}=1 \,\middle|\, \mathcal{F}, \mathcal{E}\right)\neq 1/3$ as in Fig. 13.2, or $\Pr\left(Z_{ij}=1 \,\middle|\, \mathbf{S}=\mathbf{s}, \mathcal{F}, \mathcal{E}\right)\neq 1/2$ as in Fig. 13.3, or both.

Write $\lambda_{ij}=\Pr\left(S_{ij}=1 \,\middle|\, \mathcal{F}, \mathcal{E}\right)$, so $1=\sum_{j=1}^{3}\lambda_{ij}$ for each i. Write $\theta_{\mathbf{s}ij}=\Pr\left(Z_{ij}=1 \,\middle|\, \mathbf{S}=\mathbf{s}, \mathcal{F}, \mathcal{E}\right)$, so $\theta_{\mathbf{s}ij}=0$ if $s_{ij}=1$ and $1=\sum_{j=1}^{3}\theta_{\mathbf{s}ij}$ for each $\mathbf{s}$ and i. The sensitivity model is the model from Chap. 8 used twice, namely, for $\Upsilon\geq 1$ and $\Gamma\geq 1$:

$$\frac{1}{\Upsilon}\leq\frac{\lambda_{ij}}{\lambda_{ij'}}\leq\Upsilon \text{ and } \frac{1}{\Gamma}\leq\frac{\theta_{\mathbf{s}ij}}{\theta_{\mathbf{s}ij'}}\leq\Gamma \text{ if } s_{ij}=s_{ij'}=0. \tag{13.4}$$

Then randomized allocation to groups is $(\Gamma, \Upsilon)=(1,1)$, Fig. 13.2 has $(\Gamma, \Upsilon)=(1,3)$ and Fig. 13.3 has $(\Gamma, \Upsilon)=(3,1)$.

Using (8.12), at the unknown but true values of λ_{ij} and $\theta_{\mathbf{s}ij}$, there are two P-values, a conditional P-value, $P_{1\mathbf{s}}$, given $\mathbf{S}=\mathbf{s}$, for factor 1, and a marginal P-value, P_2, for factor 2. The marginal P-value for factor 1 is $P_{1\mathbf{S}}$; that is, $P_{1\mathbf{s}}$ is calculated from the conditional distribution $\Pr(\mathbf{Z}\mid\mathbf{S}=\mathbf{s})$, and then $P_{1\mathbf{S}}$ is the resulting value of $P_{1\mathbf{s}}$ when $\mathbf{S}=\mathbf{s}$.

If the null hypothesis H_0 of no treatment effect is true, then the vector $(P_{1\mathbf{S}}, P_2)$ is stochastically larger than $\mathbf{U}=(U_1, U_2)$, where U_1 and U_2 are independent uniform random variables. Consequently, $(P_{1\mathbf{S}}, P_2)$ may be combined by a monotone increasing function $g(P_{1\mathbf{S}}, P_2)$, such as Fisher's $g(P_{1\mathbf{S}}, P_2)=P_{1\mathbf{S}}\times P_2$, to produce a single P-value. In Sect. 13.3, this was done in the special case of randomized group assignment with $\lambda_{ij}=1/3$ and $\theta_{\mathbf{s}ij}=1/2$ if $s_{ij}=0$ or $\theta_{\mathbf{s}ij}=0$ if $s_{ij}=1$. Of course, for $\Gamma>1$ and $\Upsilon>1$, these true P-values are unknown, because the true values of λ_{ij} and $\theta_{\mathbf{s}ij}$ are unknown.

Using the methods in Chap. 8 and (8.13) conditionally given $\mathbf{S}=\mathbf{s}$, calculate an upper bound $\overline{P}_{1\Gamma\mathbf{s}}$ on $P_{1\mathbf{s}}$ for all $\theta_{\mathbf{s}ij}$ that satisfy (13.4). Using the methods in Chap. 8 and (8.13) with S_{ij} in place of Z_{ij}, calculate an upper bound $\overline{P}_{2\Upsilon}$ on P_2 for all λ_{ij} that satisfy (13.4). If the true values of λ_{ij} and $\theta_{\mathbf{s}ij}$ satisfy (13.4), then (i) $\overline{P}_{2\Upsilon}\geq P_2$ and (ii) $\overline{P}_{1\Gamma\mathbf{s}}\geq P_{1\mathbf{s}}$ for each $\mathbf{s}$, so $\overline{P}_{1\Gamma\mathbf{S}}\geq P_{1\mathbf{S}}$. Consequently, if H_0 is true, then $\left(\overline{P}_{1\Gamma\mathbf{S}}, \overline{P}_{2\Upsilon}\right)$ is stochastically larger than $(P_{1\mathbf{S}}, P_2)$, which is stochastically larger than $\mathbf{U}=(U_1, U_2)$; so, $\left(\overline{P}_{1\Gamma\mathbf{S}}, \overline{P}_{2\Upsilon}\right)$ is stochastically larger than $\mathbf{U}=(U_1, U_2)$, and $g\left(\overline{P}_{1\Gamma\mathbf{S}}, \overline{P}_{2\Upsilon}\right)$ is stochastically larger than $g(U_1, U_2)$, for monotone increasing $g(\cdot)$. In other words, referring $g\left(\overline{P}_{1\Gamma\mathbf{S}}, \overline{P}_{2\Upsilon}\right)$ to the known distribution of $g(U_1, U_2)$

yields an upper bound on the combined P-value when H_0 is true and the inequalities in (13.4) hold. This is the simplest case of a general method [55].

Sensitivity Analysis in the Binge Drinking Example

In Sect. 13.3, the binge drinking and blood pressure comparison from Sect. 1.5 was analyzed as if it were a randomized experiment, for both evidence factors, for "B versus N" and for "P versus B∪N," as depicted in Fig. 13.1. Both evidence factors rejected the null hypothesis of no effect with very small P-values, and these combined using the truncated product to a single even smaller P-value. The randomization analysis is the same as a sensitivity analysis with $(\Gamma, \Upsilon) = (1, 1)$. How sensitive are these comparisons to unmeasured bias in either factor?

Table 13.2 shows the corresponding sensitivity analysis. If $(\Gamma, \Upsilon) = (1.75, 1.75)$, each factor has a P-value upper bound below 0.05, and their combination is 0.012. At $(\Gamma, \Upsilon) = (1.90, 1.90)$, neither factor has a P-value bound below 0.05, but their combined P-value is 0.038. So, the two factors together are mutually supporting: together they are insensitive to a larger bias than either one is on its own. In Sect. 8.7, a bias of $\Gamma = 1.75$ amplifies to $(\Lambda, \Psi) = (3.00, 3.40)$, but $\Gamma = 1.90$ amplifies to $(\Lambda, \Psi) = (3.00, 4.27)$.

Also in Table 13.2, each factor is insensitive to a bias of 1.5 even if the other factor is infinitely biased: the combined P-values for $(\Gamma, \Upsilon) = (1.50, \infty)$ and $(\Gamma, \Upsilon) = (\infty, 1.50)$ are both 0.036 or less. In other words, total invalidation of either factor leaves another factor that is insensitive to small and moderate unmeasured biases. In Sect. 8.7, a bias of $\Gamma = 1.5$ amplifies to $(\Lambda, \Psi) = (2, 4)$ and to $(\Lambda, \Psi) = (4, 2)$, so $\Gamma = 1.5$ is far from a trivial unmeasured bias.

In brief, there are two senses in which a second control group—here, group P—increases insensitivity to unmeasured bias. In a quantitative sense, each factor in Table 13.2 is sensitive to a bias of $(\Gamma, \Upsilon) = (1.80, 1.80)$, but together they are insensitive to $(\Gamma, \Upsilon) = (1.90, 1.90)$. The qualitative sense is equally important.

Table 13.2 Sensitivity analysis for the binge drinking and blood pressure data in two evidence factors, "B versus N" and "P versus B ∪ N," using the statistic U868. The table contains upper bounds on one-sided P values testing the hypothesis of no effect. The combined P-value bound applies the truncated product of P-values with truncation 0.2

(Γ, Υ)	B versus N	P versus B ∪ N	Combined
(1.00, 1.00)	0.000	0.000	0.000
(1.75, 1.75)	0.048	0.046	0.012
(1.80, 1.80)	0.062	0.060	0.019
(1.90, 1.90)	0.099	0.095	0.038
(2.00, 1.85)	0.147	0.076	0.043
(1.85, 2.00)	0.079	0.140	0.043
(2.00, 2.00)	0.147	0.140	0.067
(1.50, ∞)	0.008	1.000	0.035
(∞, 1.50)	1.000	0.009	0.036

Even infinite biases that completely invalidate either factor alone are insufficient to explain away the association between binge drinking and high blood pressure. Rather, an infinite bias in one factor must combine with a moderately large bias in the other to explain this association. Of course, both factors could be severely biased; so, this qualitative sense is less than we might prefer, but it is more than a sensitivity analysis with a single control group can do on its own.

13.5 A Better Test Statistic for the Second Control Group

Is U868 a Good Statistic for the Second Evidence Factor?

In Chaps. 9 and 11, the U-statistics U868 and U878 were found to have reasonably high design sensitivity and Bahadur efficiency when comparing one treated individual to $J - 1$ controls in blocks of size J, in a favorable situation consisting of a conventional linear model for a block design with additive treatment and block effects and normal errors or errors from a t-distribution with 5 degrees of freedom. In the previous subsection, U868 was used for both evidence factors. Was this wise?

It seems reasonable to use U868 for factor 1, the comparison of the treated group B and the first control group N, because for $J = 2$ this is similar to the situation evaluated in Chaps. 10 and 11. Continuing to use the same additive block model, this section compares statistics for the second evidence factor on the right side of Fig. 13.1, where the treated group, B, has been merged with the first control group, N, in comparison with the second control group P.

Was U868 a wise choice of test statistic for the second evidence factor, the comparison of B∪N and P? The answer is not obvious from the comparisons in Chaps. 9 and 11. In each block i in the same favorable situation, group B∪N contains one treated individual and one untreated control; so, we expect one individual from B∪N to have elevated blood pressure due to binge drinking and the other individual to exhibit no effect from binge drinking. In that sense, comparing B∪N and P is unlike comparing a treated individual to a control. Only half of B∪N is expected to respond to the treatment, binge drinking, because only half were exposed to it.

In the discussion of "large but rare treatment effects" in Sect. 9.6, it was noted that statistics of the form $(m, \underline{m}, \overline{m}) = (m, m, m)$ in (9.11) have attractive properties when only a fraction of treated individuals respond to treatment. Specifically, developing an idea of Erich Lehmann [33], William Conover and David Salsburg [11] found the locally most powerful two-sample rank test when only a fraction of the population responds to treatment. Motivated by different considerations, Robert Stephenson [62] had proposed rank scores that are very similar to the Conover-Salsburg ranks in large samples [47]. Specifically, Stephenson [62] created a U-statistic in the following way. He focused on matched pairs, $J = 2$, looking at all $\binom{I}{m}$ subsets of m of the I pairs, scoring a 1 if the largest absolute pair difference in outcomes, $|R_{i1} - R_{i2}|$, in these m pairs was a positive treated-minus-control difference, $(Z_{i1} - Z_{i2})(R_{i1} - R_{i2}) > 0$. The mean of Stephenson's $\binom{I}{m}$ scores is a U-statistic and a linear rank statistic; see

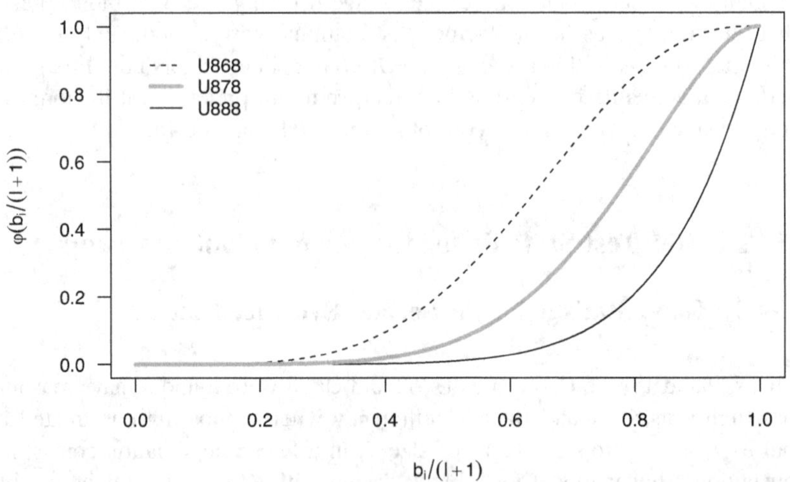

Fig. 13.4 Comparison of the score functions $\varphi(\cdot)$ for block ranges for U888, U878, and U868

the discussion of Fig. 9.1 in Chap. 9. The formula (9.11) with $\left(m, \underline{m}, \overline{m}\right) = (m, m, m)$ closely approximates Stephenson's rank scores [50, Lemma 1]. In addition to maximizing local power in large samples, these rank scores also have good design sensitivity, $\widetilde{\Gamma}$, when only some treated individuals respond to treatment [54, Ch. 17]. Figure 13.4 compares U888 or $\left(m, \underline{m}, \overline{m}\right) = (8, 8, 8)$ to U868 and U878. Notably, of these three statistics, the φ-function for U888 pays the least attention to blocks that seem homogeneous in R_{ij}, with small ranks b_i of their within-block ranges (2.11). Design sensitivities, $\widetilde{\Gamma}$, of $\left(m, \underline{m}, \overline{m}\right) = (5, 5, 5)$, (8,8,8), and (20,20,20) have been calculated for various favorable situations [50, Table 3].

Is U868 a good statistic for the second evidence factor, comparing P and B∪N? Here, the null hypothesis says there is no treatment effect, and the right side of Fig. 13.1 is produced by selection bias. The alternative hypothesis is a favorable situation with no selection bias and a treatment effect that increases the responses of treated individuals. How do we decide whether U868 is a good statistic for the second evidence factor? From first principles, we compare U868 to other statistics in terms of its design sensitivity and its Bahadur efficiency in a sensitivity analysis.

Comparing Forty Test Statistics

Examination of forty test statistics in terms of design sensitivity and Bahadur efficiency yielded a better test statistic [56, Tables 2 and 3]. The forty statistics formed a $5 \times 4 \times 2$ factorial arrangement. All were weighted rank statistics of the type in

Sect. 2.6, $T^* = \sum_{i=1}^{I}\sum_{j=1}^{3} S_{ij}\, q_{ij}$ with $q_{ij} = \rho\left(q_{ij}^*\right)\, \varrho\{b_i/(I+1)\}$. There were five ϱ-functions defined by $(m, \underline{m}, \overline{m})$ in (9.11) to score between-block ranks, b_i, and four ϱ-functions to transform the within-block ranks, $\varrho\left(q_{ij}^*\right)$, making $5 \times 4 = 20$ combinations. The third factor, the two-level factor, ranked either the within-block ranges, $\left|R_{i(3)} - R_{i(1)}\right|$, or the within-block gaps $\left|R_{i(3)} - \left\{R_{i(1)} + R_{i(1)}\right\}/2\right|$, where $R_{i(1)} \le R_{i(2)} \le R_{i(3)}$ are the order statistics in block i. In terms of design sensitivity and Bahadur efficiencies, the best statistic of the 40 statistics[9] used $(m, \underline{m}, \overline{m}) = (8, 8, 8)$ with the rank b_i of the gap, scoring the within-block ranks $\rho(1) = 1$, $\rho(2) = 2$, and $\rho(3) = 5$.[10] With obvious notation, this statistic is called "U888gap125," whereas the analysis in Sect. 13.4 used "U868range123."

This statistic, $T^* = \sum_{i=1}^{I}\sum_{j=1}^{3} S_{ij}\, q_{ij}$ with $q_{ij} = \rho\left(q_{ij}^*\right)\, \varrho\{b_i/(I+1)\}$, emphasizes blocks with large gaps and rejects H_0 when T^* is small. In other words, H_0 is rejected when the second control, with $S_{ij} = 1$, has a small score, $\sum_{j=1}^{3} S_{ij}\, q_{ij}$, for many blocks i. When is $\sum_{j=1}^{3} S_{ij}\, q_{ij}$ small? Essentially, $\sum_{j=1}^{3} S_{ij}\, q_{ij}$ is small when it is not large, and given that $(m, \underline{m}, \overline{m}) = (8, 8, 8)$ in Fig. 13.4, $\sum_{j=1}^{3} S_{ij}\, q_{ij}$ is large only if the gap, $\left|R_{i(3)} - \left\{R_{i(1)} + R_{i(1)}\right\}/2\right|$, is quite large and the second control, with $S_{ij} = 1$, has rank $q_{ij}^* = 3$ in block i. That is, $\sum_{j=1}^{3} S_{ij}\, q_{ij}$ is large if b_i is large and $\sum_{j=1}^{3} S_{ij}\, q_{ij} = \sum_{j=1}^{3} S_{ij}\, \rho\left(q_{ij}^*\right)\, \varrho\{b_i/(I+1)\}$ is $5 \cdot \varrho\{b_i/(I+1)\}$. In other words, $T^* = \sum_{i=1}^{I}\sum_{j=1}^{3} S_{ij}\, q_{ij}$ is small, leading to rejection of H_0, if the second control rarely has the largest response, R_{ij}, in blocks i with large gaps.

Consider the case of a treatment effect in the block model (9.9) that is half the standard deviation of a treated-minus-control matched-pair difference with normal errors. Group B experiences this effect, groups N and P do not, but factor 2 compares group P to the merged group B∪N, so this effect is diluted in B∪N by the presence of unaffected controls from group N. In factor 2, the design sensitivities, $\widetilde{\Upsilon}$, of U878range123 and U888range123 using the range with $\rho(1) = 1$, $\rho(2) = 2$, and $\rho(3) = 3$ are close, 2.23 and 2.36, respectively [56, Table 2]. In contrast, the design sensitivities, $\widetilde{\Upsilon}$, of U878gap125 and U888gap125 using the gap with $\rho(1) = 1$, $\rho(2) = 2$, and $\rho(3) = 5$ are quite a bit higher and somewhat different, 2.90 and 3.27, respectively.

Consider the Bahadur relative efficiencies [56, Table 3] of sensitivity analyses performed at an $\Upsilon < \widetilde{\Upsilon}$. In a sensitivity analysis performed with $\Upsilon = 2$, the Bahadur efficiencies relative to U888gap125 are 0.11 for U878range123, 0.18 for U888range123, 0.82 for U878gap125, and, of course, 1.00 for U888gap125. The

[9] There was no uniformly best statistic [56, Tables 2 and 3]. This statistic was consistently either the best or reasonably close to it, in terms of design sensitivity or Bahadur efficiency, for normal or logistic error distributions and treatment effects that were either half or a third of the standard deviation of a single matched pair difference in outcomes. For error distributions with longer tails than the logistic distribution, replacing $(m, \underline{m}, \overline{m}) = (8, 8, 8)$ by $(m, \underline{m}, \overline{m}) = (8, 7, 8)$ and $\rho(3) = 5$ by $\rho(3) = 4$ may be advantageous; however, this change will degrade performance with normal errors.

[10] The statistic is implemented in the `ef2c` function of the `weightedRank` package in R.

poor relative efficiencies of U878range123 and U888range123 are consistent with the observation that their design sensitivities, $\widetilde{\Upsilon}$, of 2.23 and 2.36, are only slightly greater than $\Upsilon = 2$. As always, the Bahadur efficiency drops to zero as $\Upsilon \rightarrow \widetilde{\Upsilon}$.

The statistic U888gap125 twice emphasizes the tail of the distribution of R_{ij}, once between blocks using U888 and once within blocks using $\rho(3) = 5$. It performed well with the short-tailed normal distribution. Does it continue to perform well when the tails are longer? Consider the corresponding situation with logistic rather than normal errors. The design sensitivities are 2.15 for U878range123, 2.22 for U888range123, 2.77 for U878gap125, and 3.02 for U888gap125. Bahadur efficiency is computed relative to U888gap125. At $\Upsilon = 2$, both U878gap125 and U888gap125 have relative efficiency 1.00, whereas U878range123 has relative efficiency 0.09 and U888range123 has relative efficiency 0.18. Again, the Bahadur efficiencies are consistent with the design sensitivities: efficiency is positive but poor when Υ is below but close to $\widetilde{\Upsilon}$.

The statistic U888gap125 has attractive design sensitivity, $\widetilde{\Upsilon}$, and Bahadur efficiency for factor 2 under a conventional block model (9.9) with normal or logistic errors. How does U888gap125 perform in the blood pressure example?

Reanalysis of Binge Drinking and Blood Pressure

Table 13.3 is similar to Table 13.2, except that this new statistic has been substituted for U868 in the second evidence factor on the right side of Fig. 13.1. The P-values from the first factor are unaffected, but the combined P-value is affected.

Unlike Table 13.2, in Table 13.3 the second evidence factor is insensitive to $\Upsilon = 2$, and the combined analysis is insensitive to $(\Gamma, \Upsilon) = (2.0, 2.3)$. As suggested by its design sensitivity and Bahadur relative efficiency, the second evidence factor reports greater insensitivity to unmeasured bias if U888gap125 is used as the test statistic.

Table 13.3 Sensitivity analysis for the binge drinking and blood pressure data in two evidence factors, "B versus N" using the statistic U868 and "P versus B ∪ N," using the statistic U888/Gap/125. The table contains upper bounds on one-sided P values testing the hypothesis of no effect. The combined P-value bound applies the truncated product of P-values with truncation 0.2. Above the double line, (Γ, Υ) are as in Table 13.2, but the P-values for the second factor and the combination are smaller. Below the double line, the (Γ, Υ) values are larger than in Table 13.2

(Γ, Υ)	B versus N	P versus B ∪ N	Combined
(1.00, 1.00)	0.000	0.000	0.000
(1.75, 1.75)	0.048	0.026	0.007
(1.80, 1.80)	0.062	0.030	0.010
(1.90, 1.90)	0.099	0.039	0.019
(2.00, 1.85)	0.147	0.034	0.023
(1.85, 2.00)	0.079	0.050	0.019
(2.00, 2.00)	0.147	0.050	0.031
(1.90, 2.50)	0.099	0.122	0.046
(2.00, 2.30)	0.147	0.089	0.049

13.6 Other Aspects of Evidence Factors

This chapter has considered the simplest example of evidence factors, namely, a second evidence factor to isolate the information added by a second control group [56]. There are many other types of evidence factors, and there are various conceptual and practical issues that arise in using them in practice [55, Parts I and II]. A few of these issues are briefly mentioned here.

The example in Fig. 13.1 refers to two factors, or two comparisons, inside each of I blocks. Some other evidence factors entail one comparison within blocks and another comparison between blocks. For example, the right side of Fig. 10.2 has two factors. In the HDL cholesterol data in Fig. 10.2, there are $I = 603 = 406 + 197$ pairs of a regular drinker and a never-drinker. Of these 603 pairs, 406 contain a daily drinker, and 197 contain someone who drinks on two or three days each week. There are two essentially independent evidence factors in Fig. 10.2. One factor compares regular drinkers to never drinkers within 603 pairs, ignoring the distinction between daily and less frequent drinking. The other factor compares the 406 treated-minus-control pair differences in HDL cholesterol for daily drinkers to the 197 treated-minus-control pair differences for less frequent drinkers. So, one comparison is within 603 pairs and the other is between two groups of pairs. The between-pair comparison conditions upon the treatment assignment within pairs, while the within-pair comparison ignores the distinction between daily and less frequent drinkers. So the within-pair comparison depends upon one treatment assignment within pairs, say $\mathbf{S}$, and the between-pair comparison depends upon two treatment assignments, within and between pairs, say $(\mathbf{Z}, \mathbf{S})$, but uses the conditional distribution of $\mathbf{Z}$ given $\mathbf{S}$. The between-pair comparisons might have a continuous dose instead of two categories, and in either case straightforward evidence factor analyses are possible [55, §5.3].

Of course, there can be more than two evidence factors [55, §4.4]. There can be several comparisons within blocks, together with several comparisons between blocks, perhaps in a nested hierarchy of block structures. A comparison of treated and control groups may form one factor, and doses of treatment may be compared with outcomes for treated individuals, where there are no doses for controls [55, §4.5].

An evidence factor analysis may play a supporting role. A primary analysis may use information from both factors. Indeed, in focusing on daily drinkers in Sect. 1.4 in the study of HDL cholesterol, most of the analyses in this book have used only the daily drinkers, not the less frequent drinkers; that is, in the notation just above, the analyses used $(\mathbf{Z}, \mathbf{S})$ jointly, not $\mathbf{S}$ and $\mathbf{Z}$-given-$\mathbf{S}$ separately. A focus on daily drinkers was motivated by the consideration in Sect. 10.3, namely, including diluted doses of treatment reduces design sensitivity. Similarly, the main analyses in this book of binge drinking and blood pressure in Sect. 1.5 compared binge drinkers B to both controls, N and P, so again these analyses used $(\mathbf{Z}, \mathbf{S})$ jointly, not $\mathbf{S}$ and $\mathbf{Z}$-given-$\mathbf{S}$ separately. A focus on comparing B to two controls, both N and P, was motivated by the consideration in Sect. 10.2, namely, 2-to-1 blocked comparisons typically have larger design sensitivities than 1-to-1 paired comparisons. In both cases, the primary analysis was planned for a study design likely to secure a large design sensitivity. It is possible to combine a primary analysis without evidence factors and a supporting analysis with evidence factors while controlling the family-wise error rate [55, §6.3]; typically, this involves some variant of closed testing [36] or ordered testing [48].

Each of two evidence factors provides point estimates and confidence intervals, and may provide equivalence tests. These may be integrated into a single estimate, interval or test [55, §6.2].

13.7 *Further Reading

Multiple control groups: Introduced by Donald Campbell [7,8], multiple control groups are a standard device in quasi-experiments [2,17,23,35,39,43,61,63] with a variety of statistical properties [44,45,56,64]. Applications of the device are common [31,42,65,68].

Computerized construction of multiple control groups: Several algorithms have been proposed for matching with multiple control groups, including approximation algorithms [28], the construction of a balanced incomplete block design [34], randomized rounding to compare groups of very different sizes [6], and control groups constructed to attenuate unmeasured bias [40].

Bracketing using two control groups: Bracketing is a step beyond control by systematic variation [7,8]. In bracketing, an attempt is made to find two control groups, one higher, the other lower, than the treated group in terms of the distribution of an unmeasured covariate. Aspects of bracketing are discussed by Raiden Hasegawa and colleagues [18] and Ting Ye and colleagues [67].

Evidence factors: The statistical literature contains various methods for extracting two independent or uncorrelated statistics from reanalysis of the same data [1,14, 19,20,37,41,57,66]. Evidence factors use related ideas to provide insight into unmeasured biases in observational studies. Evidence factors for rank statistics [49] were extended to general statistics and situations with sensitivity analyses [51,52, 55]. Bikram Karmakar and others [26,56] discuss the Bahadur efficiency of joint analyses of several evidence factors. With three or more evidence factors, there is the possibility that two or more factors concur, and Bikram Karmakar and Dylan Small [27] examine this possibility using the concept of a partial conjunction hypothesis introduced by Yoav Benjamini and Ruth Heller [3]. Evidence factors have been applied to biomarkers of exposure to treatment [29] and to case-control studies [25]. Instead of assuming that several instruments are valid, evidence factors have been used to examine the extent to which instruments valid under different assumptions provide mutually supporting information [30,70]. Recent reviews of evidence factors are available [24,55].

Problems

13.1 Univariate Stochastic Order

Section 8.5 defined stochastic ordering of random variables in terms of their cumulative distribution functions. In a different way, Sect. 13.3 defined stochastic ordering of K-dimensional random vectors in terms of expectations of monotone increasing functions. View a random variable as a $K = 1$ dimensional random vector. Show that if scalar random variable V is stochastically larger than V^* in the sense of Sect. 13.3 if and only if it is stochastically larger in the sense of Sect. 8.5. (This is not difficult; see Marshall and Olkin [38, Proposition 17.A.1].)

13.2 Multivariate Stochastic Order

Give a counterexample showing that

$$\Pr(X_1 > a, X_2 > b) \leq \Pr(Y_1 > a, Y_2 > b)$$

for all a and b does **not** imply that $\mathbf{Y} = (Y_1, Y_2)$ is stochastically larger than $\mathbf{X} = (X_1, X_2)$ in the sense of Sect. 13.3. (Hint: Let the Xs be independent flips of two fair coins. Use infinitely thin, mathematical Scotch tape to tape those coins together, so the taped coins fairly come up heads together or tails together. From Marshall and Olkin [38, Example 17.A.2].)

13.3 Fisher's Product of P-Values

Let $\mathbf{U}$ be a K-dimensional vector whose coordinates are independent and uniformly distributed on the unit interval. Determine the probability that $\prod_{k=1}^{K} U_k \leq a$. (Hint: Consider the probability that $-\sum \log(U_k) \geq -\log(a)$. If U_k is uniform, what is the distribution of $-\log(U_k)$? What then is the distribution of $-\sum \log(U_k)$?) (Solution: [58, Example 7.15].)

13.4 Truncated Product of P-Values

Let $\mathbf{U}$ be a K-dimensional vector whose coordinates are independent and uniformly distributed on the unit interval. As noted in Sect. 13.3, Zahkin and colleagues [69] combine independent P-values by taking the product of those P-values that are less than or equal to a threshold, ι. They obtain the distribution of the truncated product by a calculus argument. Obtain the same distribution as a binomial mixture of gamma distributions. (Solution [21, §3.1].)

13.5 Truncation Point for the Truncated Product of P-Values

Use either `truncatedP` or `truncatedPbg` from the R package `sensitivitymv` for this problem.

(i) What is the combined P-value from P-values (0.0136, 1.0000) if the truncated product of P-values is used with truncation point $\iota = 0.2$? How does that change with P-values (0.0136, 0.2001)? With P-values (0.0136, 0.2000)?
(ii) What is the combined P-value from P-values (0.0136, 1.0000) if the truncated product of P-values is used with truncation point $\iota = 0.1$? What is the combined P-value from P-values (0.022, 1.0000) if the truncated product of P-values is used with truncation point $\iota = 0.1$? What is the Bonferroni-adjusted P-value if the two P-values are (0.0136, 1.0000)? What is the Bonferroni-adjusted P-value if the two P-values are (0.022, 1.0000)?
(iii) What is the combined P-value from P-values (0.068, 0.2) if the truncated product of P-values is used with truncation point $\iota = 0.2$? What is the Bonferroni-adjusted P-value if the two P-values are (0.068, 0.2)?
(iv) Fisher's method is the same as the truncated product with $\iota = 1$. Using Fisher's method, what is the combined P-value if the two P-values are (0.068, 0.2)? If two P-values are (0.068, 1)? If two P-values are (0.0136, 1)?
(v) You have explored several methods for combining two P-values. What conclusions would they produce with the P-values in Table 13.2?

13.6 Do an Evidence Factor Analysis for the HDL Cholesterol Data
Return to the HDL cholesterol data from Sect. 1.4, which is `aHDL` in the `weightedRank` package in `R`. Use the treated group D=daily drinking, N=never, and B=past binge drinker (omitting group R=rare). Use the function `ef2C` in this package to compare two evidence factors, D-vs-N and B-vs-(DUN). Use the default settings for `ef2C` while adjusting gamma and upsilon. Together, are the two factors jointly insensitive to a bias of $\Gamma = 4$ and $\Upsilon = 3.75$? Is factor 1 alone sensitive to a bias of $\Gamma = 4$? Is factor 2 alone sensitive to a bias of $\Upsilon = 3.75$? What happens if you change the default setting from `scores=c(1,2,5)` to `scores=c(1,2,6)`? To `scores=c(1,2,7)`? To `scores=c(1,2,3)`?

References

1. Alam, K.: Some nonparametric tests of randomness. J. Am. Stat. Assoc. **69**(347), 738–739 (1974)
2. Battistin, E., Rettore, E.: Ineligibles and eligible non-participants as a double comparison group in regression-discontinuity designs. J. Economet. **142**(2), 715–730 (2008)
3. Benjamini, Y., Heller, R.: Screening for partial conjunction hypotheses. Biometrics **64**(4), 1215–1222 (2008)
4. Berk, R.H., Cohen, A.: Asymptotically optimal methods of combining tests. J. Am. Stat. Assoc. **74**(368), 812–814 (1979)
5. Bitterman, M.E.: Phyletic differences in learning. Am. Psychologist **20**(6), 396 (1965)
6. Brumberg, K., Ellis, D.E., Small, D.S., Hennessy, S., Rosenbaum, P.R.: Using natural strata when examining unmeasured biases in an observational study of neurological side effects of antibiotics. J. Roy. Stat. Soc. C (Appl. Stat.) **72**(2), 314–329 (2023)
7. Campbell, D.T.: Prospective: Artifact and control. In: R. Rosenthal, R. Rosnow (eds.) Artifacts in Behavioral Research. Academic Press, New York (1969). Reprinted in Campbell 1988, pp. 167–190

8. Campbell, D.T.: Methodology and Epistemology for Social Science: Selected Papers. University of Chicago Press, Chicago (1988)
9. Cochran, W.G.: The comparison of percentages in matched samples. Biometrika **37**(3/4), 256–266 (1950)
10. Cohen, A., Sackrowitz, H.B.: On stochastic ordering of random vectors. J. Appl. Probab. **32**(4), 960–965 (1995)
11. Conover, W.J., Salsburg, D.S.: Locally most powerful tests for detecting treatment effects when only a subset of patients can be expected to "respond" to treatment. Biometrics **44**, 189–196 (1988)
12. Dantzig, G.B.: The diet problem. Interfaces **20**(4), 43–47 (1990)
13. Dudbridge, F., Koeleman, B.P.C.: Rank truncated product of p-values, with application to genomewide association scans. Genetic Epidemiol. **25**(4), 360–366 (2003)
14. Dwass, M.: Some k-sample rank-order tests. In: Contributions to Probability and Statistics: Essays in Honor of Harold Hotelling. Stanford University Press, Redwood City (1960)
15. Fisher, R.A.: Statistical Methods for Research Workers. Oliver and Boyd, Edinburgh (1928)
16. Friedman, M.: The use of ranks to avoid the assumption of normality implicit in the analysis of variance. J. Am. Stat. Assoc. **32**(200), 675–701 (1937)
17. Gangl, M.: Causal inference in sociological research. Annu. Rev. Sociol. **36**, 21–47 (2010)
18. Hasegawa, R.B., Webster, D.W., Small, D.S.: Evaluating missouri's handgun purchaser law: a bracketing method for addressing concerns about history interacting with group. Epidemiology **30**(3), 371–379 (2019)
19. Hogg, R.V.: Iterated tests of the equality of several distributions. J. Am. Stat. Assoc. **57**(299), 579–585 (1962)
20. Hollander, M.: Certain uncorrelated nonparametric test statistics. J. Am. Stat. Assoc. **63**(322), 707–714 (1968)
21. Hsu, J., Small, D., Rosenbaum, P.R.: Effect modification and design sensitivity in observational studies. J. Am. Stat. Assoc. **108**(501), 135–148 (2013)
22. Hume, D.: An Enquiry Concerning Human Understanding. Oxford University Press, New York (2007)
23. Imbens, G.W., Wooldridge, J.M.: Recent developments in the econometrics of program evaluation. J. Econ. Literat. **47**(1), 5–86 (2009)
24. Karmakar, B.: Evidence factors. In: J.R. Zubizarreta, E.A. Stuart, D.S. Small, P.R. Rosenbaum (eds.) Handbook of Matching and Weighting Adjustments for Causal Inference, pp. 583–610. Chapman and Hall/CRC, Boca Raton, FL (2023)
25. Karmakar, B., Doubeni, C.A., Small, D.S.: Evidence factors in a case-control study with application to the effect of flexible sigmoidoscopy screening on colorectal cancer. Ann. Appl. Stat. **14**(2), 829–849 (2020)
26. Karmakar, B., French, B., Small, D.: Integrating the evidence from evidence factors in observational studies. Biometrika **106**(2), 353–367 (2019)
27. Karmakar, B., Small, D.S.: Assessment of the extent of corroboration of an elaborate theory of a causal hypothesis using partial conjunctions of evidence factors. Ann. Stat. **48**(6), 3283–3311 (2020)
28. Karmakar, B., Small, D.S., Rosenbaum, P.R.: Using approximation algorithms to build evidence factors and related designs for observational studies. J. Comput. Graph. Stat. **28**(3), 698–709 (2019)
29. Karmakar, B., Small, D.S., Rosenbaum, P.R.: Using evidence factors to clarify exposure biomarkers. Am. J. Epidemiol. **189**(3), 243–249 (2020)
30. Karmakar, B., Small, D.S., Rosenbaum, P.R.: Reinforced designs: Multiple instruments plus control groups as evidence factors in an observational study of the effectiveness of catholic schools. J. Am. Stat. Assoc. **116**(533), 82–92 (2021)
31. Lavy, V.: Effects of free choice among public schools. Rev. Econ. Stud. **77**(3), 1164–1191 (2010)
32. Lehmann, E.: Ordered families of distributions. Ann. Math. Stat. **26**(3), 399–419 (1955)
33. Lehmann, E.L.: The power of rank tests. Ann. Math. Stat. **24**, 23–43 (1953)

34. Lu, B., Rosenbaum, P.R.: Optimal pair matching with two control groups. J. Comput. Graph. Stat. **13**(2), 422–434 (2004)
35. Lu, X., White, H.: Robustness checks and robustness tests in applied economics. J. Economet. **178**, 194–206 (2014)
36. Marcus, R., Peritz, E., Gabriel, K.R.: On closed testing procedures with special reference to ordered analysis of variance. Biometrika **63**(3), 655–660 (1976)
37. Marden, J.I.: Use of nested orthogonal contrasts in analyzing rank data. J. Am. Stat. Assoc. **87**(418), 307–318 (1992)
38. Marshall, A.W., Olkin, I.: Inequalities: Theory of Majorization and Its Applications. Academic Press, New York (1979)
39. Meyer, B.D.: Natural and quasi-experiments in economics. J. Bus. Econ. Stat. **13**(2), 151–161 (1995)
40. Pimentel, S.D., Small, D.S., Rosenbaum, P.R.: Constructed second control groups and attenuation of unmeasured biases. J. Am. Stat. Assoc. **111**(515), 1157–1167 (2016)
41. Randles, R.H., Hogg, R.V.: Certain uncorrelated and independent rank statistics. J. Am. Stat. Assoc. **66**(335), 569–574 (1971)
42. Ray, W.A., Murray, K.T., Hall, K., Arbogast, P.G., Stein, C.M.: Azithromycin and the risk of cardiovascular death. New Engl. J. Med. **366**(20), 1881–1890 (2012)
43. Reichardt, C.S.: Quasi-experimentation: A Guide to Design and Analysis. Guilford Publications, New York (2019)
44. Rosenbaum, P.R.: The role of a second control group in an observational study. Stat. Sci. **2**(3), 292–306 (1987)
45. Rosenbaum, P.R.: On permutation tests for hidden biases in observational studies. Ann. Stat. **17**(2), 643–653 (1989)
46. Rosenbaum, P.R.: Observational Studies, 2nd edn. Springer, New York (2002)
47. Rosenbaum, P.R.: Confidence intervals for uncommon but dramatic responses to treatment. Biometrics **63**(4), 1164–1171 (2007)
48. Rosenbaum, P.R.: Testing hypotheses in order. Biometrika **95**(1), 248–252 (2008)
49. Rosenbaum, P.R.: Evidence factors in observational studies. Biometrika **97**(2), 333–345 (2010)
50. Rosenbaum, P.R.: A new U-statistic with superior design sensitivity in matched observational studies. Biometrics **67**(3), 1017–1027 (2011)
51. Rosenbaum, P.R.: Some approximate evidence factors in observational studies. J. Am. Stat. Assoc. **106**(493), 285–295 (2011)
52. Rosenbaum, P.R.: The general structure of evidence factors in observational studies. Stat. Sci. **32**(4), 514–530 (2017)
53. Rosenbaum, P.R.: Observation and Experiment: An Introduction to Causal Inference. Harvard University Press, Cambridge, MA (2017)
54. Rosenbaum, P.R.: Design of Observational Studies, 2nd edn. Springer, New York (2020)
55. Rosenbaum, P.R.: Replication and Evidence Factors in Observational Studies. Chapman and Hall/CRC, New York (2021)
56. Rosenbaum, P.R.: A second evidence factor for a second control group. Biometrics **79**, 3968–3980 (2023)
57. Savage, I.R.: On the independence of tests of randomness and other hypotheses. J. Am. Stat. Assoc. **52**(277), 53–57 (1957)
58. Severini, T.A.: Elements of Distribution Theory. Cambridge University Press, New York (2005)
59. Shaked, M., Shanthikumar, J.G.: Stochastic Orders. Springer, New York (2007)
60. Snedecor, G.W., Cochran, W.G.: Statistical Methods, 8th edn. Iowa State University Press, Ames, Iowa (1989)
61. Sobel, M.E.: An introduction to causal inference. Sociol. Methods Res. **24**(3), 353–379 (1996)
62. Stephenson, W.R.: A general class of one-sample nonparametric test statistics based on subsamples. J. Am. Stat. Assoc. **76**(376), 960–966 (1981)
63. Steventon, A., Grieve, R., Sekhon, J.S.: A comparison of alternative strategies for choosing control populations in observational studies. Health Serv. Outcomes Res. Methodol. **15**, 157–181 (2015)

64. Stuart, E.A., Rubin, D.B.: Matching with multiple control groups with adjustment for group differences. J. Educ. Behav. Stat. **33**(3), 279–306 (2008)
65. Van Staa, T., Leufkens, H., Cooper, C.: Use of inhaled corticosteroids and risk of fractures. J. Bone Mineral Res. **16**(3), 581–588 (2001)
66. Wolfe, D.A.: Some general results about uncorrelated statistics. J. Am. Stat. Assoc. **68**(344), 1013–1018 (1973)
67. Ye, T., Keele, L., Hasegawa, R., Small, D.S.: A negative correlation strategy for bracketing in difference-in-differences. J. Am. Stat. Assoc. (2024). https://doi.org/10.1080/01621459.2023.2252576
68. Yoon, F.B., Huskamp, H.A., Busch, A.B., Normand, S.L.T.: Using multiple control groups and matching to address unobserved biases in comparative effectiveness research: an observational study of the effectiveness of mental health parity. Stat. Biosci. **3**(1), 63–78 (2011)
69. Zaykin, D.V., Zhivotovsky, L.A., Westfall, P.H., Weir, B.S.: Truncated product method for combining p-values. Genetic Epidemiol. **22**(2), 170–185 (2002)
70. Zhao, A., Lee, Y., Small, D.S., Karmakar, B.: Evidence factors from multiple, possibly invalid, instrumental variables. Ann. Stat. **50**(3), 1266–1296 (2022)

Chapter 14
Tightened Blocks for Complementary Analyses

> Rationality . . . is most plausibly identified as argument and counterargument, with the just and fair weighing of conflicts of evidence.
>
> Stuart Hampshire [11, p. 45]

Abstract A complementary analysis is a planned analysis that supports a primary analysis by providing evidence relevant to counterclaims that might be raised concerning the primary analysis. A complementary analysis sheds light on counterclaims. A compelling observational study is often composed of a strong primary analysis protected by a bodyguard of strong complementary analyses. When the primary analysis is based on a block design, a complementary analysis may be based on tightened blocks—that is, a smaller block design formed by either removing some controls from a block or some entire blocks or both, in an effort to address particular counterclaims.

14.1 What Is a Complementary Analysis?

In most observational studies, a primary analysis compares the outcomes in treated and control groups after adjustment for measured covariates. In parallel with a randomized clinical trial, this primary analysis is a planned analysis—that is, an analysis described in detail before any outcome data are examined. Typically, the description of the primary analysis is recorded in the grant proposal that funded the research and possibly also in a study protocol. The plan identifies the primary outcome or

© The Author(s), under exclusive license to Springer Nature Switzerland AG 2025
P. R. Rosenbaum, *An Introduction to the Theory of Observational Studies*,
Springer Texts in Statistics, https://doi.org/10.1007/978-3-031-90494-3_14

outcomes; the covariates for which adjustments will be made; the methods of adjustment, as in Chaps. 5–7; the analytic methods to be used in the primary analysis and its sensitivity analyses, as in Chap. 8; and any quasi-experimental devices that will be employed, as in Chaps. 12–13.

A complementary analysis is also a planned analysis, but not one that means much on its own in the absence of the primary analysis. A complementary analysis addresses some plausible concern about the primary analysis, perhaps weakening the primary analysis by finding that the concern has merit, or perhaps strengthening the primary analysis by finding that the concern has little or no merit. In other words, the complementary analysis investigates counterclaims or objections that the investigator anticipates will be raised about the claims made by the primary analysis [32]. Often, a compelling observational study has a strong primary analysis protected by a strong bodyguard of complementary analyses. The obvious objections to the primary analysis are rebutted before they are spoken. To be effective, a bodyguard must stay close to the guarded body—a complementary analysis must change some critical component while staying close to the primary analysis, so that this critical component is seen with clarity.

In block designs, complementary analyses are often formed by tightening blocks. A tightened block design is a new block design formed as part of an existing block design: it retains the block structure—who is blocked or matched with whom—but it removes some people from each block or some entire blocks. Because a tightened block design uses the same analytic procedures with a subset of the same people in almost the same design, it is usually clear that any shift in conclusions reflects the tightening—the deliberate, explicit, and purposeful removal of some people or some whole blocks. In contrast, a complementary analysis that arbitrarily changes many things—one that changes the population studied, the analytical methods, the adjustments for covariates, and so on—will raise doubts about which of these many things is responsible for any changes in conclusions.

14.2 Affected Concomitant Variables

Should Adjustments Be Made for Obesity?

In studying the effects caused by alcohol, should an adjustment be made for the body mass index (BMI), a measure of obesity? In the blood pressure example in Sect. 1.5, treated and control groups were matched for BMI, but in the cholesterol example in Sect. 1.4 there was no adjustment for BMI. In this book, that decision was made for pedagogical reasons: the example in Sect. 1.4 is closely matched for several covariates and represents matching conceptually, but the example in Sect. 1.5 represents modern multivariate matching methods that can balance many covariates in Chaps. 5 and 6. Setting pedagogy aside, ask: What should be done with BMI?

In the HDL cholesterol example in Sect. 1.4, BMI is not matched in the $I = 406$ blocks comparing four groups, D = daily drinker, N = never drinker, R = rare drinker, and B = past binge drinker. If we apply Friedman's [9] test to the unmatched BMI levels, then the four groups differ significantly, with P-value 2.2×10^{-9}. Whatever the pattern of BMIs means, it certainly is not an accident.

If BMI were a covariate, then it would be reasonable to match or adjust for it. Is current BMI a covariate for alcohol consumption in the past year? By definition, a covariate is a variable measured prior to treatment and hence unaffected by the assignment of an individual to treatment or control; so, a covariate exists in a single version, $\mathbf{x}_{ij}$. In this sense, a covariate is different from an outcome: an outcome may be affected by the treatment, so it exists in two versions, (r_{Tij}, r_{Cij}), where r_{Tij} is observed under treatment, $Z_{ij} = 1$, and r_{Cij} is observed under control, $Z_{ij} = 0$. The matching in Sect. 1.4 controlled for age, sex, and education. Age and sex are covariates; they are not affected by daily light alcohol consumption in the past year. For most people in Sect. 1.4, education was completed many years ago and so is a covariate; moreover, even for a few people who are in school or recent graduates, light daily alcohol consumption is likely to have little or no effect on years of education. In contrast, ask: Is BMI a covariate?

The US Department of Agriculture (USDA) says that a 5-ounce glass of wine has 125 calories [46]. Two glasses of wine each day for a year has $365 \times 125 \times 2 = 91250$ calories. The US Centers for Disease Control (CDC) says that a pound of body fat stores 3500 calories [45]. Long division yields that two glasses of wine per day for a year could be stored in $91250/3500 = 26$ pounds of added body fat. The biology, psychology, and sociology of eating and drinking are, no doubt, more complex than long division, but it is certainly possible that consuming alcohol has an effect on BMI. It is certainly possible that both HDL cholesterol and BMI are outcomes affected by drinking daily. Write (r_{Tij}, r_{Cij}) and $R_{ij} = Z_{ij}\, r_{Tij} + (1 - Z_{ij})\, r_{Cij}$ for HDL cholesterol, and write (s_{Tij}, s_{Cij}) and $S_{ij} = Z_{ij}\, s_{Tij} + (1 - Z_{ij})\, s_{Cij}$ for BMI.

If you act as if an affected outcome were a covariate—if you adjust one outcome R_{ij} for another outcome S_{ij}—then you may induce a bias in the estimated effect of the treatment [27]. This induced bias occurs even in randomized experiments; so, in this case, the bias is avoided simply by not adjusting for S_{ij}. The situation is more complicated in an observational study, where adjustment for an unaffected outcome, $s_{Tij} = s_{Cij}$, or a slightly affected outcome may also reduce bias from some unmeasured covariate. Under some special circumstances, analyses that adjust one outcome for another may have an interpretation [14]. In the absence of special circumstances, adjustment of one outcome R_{ij} for another outcome S_{ij} need not estimate the effect caused by any actual or possible treatment. For instance, you can describe in words a treatment that consists of adding two glasses of wine per day, making no other changes in diet or calories, making no changes in energy expenditure, and that holds BMI fixed, and you can fit a regression model that expresses that description; however, it is very doubtful that any such treatment could exist in the world we actually inhabit [12].

If drinking alcohol does affect BMI—if $s_{Tij} \neq s_{Cij}$—then what is the nature of the effect? Long division hints that drinking adds calories and increases BMI, $s_{Tij} > s_{Cij}$, but maybe the situation is more complex than long division. Perhaps a glass of beer with dinner leads you to eat more or fewer calories from food. Perhaps

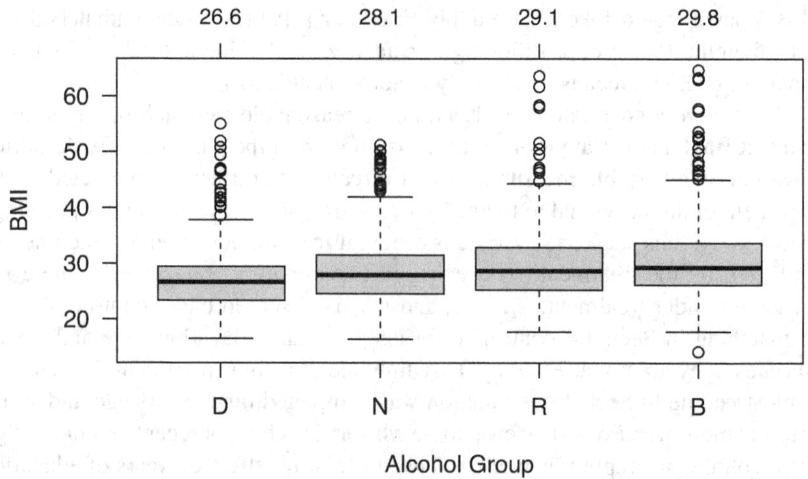

Fig. 14.1 Body mass index (BMI) in the study of HDL cholesterol and light daily alcohol consumption. Huber's M-estimate appears above each boxplot. D = daily drinking, N = never drinking, R = rare drinking, B = past binge drinking

it is uncomfortable to eat little when dining with others—perhaps it is uncomfortable to sit by and skip the appetizers and desserts that dinner partners are enjoying—but perhaps that discomfort is reduced by nursing one glass of wine through a long meal. The scientific literature says alcohol may cause, prevent, or have no effect on obesity [16, 47, 48], perhaps with different effects for men and women. What pattern do we see here?

Figure 14.1 depicts BMI by group for the $I = 406$ blocks in Sect. 1.4. As always and as seen in Sect. 1.4, the groups are matched or blocked for age, sex, and education. Despite the calories from alcohol, the daily drinkers (D) have the lowest typical BMI, and the group that engaged in frequent binge drinking in the past (B) has the highest typical BMI. Although the meaning of Fig. 14.1 is not yet clear, it sits uncomfortably with the notion that daily drinking mechanically adds 91250 calories per year and increases body fat by 26 pounds per year. There is something wrong with that notion.

A Tightened Block Comparison

The tightened block design rearranges the $IJ = 406 \times 4 = 1624$ people in the original design in Sect. 1.4. The same people are studied in the same blocks. There are still $I = 406$ blocks, and a person who was in block i is still in block i in the tightened design, for $i = 1, \ldots, I$. The daily drinking group (D) has not changed. The controls have been rearranged into group C and group O. For block i, group C contains two of the three controls from block i, selected to balance BMI between groups D and C, thereby removing the imbalance seen in Fig. 14.1. For block i, group O contains the

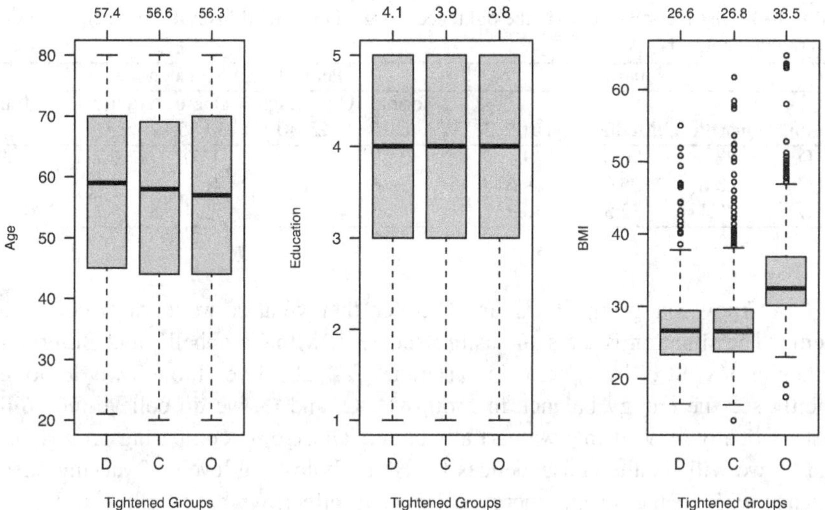

Fig. 14.2 Age, education, and BMI in the tightened block design. Also, each group is 33.7% female. Group C contains two of the original controls in each block, selected so that BMI is balanced between groups D and C. Group O contains the one omitted control from each block, and it has much higher BMIs. D = 406 daily drinkers, C = 812 tightened controls, O = 406 omitted controls. M-estimates appear above each boxplot

one remaining control from block i. The construction of the tightened block design requires some care and is described in the next subsection. To emphasize, group C does *not* consist of the two closest controls to the daily drinker; that approach does not balance BMI.

Figure 14.2 shows age, education, and BMI for the tightened block design. Not shown there, each group is 33.7% female. By design, groups D, C, and O look similar in terms of age, education, and sex, and groups D and C look similar in terms of BMI. Group O has much higher BMIs. Although Figs. 14.1 and 14.2 contain the same $IJ = 406 \times 4 = 1624$ people in the same $I = 406$ blocks, Fig. 14.2 presents a starker comparison in terms of BMI: two groups are very similar and one is very different. Table 14.1 shows the BMIs in greater detail.

Groups D, C, and O clearly differ. Obviously, group O is visibly different from the other two groups because their BMIs are higher. Groups D and C must differ also in ways we do not see, because they have similar BMIs despite added calories from daily drinking in group D. One common view—perhaps merely one common but crude approximation—sees BMI as reflecting "energy balance," or the difference between calories consumed in food or drink and calories burned in metabolism and activity [12]. On this view, groups D and C can have the same distribution of BMIs despite their difference in alcohol consumption only if group D either consumes fewer calories from other sources or burns more calories in activities or both. On this same view, groups C and O must differ in energy balance.

Table 14.1 Distribution of BMI in the tightened design. D = daily drinker, C = tightened controls, O = omitted controls

	Quartiles			Percents in BMI categories				
				Normal	Overweight	Obese	Higher	Total
Group	Quartile 1	Median	Quartile 3	< 25	25-30	30-35	≥ 35	
D	23.3	26.6	29.4	36.9	40.4	16.0	6.7	100.0%
C	23.8	26.6	29.6	34.6	41.7	16.1	7.5	100.0%
O	30.1	32.5	36.9	2.0	22.4	39.4	36.2	100.0%

If we know that groups D, C, and O differ, then what do we learn by comparing them? The situation is the same as in Sect. 13.1, with Campbell's and Bitterman's principle of control by systematic variation [2–4, 28]. Even though we do not explicitly see the energy balance in groups D, C, and O, we do believe they differ systematically in ways that we partially understand. So, in comparing groups D, C, and O, we will see the consequences for HDL cholesterol levels of varying energy balance without measuring energy balance. In effect, we have built a useful situation with systematic variation that is analogous to multiple control groups by an algorithmic process that used measured variables, in this case BMI [24].

When we compare groups D, C, and O, many patterns are possible. If groups D and C had similar HDL cholesterol levels and group O had much lower HDL cholesterol levels, then that might suggest an important role for BMI or energy balance, perhaps with light alcohol consumption helping some people to consume fewer calories from food. That pattern is also compatible with a simple bias in who drinks daily, perhaps with greater physical activity predicting lower BMI and higher HDL cholesterol, perhaps in the absence of any effect caused by alcohol. Alternatively, if group D has much higher HDL cholesterol levels than both groups C and O, with groups C and O having very similar cholesterol levels, then that is not inconsistent with a primary role for alcohol itself, with little or no role for BMI or energy balance. As is true in observational studies generally, the situation here is not identified by observable distributions, so several explanations of the observable distributions are often possible; however, observable distributions do place constraints on what is possible.

Figure 14.3 compares HDL cholesterol levels in groups D, C, and O. The left side of Fig. 14.3 depicts the cholesterol levels, ignoring the blocks. Groups D and O each contain $I = 406$ individuals, while group C contains $2I = 812$ individuals. The right side of Fig. 14.3 shows the within-block pair differences in cholesterol levels. For D-minus-O, there are $I = 406$ pair differences within the $I = 406$ blocks. For D-minus-C, there are $2I = 812$ differences, two from each block; they share the same daily drinker, but have different controls.

In Fig. 14.3, the daily drinkers in group D have decidedly higher HDL cholesterol levels that the individuals in groups C and O, but cholesterol levels are somewhat higher in group C than in group O. If we momentarily acted as if BMI were a covariate with $s_{Tij} = s_{Cij}$, then the blocked comparison of HDL cholesterol levels in groups D and C yields a one-sided P-value bound of 0.044 at $\Gamma = 4.1$ using U878; so, there is fairly strong evidence of an effect of alcohol on HDL cholesterol when comparing

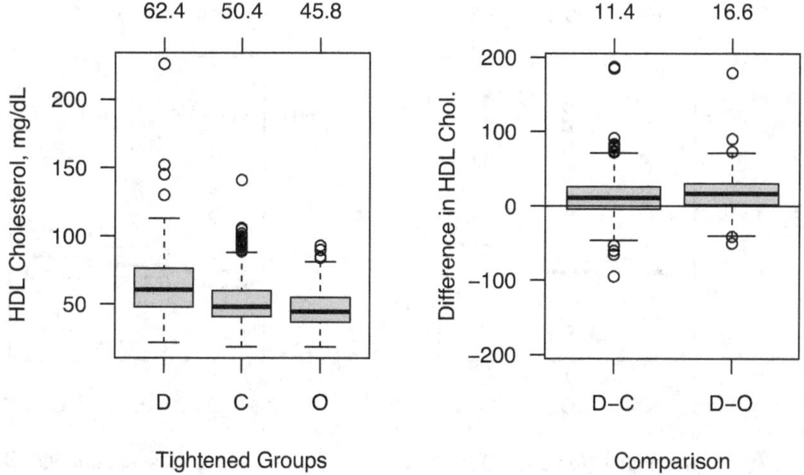

Fig. 14.3 HDL cholesterol in the tightened design. D = 406 daily drinkers, C = 812 tightened controls, O = 406 omitted controls. The right side shows within-block treated-minus-control pair differences, 812 D-minus-C differences, and 406 D-minus-O differences. M-estimates of location appear above each boxplot

groups constructed to have similar BMIs. It is unclear whether the comparison of D and C has removed a bias due to differences in BMI, or whether it has removed part of the actual effect of alcohol in which daily drinking reduces BMI, or whether it has done both of these things [27]. It is clear that HDL cholesterol tracks light daily alcohol consumption, whether BMI is forced to balance or is allowed to do what it naturally does. Despite a large difference in BMI, groups C and O differ much less in terms of HDL cholesterol than do groups D and C.

The difference is larger and insensitive to larger biases when comparing groups D and O, with a *P*-value bound of 0.047 at $\Gamma = 7.5$ using U878. This speaks, at least, against the thought that the added calories in alcoholic beverages are a decisive consideration. After all, group D consumed extra calories from daily alcohol, perhaps 90000 extra calories per year, yet is leaner than group O which consumed little alcohol, and group D has decidedly higher HDL cholesterol levels.

Constructing the Tightened Design

The tightened design picks two of the three controls in each block i for group C, placing the remaining control in group O. It might seem natural to pick for group C the two controls in block i whose BMIs are closest to the BMI of the treated individual in block i; however, this would be a mistake. In the third or right panel of Fig. 14.2, groups D and C had similar BMIs and groups C and O had very different BMIs, making for a desirably stark comparison, a clearer comparison than

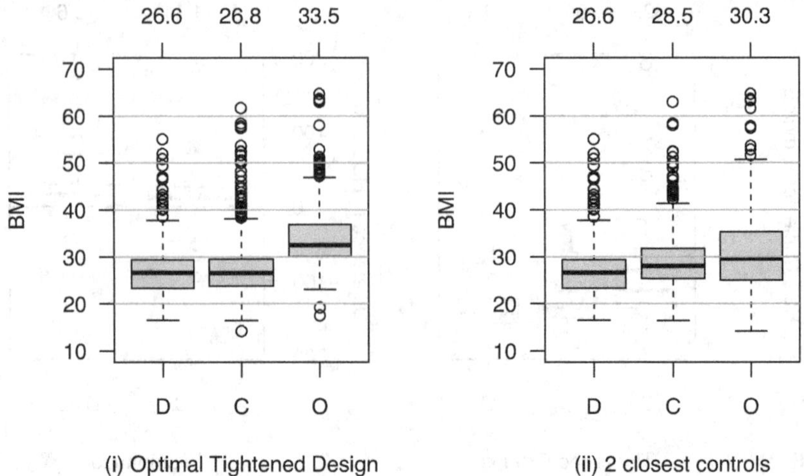

Fig. 14.4 Comparison of two tightened designs. The left side depicts BMI in the design in Fig. 14.2: it was built using optimal fine balance for BMI. The right side depicts the inadequate design that simply picked for group C the two controls whose BMIs were closest to the daily drinker (D) in that block. On the left, as desired, groups D and C are closer, and groups C and O are further apart. Huber's M-estimates appear above each boxplot

in Fig. 14.1; however, this stark pattern requires the use of fine balance for BMI in Sects. 5.3 and 5.4, not the close pairing for BMI in Sect. 5.2. In forming group C, we need to balance BMI across blocks in ways that cannot be accomplished by balancing BMI within blocks.

Figure 14.4(i) reproduces the third panel of Fig. 14.2, while Fig. 14.4(ii) depicts the balance for BMI obtained by simply picking the two closest controls in each block. Panel (ii) of Fig. 14.4 is clearly not what we want: (a) we want groups D and C to have similar distributions of BMI, and (b) for a stark comparison, we want groups C and O to have very different distributions of BMI. Both sides of Fig. 14.4 contain the same $IJ = 406 \times 4 = 1624$ people, and group D has not changed; only the division of the $I(J-1) = 406 \times 3 = 1218$ controls into groups C and O has changed from Fig. 14.4(i) to Fig. 14.4(ii). Also, on both sides of Fig. 14.4, the same four people are in block i for $i = 1, \ldots, I = 406$.

Consider one block as an example. In block $i = 16$, the daily drinker had a BMI of 46.8, and the three controls had BMIs of 25.9, 34.7, and 36.8. The inadequate design on the right in Fig. 14.4(ii) picked the closest two of the three controls, so it picked the controls with BMIs of 34.7 and 36.8. This is a mistake. We are trying to correct an overall imbalance in BMIs in which treated individuals typically have lower BMIs than controls. True, this overall imbalance is not evident in block $i = 16$, but that means that block i offers a small opportunity to take a step in correcting the overall imbalance in BMI. By selecting the two controls with BMIs of 25.9 and 34.7, the balanced design in Fig. 14.4(i) reduced the imbalance in BMI between groups D and C, even though $|46.8 - 25.9| > |46.8 - 36.8|$. The close balance in groups D and

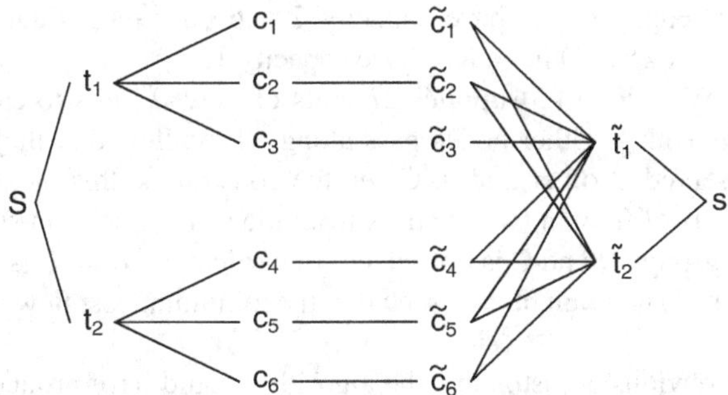

Fig. 14.5 Network for optimal tightening of an existing block design. This network resembles Fig. 5.5 for two-criteria matching [51], except on the left, a treated individual, say t_i is connected only to controls in block i, here to 3 controls. To pick 2 controls from each block, $2I$ units of flow leave the source, S, and are absorbed by the sink, s, and each edge involving the source or the sink has capacity to carry two units of flow. Balancing occurs on the right where edges can cross blocks

C in Fig. 14.4(i) reflects many carefully chosen steps towards balancing BMI, and these were implemented using fine balance in Sect. 5.3 and two-criteria matching in Sect. 5.4.[1]

The design in Fig. 14.2 and Fig. 14.4(i) was built as follows. Because this is a tightening of an existing block design, only the $IJ = 406 \times 4 = 1624$ individuals in the existing block design were eligible for matching; so, only these IJ individuals appear in the matching network. The network in Fig. 14.5 is analogous to the network for two-criteria matching [51] in Fig. 5.5; however, there are $I = 406$ treated individuals, $t_1, \ldots, t_I$, and $I(J-1) = 406 \times 3 = 1218$ controls, $c_1, \ldots, c_{3I}$. For notational simplicity, assume that the first block in the original design is (t_1, c_1, c_2, c_3), the second block is (t_2, c_4, c_5, c_6), and so on.

The treated individual in block i is paired to two of the three controls in block i. We can require this in either of two ways, either by removing edges or by penalizing edges. In the first way, on the left side of Fig. 14.5, treated individual t_i is connected only to the $J - 1 = 3$ controls from block i; for instance, on the left in Fig. 14.5, t_1 is connected only to c_1, c_2 and c_3; t_2 is connected only to c_4, c_5 and c_6. In the second way, in Fig. 5.5, the cost of an edge that connects t_i to a control c_ℓ who is not in block i is greatly increased—is penalized—so that a minimum cost flow avoids these edges.

In contrast, on the right side of Fig. 14.5, no edges are removed or penalized because of block membership. That is, an edge connects $\bar{t}_i$ to $\bar{c}_\ell$ for $i = 1, \ldots, I$ and $\ell = 1, \ldots, I(J-1)$. These edges $\left(\bar{t}_i, \bar{c}_\ell\right)$ have costs that work to balance BMI across blocks.

[1] For access to the data, complete details of the match, and its replication, see the documentation for the R package `tightenBlock` and the replication appendix for reference [36]. The details are slightly more complex than is described here. In particular, fine balance used narrow but discrete BMI categories, so that the entire distributions of BMI are balanced, not just their means.

In Fig. 14.5, edges (S, t_i) have capacity 2 and cost zero. Edges $(\bar{t}_i, s)$ have capacity 2 and cost zero. Other edges have capacity 1.

The source S in Fig. 14.5 supplies $2I$ units of flow, 2 units to each t_i, that are collected by the sink s. Other nodes pass along all the flow that they receive; that is, flow is conserved at other nodes. Given the constraints, this means that each t_i deposits two units of flow in two controls from the same block i in such a way that balance across groups D and C is optimized. In particular, group C is defined by the two controls, say ℓ and m, in block i such that the minimum cost flow has $f_{(t_i, c_\ell)} = 1$ and $f_{(t_i, c_m)} = 1$.

With minor obvious adjustments, the algorithm could have produced a group C of size I and a group O of size $2I$. Other patterns are possible for larger block sizes, $J > 4$; for instance, for $J = 5$, one could construct two groups, C and O, each of size $2I$. Tightening blocks can use the full array of matching tactics in Chap. 5 and elsewhere in the literature [19, 21–23, 34, 35, 51–53]. Tightening blocks can also provide a complementary analysis that explores the possibility of attenuating unmeasured bias by allowing a possibly irrelevant covariate to fluctuate freely in the O group [24].

14.3 Differential Effects and Generic Unmeasured Biases

Unmeasured Biases That Promote Several Treatments

In Table 13.1, which refers to the study of alcohol and HDL cholesterol, we saw that people in daily drinking group (D) were more likely than controls to have been to the dentist in the past year. What should we make of this association?

The overall impression is that the four variables in Table 13.1 reflect different attitudes in groups D = daily, N = never, R = rarely, and B = past binge drinker. Groups N and R avoided cocaine, heroin, and methamphetamine, and group N also avoided marijuana and hashish, while groups D and B are much more likely to have, at least, tried these drugs. That is, alcohol use at present or in the past seems to occur with having tried various drugs. From their methylmercury levels, it appears that group D eats more fish than the other groups. It is at least possible that eating fish, visiting the dentist, and light daily drinking are perceived by daily drinkers, perhaps correctly, as beneficial to health. The lower BMIs of daily drinkers fit the same pattern. For instance, Walter Willett and colleagues [50] speak favorably of fish and light alcohol as components of a healthy diet, and similar statements are in news reports. Could someone reasonably dismiss the association between light daily drinking and higher HDL cholesterol levels, arguing that group D takes various actions to promote health, presumably more actions than eating fish, going to the dentist, maintaining a lower BMI, and light daily drinking; so, higher HDL cholesterol levels could be a by-product of a healthy lifestyle whose full extent is not evident in the data? Or are higher HDL cholesterol levels specific to light alcohol consumption [49]?

An unmeasured attitude or disposition that promotes several or many treatments is said to be a "generic unmeasured bias." It is generic in not being specific to one treatment. We associate generic biases with so-called "lifestyle choices" and similar situations. Although generic biases leave visible traces in patterns of treatments received or avoided, we should be cautious in characterizing such dispositions. Perhaps eating fish, going to the dentist, and light daily drinking aim at a healthy lifestyle, but perhaps trying cocaine, heroin, or methamphetamine suggests a more nuanced description of this disposition.

The are two facts. First, if a general attitude or disposition promotes many treatments, then adjusting for a few of those treatments as if they were covariates invariably underadjusts for the general disposition and its other manifestations [13, Thm. 6]. Second, under certain conditions, certain analyses can remove unmeasured generic biases when studying the differential effect of two treatments [29,31]. These analyses overadjust for, say, having been to the dentist in an effort to adequately adjust for the general disposition. This second fact is the focus of the current section.

A 2 × 2 Factorial Design

Suppose that, instead of one binary treatment, Z, there are two binary treatments, (Z, Z'), making a 2×2 factorial arrangement, $Z \times Z'$. There are then four potential outcomes, $\mathbf{r} = (r_{11}, r_{10}, r_{01}, r_{00})$ where r_{ab} is observed if $(Z, Z') = (a, b)$. Of course, we observe only (R, Z, Z') where

$$R = Z\, Z'\, r_{11} + Z\, (1 - Z')\, r_{10} + (1 - Z)\, Z'\, r_{01} + (1 - Z)\, (1 - Z')\, r_{00}.$$

By analogy with Chap. 4, define (i) $\zeta_{ab} = \zeta_{ab}(\mathbf{r}, \mathbf{x}) = \Pr(Z = a,\, Z' = b \mid \mathbf{r}, \mathbf{x})$ and $\boldsymbol{\zeta}(\mathbf{r}, \mathbf{x}) = \boldsymbol{\zeta} = (\zeta_{11}, \zeta_{10}, \zeta_{01}, \zeta_{00})$, where $1 = \zeta_{11} + \zeta_{10} + \zeta_{01} + \zeta_{00}$, and (ii) $e_{ab} = e_{ab}(\mathbf{x}) = \Pr(Z = a,\, Z = b \mid \mathbf{x})$ and $\mathbf{e} = (e_{11}, e_{10}, e_{01}, e_{00})$, where $1 = e_{11} + e_{10} + e_{01} + e_{00}$. Let $\mathbf{w} = (w_{11}, w_{10}, w_{01}, w_{00})$ be four fixed numbers, not all zero.

Suppose that we want to estimate the expectation given $\mathbf{x}$ of a causal comparison $\mathbf{w}^T\mathbf{r} = w_{11}\, r_{11} + w_{10}\, r_{10} + w_{01}\, r_{01} + w_{00}\, r_{00}$; that is, we want to estimate the regression $\mathrm{E}\left(\mathbf{w}^T\mathbf{r} \,\middle|\, \mathbf{x}\right)$. If $\mathbf{w} = (1, 1, -1, -1)$, then $\mathrm{E}\left(\mathbf{w}^T\mathbf{r} \,\middle|\, \mathbf{x}\right)$ is a main effect of treatment Z, $\mathbf{w} = (1, -1, 1, -1)$ refers to a main effect of Z', and $\mathbf{w} = (1, -1, -1, 1)$ refers to an interaction of Z and Z', or equivalently to a difference-in-differences, specifically the difference in the effect of Z at the two levels of Z'.

If

$$0 < \zeta_{ab}(\mathbf{r}, \mathbf{x}) = e_{ab}(\mathbf{x}) < 1 \text{ for } a = 0,\ 1,\ b = 0,\ 1, \tag{14.1}$$

then reasoning analogous to Chap. 4 shows [15,38]

$$\mathbf{r} \perp\!\!\!\perp (Z, Z') \mid \mathbf{x}$$

and

$$\mathrm{E}\left(\mathbf{w}^T\mathbf{r}\,\middle|\,\mathbf{x}\right) = \sum_{a=0}^{1}\sum_{b=0}^{1}\mathrm{E}\left(w_{ab}\,r_{ab}\mid\mathbf{x}\right) = \sum_{a=0}^{1}\sum_{b=0}^{1} w_{ab}\,\mathrm{E}\left(r_{ab}\mid Z=a,\ Z'=b,\ \mathbf{x}\right),$$

where $\mathrm{E}\left(r_{ab}\mid Z=a,\ Z'=b,\ \mathbf{x}\right)$ is a regression involving observable quantities, namely, the regression of r_{ab} on $\mathbf{x}$ in the subpopulation with $(Z=a,\ Z'=b)$. Stated concisely, if treatment assignment is ignorable given $\mathbf{x}$ in the sense of (14.1), with the principal unobserved covariate $\zeta_{ab}(\mathbf{r}, \mathbf{x})$ equal to the propensity score $e_{ab}(\mathbf{x})$, then any comparison among treatments $\mathrm{E}\left(\mathbf{w}^T\mathbf{r}\,\middle|\,\mathbf{x}\right)$ is estimable.

Differential Effects Immune to Generic Unmeasured Biases

A slightly less familiar comparison is $\mathbf{w} = (0, 1, -1, 0)$ or $\mathbf{w}^T\mathbf{r} = r_{10} - r_{01}$; it is the differential effect of giving treatment Z in lieu of giving treatment Z', or the effect of $(Z=1,\ Z'=0)$ instead of $(Z=0,\ Z'=1)$. The differential effect may or may not be an interesting effect; that depends upon the two treatments and the context. The differential effect is often of interest in clinical medicine. For instance, we may be interested in whether surgical technique A leads to faster recovery than technique B, in a context in which the patient clearly needs surgery, and applying both techniques A and B is conceptually possible but surgically absurd. The same issue often arises when studying the intended effects or unintended side effects of two drugs [10, 40], and in various other contexts [33, Ch. 12].

In observational studies, the differential effect has a curious, and often useful, property. The differential effect, $\mathrm{E}\left(\mathbf{w}^T\mathbf{r}\,\middle|\,\mathbf{x}\right)$ with $\mathbf{w} = (0, 1, -1, 0)$, is identified and estimable under certain conditions in which treatment assignment is affected by unmeasured biases, so that ignorability given $\mathbf{x}$ in (14.1) is false. This happens when unmeasured covariates promote treatment Z, and they also promote treatment Z', but only measured covariates favor treatment Z over Z'. In the previous paragraph, whether or not a patient is judged to need surgery may be biased by unmeasured covariates, but given that a patient does need surgery, the choice between technique A and technique B may not be biased by unmeasured covariates.

If $\{\zeta_{11}(\mathbf{r}, \mathbf{x}),\ \zeta_{10}(\mathbf{r}, \mathbf{x}),\ \zeta_{01}(\mathbf{r}, \mathbf{x}),\ \zeta_{00}(\mathbf{r}, \mathbf{x})\}$ depends on $\mathbf{r}$, then (14.1) is false; however, in the sense of Definition 14.1, the unmeasured biases may be generic [29, Def. 1].

Definition 14.1 There are only generic unmeasured biases if the ratio $\psi(\mathbf{r}, \mathbf{x}) = \zeta_{10}(\mathbf{r}, \mathbf{x}) / \zeta_{01}(\mathbf{r}, \mathbf{x})$ does not depend upon $\mathbf{r}$ and $0 < \psi(\mathbf{r}, \mathbf{x}) < \infty$. When there are only generic unmeasured biases, write $\psi^{\dagger}(\mathbf{x})$ for $\psi(\mathbf{r}, \mathbf{x})$.

Definition 14.1 holds, yet (14.1) is false, under a variety of familiar models for treatment assignment $(Z,\ Z')$. These models describe the conditional distribution of $(Z,\ Z')$ given either $(\mathbf{x}, \mathbf{r})$ or $(\mathbf{x}, u)$ for an unobserved covariate u, and the model may change in any way at all as $\mathbf{x}$ changes, but the model has a specific structure as

$\mathbf{r}$ or u changes with $\mathbf{x}$ fixed. The models include a Rasch model [25, 26] for (Z, Z') given an unmeasured covariate u; certain preference-tree models for hierarchical choice among the four possible values, $(0, 0)$, $(0, 1)$, $(1, 0)$, and $(1, 1)$ of (Z, Z') [44]; and certain symmetric multinomial logit models [29, §3.3].

There is a key fact about generic unmeasured biases: they do not bias differential comparisons of receiving treatment Z in lieu of treatment Z'. A person is in the differential comparison if and only if $Z + Z' = 1$, so that $(Z, Z') = (1, 0)$ or $(Z, Z') = (0, 1)$. Then, for the differential comparison,

$$\Pr(Z = 1, Z' = 0 \mid Z + Z' = 1, \mathbf{r}, \mathbf{x})$$
$$= \frac{\Pr(Z = 1, Z' = 0 \mid \mathbf{r}, \mathbf{x})}{\Pr(Z = 1, Z' = 0 \mid \mathbf{r}, \mathbf{x}) + \Pr(Z = 0, Z' = 1 \mid \mathbf{r}, \mathbf{x})}$$
$$= \frac{\zeta_{10}(\mathbf{r}, \mathbf{x})}{\zeta_{10}(\mathbf{r}, \mathbf{x}) + \zeta_{01}(\mathbf{r}, \mathbf{x})} = \frac{\psi(\mathbf{r}, \mathbf{x})}{\psi(\mathbf{r}, \mathbf{x}) + 1}; \tag{14.2}$$

so, $\Pr(Z = 1, Z' = 0 \mid Z + Z' = 1, \mathbf{r}, \mathbf{x}) = \psi^{\dagger}(\mathbf{x}) / \{\psi^{\dagger}(\mathbf{x}) + 1\}$ does not depend upon $\mathbf{r}$ if there are only generic unmeasured biases, even if $\zeta_{10}(\mathbf{r}, \mathbf{x})$ and $\zeta_{01}(\mathbf{r}, \mathbf{x})$ do depend upon $\mathbf{r}$. Consequently, the differential comparison of $(Z, Z') = (1, 0)$ or $(Z, Z') = (0, 1)$ is ignorable given $\mathbf{x}$ whenever there are only generic unmeasured biases, and $\psi^{\dagger}(\mathbf{x}) / \{\psi^{\dagger}(\mathbf{x}) + 1\}$ is its propensity score.

Of course, there may be differential unmeasured biases, not just generic unmeasured biases, so that $\psi(\mathbf{r}, \mathbf{x})$ does depend upon $\mathbf{r}$. Then $\psi(\mathbf{r}, \mathbf{x}) / \{\psi(\mathbf{r}, \mathbf{x}) + 1\}$ is what is left of $\zeta(\mathbf{r}, \mathbf{x})$ having removed the generic component by restricting attention to individuals with $Z + Z' = 1$. Once the generic biases are removed by focusing on the differential comparison, the sensitivity analysis in Chap. 8 applies to the differential comparison and refers to any differential biases that may remain [29, §3.4].

A Tightened Block Design for a Differential Comparison

Consider a tightened design that examines the differential effect of light daily alcohol consumption ($Z = 1$, $Z' = 0$) in lieu of visiting the dentist in the last year ($Z = 0$, $Z' = 1$). This comparison does not adjust for going to the dentist, Z'; rather, it overadjusts for Z'. The comparison discards people who take two possibly health-promoting steps, ($Z = 1$, $Z' = 1$) or $Z + Z' = 2$, and also people who take none, ($Z = 0$, $Z' = 0$) or $Z + Z' = 0$, to focus on ambivalent people who take one step but not the other, $Z + Z' = 1$.

The differential comparison is immune to a generic bias, in the sense of Definition 14.1, that promotes both Z and Z'. If visits to the dentist do not cause an increase in HDL cholesterol, then we would expect the differential effect to tell us about the effect of light daily alcohol consumption, with the generic bias removed. Conversely, if going to the dentist seems as, or more, effective than daily alcohol for

Table 14.2 Relationship between light daily alcohol consumption and dental visits in the past year for the $I \times J = 406 \times 4 = 1624$ individuals in the study of HDL cholesterol. The odds ratio in this table is 1.72 and it differs significantly from 1 in Fisher's exact test with P-value 5.8×10^{-6}. There are 133 light daily drinkers who might be included in the differential comparison

	Dental visit	No dental visit	Total
Daily alcohol	273	133	406
Control	663	555	1218
Total	936	688	1624

raising HDL cholesterol, you would be left wondering whether alcohol is correctly labeled as the lifestyle component that actually causes a change in HDL cholesterol.[2]

Table 14.2 describes the relationship between Z and Z' among the $I \times J = 406 \times 4 = 1624$ individuals in Sect. 1.4. Notably, daily alcohol and visiting the dentist are positively associated, and there are 133 daily drinkers with $(Z = 1,\ Z' = 0)$ who might be used in a differential comparison. Of these 133 daily drinkers, 118 are in the same block with at least one control who did visit the dentist; so, at most 118 differential matched pairs can be obtained. In 53 of the 118 blocks, there is only one control who visited the dentist; in 51 blocks, there are two eligible controls, and in 14 blocks there are three eligible controls. From the 118 eligible blocks, the goal is to extract as many $(Z = 1,\ Z' = 0)$-versus-$(Z = 0,\ Z' = 1)$ pairs as possible while maintaining covariate balance. The maximum number of pairs is 118, but an option is to improve within-pair covariate distance and covariate balance using fewer than 118 pairs, selected by optimal subset matching [20, 30, 36].

Table 14.3 compares three matched samples, M1, M2, and M3, in terms of balance for education. The balance is slightly off in M1 which uses all 118 eligible blocks, particularly for "Less Than 9th Grade Education" and in the opposite direction for "Some College." The balance is perfect in M3 which uses 105 blocks. Match M2 is an attractive compromise with 112 blocks: the balance is almost perfect at the cost of 6 blocks, rather than 13 blocks for M3. Figure 14.6 depicts the balance for age and education in match M2, where in addition both groups are 26.8% female. Match M2 has balanced (or rebalanced) covariates, but M2 differs from the $IJ = 1624$ people in the untightened block design in Sect. 1.4; for instance, in Sect. 1.4, each group was 33.7% female, not 26.8% female.

In the differential comparison, Fig. 14.7 examines two outcomes, the primary outcome, HDL cholesterol, and also BMI which was briefly considered in Sect. 14.2. Evidently, adjustment for a generic bias that promotes both daily drinking and dental visits does not greatly alter earlier analyses: the differential effect of daily drinking in lieu of visiting the dentist is almost as large as the main effect in the primary analysis.

---

[2] It is not inconceivable that dental health and cardiovascular health are connected in ways besides a disposition to engage in activities imagined to promote good health [17]. Nonetheless, the differential comparison is still of interest. If it were true that dental visits cause an increase in HDL cholesterol and so does light daily alcohol consumption, so that the differential effect was zero, then that would argue for visiting the dentist, because dental visits also benefit teeth and are not carcinogenic.

Table 14.3 Balance for education in three differential matched samples, where M1 uses all 118 possible blocks, M2 uses 112 better balanced blocks, and M3 uses 105 perfectly balanced blocks

	< 9th	9th–11th	High school	Some college	BA+	Total
M1: alcohol/no dentist	4	12	30	42	30	118
M1: no alcohol/dentist	9	12	31	37	29	118
M2: alcohol/no dentist	4	10	30	38	30	112
M2: no alcohol/dentist	6	10	30	37	29	112
M3: alcohol/no dentist	4	8	28	36	29	105
M3: no alcohol/dentist	4	8	28	36	29	105

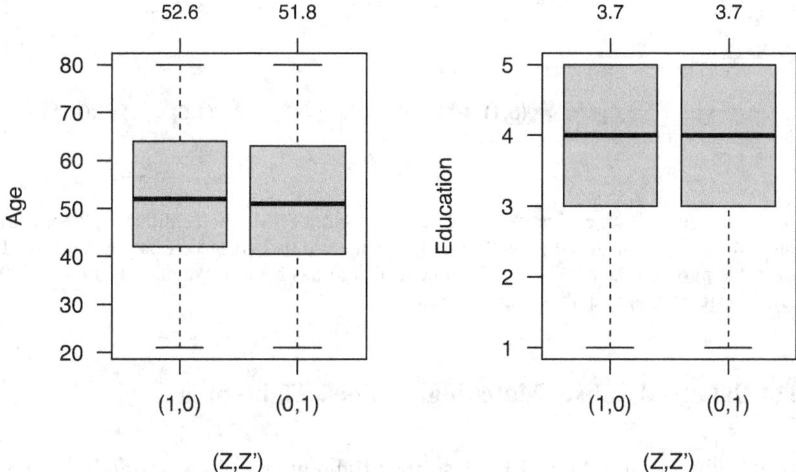

Fig. 14.6 Balance for age and education in differential match M2 with 112 matched pairs. In addition, both groups are 26.8% female. Here, (1,0) denotes a daily drinker who has not visited the dentist in the past year, and (0,1) denotes a control who has been to the dentist in the past year. Covariate means appear above the boxplots

A randomization inference for HDL cholesterol in Fig. 14.7 using U868 yields an estimated differential effect of 10.5, with 95% confidence interval [6, 15], and one-sided P-value testing no effect of 1.02×10^{-7}. At $\Gamma = 3$, the P-value bound is 0.047.[3] The differential comparison removes generic biases in the sense of Definition 14.1, and rejection of the hypothesis of no differential effect is insensitive to differential biases no larger than $\Gamma = 3$.

[3] Replication of the match is done in the example for the documentation for the `tighten` function in the `tightenBlock` package in R. The analyses use the `weightedRank` package and are given in a replication file [36, Online appendix]. The sensitivity analysis in Chap. 8 may be applied directly to the differential comparison and refers to any differential biases that remain now that generic biases have been removed [29, §3.4].

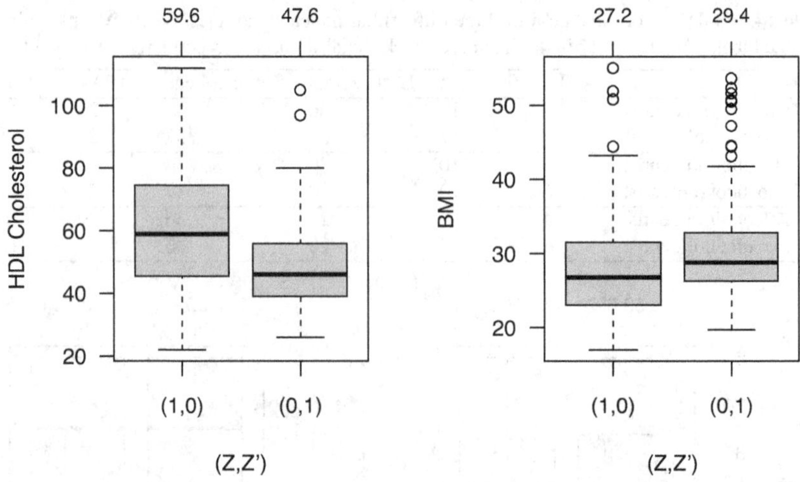

Fig. 14.7 Outcomes HDL cholesterol and body mass index (BMI) in the differential comparison in match M2 with 112 matched pairs. Here, (1,0) denotes a daily drinker who has not visited the dentist in the past year, and (0,1) denotes a control who has been to the dentist in the past year. Huber's M-estimates appear above each boxplot

Use of Balanced Subset Matching in Block Tightening

The final subsection of Sect. 14.2 described tightening a block design by removing some controls from each block. In the current section, this activity was combined with the optimal removal of 6 blocks to produce 112 pairs in match M2. Removing a block reduces the number of treated individuals, but no treated individual was removed when reducing the number of controls in each block from 3 to 2 in Sect. 14.2. For this reason, removing blocks would typically be considered only when constructing matched pairs; so, the discussion will focus on this case. For pairs, edges of the form (S, t_i) and $(\overline{t}_i, s)$ have capacity one and cost zero.

One approach specifies the desired number of pairs, say 112 pairs of the 118 possible pairs. In this case, in Fig. 14.5, the flow supplied by the source S and the flow absorbed by the sink s are both set to the desired number of pairs, here 112 pairs.

An alternative approach specifies a criterion for removing blocks and lets the algorithm decide how many pairs to remove [30, §2.2]. In this case, S supplies 118 units of flow and s absorbs 118 units of flow, but some units of flow bypass the controls. Suppose that we want to remove a block only if its inclusion would increase the average cost per used block by more than $\lambda > 0$. Then add to Fig. 14.5 the dashed bypass edges in Fig. 14.8 that connect t_i directly to $\overline{t}_i$ with capacity one and cost λ. If the minimum cost flow sends a unit of flow along a bypass edge, then that block is

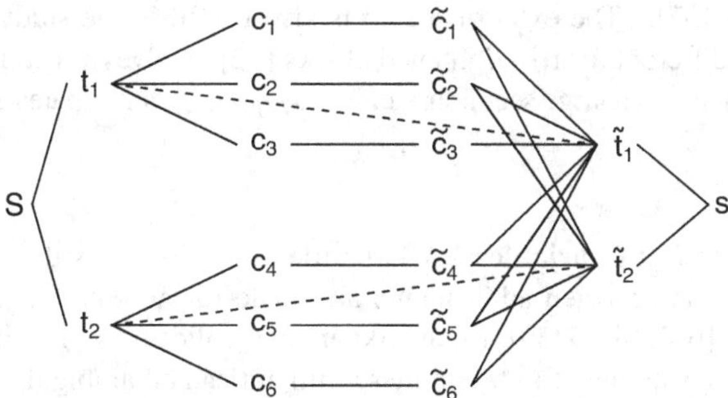

Fig. 14.8 A network for optimal tightening of an existing $K \times J$ block design into pairs with the possible removal of some of the K blocks, where $K = 118$ in Table 14.3. This figure resembles Fig. 14.5, except there are now dashed bypass edges with capacity one for use in optimal subset matching [30]. If the minimum cost flow sends flow along a bypass edge, then that block is removed. To form matched pairs, K units of flow leave the source, S, and are absorbed by the sink, s, and each edge involving the source or the sink has capacity to carry one unit of flow. Decreasing the cost of the bypass edges will result in fewer pairs that are closer and better balanced

removed, on the grounds that including it would increase the average cost per block used by more than λ.[4]

14.4 *Further Reading

Tightened blocks: Tightened blocks are one transparent way, but not the only way, to implement a complementary analysis. A recent article discusses optimization of tightened blocks [36]. A different strategy first builds a block design for a primary analysis and then tacks on an additional comparison group to existing blocks that are used only in complementary analyses; see Samuel Pimentel and colleagues [24, §5.3]. By tacking on a control group to an existing design, the tacked-on controls have a slightly unnatural aspect: they are selected from controls previously rejected for the primary analysis. Pimentel et al. make the case that these rejected controls can provide some useful complementary analyses. Shoshana Daniel and colleagues [7] form two control groups with different properties by optimally splitting a single control population. Yet another approach uses naturally occurring but overlapping control groups—i.e., one person may be in two control groups—eliminating the overlap when comparing control groups—as in Fig. 14.3—using a device called the

[4] One could consider every possible number of pairs, say 118 pairs, 117 pairs, and so on. One could instead consider every possible $\lambda > 0$. In either case, one would produce the same set of Pareto optimal matched designs—that is, designs whose average cost per used pair can only be lowered by reducing the number of used pairs. The two approaches are different ways of exploring the Pareto optimal designs.

exterior match [37].[5] The exterior match is also useful in the study of disparities [37,41–43]. A different form of tightened blocks [32] involves a secondary outcome, (s_{Tij}, s_{Cij}), such that a large secondary effect, $s_{Tij} - s_{Cij}$, anticipates a large primary effect, $r_{Tij} - r_{Cij}$.

Affected concomitant variables: A large literature discusses the difficulties and ambiguities that arise when adjustments are made for an outcome as if it were a covariate; e.g., [6, 8, 14, 27, 39]. Bijan Niknam and colleagues [18] dissect a particularly egregious example. Too often, these difficulties and ambiguities are resolved simply by assuming they are absent. Opposed to this, complementary analyses at least allow the data to speak to the issue.

Generic biases: Differential effects and generic biases are discussed in several articles [29,31]. A book chapter offers motivation and numerous examples [33, Ch. 12].

Isolation: When treatments are received at various times, the timing of treatment may be biased by unmeasured covariates, while only generic biases affect the specific treatment received at that time. For instance, a mother may carefully decide the number and timing of the births of her children, but whether she has a single child or twins may be little more than luck [1]. Similarly, certain brands of cars are known for their safety, others for their acceleration, so that the physical safety of the vehicle may be confounded with the manner in which it is driven; however, all of this matters less conditionally given that two vehicles have in fact collided [55]. Study designs that exploit these situations are said to employ "isolation," meaning differential effects in a risk-set match [54, 55].

Problems

14.1 Reproduce a Block Tightening

Use the example in the documentation for the function `tighten` in the `tightenBlock` package in R to reproduce the 406×3 tightened block design in Sect. 14.3.

14.2 Reproduce Another Block Tightening

Use the example in the documentation for the function `tighten` in the `tightenBlock` package in R to reproduce the three matched pairs designs in Table 14.3 of Sect. 14.2.

14.3 The Need for an Exterior Match

The exterior match [37] was mentioned in the Further Reading section. It is used, for example, in disparities research [37, 41–43], but it could also be used to create two matched control groups, one matched for a possibly affected outcome like BMI

[5] Implemented in R package `exteriorMatch`

and the other not matched for BMI. There are many related applications in which you match for more or different covariates in one control group than in another. An important decision is whether or not to allow the two control groups to overlap. There are two issues: (i) if you do not allow overlap, you may not have enough controls to balance covariates, and (ii) if you do not allow overlap, you may distort the second control group because of the controls you removed in forming the first control group. This problem looks at the simplest aspect of the problem of overlap. The exterior match [37] is used in inference when two control groups are allowed to overlap.
(i) Suppose that a treated group contains 50 women and 200 men. Suppose that the available controls consist of 75 women and 600 men. You want to create two control groups, each pair-matched to the treated group with the maximum number of pairs matched exactly for sex. The first control group will be matched for sex but not for BMI, while the second control group will be matched for both sex and BMI, say for BMI < 30 versus BMI ≥ 30. You create the first pair-matched control group and then try to create the second pair-matched control group using the controls who were not matched in forming the first pair-matched control group. What will the distribution of sex be in the first matched control group? What will the distribution of sex be in the second matched control group?
(ii) Instead, suppose you match the two control groups separately. In this case, can both control groups perfectly balance sex? Will the control groups overlap? Overlap means that at least one control is in both control groups.
(iii) So far, we have not discussed BMI. Suppose BMIs tend to be lower in the treated group than among available controls. If you forbid overlap, does it matter whether you match first for sex in group 1 and then for sex and BMI in group 2, or instead reverse the order and match first for sex and BMI and later for sex alone? If you match first for sex and BMI, which BMIs will disproportionately be removed in forming the first control group, and what is the consequence for a second control group built from the remaining unmatched controls? If overlap is permitted, does it make any difference which control group is matched first? If the control groups are defined a priori so they do not overlap, as in Sects. 1.4 and 1.5, does it make any difference which control group is matched first?
(iv) Issues of the kind in this problem seem to be absent when regression is used instead of matching to adjust for covariates. In fact, the problem is present but hidden from view. Ambarish Chattopadhyay and José Zubizarreta [5] show that a covariance adjustment model creates an implied control group via an implicit weighting of controls: change the model or its covariates and you change the implied control group. Read their article to gain more insight into this topic. Consider the possibility that the weighting of controls should be explicit, transparent and sensible, rather than implicit and automatic.

14.4 Structure of the Exterior Match

This problem uses elementary (undirected) graph theory, and it is therefore **optional**.[6] The problem introduces the structure of the exterior match [37]. Suppose that you

[6] The networks in matching, like Fig. 14.5, are directed graphs: edges are ordered pairs of nodes and flow can only move from the first node to the second node. In an undirected graph, an edge is

have pair-matched two control groups to one treated group, but you have permitted the two control groups to overlap, as in Problem 14.3. To emphasize, if Harry is a potential control, then possibly: (a) Harry is picked for neither control group, or (b) Harry is picked for the first control group but not the second, or (c) Harry is picked for the second control group but not the first, or (d) Harry is picked for both control groups. Harry appears at most once in each control group, and in case (d) he is part of the overlap and appears once in both control groups. Before we can use statistical methods to ask whether the two control groups differ from each other in terms of outcomes, we had better remove Harry if he is in both control groups, because Harry is not likely to differ significantly from Harry. If you are matching for different covariates in the two control groups and if Harry is duplicated, then it is quite possible that he will be matched to different treated individuals when he appears in the two control groups. For example, think about matching for sex alone in one control group and for sex plus two BMI categories in the other control group. **(i)** Create a bipartite graph connecting the two control groups, as follows. On the left, list the controls in the first control group as nodes. On the right, list the controls in the second control group as nodes. Two nodes are connected by an edge if they are in different control groups but are matched to the same treated person; also, two nodes are connected if they are in different control groups but represent the same person. If Harry and Sally are matched to the same treated person, then an edge connects Harry and Sally. If Harry appears in both control groups, then his two appearances are connected. The degree of a node is the number of edges that touch that node. What are the possible degrees of the nodes in this bipartite graph? What does the degree of a node tell you about duplication?
(ii) Two nodes of a graph are connected if one can move from one node to the other along a sequence of edges. Show that "being connected" is an equivalence relation on the nodes of a graph. (The equivalence classes are called "connected components.")
(iii) Use your answer to part (i) to show that every connected component of this bipartite graph is either of the following form: (a) $n_1 - n_2 - \cdots - n_{L-1} - n_L$ where the n_ℓ are L distinct nodes connected by an edge or (b) a cycle $n_1 - n_2 - \cdots - n_{L-1} - n_1$ where the n_ℓ are $L - 1$ distinct nodes, and the first and last nodes are the same. In case (b), show that all of the nodes represent duplicated controls who appear in both control groups. In case (a), show that only n_1 and n_L are not duplicated. In case (a), n_1 and n_L are called exterior nodes, and case (b) has no exterior nodes.
(iv) The exterior match removes all the duplicates by retaining only the exterior nodes. In doing this, it breaks up some existing pairs in connected components of type (a). (Connected components of type (b) disappear entirely.) For example, if $L > 2$, show that in connected component $n_1 - n_2 - \cdots - n_{L-1} - n_L$ of type (a), the pair $n_1 - n_2$ were distinct controls in different control groups matched to the same treated person, but that pair was broken when only exterior nodes were retained. The same is true of $n_{L-1} - n_L$.
(v) To fix the broken pairs, the exterior match "re-pairs" as follows: if $L > 2$, then connected component $n_1 - n_2 - \cdots - n_{L-1} - n_L$ of type (a) becomes a pair $n_1 - n_L$

a set of two distinct nodes, and there is no direction to an edge. You can move along an undirected edge in either direction.

of unduplicated individuals. Show that if both control groups were exactly matched for sex, then the new pair $n_1 - n_L$ is exactly matched for sex.
(vi) Consider the two control groups produced by the exterior match as groups, ignoring who is matched to whom. If sex is perfectly balanced but not exactly matched—if both control groups are 37% female, but females are not always matched to females—then we may ask whether sex is also balanced in the exterior match. Is it? (Hint: If Harry is duplicated and we remove him from both control groups, do we thereby introduce an imbalance in sex?)
Remark: We do not remove duplicates when comparing the treated group to each control group separately. We remove duplicates to avoid tautologies only when comparing two control groups that overlap [37]. Obviously, if the two control groups contain exactly the same people, then the exterior match removes everyone, and that informs us that the two control groups do not differ: whatever we did—say, add control for BMI—to produce two control groups did not do anything, because the same control groups were selected. Whatever difference there is between the two control groups comes from the unduplicated parts of the control groups, and we can use statistical methods to compare the unduplicated parts. Expressed differently: do not do a t-test to see if Harry differs from Harry. A priori knowledge is not common in statistics, but that Harry does not differ from Harry is as good as it gets.

References

1. Angrist, J.D., Evans, W.: Children and their parents' labor supply: Evidence from exogenous variation in family size. Am. Econ. Rev. **88**(3), 450–77 (1998)
2. Bitterman, M.E.: Phyletic differences in learning. Am. Psychol. **20**(6), 396 (1965)
3. Campbell, D.T.: Prospective: Artifact and control. In: R. Rosenthal, R. Rosnow (eds.) Artifacts in Behavioral Research. Academic Press, New York (1969). Reprinted in Campbell 1988, pp. 167–190.
4. Campbell, D.T.: Methodology and Epistemology for Social Science: Selected Papers. University of Chicago Press, Chicago (1988)
5. Chattopadhyay, A., Zubizarreta, J.R.: On the implied weights of linear regression for causal inference. Biometrika **110**(3), 615–629 (2023)
6. Cochran, W.G.: Analysis of covariance: Its nature and uses. Biometrics **13**(3), 261–281 (1957)
7. Daniel, S.R., Armstrong, K., Silber, J.H., Rosenbaum, P.R.: An algorithm for optimal tapered matching, with application to disparities in survival. J. Comput. Graph. Stat. **17**(4), 914–924 (2008)
8. Frangakis, C.E., Rubin, D.B.: Principal stratification in causal inference. Biometrics **58**(1), 21–29 (2002)
9. Friedman, M.: The use of ranks to avoid the assumption of normality implicit in the analysis of variance. J. Am. Stat. Assoc. **32**(200), 675–701 (1937)
10. Gibbons, R.D., Amatya, A.K., Brown, C.H., Hur, K., Marcus, S.M., Bhaumik, D.K., Mann, J.J.: Post-approval drug safety surveillance. Annu. Rev. Public Health **31**(1), 419–437 (2010)
11. Hampshire, S.: Justice is Conflict. Princeton University Press, Princeton, NJ (2001)
12. Hill, J.O., Wyatt, H.R., Peters, J.C.: Energy balance and obesity. Circulation **126**(1), 126–132 (2012)
13. Holland, P.W., Rosenbaum, P.R.: Conditional association and unidimensionality in monotone latent variable models. Ann. Stat. **14**, 1523–1543 (1986)

14. Imai, K., Keele, L., Yamamoto, T.: Identification, inference and sensitivity analysis for causal mediation effects. Stat. Sci. **25**, 51–71 (2010)
15. Imai, K., Van Dyk, D.A.: Causal inference with general treatment regimes: Generalizing the propensity score. J. Am. Stat. Assoc. **99**(467), 854–866 (2004)
16. Kleiner, K.D., Gold, M.S., Frostpineda, K., Lenzbrunsman, B., Perri, M.G., Jacobs, W.S.: Body mass index and alcohol use. J. Addict. Dis. **23**(3), 105–118 (2004)
17. Mattila, K.J., Pussinen, P.J., Paju, S.: Dental infections and cardiovascular diseases: A review. J. Periodontol. **76**, 2085–2088 (2005)
18. Niknam, B.A., Arriaga, A.F., Rosenbaum, P.R., Hill, A.S., Ross, R.N., Even-Shoshan, O., Romano, P.S., Silber, J.H.: Adjustment for atherosclerosis diagnosis distorts the effects of percutaneous coronary intervention and the ranking of hospital performance. J. Am. Heart Assoc. **7**(11), e008366 (2018)
19. Niknam, B.A., Zubizarreta, J.R.: Using cardinality matching to design balanced and representative samples for observational studies. J. Am. Med. Assoc. **327**(2), 173–174 (2022)
20. Pimentel, S.D.: Large, sparse optimal matching with R package rcbalance. Observat. Stud. **2**(1), 4–23 (2016)
21. Pimentel, S.D.: Fine balance and its variations in modern optimal matching. In: J.R. Zubizarreta, E.A. Stuart, D.S. Small, P.R. Rosenbaum (eds.) Handbook of Matching and Weighting Adjustments for Causal Inference, pp. 105–134. Chapman and Hall/CRC, Boca Raton, FL (2023)
22. Pimentel, S.D., Kelz, R.R.: Optimal tradeoffs in matched designs comparing US-trained and internationally-trained surgeons. J. Am. Stat. Assoc. **115**(532), 1675–1688 (2020)
23. Pimentel, S.D., Kelz, R.R., Silber, J.H., Rosenbaum, P.R.: Large, sparse optimal matching with refined covariate balance in an observational study of the health outcomes produced by new surgeons. J. Am. Stat. Assoc. **110**(510), 515–527 (2015)
24. Pimentel, S.D., Small, D.S., Rosenbaum, P.R.: Constructed second control groups and attenuation of unmeasured biases. J. Am. Stat. Assoc. **111**(515), 1157–1167 (2016)
25. Rasch, G.: An item analysis which takes individual differences into account. Br. J. Math. Stat. Psychol. **19**(1), 49–57 (1966)
26. Rasch, G.: Probabilistic Models for Some Intelligence and Attainment Tests. University of Chicago Press, Chicago (1980)
27. Rosenbaum, P.R.: The consequences of adjustment for a concomitant variable that has been affected by the treatment. J. Roy. Stat. Soc. A **147**(5), 656–666 (1984)
28. Rosenbaum, P.R.: The role of a second control group in an observational study. Stat. Sci. **2**(3), 292–306 (1987)
29. Rosenbaum, P.R.: Differential effects and generic biases in observational studies. Biometrika **93**(3), 573–586 (2006)
30. Rosenbaum, P.R.: Optimal matching of an optimally chosen subset in observational studies. J. Comput. Graph. Stat. **21**(1), 57–71 (2012)
31. Rosenbaum, P.R.: Using differential comparisons in observational studies. Chance **26**(3), 18–25 (2013)
32. Rosenbaum, P.R.: Some counterclaims undermine themselves in observational studies. J. Am. Stat. Assoc. **110**(512), 1389–1398 (2015)
33. Rosenbaum, P.R.: Observation and Experiment: An Introduction to Causal Inference. Harvard University Press, Cambridge, MA (2017)
34. Rosenbaum, P.R.: Design of Observational Studies, 2nd edn. Springer, New York (2020)
35. Rosenbaum, P.R.: Modern algorithms for matching in observational studies. Annu. Rev. Stat. Appl. **7**, 143–176 (2020)
36. Rosenbaum, P.R.: Tightening blocks in complementary analyses of observational studies: Optimization algorithm and examples. Am. Stat. **79**, 1–9 (2025)
37. Rosenbaum, P.R., Silber, J.H.: Using the exterior match to compare two entwined matched control groups. Am. Stat. **67**(2), 67–75 (2013)
38. Rosenbaum, P.R., Zubizarreta, J.R.: Effect aliasing in observational studies. Manuscript (2024)
39. Rubin, D.B.: Direct and indirect causal effects via potential outcomes. Scand. J. Stat. **31**(2), 161–170 (2004)

40. Schneeweiss, S., Gagne, J., Glynn, R., Ruhl, M., Rassen, J.: Assessing the comparative effectiveness of newly marketed medications: methodological challenges and implications for drug development. Clin. Pharmacol. Therapeut. **90**(6), 777–790 (2011)
41. Silber, J.H., Rosenbaum, P.R., Clark, A.S., Giantonio, B.J., Ross, R.N., Teng, Y., Wang, M., Niknam, B.A., Ludwig, J.M., Wang, W., Fox, K.R.: Characteristics associated with differences in survival among black and white women with breast cancer. J. Am. Med. Assoc. **310**(4), 389–397 (2013)
42. Silber, J.H., Rosenbaum, P.R., Ross, R.N., Niknam, B.A., Ludwig, J.M., Wang, W., Clark, A.S., Fox, K.R., Wang, M., Even-Shoshan, O., Giantonio, B.J.: Racial disparities in colon cancer survival: a matched cohort study. Anna. Internal Med. **161**(12), 845–854 (2014)
43. Silber, J.H., Rosenbaum, P.R., Ross, R.N., Reiter, J.G., Niknam, B.A., Hill, A.S., Bongiorno, D.M., Shah, S.A., Hochman, L.L., Even-Shoshan, O., Fox, K.R.: Disparities in breast cancer survival by socioeconomic status despite Medicare and Medicaid insurance. Milbank Quart. **96**(4), 706–754 (2018)
44. Tversky, A., Sattath, S.: Preference trees. Psychol. Rev. **86**, 542–573 (1979)
45. US Centers for Disease Control: Session 7: Tip the calorie balance. https://www.cdc.gov/diabetes/prevention/pdf/ handout-session7.pdf, (Accessed 1 November 2023)
46. US Department of Agriculture: Fooddata Central: Alcoholic beverage, wine, table, red (2019). Https://fdc.nal.usda.gov/fdc-app.html#/food-details/173190/nutrients (Accessed 1 August 2024).
47. Wang, L., Lee, I.M., Manson, J.E., Buring, J.E., Sesso, H.D.: Alcohol consumption, weight gain, and risk of becoming overweight in middle-aged and older women. Arch. Internal Med. **170**(5), 453–461 (2010)
48. Wannamethee, S.G., Shaper, A.G.: Alcohol, body weight, and weight gain in middle-aged men. Am. J. Clin. Nutrit. **77**(5), 1312–1317 (2003)
49. Weiss, N.S.: Can the "specificity" of an association be rehabilitated as a basis for supporting a causal hypothesis? Epidemiology **13**(1), 6–8 (2002)
50. Willett, W., Skerrett, P.J., Giovannucci, E.L.: Eat, Drink, and Be Healthy: The Harvard Medical School Guide to Healthy Eating. Simon and Schuster, New York (2017)
51. Zhang, B., Small, D.S., Lasater, K.B., McHugh, M., Silber, J.H., Rosenbaum, P.R.: Matching one sample according to two criteria in observational studies. J. Am. Stat. Assoc. **118**, 1140–1151 (2022)
52. Zubizarreta, J.R.: Using mixed integer programming for matching in an observational study of kidney failure after surgery. J. Am. Stat. Assoc. **107**(500), 1360–1371 (2012)
53. Zubizarreta, J.R., Reinke, C.E., Kelz, R.R., Silber, J.H., Rosenbaum, P.R.: Matching for several sparse nominal variables in a case-control study of readmission following surgery. Am. Stat. **65**(4), 229–238 (2011)
54. Zubizarreta, J.R., Small, D.S., Rosenbaum, P.R.: Isolation in the construction of natural experiments. Ann. Appl. Stat. **8**, 2096–2121 (2014)
55. Zubizarreta, J.R., Small, D.S., Rosenbaum, P.R.: A simple example of isolation in building a natural experiment. Chance **31**(4), 16–23 (2018)

Chapter 15
A Look Back Along the Path Taken

Abstract This chapter takes a quick look backwards along the path we have taken in this introduction to the theory of observational studies.

15.1 Randomized Experiments as a Leading Case

Chapter 1 proposed randomized experiments as a "leading case" of causal inference, not a "gold standard" for causal inference. As noted previously, the *Oxford English Dictionary* defines a leading case as follows:

> **leading case**: n. *Law*. A case that has settled some important point and is frequently cited as a precedent.

What "important points" are settled by the theory and practice of randomized experimentation? In what sense is it a precedent, but not a standard? Chapter 2 offered answers.

Anything that exists is possible. What is, is possible. Flying is possible because birds do it, and that ends discussion about whether flying is possible. Causal inference is possible without identifying assumptions because causal inference is possible in randomized experiments without identifying assumptions.[1] This book has been a conversation about what is possible in observational studies, where causal inference is more difficult.

Randomization solves one problem, not all problems. Causal inference in randomized experiments is limited in various ways, and commonly observational studies are limited in parallel ways. Randomized experiments warrant causal inferences about the effects caused by a treatment on the finite population of individuals included

[1] You still sometimes hear that causal inference in randomized experiments depends upon assumptions such as "no interference between units" but that is simply untrue [8, 16]. Interference introduces complexity, not barriers.

© The Author(s), under exclusive license to Springer Nature Switzerland AG 2025
P. R. Rosenbaum, *An Introduction to the Theory of Observational Studies*,
Springer Texts in Statistics, https://doi.org/10.1007/978-3-031-90494-3_15

in the experiment. Donald Campbell [3] called this "internal validity," saying randomization conferred internal validity but not "external validity," not an ability to infer causal effects on other populations. If there is a warranted inference to other populations, then its basis comes from something other than randomized treatment assignment. Even in randomized experiments, the causal effect on one individual, $\delta_{ij} = r_{Tij} - r_{Cij}$, is not identified—this is the central problem in causal inference.

Randomized experiments are not a "gold standard," because practical or ethical barriers prevent randomized treatment assignment in many important contexts in political economy, public health, epidemiology, public policy, and other fields. Topics are selected for empirical investigation based on their importance. No sane person would refuse to study an important problem in political economy or public health merely because a randomized experiment is impractical or unethical.

15.2 The Several Distinct Roles of Assumptions

Unlike the premises of a mathematical theorem, assumptions have a variety of roles in statistical inference. Recall Tukey's [30, p. 72] remarks on this subject, as quoted in Sect. 2.8.

The innocuous use of assumptions occurs when understanding and comparing the performance of competing statistical procedures. Procedures are sought that have good performance for several reasonable models. This was the goal in Chaps. 9–11, where methods and study designs were sought that could distinguish meaningful treatment effects from nontrivial biases in treatment assignment. This was also the goal in Sect. 3.2, where it was found that Fisher's randomization test of his hypothesis of no effect is also the *only* valid test of a much weaker or broader hypothesis asserting that treated and control individuals in the same block have the same distribution of responses. These uses of assumptions are innocuous precisely because they lead to conclusions about statistical procedures and their mathematical properties—which procedures are better procedures in mathematical situations—not conclusions about treatments and policies in the world we actually inhabit.

In contrast, assumptions that play a role in scientific conclusions require close scrutiny. It is here that a false assumption can lead to a false conclusion, and an unwarranted assumption can lead to an unwarranted conclusion. Michael Polanyi [13, p. 17] wrote:

> Only explicitly formulated knowledge can be thus derived from specifiable premises according to clear rules of inference. And it is the most important function of critical thought to test such explicit processes of inference, by rehearsing their chain of reasoning in search of some weak link.

To the extent that an assumption matters for scientific conclusions, its explicit statement picks that assumption out as a weak link in inference, a link demanding close scrutiny. Sensitivity analysis in Chap. 8 assesses the quantitative degree to which an assumption matters for an inference. Quasi-experimental devices, such as multiple control groups and known effects in Chaps. 12 and 13, shed light on whether an assumption is false and on what else might be true instead. All of this is possible only if there are few such assumptions to consider and only if the study design and analytical methods have avoided pointless complexity.

15.3 Multiple Working Hypotheses

Given two probability distributions, the Neyman-Pearson lemma [10, §3.2] characterizes the best or most powerful test. Erich Lehmann and Joseph Romano [10, p. 107] write:

> The first authors to recognize that the rational choice of a test must involve consideration not only of the hypothesis but also the alternatives against which it is being tested were Neyman and Pearson [12].

The Neyman-Pearson lemma has technical uses, but it is also a metaphor. First, it says: to closely scrutinize one hypothesis, you need one or more alternative hypotheses. Second, because the lemma directs attention to the likelihood ratio, it says: all of the information that distinguishes two hypotheses comes from events that are probable under one hypothesis and improbable under the other. The metaphorical use of the Neyman-Pearson lemma is related to Tukey's [30, p. 72] endorsement in Sect. 2.8 of Chamberlain's [4] use of "multiple working hypotheses" and is also related to the following comment of Paul Feyerabend [5, pp. 14-15]:

> You can be a good empiricist only if you are prepared to work with many alternative theories, rather than a single point of view and "experience" ... The *function* of such concrete alternatives is, however, this: They provide a means of criticizing the accepted theory ... Such a plurality allows for a much sharper criticism of accepted ideas ....

Chapters 9–13 contrasted an unfavorable situation with no treatment effect and a bias in treatment assignment to a favorable situation with a treatment effect and no bias in treatment assignment. As in the Neyman-Pearson lemma, this led in Figs. 8.1 and 13.4 to statistics that emphasize events that are probable in one situation and improbable in the other.

15.4 Propensity Scores and the Principal Unobserved Covariate

The dimensionality of the observed covariates $\mathbf{x}$ did not play a critical role in causal inference in randomized experiments in Chap. 2. In a randomized experiment, adjustment for $\mathbf{x}$ might increase precision or help in locating effect modification, but it is not essential for basic causal inferences. In contrast, adjustments for observed covariates $\mathbf{x}$ are typically needed in observational studies.

In Chap. 4 also, the dimensionality of observed and unobserved covariates $\mathbf{x}$ did not play a key role. In principle, bias due to observed covariates can be summarized and removed by adjusting for the scalar propensity score, $e(\mathbf{x}) = \Pr(Z = 1 \mid \mathbf{x})$, or the conditional probability of treatment given the observed covariates. Many low-dimensional summaries of $\mathbf{x}$ are balanced in treated and control groups in randomized experiments, and this is also true in observational studies when comparing groups with the same or similar propensity scores. As in randomized experiments, gains in efficiency or insights into effect modification may result from attention paid to aspects of $\mathbf{x}$ as well as $e(\mathbf{x})$, but the dimensionality of $\mathbf{x}$ is not key when removing bias due to $\mathbf{x}$ alone.

Alas, adjustments for measured covariates do not suffice for causal inference in observational studies, because the probability of treatment may also depend upon relevant unobserved covariates. The bias due to the observed and unobserved covariates is again captured by a scalar, albeit an unobserved scalar, namely, the principal unobserved covariate $\zeta = \zeta(\mathbf{x}, r_T, r_C) = \Pr(Z = 1 \mid \mathbf{x}, r_T, r_C)$. The principal unobserved covariate is not observed because (r_T, r_C) are not jointly observed. With some caveats discussed in Chap. 4, adjustments for $\mathbf{x}$ alone would suffice to estimate causal effects if the propensity score and the principal unobserved covariate were equal—i.e., if $e(\mathbf{x}) = \Pr(Z = 1 \mid \mathbf{x}) = \Pr(Z = 1 \mid \mathbf{x}, r_T, r_C) = \zeta$—and adjustments for ζ always suffice [22, 24]. However, the basic problem remains because we have no access to ζ—this is the central problem in observational studies.

15.5 Matching and Transparency

> No theory is kind to us that cheats us of seeing.
> Henry James [9]

> The most robust statistical technique is to look at the data.
> Colin Mallows [11]

Transparency means making evidence evident [21, Ch. 6]. Transparent evidence is open to view and available for public discussion and critical debate. Too many scientific articles report some private experience that its authors had with some private data.

In an observational study, little can be seen in data before adjustments are made for measured covariates, $\mathbf{x}$. Before that, under treatment and control, you could be comparing princes to paupers and infants to the elderly. If adjustments for $\mathbf{x}$ begin by fitting a model, then you end up looking at the model, not at the data.

In a balanced matched sample, it is possible to look directly at data adjusted for $\mathbf{x}$, to plot the data from various perspectives, to summarize its many aspects using simple descriptive statistics.

Matching is properly part of the design of the study and is completed before outcomes are examined [27, 28]; so, there is no concern that investigators shopped for a preferred conclusion among many possible models. Matching is assessed by examining, depicting and displaying the distribution of $\mathbf{x}$ before and after matching in treated and control groups. This depiction shows how matching altered the distribution of $\mathbf{x}$ in the control group, and it shows that the treated and control groups look comparable in terms of observed covariates **x** after matching; see the simple displays in Sects. 1.4 and 1.5 and the greater detail in Chap. 6. Depiction of the distribution of **x** also characterizes the population under study and cautions against extrapolation of conclusions to other populations with very different distributions of **x**. If, before matching, treated and control groups exhibit limited overlap for certain regions of **x**, then this will often be apparent when covariate balance is assessed; so, any needed redefinition of the study population takes place before outcomes are examined [6, 31].

Matching does not preclude additional model-based adjustments of matched samples [25, 26]; see Chap. 7. Still, if adding model-based adjustments to a competently matched comparison greatly alters the substantive conclusions, then we should examine that model and its origins with care.

Matching creates a comparison of people who look comparable in terms of measured covariates, **x**. Attention can then turn to the central problem in observational studies, namely, whether people who look comparable actually are comparable, given that treatments were not randomly assigned.

Transparency is compatible with confidentiality. A matched comparison can be open to view in many graphs and summary statistics without revealing anything about particular individuals.

A transparent investigation is open to critical discussion. Critical discussion may be, but is not always, of high quality [1]: sometimes it is self-serving, incompetent, pointlessly argumentative, or arrogant. If the study is transparent, its audience is in a good position to judge the study and its critics. If critical discussion identifies specific and genuine ambiguities or faults, then it may stimulate other investigations to address these ambiguities or faults. If critical discussion fails to identify specific and genuine ambiguities or faults, then a transparent study enjoys the implicit endorsement of having survived critical discussion largely unscathed. Ambiguities or faults are more likely to be discovered in a transparent study than in an obscure study; so, when ambiguities or faults are not identified, we have more reason to trust the conclusions of a transparent study than an obscure one.

15.6 Rubin's Picture of Confounding and Model Misspecification

Chapter 7 presented in Fig. 7.2 one of Donald Rubin's [25, 26] theoretical examples showing that it could be difficult, even with no treatment effect, to recognize misspecification of a covariance adjustment model when the distributions of **x** are different in treated and control groups. In this example, the linear model predicts treated responses, r_T, very poorly at values of **x** where there are very few treated individuals, and hence very few observed treated responses, r_T. In this one example, the linear covariance adjustment creates the impression of a treatment effect where there is none. This led Rubin to conclude that covariance adjustment is more robust to model misspecification when it is applied to competently matched samples.

15.7 Theoretical Implications of Systematic Bias

A systematic bias is one that does not diminish in size as the sample size increases, $I \to \infty$. Randomized experimentation prevents certain systematic biases when estimating the effects caused by treatments, but systematic bias is possible, indeed likely, in observational studies. This inescapable fact is important, but not debilitating.

Uncertainty about systematic bias does not diminish as $I \to \infty$, but uncertainty from sampling variability does diminish; so, systematic bias becomes a relatively more important consideration than sampling variability as $I \to \infty$. This simple, obvious fact necessitates some adjustments in the way we think about research designs and statistical methods.

If we could trade a portion of the sample, some sampling efficiency, for a stronger statement about unmeasured bias, that trade would become increasingly attractive as $I \to \infty$. The trade requires some thought because two things are exchanged that are not commensurate. We have seen this again and again. Comparing two statistics, the statistic that is more efficient in a randomization test in a randomized block experiment may be the less efficient statistic in a sensitivity analysis in a blocked observational study, simply because the null hypothesis has changed; see Chap. 11. Local alternatives—small treatment effects—are beside the point, because every infinitely small effect is sensitive to infinitely small biases. Formally, as the effect diminishes, $\tau \to 0$, the design sensitivity diminishes, $\widetilde{\Gamma} \to 1$; see Chaps. 9–10. In observational studies, we hope to distinguish meaningful treatment effects from nontrivial unmeasured biases; there is no possibility of distinguishing infinitesimal effects from biases of unbounded magnitude, so that cannot be a correct statement of a practical problem. The efficiency of a statistic in a sensitivity analysis drops to zero as Γ increases to $\widetilde{\Gamma}$, so increasing the design sensitivity, $\widetilde{\Gamma}$, is a practical problem, solved in part through better design [21] and in part through better methods of analysis [17–19, 23]. In an observational study, an investigator who chooses to use all of the data simply because that is what everyone must do, who chooses methods that would be most efficient in the absence of systematic bias—such an investigator is not thinking carefully about the provable consequences of their choices.

A mistaken decision that leads to a lower design sensitivity, $\widetilde{\Gamma}$, means a weaker statement about unmeasured biases no matter how large the sample size I becomes. Mistakes about $\widetilde{\Gamma}$ are not self-correcting as $I \to \infty$; weak conclusions are permanent. Consequently, adaptive inference (Sect. 9.5) and sample splitting [7] may trade a diminishing part of the sample size, I, for a permanent increase in design sensitivity, $\widetilde{\Gamma}$.

15.8 Evidence About—Not Merely Evidence of—Unmeasured Biases

Every observational study is affected by unmeasured biases—the only way to not notice this is to not look—but this inescapable fact is not debilitating. Firm, important conclusions have been reached on the basis of a series of well-executed observational studies, each affected to some degree by unmeasured biases. Smoking does cause lung cancer. Seat belts do reduce fatalities in car crashes. Central control of all prices by the government ends badly or continues terribly.

Pretending there are no unmeasured biases is pretending. In statistics, we don't pretend. We design studies and plan analyses to reach the firmest conclusions that are possible, candidly describing conclusions that are less firm than we might like.

We always look for evidence about unmeasured biases. Chapters 12 and 13 considered two of the many simple, common techniques: evidence from known effects and multiple control groups [14, 15, 20]. Sometimes we unearth evidence that heightens concern about the possibility that an association between treatment and outcome is not an effect of the treatment [2, 29]. At other times, evidence from known effects or multiple control groups strengthens a causal conclusion—it increases the insensitivity of a causal conclusion to unmeasured bias—and this happened in Chaps. 12 and 13.

References

1. Bross, I.D.J.: Statistical criticism. Cancer **13**(2), 394–400 (1960). Reprinted in *Observational Studies*, Volume 4, Issue 2, 2018, with Discussion by William B. Fairley, William A. Huber, Joseph L. Gastwirth, Andrew Gelman, Jennifer Hill, Katherine J. Hoggatt, Daniel E. Ho, Charles S. Reichardt, David Rindskopf, Paul R. Rosenbaum and Dylan S. Small
2. Brumberg, K., Ellis, D.E., Small, D.S., Hennessy, S., Rosenbaum, P.R.: Using natural strata when examining unmeasured biases in an observational study of neurological side effects of antibiotics. J. Roy. Stat. Soc. C (Appl. Stat.) **72**(2), 314–329 (2023)
3. Campbell, D.T.: Relabeling internal and external validity for applied social scientists. New Direct. Program Eval. **1986**(31), 67–77 (1986)
4. Chamberlain, T.C.: The method of multiple working hypotheses. Science **15**(366), 92–96 (1890). Reprinted in Science 1965;148:754–759
5. Feyerabend, P.K.: How to be a good empiricist: A plea for tolerance in matters epistemological. In: P.H. Nidditch (ed.) The Philosophy of Science. Oxford University Press, New York (1968)
6. Fogarty, C.B., Mikkelsen, M.E., Gaieski, D.F., Small, D.S.: Discrete optimization for interpretable study populations and randomization inference in an observational study of severe sepsis mortality. J. Am. Stat. Assoc. **111**(514), 447–458 (2016)
7. Heller, R., Rosenbaum, P.R., Small, D.S.: Split samples and design sensitivity in observational studies. J. Am. Stat. Assoc. **104**(487), 1090–1101 (2009)
8. Hudgens, M.G., Halloran, M.E.: Toward causal inference with interference. J. Am. Stat. Assoc. **103**(482), 832–842 (2008)
9. James, H.: Letter to Robert Louis Stevenson, January 12, 1891. In: The Letters of Henry James. Charles Scribner's and Sons, New York (1920)
10. Lehmann, E.L., Romano, J.P.: Testing Statistical Hypotheses, 3rd edn. Springer, New York (2005)

11. Mallows, C.L., Denby, L., Landwehr, J.: A conversation with Colin L. Mallows. Int. Stat. Rev. **81**(3), 338–360 (2013)
12. Neyman, J., Pearson, E.S.: On the use and interpretation of certain test criteria for purposes of statistical inference. Biometrika **20A**, 175–240 (1928)
13. Polanyi, M.: The Study of Man. University of Chicago Press, Chicago (1959)
14. Rosenbaum, P.R.: From association to causation in observational studies: The role of tests of strongly ignorable treatment assignment. J. Am. Stat. Assoc. **79**(385), 41–48 (1984)
15. Rosenbaum, P.R.: The role of known effects in observational studies. Biometrics **45**, 557–569 (1989)
16. Rosenbaum, P.R.: Interference between units in randomized experiments. J. Am. Stat. Assoc. **102**(477), 191–200 (2007)
17. Rosenbaum, P.R.: Design sensitivity and efficiency in observational studies. J. Am. Stat. Assoc. **105**(490), 692–702 (2010)
18. Rosenbaum, P.R.: Weighted M-statistics with superior design sensitivity in matched observational studies with multiple controls. J. Am. Stat. Assoc. **109**(507), 1145–1158 (2014)
19. Rosenbaum, P.R.: Bahadur efficiency of sensitivity analyses in observational studies. J. Am. Stat. Assoc. **110**(509), 205–217 (2015)
20. Rosenbaum, P.R.: How to see more in observational studies: Some new quasi-experimental devices. Annu. Rev. Stat. Appl. **2**, 21–48 (2015)
21. Rosenbaum, P.R.: Design of Observational Studies, 2nd edn. Springer, New York (2020)
22. Rosenbaum, P.R.: Modern algorithms for matching in observational studies. Ann. Rev. Stat. Appl. **7**, 143–176 (2020)
23. Rosenbaum, P.R.: Bahadur efficiency of observational block designs. J. Am. Stat. Assoc. **119**(547), 1871–1881 (2024)
24. Rosenbaum, P.R., Rubin, D.B.: Propensity scores in the design of observational studies for causal effects. Biometrika **110**, 1–13 (2023)
25. Rubin, D.B.: The use of matched sampling and regression adjustment to remove bias in observational studies. Biometrics **29**, 185–203 (1973)
26. Rubin, D.B.: Using multivariate matched sampling and regression adjustment to control bias in observational studies. J. Am. Stat. Assoc. **74**(366a), 318–328 (1979)
27. Rubin, D.B.: The design versus the analysis of observational studies for causal effects: parallels with the design of randomized trials. Stat. Med. **26**(1), 20–36 (2007)
28. Rubin, D.B.: For objective causal inference, design trumps analysis. Ann. Appl. Stat. **2**(3), 808–840 (2008)
29. Silber, J.H., Rosenbaum, P.R., Reiter, J.G., Jain, S., Hill, A.S., Hashemi, S., Brown, S., Olfson, M., Ing, C.: Exposure to operative anesthesia in childhood and subsequent neurobehavioral diagnoses: A natural experiment using appendectomy. Anesthesiology **141**(3), 489–499 (2024)
30. Tukey, J.W.: Sunset salvo. Am. Stat. **40**(1), 72–76 (1986)
31. Yu, R.: Evaluating and improving a matched comparison of antidepressants and bone density. Biometrics **77**(4), 1276–1288 (2021)

Some Books and Articles About Causal Inference

There are many good books concerning causal inference. Some are general; others go into depth about particular topics. A few excellent books and survey articles are mentioned here.

General books about causal inference include Angrist and Pischke [3], Brumback [7], Ding [14], Hernán and Robins [18], Imbens and Rubin [21], and Morgan and Winship [28]. In particular, Hernán and Robins [18] discuss the large and important topic of treatment regimes that vary over time; see also Diggle, Heagerty, Liang, and Zeger [13].

Books emphasizing quasi-experimental designs include Campbell and Stanley [9], Reichardt [30], and Shadish, Cook and Campbell [38]; see also Rossi, Lipsey, and Henry [35].

Aspects of natural experiments and instruments are surveyed by Angrist and Krueger [1,2]; Baiocchi, Cheng, and Small [4]; Diamond and Robinson [12]; Dunning [15]; Meyer [27]; Rosenzweig and Wolpin [34]; and Sekhon and Titiunik [37]. For Mendelian randomization as a source of natural experiments and instruments, see Burgess and Thompson [8]. For genetic transmission disequilibrium as a source of natural experiments, see Ewens and Spielman [16].

Case-control studies are important in epidemiology. They are discussed by Borgan et al. [5], Breslow and Day [6], Holland and Rubin [20], Keogh and Cox [22] and Lash, VanderWeele, Haneuse, and Rothman [23]. For related designs without controls, see Greenland [17].

The Manski-bounds under partial identification of causal effects are discussed by Manski [25,26].

Graphical models of dependence among variables and their connections to causal inference are discussed by Dawid [11]; Holland [19]; Lauritzen [24]; Pearl [29]; Rubin [36]; Spirtes, Glymour, and Scheines [39]; and VanderWeele [40].

Smoking and lung cancer played an important role in the history of causal inference. Two essays of enduring interest are Cornfield et al. [10] and White [41].

© The Author(s), under exclusive license to Springer Nature Switzerland AG 2025
P. R. Rosenbaum, *An Introduction to the Theory of Observational Studies*,
Springer Texts in Statistics, https://doi.org/10.1007/978-3-031-90494-3

References

1. Angrist, J.D., Krueger, A.B.: Empirical strategies in labor economics. In: O. Ashenfelter, D. Card (eds.) Handbook of Labor Economics, vol. 3, pp. 1277–1366. Elsevier, New York (1999)
2. Angrist, J.D., Krueger, A.B.: Instrumental variables and the search for identification: From supply and demand to natural experiments. J. Econ. Perspect. **15**(4), 69–85 (2001)
3. Angrist, J.D., Pischke, J.S.: Mostly Harmless Econometrics: An Empiricist's Companion. Princeton University Press, Princeton, NJ (2009)
4. Baiocchi, M., Cheng, J., Small, D.S.: Instrumental variable methods for causal inference. Stat. Med. **33**(13), 2297–2340 (2014)
5. Borgan, Ø., Breslow, N., Chatterjee, N., Gail, M.H., Scott, A., Wild, C.J.: Handbook of Statistical Methods for Case-Control Studies. Chapman and Hall/CRC Press, Boca Raton, FL (2018)
6. Breslow, N.E., Day, N.E.: Statistical Methods in Cancer Research, Volume I: The Analysis of Case-Control Studies. International Agency for Research on Cancer, Lyon (1980)
7. Brumback, B.A.: Fundamentals of Causal Inference. Chapman and Hall/CRC, Boca Raton, FL (2021)
8. Burgess, S., Thompson, S.G.: Mendelian Randomization: Methods for Using Genetic Variants in Causal Estimation. Chapman and Hall/CRC Press, Boca Raton, FL (2021)
9. Campbell, D.T., Stanley, J.C.: Experimental and Quasi-experimental Designs for Research. Rand McNally, Chicago (1966)
10. Cornfield, J., Haenszel, W., Hammond, E.C., Lilienfeld, A.M., Shimkin, M.B., Wynder, E.L.: Smoking and lung cancer: recent evidence and a discussion of some questions (reprint from 1959 with new Discussion by D. R. Cox, J. P. Vandenbroucke, M. Zwahlen and J. B. Greenhouse). Int. J. Epidemiol. **38**(5), 1175–91 (2009)
11. Dawid, A.P.: Beware of the DAG! In: JMLR Workshop and Conference Proceedings: NIPS 2008 Workshop on Causality, pp. 59–86. PMLR (2010)
12. Diamond, J., Robinson, J.A.: Natural Experiments of History. Harvard University Press, Cambridge, MA (2012)
13. Diggle, P., Heagerty, P., Liang, K.Y., Zeger, S.: Analysis of Longitudinal Data. Oxford University Press, New York (2013)
14. Ding, P.: A First Course in Causal Inference. Chapman and Hall/CRC, Boca Raton, FL (2024)
15. Dunning, T.: Natural Experiments in the Social Sciences: A Design-Based Approach. Cambridge University Press, New York (2012)
16. Ewens, W.J., Spielman, R.S.: The transmission/disequilibrium test. In: Handbook of Statistical Genetics, pp. 507–518. Wiley, New York (2001)
17. Greenland, S.: A unified approach to the analysis of case-distribution (case-only) studies. Stat. Med. **18**(1), 1–15 (1999)
18. Hernán, M.A., Robins, J.M.: Causal Inference. Chapman and Hall/CRC, Boca Raton, FL (2010)
19. Holland, P.W.: Causal inference, path analysis, and recursive structural equations models. Sociol. Methodol. **18**, 449–484 (1988)
20. Holland, P.W., Rubin, D.B.: Causal inference in retrospective studies. Evaluat. Rev. **12**(3), 203–231 (1988)
21. Imbens, G.W., Rubin, D.B.: Causal Inference in Statistics, Social, and Biomedical Sciences. Cambridge University Press, New York (2015)
22. Keogh, R.H., Cox, D.R.: Case-Control Studies. Cambridge University Press, New York (2014)
23. Lash, T.L., VanderWeele, T.J., Haneuse, S., Rothman, K.J.: Modern Epidemiology. Wolters Kluwer, Philadelphia (2021)
24. Lauritzen, S.L.: Graphical Models. Oxford University Press, New York (1996)
25. Manski, C.F.: Identification Problems in the Social Sciences. Harvard University Press, Cambridge, MA (1995)
26. Manski, C.F.: Partial Identification of Probability Distributions. Springer, New York (2003)

27. Meyer, B.D.: Natural and quasi-experiments in economics. J. Bus. Econ. Stat. **13**(2), 151–161 (1995)
28. Morgan, S.L., Winship, C.: Counterfactuals and Causal Inference. Cambridge University Press, New York (2015)
29. Pearl, J.: Causality. Cambridge University Press, New York (2009)
30. Reichardt, C.S.: Quasi-experimentation: A Guide to Design and Analysis. Guilford Publications, New York (2019)
31. Rosenbaum, P.R.: Observational Studies, 2nd edn. Springer, New York (2002)
32. Rosenbaum, P.R.: Observation and Experiment: An Introduction to Causal Inference. Harvard University Press, Cambridge, MA (2017)
33. Rosenbaum, P.R.: Design of Observational Studies, 2nd edn. Springer, New York (2020)
34. Rosenzweig, M.R., Wolpin, K.I.: Natural "natural experiments" in economics. J. Econ. Literat. **38**(4), 827–874 (2000)
35. Rossi, P.H., Lipsey, M.W., Henry, G.T.: Evaluation: A Systematic Approach. Sage Publications, New York (2018)
36. Rubin, D.B.: Direct and indirect causal effects via potential outcomes. Scand. J. Stat. **31**(2), 161–170 (2004)
37. Sekhon, J.S., Titiunik, R.: When natural experiments are neither natural nor experiments. Am. Polit. Sci. Rev. **106**(1), 35–57 (2012)
38. Shadish, W., Cook, T.D., Campbell, D.T.: Experimental and Quasi-experimental Designs for Generalized Causal Inference. Houghton Mifflin Boston, MA (2002)
39. Spirtes, P., Glymour, C., Scheines, R.: Causation, Prediction, and Search. MIT Press, Cambrige, MA (2001)
40. VanderWeele, T.: Explanation in Causal Inference: Methods for Mediation and Interaction. Oxford University Press, New York (2015)
41. White, C.: Research on smoking and lung cancer: A landmark in the history of chronic disease epidemiology. Yale J. Biol. Med. **63**(1), 29 (1990)

Notation

Finding the Meaning of a Symbol

Notation is defined as it is introduced. In the index, a **bold** page number indicates a definition. Some symbols are used in a single way throughout the book, including i, j, r_{Tij}, r_{Cij}, R_{ij}, Z_{ij}, z_{ij}, u_{ij}, δ_{ij}, δ_{0ij}, $R_{ij}^{\delta_0}$, q_{ij}, q_{ij}^*, θ_{ij}, $\overline{\theta}_{ij}$, $i = 1, \ldots, I$, $j = 1, \ldots, J$, and various **bold** matrices of dimension $I \times J$ that contain these quantities. Other important symbols that retain their meanings are $\mathcal{Z}$, $\mathcal{F}$, $\mathbf{x}_{ij}$, Γ, $\widetilde{\Gamma}$, $\Phi(\cdot)$, $\Phi^{-1}(\cdot)$. Symbols that are used in a single way throughout the book appear in the index and are discussed below.

Many other symbols change their meaning from one chapter to the next, including A, a, B, b, D, d, V, v, W, w, ι, ρ, and ω; so, they are not in the book's index, and you should look locally in the current chapter to find the meaning of these symbols. The symbol μ is an expectation, and σ^2 is a variance, but they will be expectations and variances of different things in different chapters; so, again, look locally in the current chapter for the precise definition. In the same way, ϵ and ε are random errors of some sort, but look locally to find their precise meaning.

The transpose of a matrix $\mathbf{a}$ is denoted $\mathbf{a}^T$. In contrast, no matter what A is, the symbols A', A'', A^*, $A^\dagger$, and $A^\ddagger$ are siblings of A whose exact meaning is defined locally.

Specific Symbols That Maintain Their Meaning

0 and 1: A vector or matrix of 0s or 1s of appropriate dimension, typically an $I \times J$ matrix.

$|\mathcal{S}|$: If $\mathcal{S}$ is a finite set, then $|\mathcal{S}|$ is the number of elements in $\mathcal{S}$. If $\mathcal{S} = \{1, 7, 21\}$, then $|\mathcal{S}| = 3$; see Sect. 2.1.

© The Author(s), under exclusive license to Springer Nature Switzerland AG 2025

P. R. Rosenbaum, *An Introduction to the Theory of Observational Studies*,
Springer Texts in Statistics, https://doi.org/10.1007/978-3-031-90494-3

$\boldsymbol{\delta_{ij}}$**:** The causal effect, $\delta_{ij} = r_{Tij} - r_{Cij}$ for person j in block i; see Sect. 2.2.

A · in a function, e.g., $\boldsymbol{f(\cdot)}$**:** Where $f(x)$ denotes the value of the function at x, the notation $f(\cdot)$ refers to the function itself, not its value at a particular x; see, for instance, $F_T(\cdot)$ in Sect. 2.4.

$\boldsymbol{\mathcal{F}}$**:** Defined in (2.3), $\mathcal{F}$ contains the potential outcomes, (r_{Tij}, r_{Cij}), observed and unobserved covariates, $(\mathbf{x}_{ij}, u_{ij})$, for the IJ individuals ij in the block design with I blocks and J individuals per block; see Sect. 2.2. Later, in Sect. 4.5, we realize that the only unmeasured covariate that matters is the principle unobserved covariate, $\zeta = \zeta(r_T, r_C, \mathbf{x}) = \Pr(Z = 1 \mid r_T, r_C, \mathbf{x})$, which is a function of $(r_T, r_C, \mathbf{x})$ that is already in $\mathcal{F}$; so, the explicit appearance of u_{ij} in $\mathcal{F}$ could be viewed as redundant.

$\boldsymbol{\kappa}$**:** Beginning in Chap. 9, the symbol κ is the finite maximum value of $\varphi(\cdot)$ in (9.11) over its domain $[0, 1]$. Here and there, it is important that $\varphi(\cdot)$ in (9.11) is continuous and bounded on its domain. Also, in plots of $\varphi(\cdot)$ in (9.11) comparing different $(m, \underline{m}, \overline{m})$, it is helpful to plot $\varphi(\cdot)/\kappa$ rather than $\varphi(\cdot)$.

$\boldsymbol{i, j, ij, I, J}$**:** This book makes frequent reference to a block design with I blocks, $i = 1, \ldots, I$, each block containing J distinct people, $j = 1, \ldots, J$, where no person appears in more than one block. "For all i" means for all I blocks. "For all ij" means for all IJ people in the block design. "For all j in block i" means for all J people in a particular block i. To speak of ij and ij' with $j \neq j'$ is to speak of two different people, namely, $j \neq j'$, in the same block i. See Sect. 2.1.

$\boldsymbol{\Phi(\cdot), \Phi^{-1}(\cdot)}$**:** The functions $\Phi(\cdot)$ and $\Phi^{-1}(\cdot)$ are the cumulative distribution function and its inverse for the standard normal distribution, respectively. The standard normal distribution has expectation zero and variance one. For a random variable A that has the standard normal distribution, $\Pr(A \leq a) = \Phi(a)$ for any $a \in (-\infty, \infty)$ and $\Pr\{A \leq \Phi^{-1}(b)\} = b$ for any $b \in (0, 1)$.

$\boldsymbol{\varphi(\cdot), \kappa}$**:** The function $\varphi(\cdot)$ is an aspect of a weighted rank statistic; see Sect. 2.6. For $\varphi(\cdot)$ given by (9.11), κ is its maximum value over $[0, 1]$.

$\boldsymbol{\Re, \Re^K, \Re_+}$**:** $\Re$ is the real line and $\Re^K$ is K-dimensional Euclidean space. The strictly positive real numbers are $\Re_+$.

$\boldsymbol{(r_{Tij}, r_{Cij})}$**:** Potential outcomes of individual j in block i under treatment, T, or control C; see Sect. 2.2.

$\boldsymbol{R_{ij}}$**:** The observed outcome of individual j in block i under the treatment this individual did receive, $R_{ij} = r_{Tij}$ if $Z_{ij} = 1$ or $R_{ij} = r_{Cij}$ if $Z_{ij} = 0$; see Sect. 2.2.

$\boldsymbol{\overline{R}_t}$ **and** $\boldsymbol{\overline{R}_c}$**:** $\overline{R}_t$ is the mean response observed from the I treated individuals and $\overline{R}_c$ is the mean response from the $I(J-1)$ controls in the block design with IJ individuals; see Sect. 2.2.

$\boldsymbol{\theta, \overline{\theta}}$**:** The $I \times J$ matrix of treatment assignment probabilities θ_{ij} is $\boldsymbol{\theta}$, where these probabilities sum to 1 in each of the I rows of $\boldsymbol{\theta}$. In a randomized block experiment, the treatment assignment probabilities are $\overline{\boldsymbol{\theta}}$, where $\overline{\theta}_{ij} = 1/J$ for every ij. See Sect. 8.2.

$\mathbf{Z}_{ij}$**:** The treatment received by person j in block i, $Z_{ij} = 1$ for treatment T or $Z_{ij} = 0$ for control C; see Sect. 2.2.

$\mathcal{Z}$**:** The set $\mathcal{Z}$ contains the J^I possible assignments $\mathbf{z}$ for the IJ individuals in a block design with I blocks and J individuals in each block, one of whom is treated; see Sect. 2.1. With a slight abuse of notation, conditioning on the event $\mathbf{Z} \in \mathcal{Z}$ is abbreviated as conditioning on $\mathcal{Z}$; see Sect. 2.3.

Glossary

Adjusted *P*-value See Holm's procedure.

A priori In statistics, we know something a priori if we know it before examining any data from the current investigation. For example, in connection with adaptive inference in Sect. 9.5, we might say: "An omniscient investigator would know that test statistic T_1 has larger design sensitivity than test statistic T_2, but since we are not omniscient we cannot know this a priori; so, we must pay a price for multiple testing for discovering this in the data." Or we might say: "The one primary analysis was specified a priori in the grant proposal before any data were collected, but we also report one exploratory analysis suggested by the data; however, exploratory analyses must be viewed with appropriate skepticism."

Bonferroni procedure See Holm's procedure.

Central problem of causal inference The effect δ_{ij} of a treatment on individual ij is the comparison of the potential response r_{Tij} of ij under treatment and the potential response r_{Cij} of ij under control—that is, $\delta_{ij} = r_{Tij} - r_{Cij}$—but we see r_{Tij} only if individual ij receives treatment with $Z_{ij} = 1$, and we see r_{Cij} only if individual ij receives the control with $Z_{ij} = 0$; so, we never see a causal effect, δ_{ij}.

Central problem of observational studies Randomized treatment assignment permits certain inferences about a collection of causal effects, δ_{ij}; however, treatments are not randomly assigned in an observational study. In drawing inferences about causal effects, it would suffice to adjust for observed covariates **X** in an observational study if treatment assignment Z were ignorable (or unconfounded) given **X**—that is, if

$$0 < \zeta = \Pr(Z = 1 \mid \mathbf{X}, r_T, r_C) = \Pr(Z = 1 \mid \mathbf{X}) = e(\mathbf{X}) < 1; \qquad (15.1)$$

© The Author(s), under exclusive license to Springer Nature Switzerland AG 2025

P. R. Rosenbaum, *An Introduction to the Theory of Observational Studies*, Springer Texts in Statistics, https://doi.org/10.1007/978-3-031-90494-3

however, only randomized treatment assignment can guarantee that (15.1) is true. In (15.1), $\zeta = \Pr(Z = 1 \mid \mathbf{X}, r_T, r_C)$ is the principal unobserved covariate and $e(\mathbf{X}) = \Pr(Z = 1 \mid \mathbf{X})$ is the propensity score.

Composite null hypothesis See simple null hypothesis.

Conservative test See level of a test.

Convergence in probability; consistent estimate If $\widehat{\tau}_I$ is a random variable, perhaps an estimator, computed from the first I observations, and τ is a constant, perhaps a parameter to be estimated, then $\widehat{\tau}_I$ converges in probability to τ if $\lim_{I\to\infty} \Pr(|\widehat{\tau}_I - \tau| > \epsilon)$ exists and equals 0 for all $\epsilon > 0$. In this case, an estimator $\widehat{\tau}_I$ is said to be consistent for a parameter τ.

Exchangeable distribution A bivariate distribution of (W_1, W_2) is exchangeable if $\Pr(W_1 \leq a, W_2 \leq b) = \Pr(W_1 \leq b, W_2 \leq a)$ for all a and b. If (W_1, W_2) are exchangeable, then they have the same marginal distribution, $\Pr(W_1 \leq a) = \Pr(W_2 \leq a)$ for all a. In a straightforward way, the concept of exchangeable distributions extends from bivariate distributions to multivariate distributions with more than two variables [4, §2.5].

Family-wise error rate When testing several hypotheses, $H_1, \ldots, H_K$, strong control of the family-wise error rate at level α means that, no matter which hypotheses are true or false, the probability that at least one true hypothesis is falsely rejected is at most α. Weak control is a less adequate, less useful concept; so, it is little discussed. Weak control of the family-wise error rate means that if $H_1, \ldots, H_K$ are *all* true, then the probability that at least one of $H_1, \ldots, H_K$ is falsely rejected is at most α. If H_1 is false but $H_2, \ldots, H_K$ are true, then weak control makes no promises about falsely rejecting $H_2, \ldots, H_K$, whereas strong control makes a strong promise. Holm's procedure in this glossary provides strong control of the family-wise error rate.

Holm's procedure Holm's [1] procedure is a method for testing K null hypotheses with probability at most α of rejecting at least one true hypothesis. Holm's procedure is an improvement on the more familiar Bonferroni procedure. It is an improvement in the sense that (i) both procedures run at most an α chance of rejecting at least one true hypothesis, but (ii) Holm's procedure rejects every hypothesis rejected by the Bonferroni procedure and may also reject additional hypotheses. Suppose that we wish to test K null hypotheses, $k = 1, \ldots K$, and K tests of these hypotheses have produced valid P-values, $P_1, \ldots P_K$. These K P-values need not be statistically independent. The Bonferroni procedure then rejects hypothesis k if $P_k \leq \alpha/K$, or equivalently it reports an adjusted P-value for hypothesis k of $\min(1, K \times P_k)$. The first step of Holm's procedure is the same: the smallest of the K P-values is compared to α/K, and the corresponding hypothesis is rejected if this smallest P-value is $\leq \alpha/K$. Only if this hypothesis is rejected, the second smallest P-value is compared to $\alpha/(K - 1)$. Only if this second hypothesis is also rejected, the third smallest P-value is compared to $\alpha/(K - 2)$, and so on. The smallest α that would lead to rejection of the kth hypothesis is the adjusted P-value for that hypothesis [5]. For discussion of graphical displays of multiple comparisons, see Xi and Bretz [7].

Identified, identification, partial identification A parameter, τ, is identified if different values of the parameter, say $\tau = 2$ and $\tau = 3$, imply different probability distributions for observable data. If $\tau = 2$ and $\tau = 3$ yield the same distribution for the observable data, then the observable data are inadequate to distinguish $\tau = 2$ from $\tau = 3$ no matter how large the sample size becomes. Partial identification is possible, perhaps typical: we may be able to distinguish $\tau = 5$ from the logical disjunction ($\tau = 2$ or $\tau = 3$), yet be unable to distinguish $\tau = 2$ from $\tau = 3$. Typically, a fractional factorial experiment is partially identified, because certain higher-order interactions cannot be distinguished from lower-order interactions [6]. Aspects of identification in causal inference are discussed by Charles Manski [2,3].

Level of a test A test of a null hypothesis H_0 has level α if, whenever H_0 is true, the probability of rejecting H_0 is at most α. A common convention takes $\alpha = 0.05$, but that is a convention and nothing more. Compare with the *power of a test*. The size of a test is the probability the test will reject the null hypothesis when the null hypothesis is true. So, a level-α test has size that is less than or equal to α. A test is conservative if its size is strictly less than its level.

Power of a test When alternative hypothesis H_1 is true, the power is the probability that a test of a null hypothesis H_0 will reject H_0. Ideally, a test is unlikely to reject H_0 when H_0 is true and is likely to reject H_0 when H_0 is false. A level-α test rejects H_0 when H_0 is true with probability at most α. The power is the probability that the test rejects H_0 when H_1 is true. Ideally, the level is low and the power is high. The power depends upon the alternative hypothesis: often, if H_1 is close to H_0, then it is difficult to tell them apart and the power is low, but often if H_1 is far from H_0, then it is easy to tell them apart and the power is high.

Simple null hypothesis The phrase "simple null hypothesis" is a standard, but not entirely enlightening technical term. One might expect that a simple null hypothesis would contrast with a complicated null hypothesis, but that is not the intended contrast. Some simple null hypotheses sound more complicated than some related hypotheses that are not simple. "The treatment effect is 4.8732" may sound more complicated than "the treatment effect is positive," but again the contrast is not between simple and complicated. A simple null hypothesis contrasts with a composite null hypothesis. A simple null hypothesis specifies a single probability distribution for the data when the null hypothesis is true. For example, if Y is normal with expectation μ and variance 1, then $H_0 : \mu = 0$ is a simple null hypothesis. A composite null hypothesis is composed of many—often infinitely many—simple null hypotheses. A composite null hypothesis is true if any of its components is true. For example, if Y is normal with expectation μ and variance 1, then $H_0 : \mu \leq 0$ is a composite null hypothesis, and $H_0 : \mu = 0$ and $H_0 : \mu = -1$ are two of its infinitely many simple components. If Y is normal with expectation μ and variance σ^2, with σ^2 unknown, then $H_0 : \mu = 0$ is a composite null hypothesis, and $H_0 : (\mu = 0, \sigma^2 = 1)$ and $H_0 : (\mu = 0, \sigma^2 = 2)$ are two of its infinitely many components. To reject a composite null hypothesis is to reject each of its simple components, and this might be done in various ways. The t-test for a normal mean is one familiar test of a composite null hypothesis that employs an independent estimate of the unknown σ^2. See Sects. 2.5, 2.8, and 2.9.

Size of a test See level of a test.

Unbiased estimator An estimator, say $\widehat{\tau}$, is unbiased for a parameter, say τ, if the expectation of $\widehat{\tau}$ is τ, that is, if $\mathrm{E}(\widehat{\tau}) = \tau$; see, for instance, Sect. 2.4. All of this presupposes that $\widehat{\tau}$ has an expectation.

Valid test, valid confidence interval The word "valid" is a common word in English with a variety of overlapping meanings. The word "valid" is employed in a variety of technical contexts with a variety of well-defined and distinct meanings. In particular, a level-α statistical test of a null hypothesis H_0 is valid if the probability is at most α that H_0 will be rejected when H_0 is true. A valid test need not be a good test; for instance, it may have less power than some other valid test. A $1 - \alpha$ confidence interval for a parameter or random variable is valid if the random confidence interval covers its target with probability at least $1-\alpha$. Again, a valid confidence interval may not be a good confidence interval; for instance, there may be other valid confidence intervals whose expected length is shorter. Valid tests and confidence intervals are closely connected because a confidence interval is a set of hypotheses not rejected by a test. Admittedly, one might reasonably argue that an invalid level-α test simply is not a level-α test, as one might reasonably argue that a dishonest bank simply is not a bank; yet, these slightly redundant phrases do seem to have their uses. See also Sect. 2.8 and Tukey's remarks about assumptions that affect validity.

References

1. Holm, S.: A simple sequentially rejective multiple test procedure. Scand. J. Stat. **6**, 65–70 (1979)
2. Manski, C.F.: Identification Problems in the Social Sciences. Harvard University Press, Cambridge, MA (1995)
3. Manski, C.F.: Partial Identification of Probability Distributions. Springer, New York (2003)
4. Severini, T.A.: Elements of Distribution Theory. Cambridge University Press, New York (2005)
5. Wright, S.P.: Adjusted p-values for simultaneous inference. Biometrics **48**, 1005–1013 (1992)
6. Wu, C.F.J., Hamada, M.S.: Experiments: Planning, Analysis, and Optimization. Wiley, New York (2021)
7. Xi, D., Bretz, F.: Graphical approaches for multiple comparison procedures. In: Handbook of Multiple Comparisons, pp. 91–119. Chapman and Hall/CRC, Boca Raton, FL (2021)

Solutions to Selected Problems

Selected Problems of Chap. 1

1.1 (a) The least squares unbiased estimate of

$$\mu_1 - \frac{(\mu_2 + \cdots + \mu_J)}{J-1} \text{ is } \overline{y}_1 - \frac{(\overline{y}_2 + \cdots + \overline{y}_J)}{J-1}$$

with variance

$$\sigma^2 \left\{ \frac{1}{n_1} + \left(\frac{1}{J-1} \right)^2 \left(\frac{1}{n_2} + \cdots + \frac{1}{n_J} \right) \right\}. \tag{15.2}$$

The variance (15.2) of the estimate tends to zero as $\min_{1 \le j \le J} (n_j) \to \infty$, but (15.2) does not tend to zero if $\min_{2 \le j \le J} (n_j) \to \infty$ with n_1 fixed. That is, if the treated group is of limited size, n_1, then using large numbers of controls is of limited benefit.
(b) $0.00328 \times \sigma^2$
(c) $0.00275 \times \sigma^2$
(d) 1.093
(e) 0.397
(f) The matched sample uses about 40% of the data, but its standard error is only 1.093 times larger than using 100% of the data. This ignores the fact that the matched sample is removing bias from age, sex, and education, and it ignores also the possibility that matching reduces the variance of Y_{ij} by controlling variation from age, sex, and education, as in Problem 1.2.
(g) 1.070. Although doubling the size of the N control group is practical in this example, it reduces the ratio of the standard errors from 1.093 in part (f) to 1.070 in part (g). If the number n_1 of treated individuals is fixed, then once you have 3, 4, or 5 controls per treated individual, large reductions in the standard error are difficult to obtain by increasing the number of controls.

© The Author(s), under exclusive license to Springer Nature Switzerland AG 2025

P. R. Rosenbaum, *An Introduction to the Theory of Observational Studies*, Springer Texts in Statistics, https://doi.org/10.1007/978-3-031-90494-3

Remarks about Problem 1.1: (i) It is possible to match while using 100% of the controls in matched sets of unequal sizes [4], but weights are then needed, so that the resulting variance is larger than (15.2). (ii) Huber [3, Lemma 2.1] gives a necessary and sufficient condition for a least squares estimate of a contrast to be asymptotically normal when the linear model is true with errors that are independent, identically distributed, with zero expectation, constant variance, and a distribution that is not normal. Consider the contrast estimate whose variance you determined to be (15.2). If $\min_{2 \le j \le J} (n_j) \rightarrow \infty$ with n_1 fixed, then this contrast estimate is a very simple example of a linear contrast estimator that does not satisfy Huber's condition and hence is not asymptotically normal. (iii) Part (g) contemplated doubling the size of the N control group, finding only a small reduction—a small improvement—in the standard error of the estimate. If you doubled the size of the N control group while matching for observed covariates, the average proximity of treated and control individuals in the same block would deteriorate. This topic will be explored further in Chap. 5.

1.2 The contrast estimate is unbiased, and its variance is not increased by σ_β^2, because the β_i's cancel in the estimator.

1.5 (b) Plot $Y_{ij} - Y_{ij'} = \mu_j - \mu_{j'} + \epsilon_{ij} - \epsilon_{ij'}$ for $j \neq j'$, which is free of the block terms β_i. You can plot a single pair of groups, $j \neq j'$, as in part (d) of this problem, or six boxplots for all six pairs of two distinct groups from the four groups in the HDL cholesterol data, or you can have two parallel boxplots, one for treated-control differences, $Y_{i1} - Y_{ij}$ with $j \geq 2$, the other for control-control differences, $Y_{ij} - Y_{ij'}$, $j \neq j'$, $j \geq 2$, $j' \geq 2$. See [9] for examples, variations, and extensions.
(d) See Fig. 15.1. The P-value from the Shapiro-Wilk test of a normal distribution is 7.1×10^{-10}, so block terms β_i that are constant within each block do not explain the deviation from a normal distribution.

The R code is:

```
library(iTOS)
data(aHDL)
# Note carefully that aHDL is sorted so paired individuals
# are adjacent to one another.
yDN<-aHDL$hdl[aHDL$grpL=="D"]-aHDL$hdl[aHDL$grpL=="N"]
par(mfrow=c(1,2))
boxplot(yDN,xlab="D-N",ylab="D-N Difference in HDL",
main="D-N Pair Differences",las=1,
cex.main=.8,cex.axis=.8,cex.lab=.8)
abline(h=0,lty=2)
qqnorm(yDN,ylab="D-N Difference in HDL",las=1,
cex.main=.8,cex.axis=.8,cex.lab=.8)
qqline(yDN)
shapiro.test(yDN)
```

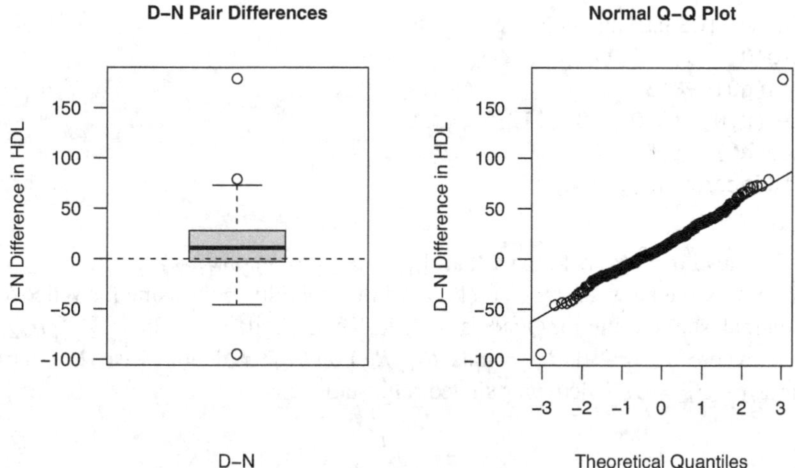

Fig. 15.1 Daily D versus never N pair differences in HDL cholesterol levels

Selected Problems of Chap. 2

2.3 For the Cauchy distribution, the difference in means is unbiased for $\overline{\delta} = \tau$ for each sample size I, but it does not converge to τ as $I \rightarrow \infty$. There is no incompatibility with Proposition 2.1, because unbiasedness for finite I and consistency as $I \rightarrow \infty$ are different things.

2.4 (a) In each block, the ranks 1, 2, and 3 occur for the treated individual with probability 1/3, and distinct blocks are independent. For $I = 2$ blocks there are $3 \times 3 = 9$ possible pairs of ranks for the two treated individuals, and each has probability $1/3 \times 1/3 = 1/9$. The two ranks sum to 4 in three ways: 1 + 3, 2 + 2, 3 + 1, each with probability 1/9, so the chance that Wilcoxon's blocked rank sum statistic equals 4 is $3/9 = 1/3$.

(b) In the `iTOS` package in R, type:

```
g0<-c(0,1/3,1/3,1/3)
names(g0)<-0:3
gconv(g0,g0)
```

(c) Either

```
round(gconv(gconv(gconv(g0,g0),g0),g0),3)
```

or

```
round(gconv(gconv(g0,g0),gconv(g0,g0)),3)
```

2.5 (a) In one block, the ranks 1, 2, and 3 occur for the treated individual with probability 1/3. In the other block, the ranks 2, 4, and 6 occur with probability 1/3. The chance that Quade's statistic is $3 = 1 + 2$ is $1/9 = 1/3 \times 1/3$, etc. Note that there are two ways to get a total of 5, namely, $5 = 1 + 4$ and $5 = 2 + 3$.

(b) In the iTOS package in R, type:

```
g0<-c(0,1/3,1/3,1/3)
names(g0)<-0:3
h0<-c(0,0,1/3,0,1/3,0,1/3)
names(h0)<-0:6
round(gconv(h0,g0),3)
```

2.6 Because $J = 2$, it follows that $|R_{i1} - R_{i2}| = \max_{1 \le j \le 2} R_{ij} - \min_{1 \le j \le 2} R_{ij}$ in (2.11); so, the between-block rank, b_i, of this quantity is the same for Wilcoxon's signed rank statistic and for Quade's statistic. Then Quade's statistic is $\sum_{i=1}^{I} b_i \sum_{j=1}^{2} q_{ij}^* Z_{ij}$, where $q_{ij}^* = 2$ if $R_{ij} = \max(R_{i1}, R_{i2})$ and $q_{ij}^* = 1$ otherwise. In contrast, using $Z_{i1} + Z_{i2} = 1$, Wilcoxon's signed rank statistic is

$$\sum_{i=1}^{I} b_i \sum_{j=1}^{2} (q_{ij}^* - 1) Z_{ij} = \sum_{i=1}^{I} b_i \sum_{j=1}^{2} q_{ij}^* Z_{ij} - \sum_{i=1}^{I} b_i$$

where $\sum_{i=1}^{I} b_i = 1 + 2 + \cdots + I = I(I+1)/2$.

2.9

(vii) In general, providing the needed expectations exist, $\mathrm{E}(A) = \mathrm{E}\{\mathrm{E}(A|B)\}$. Taking $A = \overline{R}_t - \overline{R}_c$ and $B = \mathcal{F}$ yields

$$\begin{aligned} \mathrm{E}(\overline{R}_t - \overline{R}_c | \mathcal{Z}) &= \mathrm{E}\{\mathrm{E}(\overline{R}_t - \overline{R}_c | \mathcal{Z}, \mathcal{F}) \,|\, \mathcal{Z}\} \\ &= \mathrm{E}(\overline{\delta} | \mathcal{Z}) = \tau, \end{aligned}$$

where $\mathcal{Z}$, or equivalently $\mathbf{Z} \in \mathcal{Z}$, is fixed throughout by the randomized block design.

(viii) In general, providing the needed moments exist,

$$\mathrm{var}(A) = \mathrm{E}\{\mathrm{var}(A|B)\} + \mathrm{var}\{\mathrm{E}(A|B)\},$$

so

$$\mathrm{var}(A) \ge \mathrm{E}\{\mathrm{var}(A|B)\}.$$

Therefore,

$$\begin{aligned} \mathrm{var}(\overline{R}_t - \overline{R}_c \,|\mathcal{Z}) &= \mathrm{E}\{\mathrm{var}(\overline{R}_t - \overline{R}_c \,|\, \mathcal{F}, \mathcal{Z}) \,|\, \mathcal{Z}\} + \mathrm{var}\{\mathrm{E}(\overline{R}_t - \overline{R}_c \,|\, \mathcal{F}, \mathcal{Z}) \,|\, \mathcal{Z}\} \\ &\ge \mathrm{E}\{\mathrm{var}(\overline{R}_t - \overline{R}_c \,|\, \mathcal{F}, \mathcal{Z}) \,|\, \mathcal{Z}\}. \end{aligned}$$

If $\rho = 1$, then $\tau = \delta_{ij} = r_{Tij} - r_{Cij}$, and

$$\mathrm{E}(\overline{R}_t - \overline{R}_c \,|\, \mathcal{F}, \mathcal{Z}) = \tau$$

for every $\mathcal{F}$ and $\mathcal{Z}$, so that

$$\text{var}\{\text{E}(\overline{R}_t - \overline{R}_c \mid \mathcal{F}, \mathcal{Z}) \mid \mathcal{Z}\} = 0,$$

and

$$\text{var}(\overline{R}_t - \overline{R}_c \mid \mathcal{Z}) = \text{E}\{\text{var}(\overline{R}_t - \overline{R}_c \mid \mathcal{F}, \mathcal{Z}) \mid \mathcal{Z}\}.$$

The bootstrap estimates the super-population variance, $\text{var}(\overline{R}_t - \overline{R}_c \mid \mathcal{Z})$; that is, the variance in the population from which the I blocks were sampled. See also parts (x) and (xi) of this problem.

Let us repeat all of this in words. (a) Variability in $\overline{R}_t - \overline{R}_c$ given $(\mathcal{F}, \mathcal{Z})$ is due to the random assignment of treatments, that is, the random choice of one treatment assignment $\mathbf{Z} \in \mathcal{Z}$ for a finite population in which $\mathcal{F}$ is fixed. (b) Variability in $\overline{R}_t - \overline{R}_c$ given $\mathcal{Z}$ is larger (i.e., at least as large) in expectation, because it reflects both the random assignment of treatments, $\mathbf{Z} \in \mathcal{Z}$, and also the random sampling of I blocks from the infinite super-population to yield $\mathcal{F}$. (c) If $\rho = 1$, then the treatment effect is constant, $\tau = \delta_{ij}$ for all i, j, and the expected variability in (a) equals the variability in (b). In expectation, the case $\rho = 1$ and $\tau = \delta_{ij}$ is the "worst" case for randomization inference, because an inference to the finite population $\mathcal{F}$ is expected to be no easier than an inference to the super-population from which $\mathcal{F}$ was drawn. (d) Of course, by part (iv) of this problem, there is nothing in the observable data, (R_{ij}, Z_{ij}), that distinguishes $\rho = 1$ from $\rho < 1$; so, unless we have external evidence that $\rho < 1$, valid inference must allow for the possibility that we are in the worst case, namely, that $\rho = 1$ and $\tau = \delta_{ij}$. One might compare this with Proposition 2.4 and Corollary 2.1, where, in a different way, it was hardest to reject hypotheses that assert the treatment effect is constant. All of this refers to the Gaussian block model in this problem, and to similar models, in which heterogeneity in the δ_{ij} leaves no visible trace in observable data, (R_{ij}, Z_{ij}).

Selected Problems of Chap. 4

4.2 Proof of Lemma 4.1

Proof Clearly, $\Pr\{Z = 1 \mid \mathbf{X}, \mathbf{b}(\mathbf{X})\} = \Pr\{Z = 1 \mid \mathbf{X}\}$ because $\mathbf{b}(\mathbf{X})$ is a function of $\mathbf{X}$. Using this,

$$\begin{aligned}
\Pr\{Z = 1 \mid \mathbf{b}(\mathbf{X})\} &= \text{E}[\Pr\{Z = 1 \mid \mathbf{X}, \mathbf{b}(\mathbf{X})\} \mid \mathbf{b}(\mathbf{X})] \\
&= \text{E}\{\Pr(Z = 1 \mid \mathbf{X}) \mid \mathbf{b}(\mathbf{X})\} \\
&= \text{E}\{e(\mathbf{X}) \mid e(\mathbf{X}), \mathbf{f}(\mathbf{X})\} \\
&= e(\mathbf{X}) = \Pr(Z = 1 \mid \mathbf{X}).
\end{aligned}$$

□

Selected Problems of Chap. 5

5.1 (iii) A penalty for `female` on the left tries to pair for sex, whereas a penalty for `female` on the right tries to balance sex. If you pair exactly for `female`, then you also balance sex; however, the converse is not true. Before examining any outcomes, we generally adjust the distance matrices to produce a good match defined in terms of pairing and covariate balance. There are many small tactics for improving covariate balance in a matched comparison [7, 8], and like adding interaction or quadratic terms to a linear model, these tactics become second nature with a little practice. See Bo Zhang et al. [11] for more about two-criteria matching.

Selected Problems of Chap. 6

6.3

```
B<-bingeM$age[bingeM$AlcGroup=="B"]
P<-bingeM$age[bingeM$AlcGroup=="P"]
t.test(B,P)
t.test(B-P)
wilcox.test(B,P,conf.int=TRUE)
wilcox.test(B-P,conf.int=TRUE)
```

In all cases above, the two-sample tests, point estimates and confidence intervals suggest that the typical ages in groups B and P differ by at most a few years, yet the *P*-values from the difference tests, B-P, are small. Should we be worried?

Consider near-perfect matching, always off by $\epsilon = 0.0001$ years, or about a third of one day.

```
eps<-0.0001
t.test((B+eps),(B-eps))
```

t-Statistic is 0.00013593, *P*-value is 0.9999, and mean ages are almost identical in the two groups.

```
t.test((B+eps)-(B-eps))
```

t-Statistic is 1.0059×10^{12}, *P*-value is 2.2×10^{-16}, and mean age difference is almost zero.

Selected Problems of Chap. 9

9.2 Note that $I = 10^7$ and the seed is 1. You are checking that $\widetilde{\Gamma} = 4.97$ for Noether's statistic with $f = 2/3$ for $Y_i \sim N(1/2, 1)$, so try $\Gamma = 4.9$ and $\Gamma = 5.1$. What should happen to the bound on the *P*-value between $\Gamma = 4.9$ and $\Gamma = 5.1$?

```
set.seed(1)
```

```
y<-rnorm(10000000)+.5
ay<-rank(abs(y))/length(y)
ny<-y[ay>=(2/3)]
lny<-length(ny)
binom.test(sum(ny>0),lny,4.9/(1+4.9),alternative="greater")
binom.test(sum(ny>0),lny,5.1/(1+5.1),alternative="greater")
```

9.3 This problem is a straightforward calculation using (9.8), but you do need to be a bit careful. From the standardized effect τ, you need to calculate the shift, $\varsigma = \tau\sqrt{d/(d-2)}$, where d is the degrees of freedom. You need to remember that ς shifts the central t-distribution, but is not a noncentrality parameter for a noncentral t-distribution. Then, in R, $L(y)$ is $pt(y-\varsigma, d) - pt((-y)-\varsigma, d)$, and you will need to numerically calculate $\xi = L^{-1}(f)$, perhaps using `uniroot` from the standard `stats` package in R. The plot in Fig. 15.2 applies (9.8) repeatedly. In the plot, the normal distribution wants $f \longrightarrow 1$, but you see from the t-distributions in the same plot that $f \doteq 1$ is a bad idea for $d = 5$ or $d = 3$ and even a bad idea for the normal as it uses only $(1-f)I$ of the I pairs. Note that $f = 2/3$ is a decent fixed choice, using 1/3 of the pairs, with a fairly high $\widetilde{\Gamma}$ in all four distributions. Figure 15.2 makes a case for adaptive inference.

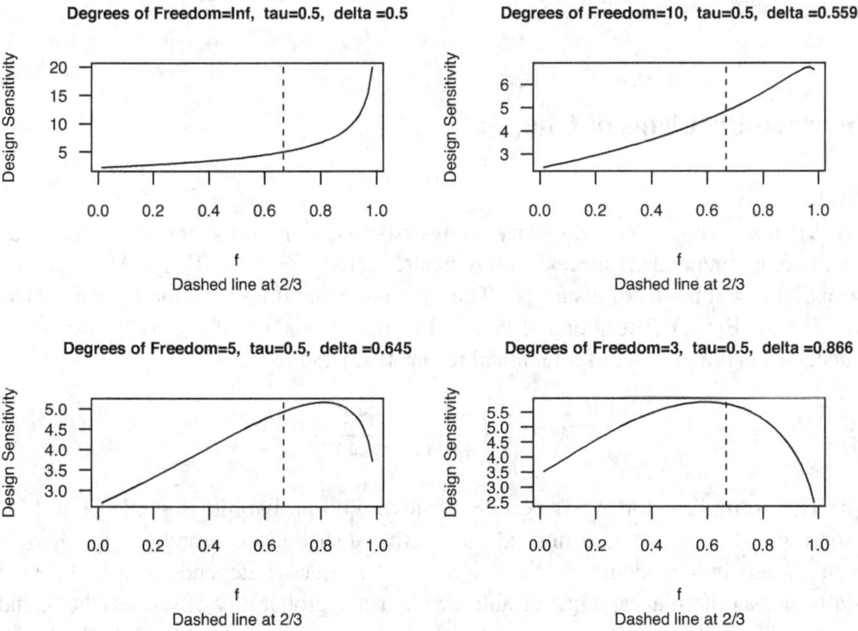

Fig. 15.2 For Problem 9.3: the design sensitivity of Noether's statistic for $J = 2$, $\tau = 1/2$ and degrees of freedom ∞, 10, 5, and 3

Selected Problems of Chap. 10

10.1

```
set.seed(1)
yHalf<-rnorm(100,mean=1/2,sd=1/2)
yOne<-rnorm(400,mean=1/2,sd=1)
library(DOS2)
senWilcox(yHalf,gamma=3.3)
senWilcox(yOne,gamma=3.3)
```

10.3

```
set.seed(1)
yHalf<-rnorm(1000,mean=1/2,sd=1/2)
yOne<-rnorm(4000,mean=1/2,sd=1)
library(DOS2)
senU(yHalf,m=8,m1=7,m2=8,gamma=10)
senU(yOne,m=8,m1=7,m2=8,gamma=10)
```

Both the choice of test statistic and the heterogeneity of the Y_i affect the degree of sensitivity to bias when there is a treatment effect and there is actually no unmeasured bias. The combined impact of the choice of test statistic and the reduction in heterogeneity is substantial.

Selected Problems of Chap. 11

11.2

(i) Write $n = |\mathcal{N}|$. The sensitivity analysis bound is found at the $\boldsymbol{\theta}$ in (8.20), so there are n independent success/failure trials, scored 1 or 0, say V_i, $i \in \mathcal{N}$, each with probability $\Gamma/(1+\Gamma)$ of a success. The moment generating function of one trial V_i is $M_i(t) = \text{E}(t\, V_i)$. The moment generating function $M(t)$ of the total number of successes is the product of n identical terms $M_i(t)$ and is

$$M(t) = \left(\frac{1}{1+\Gamma} + \frac{e^t\,\Gamma}{1+\Gamma}\right)^n .$$

(ii) The normal random variable Y_i is positive with probability $1 - \Phi(-\tau) = \Phi(\tau)$ where $\Phi(\cdot)$ is the standard normal cumulative distribution. Moreover, the Y_i, $i = 1, \ldots, I$ are independent; so, their signs, V_i, are also independent. So, the sign statistic is a binomial random variable with I trials, probability of success $\Phi(\tau)$, and expectation $I\,\Phi(\tau)$. For the sign statistic, the Bahadur slope is the standard calculation when testing the null hypothesis that a binomial random variable has probability $\Gamma/(1+\Gamma)$ of success against the alternative hypothesis that the probability of success is $\Phi(\tau)$. The design sensitivity, $\widetilde{\Gamma}$, is the solution in Γ to the equation $\Phi(\tau) = \Gamma/(1+\Gamma)$,

at which point the Bahadur slope is zero.
(iii) There are a few standard steps from the moment generating function to the Bahadur slope. See either van der Vaart [10, §14.4] or [6].
(iv) Either examine Example 14.24 in van der Vaart [10] or skip to the general approach in Problem 10.3.

11.3
(i) The moment generating function is

$$M(t) = \prod_{i=1}^{I} \left(\frac{1}{1+\Gamma} + \frac{e^{t\,a_i}\,\Gamma}{1+\Gamma} \right).$$

Compare this with the solution to Problem 11.2(i).
(ii) Set $a_i = 1$ for $i \in \mathcal{N}$ and $a_i = 0$ otherwise.
(iii) For the solution to this optional problem, see references [2, Theorem 3.2] and [6].

11.4
(i) Under H_0 at the $\boldsymbol{\theta}$ given in (8.20), $T_1 - T_2$ and T_2 are independent binomials with sample sizes $(I - \lceil f_1 I \rceil) - (I - \lceil f_2 I \rceil)$ and $I - \lceil f_2 I \rceil$ and probability of success $\Gamma/(1+\Gamma)$. In R, the exact joint distribution of $T_1 - T_2$ and T_2 is obtained by calculating binomial probabilities using `dbinom` and taking their outer product using `outer`. The joint distribution of T_1 and T_2 is determined from this matrix.
(ii) Again, $T_1 - T_2$ and T_2 are independent binomials; so, straightforward manipulations yield the joint distribution of T_3 and T_2.
(iii) Adaptive inference yields the larger of the two component design sensitivities and the larger of the two Bahadur efficiencies. Though based on two binomials, the resulting adaptive statistic is competitive [5]. If $f_1 = 1/3$ and $f_2 = 2/3$, then Noether's T_2 often has excellent design sensitivity, and T_3 is Brown's [1] statistic which is competitive with Wilcoxon's signed rank statistic.

Selected Problems of Chap. 12

12.1
```
library(weightedRank)
library(iTOS)
data(aHDL)
aMM<-aHDL[!is.na(aHDL$mmercury),]
nMM<-(dim(aMM)[1])/4
hdl<-t(matrix(aMM$hdl,4,nMM))
wgtRank(hdl,phi="quade",gamma=3.614)
```

Selected Problems of Chap. 13

13.6

```
library(weightedRank)
data(aHDL)
y<-t(matrix(aHDL$hdl,4,406))
colnames(y)<-c("D","N","R","B")
ef2C(y[,c(1,2,4)],gamma=4,upsilon=3.5)
```

Selected Problems of Chap. 14

14.4

(i) Each node has degree 1 or 2. A node, say Harry, with degree 1 is connected to one control from the other control group because they are both matched to the same treated individual. There are two possibilities: (a) that other control is someone else, not Harry, and in this case Harry is not duplicated; otherwise, (b) that other control is also Harry, and both Harry's are removed when duplicates are removed—Harry's two nodes form a connected component that is a very short cycle of the form $n_1 - n_1$. A node, say Sally, with degree 2 is connected to two nodes in the other control group: the control who is matched to the same treated individual and Sally's duplicate node in the other control group.

(ii) You do not travel far to get from n_1 to n_1; take the path n_1. If you can travel from n_1 to n_L on the path $n_1 - n_2 - \cdots - n_L$, then you can travel back from n_L to n_1 along the same (undirected!) path. If you can travel from n_1 to n_L on the path $n_1 - n_2 - \cdots - n_L$ and from n_L to n_M on the path $n_L - n_{L+1} - \cdots - n_M$, then you can travel from n_1 to n_M on the path $n_1 - n_2 - \cdots - n_M$.

(iii) The key is that every node has degree 1 or 2. Pick any node, say n_0. If n_0 has degree 1, start a path $n_0 - n_1$, where n_1 is the only node connected to n_0. If n_1 has degree 1, then stop. Otherwise, if n_1 has degree 2, then lengthen the path to $n_0 - n_1 - n_2$ where n_2 is the one other node connected to n_1. This process must stop because there are finitely many nodes. Proceed in this way until you end with a component of type (a). (It cannot be a cycle of type (b) because n_0 has degree 1.) If, instead, n_0 has degree 2, then grow the path in both directions, $n_{-1} - n_0 - n_1$, and so on. This process may end in a component of type (a) or of type (b).

(iv) In the connected component $n_1 - n_2 - \cdots - n_L$ with $L > 2$ and $n_1 \neq n_L$, node n_1 has degree 1 and node n_2 has degree 2; so n_1 and n_2 must represent different controls, where n_2 represents a duplicated control who is in both control groups, and n_1 represents an unduplicated control who is in only one control group. Removing the duplicates removes n_2 and breaks up the one pair containing n_1.

(v) In $n_1 - n_2 - \cdots - n_L$, if n_1 has the same sex as n_2, and n_2 has the same sex as $n_3, \ldots,$ and n_{L-1} has the same sex as n_L, then n_1 has the same sex as n_L.

(v) If both control groups have 47 women and 53 men, and I remove Harry from both control groups, then both control groups now have 47 women and 52 men; so sex is still perfectly balanced. For balance, it does not matter to whom Harry is matched.

References

1. Brown, B.M.: Symmetric quantile averages and related estimators. Biometrika **68**(1), 235–242 (1981)
2. Groeneboom, P., Oosterhoff, J.: Bahadur efficiency and probabilities of large deviations. Statistica Neerlandica **31**(1), 1–24 (1977)
3. Huber, P.J.: Robust regression: Asymptotics, conjectures and Monte Carlo. Ann. Stat. **1**(5), 799–821 (1973)
4. Rosenbaum, P.R.: A characterization of optimal designs for observational studies. J. Roy. Stat. Soc. B (Methodological) **53**(3), 597–610 (1991)
5. Rosenbaum, P.R.: An exact adaptive test with superior design sensitivity in an observational study of treatments for ovarian cancer. Ann. Appl. Stat. **6**, 83–105 (2012)
6. Rosenbaum, P.R.: Bahadur efficiency of sensitivity analyses in observational studies. J. Am. Stat. Assoc. **110**(509), 205–217 (2015)
7. Rosenbaum, P.R.: Design of Observational Studies, 2nd edn. Springer, New York (2020)
8. Rosenbaum, P.R.: Modern algorithms for matching in observational studies. Annu. Rev. Stat. Appl. **7**, 143–176 (2020)
9. Rosenbaum, P.R.: A new transformation of treated-control matched-pair differences for graphical display. Am. Stat. **76**(4), 346–352 (2022)
10. van der Vaart, A.W.: Asymptotic Statistics. Cambridge University Press, New York (2000)
11. Zhang, B., Small, D.S., Lasater, K.B., McHugh, M., Silber, J.H., Rosenbaum, P.R.: Matching one sample according to two criteria in observational studies. J. Am. Stat. Assoc. **118**, 1140–1151 (2022)

Some Comments for Instructors

In the preface, I wrote: "This book is a quick jog along one useful and attractive path offering brief but good views of the theory of causal inference in observational studies [... picking ...] topics and methods that offer easy access to grand vistas." An instructor might naturally want to take some steps away from this path. This brief section mentions various generalizations, additional topics and excursions that are possible.

By and large, the discussion has focused on block designs, with I blocks, J individuals per block, one treated individual and $J - 1$ controls, with continuous responses, R_{ij}, often considering what happens as $I \to \infty$. Close attention has been given to distribution-free rank statistics, particularly weighted rank statistics, and their associated tests, confidence intervals, and Hodges-Lehmann point estimates. The weighted rank statistics generalize one of the most widely used permutation tests, namely, Wilcoxon's signed rank statistic. Within this framework, a wide variety of topics in causal inference have been examined and exemplified.

Each feature of the previous paragraph simplifies something somewhere in the book, but no feature is essential, and most features provide only small simplifications. There is also simplification from discussing one situation, rather than many parallel situations. The general theory has nothing to do with the stated block structure—I blocks with one treated individual and $J - 1$ controls per block—and so the general theory can easily drop this structure with minor changes, aside from a bit more complexity in the technical details [20, 26, 30].

A simple way to dip one toe briefly into unbalanced designs with weights is to discuss Katherine Brumberg's [5] triples design, in which each block has either one treated individual and two controls or one control and two treated individuals. This design has only two weights, essentially 1 and 2, thereby encouraging graphical analysis, and it can be used to introduce the concept of the "entire number" of Pimentel, Yoon, and Keele [14]. The triples design also increases design sensitivity, $\widetilde{\Gamma}$, when compared to the matched pairs design, $J = 2$, in parallel with 1-to-2

© The Author(s), under exclusive license to Springer Nature Switzerland AG 2025

P. R. Rosenbaum, *An Introduction to the Theory of Observational Studies*, Springer Texts in Statistics, https://doi.org/10.1007/978-3-031-90494-3

matching or $J = 3$, as discussed in Sect. 10.2. Continuous inverse-probability weighting could also be introduced in connection with the propensity score [16].

The general theory also has nothing to do with rank statistics—weighted, distribution-free or otherwise—and can be developed for means or robust M-estimates and many other statistics. To fully discuss means, one needs to add somewhat tedious regularity conditions to ensure their good behavior as $I \to \infty$, and as means are not robust, they are not ideal for use in practice anyway. For Huber's M-statistics, one must make a small edit to the familiar theory in the choice of scale factor, as first proposed by Maritz [13] for randomization inference; however, with that small edit, most topics proceed as with rank statistics [23, 25]. Due to the scale factor needed for any M-estimate, the calculation of design sensitivity $\widetilde{\Gamma}$ for an M-statistic requires a small additional technical step [25, Expression (10)], a step that is not needed for rank statistics. If the responses, R_{ij}, are not continuous, then the theory applies to familiar permutation tests for binary outcomes or for outcomes given as a few integer scores [4, 10, 11], as discussed in [18–20, 31]. Similarly, the theory applies to permutation tests for censored outcomes [20, §2.8.2].

It can be slightly easier to explain evidence factors in terms of rank tests, as in Chap. 13, because (i) in simple cases, distinct factors are exactly independent, rather than merely yielding joint P-values that are stochastically larger than uniform on the unit square or unit cube, and (ii) there is a large and related literature about independent rank statistics [1, 6, 9, 12, 15, 32]. However, the theory is general and can be developed without reference to rank statistics [24, 27].

Weighted rank statistics perform well in terms of design sensitivity, $\widetilde{\Gamma}$, and they are technically convenient in a few places. In particular, weighted rank statistics facilitate adaptive inference in block designs with $J > 2$ in Sect. 9.5, and in Chapter 11 it is convenient that they have an exact moment generating function useful in Bahadur efficiency calculations [28]. There are, however, statistics with larger design sensitivities [29].

Case-control studies, case-case studies, and instruments (or instrumental variables) play a large role in some fields of application and a small role in other fields. For a class with suitable interests, these topics could be integrated into the discussion of causal effects, sensitivity analysis, design sensitivity, efficiency, or multiple control groups [2, 3, 7, 8, 17, 21, 22].

References

1. Alam, K.: Some nonparametric tests of randomness. J. Am. Stat. Assoc. **69**(347), 738–739 (1974)
2. Angrist, J.D., Imbens, G.W., Rubin, D.B.: Identification of causal effects using instrumental variables. J. Am. Stat. Assoc. **91**(434), 444–455 (1996)
3. Baiocchi, M., Small, D.S., Lorch, S., Rosenbaum, P.R.: Building a stronger instrument in an observational study of perinatal care for premature infants. J. Am. Stat. Assoc. **105**(492), 1285–1296 (2010)
4. Birch, M.W.: The detection of partial association, i: the 2×2 case. J. Roy. Stat. Soc. B **26**(2), 313–324 (1964)

5. Brumberg, K., Small, D.S., Rosenbaum, P.R.: A new design for observational studies applied to the study of the effects of high school football on cognition late in life. Ann. Appl. Stat. **18**, 3507–3527 (2024)
6. Dwass, M.: Some k-sample rank-order tests. In: Contributions to Probability and Statistics: Essays in Honor of Harold Hotelling. Stanford University Press, Redwood City (1960)
7. Ertefaie, A., Small, D.S., Rosenbaum, P.R.: Quantitative evaluation of the trade-off of strengthened instruments and sample size in observational studies. J. Am. Stat. Assoc. **113**(523), 1122–1134 (2018)
8. Heng, S., Small, D.S., Rosenbaum, P.R.: Finding the strength in a weak instrument in a study of cognitive outcomes produced by Catholic high schools. J. Roy. Stat. Soc. A **183**(3), 935–958 (2020)
9. Hogg, R.V.: Iterated tests of the equality of several distributions. J. Am. Stat. Assoc. **57**(299), 579–585 (1962)
10. Mantel, N.: Chi-square tests with one degree of freedom: Extensions of the Mantel-Haenszel procedure. J. Am. Stat. Assoc. **58**(303), 690–700 (1963)
11. Mantel, N., Haenszel, W.: Statistical aspects of the analysis of data from retrospective studies of disease. J. Natl. Cancer Inst. **22**(4), 719–748 (1959)
12. Marden, J.I.: Use of nested orthogonal contrasts in analyzing rank data. J. Am. Stat. Assoc. **87**(418), 307–318 (1992)
13. Maritz, J.S.: A note on exact robust confidence intervals for location. Biometrika **66**(1), 163–170 (1979)
14. Pimentel, S.D., Yoon, F., Keele, L.: Variable-ratio matching with fine balance in a study of the peer health exchange. Stat. Med. **34**(30), 4070–4082 (2015)
15. Randles, R.H., Hogg, R.V.: Certain uncorrelated and independent rank statistics. J. Am. Stat. Assoc. **66**(335), 569–574 (1971)
16. Rosenbaum, P.R.: Model-based direct adjustment. J. Am. Stat. Assoc. **82**(398), 387–394 (1987)
17. Rosenbaum, P.R.: Sensitivity analysis for matched case-control studies. Biometrics **47**, 87–100 (1991)
18. Rosenbaum, P.R.: Effects attributable to treatment: Inference in experiments and observational studies with a discrete pivot. Biometrika **88**(1), 219–231 (2001)
19. Rosenbaum, P.R.: Attributing effects to treatment in matched observational studies. J. Am. Stat. Assoc. **97**(457), 183–192 (2002)
20. Rosenbaum, P.R.: Observational Studies, 2nd edn. Springer, New York (2002)
21. Rosenbaum, P.R.: The case-only odds ratio as a causal parameter. Biometrics **60**(1), 233–240 (2004)
22. Rosenbaum, P.R.: Attributable effects in case^2 studies. Biometrics **61**(1), 246–253 (2005)
23. Rosenbaum, P.R.: Sensitivity analysis for M-estimates, tests, and confidence intervals in matched observational studies. Biometrics **63**(2), 456–464 (2007)
24. Rosenbaum, P.R.: Some approximate evidence factors in observational studies. J. Am. Stat. Assoc. **106**(493), 285–295 (2011)
25. Rosenbaum, P.R.: Impact of multiple matched controls on design sensitivity in observational studies. Biometrics **69**(1), 118–127 (2013)
26. Rosenbaum, P.R.: Sensitivity analysis for stratified comparisons in an observational study of the effect of smoking on homocysteine levels. Ann. Appl. Stat. **12**(4), 2312–2334 (2018)
27. Rosenbaum, P.R.: Replication and Evidence Factors in Observational Studies. Chapman and Hall/CRC, New York (2021)
28. Rosenbaum, P.R.: Bahadur efficiency of observational block designs. J. Am. Stat. Assoc. **119**(547), 1871–1881 (2024)
29. Rosenbaum, P.R.: A conditioning tactic that increases design sensitivity in observational block designs. J. Roy. Stat. Soc. B (2025). https://doi.org/10.1093/jrsssb/qkaf007
30. Rosenbaum, P.R., Krieger, A.M.: Sensitivity of two-sample permutation inferences in observational studies. J. Am. Stat. Assoc. **85**(410), 493–498 (1990)
31. Rosenbaum, P.R., Small, D.S.: An adaptive Mantel–Haenszel test for sensitivity analysis in observational studies. Biometrics **73**(2), 422–430 (2017)
32. Wolfe, D.A.: Some general results about uncorrelated statistics. J. Am. Stat. Assoc. **68**(344), 1013–1018 (1973)

Index

© The Author(s), under exclusive license to Springer Nature Switzerland AG 2025

P. R. Rosenbaum, *An Introduction to the Theory of Observational Studies*, Springer Texts in Statistics, https://doi.org/10.1007/978-3-031-90494-3